Pharmaceutical Preformulation and Formulation

A Practical Guide from Candidate Drug Selection to Commercial Dosage Form

Edited by Mark Gibson

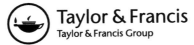

Taylor & Francis
Taylor & Francis Group

Boca Raton   London   New York   Singapore

A CRC title, part of the Taylor & Francis imprint, a member of the
Taylor & Francis Group, the academic division of T&F Informa plc.

Library of Congress Cataloging-in-Publication Data

Catalog record is available from the Library of Congress

Visit the CRC Press Web site at www.crcpress.com

No claim to original U.S. Government works
International Standard Book Number 1-57491-120-1
Printed in the United States of America   2 3 4 5 6 7 8 9 0
Printed on acid-free paper

CONTENTS

PREFACE

In my industrial career, I have gained broad experience working on many different pharmaceutical development projects and dosage forms, spanning candidate drug selection through technology transfer to production and subsequent launch. With this background and with Gerry Steele's encouragement and rich experience in preformulation studies, I planned a book that would emphasize what practical studies need to be undertaken, for what reasons and during what key stages of the drug development process. In addition to preformulation, I considered it essential to include biopharmaceutics (an area of emerging importance) as well as formulation aspects. I soon realized I could not commit the time to writing all the chapters in such a book, and, indeed, I considered the book would be more comprehensive by involving other contributors and adding their special knowledge and experiences.

I am extremely grateful to all the contributors in this book, who have given up so much of their time to create their specialised chapters. I would specially like to thank Anna-Lena Ungell and Bertil Abrahammson for the two biopharmaceutics chapters, and also Jo Broadhead for stepping in at the final hour and writing the chapter on parenterals. Without these chapters, the book would have been incomplete.

In the past few years, I have written internal company guidelines and given seminars externally on a logical approach to product development and technology transfer. This approach emphasises the importance of starting development of an NCE with product design prior to commencing product and process optimisation, scale-up and technology transfer. Two people I would particularly like to thank for their input and support for these concepts are Gordon France and Mike Dey. This logical approach to ensure that products are developed efficiently and moved speedily to market is part of my own contribution to the chapters in this book.

Preparing this book took longer than anticipated, and it contains more pages than expected. I have many vivid memories of one-finger typing on my laptop in airport lounges and hotel rooms and at home late in the evenings or on weekends. While my typing has become considerably faster, I hasten to add that I have progressed only to two-finger typing! I am indebted to my secretarial support, particularly Hayley Pruden, who has much better typing skills than I, to complete the figures and tables for this book.

This book should prove to be a useful guide to practitioners working in the pharmaceutical industry, including R&D scientists, technicians and managers. In the words of Francis Bacon (1561–1626):

> Some books are to be tasted, others to be swallowed, and some few to be chewed and digested: that is, some books are to be read only in parts; others to be read but not curiously; and some few to be read wholly, and with diligence and attention.

I would like to think that this book might fit any of the above descriptions, depending on the reader's need.

Finally, I would like to thank my wife Alison for her love, understanding and support over the time I have spent preparing this book. Now that the book is finished, I should have more time to spend with her and my three children, Laura, Joanna and David.

Mark Gibson
May 2001

Contributors

MARK GIBSON

Mark Gibson, BPharm, PhD, CChem, MRSC, MRPharmS, is currently responsible for parenteral and oral solid dosage form development at AstraZeneca R&D Charnwood, which is a division of AstraZeneca. His experience includes formulation and preformulation development, both as a bench scientist and a manger, at Cyanamid (Lederle) for six years, Fisons Pharmaceuticals for six years, Astra Pharmaceuticals for four years and AstraZeneca for two years. He has worked on a variety of dosage forms and routes of delivery, including inhalation, oral, nasal, ophthalmic, parenteral and transdermal, resulting in some patents or marketable products. Dr. Gibson is a member of the UK Academy of Pharmaceutical Sciences, the Parenteral Society and the Aerosol Society.

BERTIL ABRAHAMSSON

Bertil Abrahamsson, PhD, leads pharmaceutical and analytical research and development at AstraZeneca R&D Mölndal. His experience is in *in vitro/in vivo* correlations, *in vitro* dissolution, *in vivo* imaging of dosage forms and drug absorption. Dr. Abrahamsson has published more than 20 articles in clinical pharmacology.

KEITH R. BRAIN

Keith Brain, BPharm, PhD, is head of the drug delivery research group at Cardiff University. His major responsibilities are in molecular recognition research and skin research. He is also CEO of An-eX, a university-based spinoff company formed in 1988, which specialises in confidential contract research and development for international clients. He has organized several international conferences on skin research and workshops on molecular imprinting.

JOANNE BROADHEAD

Joanne Broadhead, PhD, MRPharmS, manages a small team of formulation scientists at AstraZeneca R&D Charnwood in the development of solid and parenteral products. Her experience includes two years as a formulation scientist for creative BioMolecules (Hopkinton, Mass., USA) prior to joining AstraZeneca in 1996. Dr. Broadhead is a member of the American Association of Pharmaceutical Scientists, the Parenteral Drug Association and the Parenteral Society.

PETER DAVIES

Peter Davies, BPharm, MRPharmS, PhD, is currently the formulation team leader in drug delivery sciences at Roche Discovery Welwyn. At Roche for 18 years, his principal areas of interest are preformulation and formulation of solid dosage forms.

NIGEL DAY

Nigel H. Day, BSc, MSc, PhD, is a team manager in product development at AstraZeneca R&D Charnwood (formerly Fisons R&D and Astra Charnwood). He has wide experience in the development of solid, liquid and inhalation formulations. His professional experience includes a postdoctoral research fellowship at the University of Bradford and seven years in the Hoffman-La Roche UK R&D Laboratories. Dr. Day is a member of the UK Academy of Pharmaceutical Sciences.

GERRY STEELE

Gerry Steele, BSc, MSc, PhD, CChem, MRSC, is a team manager at AstraZeneca R&D Charnwood. His research experience includes preformulation work and characterization and the surface rheology of phospholipid monolayers using photon correlation spectroscopy. Prior to joining AstraZeneca R&D Charnwood, he spent seven years with Fisons plc and a year at Inversesk Research International. Dr. Steele is a member of the Royal Society of Chemistry and the Academy of Pharmaceutical Scientists (of the Royal Pharmaceutical Society of Great Britain).

ANNA-LENA UNGELL

Anna-Lena Ungell, PhD, is associate director of DMPK and bioanalytical chemistry at AstraZeneca R&D Mölndal. She supports preclinical and pharmaceutical projects relating to absorption as well as the gastrointestinal absorption of drugs. Her experience includes absorption models, mechanisms of drug absorption from the intestinal tract, substance evaluation and basic formulation development. Dr. Ungell has four patents and has written numerous research articles and reviews.

KENNETH A. WALTERS

Kenneth A. Walters, PhD, is director of An-eX Analytical Services Ltd and an honorary lecturer in pharmaceutical chemistry at the Welsh School of Pharmacy. His research interests are biological membrane penetration enhancement and retardation, particularly with respect to skin. He has experience at Fisons Pharmaceuticals, Eastman Pharmaceuticals (a division of Eastman Kodak Company) and Controlled Therapeutics Ltd. (Scotland). Dr. Walters has published many articles and reviews and has co-edited two volumes on skin penetration enhancement and dermal toxicity. He is a charter member of the American Association of Pharmaceutical Scientists and also a member of the Society of Investigative Dermatology, the Controlled Release Society, the Society of Toxicology and the Society of Cosmetic Scientists.

PAUL WRIGHT

Paul Wright is an associate director within product development at AstraZeneca. He has inhalation development responsibilities at both the Charnwood (UK) site and the Lund (Sweden) site. Mr. Wright has extensive experience in major respiratory dosage forms and is a committee member of several industry groups.

1

Introduction and Perspective

Mark Gibson

AstraZeneca R&D Charnwood
Loughborough, United Kingdom

This book is intended to be a practical guide to pharmaceutical preformulation and formulation. It can be used as a reference source and a guidance tool for those working in the pharmaceutical industry or related industries, for example, medical devices and biopharmaceuticals, or anyone wanting an insight into this subject area. The information presented is essentially based on the extensive experiences of the editor and various other contributors who are all actively working in the industry and have learned "best practice" from their experiences.

There are various excellent books already available which cover the theoretical aspects of different types of pharmaceutical dosage forms and processes. A variety of books are also available that focus on the drug development process, business, regulatory and project management aspects. In my opinion, there has been a long-standing need for a pragmatic guide to pharmaceutical preformulation and formulation with an emphasis on what practical studies need to be undertaken, for what reasons and during what key stages of the drug development process. The important stages where preformulation, biopharmaceutics and formulation play a key role are candidate drug selection through the various stages of product development. This book has been written to try and address this need.

A logical approach to product development is described in the book, with the key stages identified and the preformulation, biopharmaceutics and formulation activities and typical issues at each stage discussed. Wherever possible, the book is illustrated with real or worked examples from contributors who have considerable relevant experience of preformulation, biopharmaceutics and formulation development.

Jim Wells' book on preformulation (Wells 1988) made a strong impact on trainees and pharmaceutical scientists (including myself) working in this field of the pharmaceutical industry when it was introduced over 10 years ago. It describes the important concepts and methods used in preformulation with the underlying theory. To his credit, Wells' book is still useful today, but sadly, the book is now out of print, and existing copies are hard to obtain. It also requires updating to include modern preformulation instrumental techniques which have emerged over the last decade, such as thermo gravimetric analysis (TGA), hot stage microscopy (HSM), X-ray powder diffraction (XRPD), raman and infra-red spectroscopy and solid-state nuclear magnetic resonance (NMR), to name a few. These techniques can be used to provide valuable information to characterise the drug substance and aid formulation development using the minimal amounts of compound.

Pharmaceutical Preformulation and Formulation: A Practical Guide from Candidate Drug Selection to Commercial Formulation covers a wider subject area than just preformulation. Topics include biopharmaceutics, drug delivery, formulation and process development aspects of product development. The book also describes a logical and structured approach to the product development process, recommending at what stages appropriate preformulation, biopharmaceutics and formulation work is best undertaken.

DRUG DEVELOPMENT DRIVERS, CHALLENGES, RISKS AND REWARDS

It is important that the reader is aware of the nature of pharmaceutical research and development (R&D) in order to appreciate the importance of preformulation and formulation in the overall process.

In simple terms, the objective of *pharmaceutical R&D* can be defined as "converting ideas into candidate drugs for development", and the objective of *product development* defined as "converting candidate drugs into products for registration and sale". In reality, these goals are extremely challenging and difficult to achieve because of the many significant hurdles a pharmaceutical company has to overcome during the course of drug development. Some of the major hurdles are listed in Table 1.1.

The high risk of failure in drug discovery and development throughout the pharmaceutical industry statistically shows that, on average, only 1 in 5,000 to 1 in 10,000 compounds screened in research will reach the market (Tucker 1984). Of those that are nominated for development, the failure rate will vary from 1 in 5 to 1 in 10 compounds that will achieve registration and reach the market-place. On top of that, there is a significant commercial risk from those that are marketed; only 3 out of 10 are likely to achieve a fair return on investment. The products which give poor return on investment are often the result of poor candidate drug selection (the compound does not have the desired properties of safety, selectivity, efficacy, potency or duration) and/or poor product development (the development programme does not establish the value of the product). The latter scenario should, and can be, avoided by careful assessment at the "product design" stage of development. Product design is discussed further in Chapter 5.

Table 1.1
Major hurdles to successful product registration and sale.

Activity	Requirements
Research	Novel compound (patentable?)
	Novel biological mechanism (patentable?)
	Unmet medical needs
	Potent and selective
Safety	High margin of safety
	Non-toxic (not carcinogenic, tetratogenic, mutagenic, etc.)
Clinical	Tolerable side-effects profile
	Efficacious
	Acceptable duration of action
Drug process	Bulk drug can be synthesised/scaled up
Pharmaceutical	Acceptable formulation/pack (meets customer needs)
	Drug delivery/product performance acceptable
	Stable/acceptable shelf-life
	Clinical trial process robust and can be scaled up
Regulatory	Quality of data/documentation
Manufacturing	Manufacturable
	Able to pass pre-approval inspection
Marketing/commercial	Competitive
	Meets customer needs
	Value for money
	Commercial return

To be successful and competitive, research-based pharmaceutical companies must ensure that new discoveries are frequently brought to the market to generate cash flow. This is required to fund the next generation of compounds to meet the therapeutic needs of patients, and of course, to benefit the shareholders. This cycle of events is sometimes referred to as the "product life cycle" and is further illustrated in Figure 1.1.

The costs of drug discovery and development to bring a New Chemical Entity (NCE) to the market are ever increasing. It is currently estimated that in excess of U.S. $500 million is required to recoup the costs of research, development, manufacturing, distribution, marketing and sales. A significant proportion of this total is for the cost of failures, or in other words, the elimination of unsuccessful compounds. R&D expenditure for an NCE tends to increase substantially as the compound progresses from drug discovery research through the various clinical trial phases of development. The pivotal Phase III patient trials are usually the largest, involving thousands of patients, and hence the most expensive. To reduce development costs,

Figure 1.1 Product life cycle.

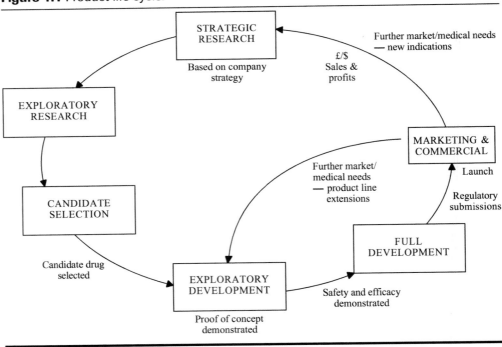

some companies selectively screen and eliminate compounds earlier in the drug development process based on results from small-scale, less expensive studies in man and progress fewer, more certain compounds to later clinical phases.

In spite of the high risks and high costs involved, there is still a huge incentive for pharmaceutical companies to seek the financial rewards from successful marketed products, and especially from the phenomenal success of the rare "blockbuster" (reaching sales of >1 billion U.S.$ per year). This can earn the company significant profits to reinvest in research and fund the product development pipeline.

Another factor, the risk of delay to registration and launch, can also have a significant impact on the financial success of a marketed product. McKinsey & Company, a management consultancy, assessed that a product that is 6 months late to market will miss out on one-third of the potential profit over the product's lifetime. In comparison, they found that a development cost overspend of 50 percent would reduce profits by just 3.5 percent, and a 9 percent overspend in production costs reduced profits by 22 percent (McKinsey & Co. 1991). The loss of product revenue is often due to competitor companies being first to market, capturing the market share and dictating the market price, in addition to the loss of effective patent life. Hence, the importance of accelerating and optimising drug discovery and development, and getting to the market first with a new therapeutic class of medicinal product, cannot be underestimated. The second product to market in the same class will usually be compared with the market leader, often unfavourably.

The average time from drug discovery to product launch is currently estimated to take 10 to 12 years. Several factors may have contributed to lengthening development times over the years, including an increase in the preclinical phase to select the candidate drug, and also an increase in the duration of the clinical and regulatory period required for marketing approval. Benchmarking studies show wide gaps between industry average or worst performance compared to what is achievable as best practice performance (Spence 1997). On average, the preclinical phase currently takes 4 to 6 years to complete, whereas the time from candidate drug nomination to regulatory submission takes on average 6 to 8 years, longer for treatments of chronic conditions. Most forward-looking pharmaceutical companies are aiming to reduce these times by re-evaluation and subsequently streamlining the development process, for example, by introducing more effective clinical programmes and more efficient data reporting systems, forward planning and conducting multiple activities in parallel. However, this, in turn, may put formulation development and clinical supplies on the critical path, with pressures to complete these activities in condensed time scales. Suggestions are offered throughout this book on how preformulation, biopharmaceutics and formulation can be conducted in the most efficient way to avoid delays in development times.

Any reduction in the total time-frame of drug discovery to market should improve the company's profitability. In a highly competitive market, product lifetimes are being eroded due to the pace of introduction of competitor products, the rapid introduction of generic products when patents expire and moves to "over-the-counter" (OTC) status. Successful pharmaceutical companies are focusing on strategies for optimum "product life cycle management" to maximise the early growth of the product on the market, sustain peak sales for as long as the product is in patent and delay the post-patent expiry decline for as long as possible. This should maximise the return on investment during a product life cycle to enable the company to recover development costs and make further investments in R&D. Figure 1.2 shows a classic cash flow profile for a new drug product developed and marketed. During development there is a negative cash flow, and it may be some time after launch before sales revenue crosses from loss to profit because of manufacturing, distribution and advertising costs. Profits continue to increase as the market is established to reach peak sales, after which sales decrease, especially after the primary patent expires and generic competition is introduced.

Throughout the life span of a product, it is in a company's interest to ensure the best patent protection in order to achieve the longest possible market exclusivity. Prior to the primary patent expiring (normally for the chemical drug substance), it is imperative to introduce new indications, formulations, manufacturing processes, devices and general technology, which are patent protected, to extend the life of the product and maintain revenue. A patent generally has a term of about 20 years, but as development times are getting longer, there will be a limited duration of protection remaining once the product is marketed (the effective patent life). A comparison of effective patent life for pharmaceutical new chemical entities in various countries around the world shows the same downward trend between the 1960s and the 1980s (Karia et al. 1992; Lis and Walker 1988).

Getting to the market quickly is a major business driving force, but this has to be balanced with the development of a product of the appropriate quality. There is a need to generate sufficient information to enable sound decisions on the selection of a candidate drug for development, as well as to develop dosage forms which are "fit for purpose" at the various stages of development. Anything more is wasting precious resources (people and drug substance), adding unnecessary cost to the programme and, more importantly, extending the development time. Perfect quality should not be the target if good quality is sufficient for the intended purpose. This can only be achieved if there is a clear understanding of the customer requirements.

Figure 1.2 Product life cycle management.

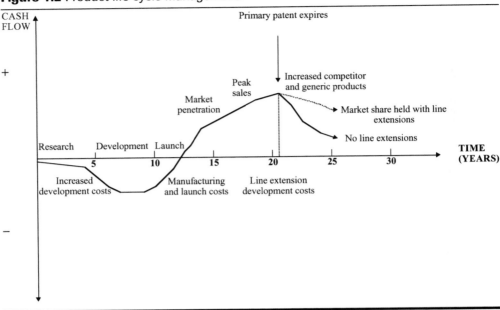

For example, if a simple, non-optimised formulation with a relatively short shelf life is acceptable for Phase I clinical studies, any further optimisation or stability testing might be considered wasteful, unless the data generated can be used later in the development programme.

There can be a significant risk associated with doing a minimum development programme and cutting corners to fast track to market. Post-launch, the cost of a retrospective fix due to poor product/process design and/or development can be extremely high. The additional financial cost from work in product/process redevelopment, manufacturing and validation, technical support, regulatory and sales and marketing (due to a product recall) can easily wipe out the profit from an early launch. This can have several unpleasant knock-on effects; it may affect the market share and the company's relationship with the regulatory authorities, and its credibility with customers (both externally and internally within the company) may be threatened. These factors need to be taken in to account when planning preformulation/formulation studies which can directly influence the progress of a product to market and final product quality.

CURRENT TRENDS IN THE PHARMACEUTICAL INDUSTRY

Increasing competition and threats to the pharmaceutical industry with respect to maintaining continued sales growth and income mean that successful companies going forward will be those which have a portfolio of products capable of showing volume growth. However, to show volume growth innovative new products are required. The cost of drug discovery and development is escalating because there are no easy targets left and the cost of development and the cost of goods sold is increasing. There have been several mergers and acquisitions of research-based pharmaceutical companies, and increased collaborations and inward licensing of products and technologies, in attempts to acquire new leads, to share costs, to reduce the time to licence and to maintain growth. Unfortunately, mergers and acquisitions also result in streamlining and job losses which improve efficiency and decrease overhead costs at the same time.

There is a changing trend in the nature of the candidate drug emerging from pharmaceutical R&D, from a low molecular weight chemical to a more complex macromolecule (biologicals), which can be a peptide, protein, enzyme, antibody, nucleic acid, genetic material or a multicomponent vaccine. Some of these compounds have been derived from biotechnological processes to produce biotechnological medicinal products that fight infection and disease. The U.S. Food and Drug Administration (FDA) and European Agency for the Evaluation of Medicinal Products (EMEA) have already approved biotechnological medicinal products for anaemia, cystic fibrosis, growth deficiency, hepatitis and transplant rejection. Many more are being developed to treat cancer, human immunodeficiency virus (HIV) infections and acquired immunodeficiency syndrome (AIDS), multiple sclerosis and stroke. A major challenge to the formulator is to develop self-administered formulations to deliver macromolecules such as proteins and polypeptides into the body, for example, by the oral or inhalation route.

More sophisticated drug delivery systems are being developed to overcome the limitations of conventional forms of drug delivery systems (e.g., tablets and intravenous [IV] solutions), to overcome problems of poor drug absorption, the non-compliance of patients and inaccurate targeting of therapeutic agents. One example of an emerging drug delivery technology is the use of low-level electrical energy to assist the transport of drugs across the skin in a process known as electrophoresis. This method could be particularly useful for the delivery of peptides and proteins which are not adequately transported by passive transdermal therapy. The drug absorption rate is very rapid and more controlled compared with passive diffusion across the skin. Another example is the improvement in inhaler technology to ensure a more efficient delivery to the lungs, with minimal drug deposition in the mouth and trachea. The use of a breath-actuated aerosol is designed to co-ordinate drug delivery with the patient's inhalation to achieve this. A third example is the use of bioerodable polymers that can be implanted or injected within the body to administer drugs from a matrix which can be formulated to degrade over a long duration from one day to six months, and do not require retrieval. Some of these specific delivery systems are explained in more detail in later chapters of this book on the various dosage forms.

Futuristic drug delivery systems are being developed which hope to facilitate the transport of a drug with a carrier to its intended destination in the body and then release it there. Liposomes, monoclonal antibodies and modified viruses are being considered to deliver "repair genes" by IV injection to target the respiratory epithelium in the treatment of cystic fibrosis. These novel drug delivery systems not only offer clear medical benefits to the patient but can also be opportunities for commercial exploitation, especially useful if a drug is approaching the end of its patent life.

There are pressures on the pharmaceutical industry which affect the way products are being developed. For example, there is a trend for more comprehensive documentation to demonstrate compliance with current Good Manufacturing Practice (cGMP) and Good Laboratory Practice (GLP) and to demonstrate that systems and procedures have been validated. The trend is for more information required for a regulatory submission, with little flexibility for changes once submitted. Therefore, the pressure is for a company to submit early and develop the product "right first time".

In spite of efforts to harmonise tests, standards and pharmacopoeias, there is still diversity between the major global markets—Europe, the United States and Japan—which have to be taken in to account in the design of preformulation and formulation programmes (Anonymous 1993). This is discussed further in Chapter 5 on product design.

Other pressures facing the pharmaceutical industry are of a political/economical or environmental nature. Some governments are trying to contain healthcare costs by introducing healthcare reforms, which may lead to reduced prices and profit margins for companies, or restricted markets where only certain drugs can be prescribed. Although the beneficial effect of drugs is not questioned in general, the pressure to contain the healthcare costs is acute. Healthcare costs are increasing partly because people are living longer and more treatments are available. This may influence the commercial price that can be obtained for a new product entering the market and, in turn, the "cost of goods (CoG) target". The industry average for the CoG target is 5 to 10 percent of the commercial price with pressure to keep it as low as possible. This may impact on the choice and cost of raw materials, components and packaging for the product and the design and cost of manufacturing the drug and product.

Environmental pressures are to use environmentally friendly materials in products and processes and to accomplish the reduction of waste emissions from manufacturing processes. A good example is the replacement of chlorofluorocarbons (CFCs) propellants in pressurised metered dose inhalers (pMDIs) with hydrofluorocarbons (HFAs). The production of CFCs in developed countries was banned by the Montreal Protocol (an international treaty) apart from "essential uses", such as propellants in pMDIs, to reduce the damage to the earth's ozone layer. However, there is increasing pressure to phase out CFCs altogether. The transition from CFC to HFA products involves a massive reformulation exercise with significant technical challenges and costs for pharmaceutical companies involved in developing pMDIs, as described in Chapter 10 "Inhalation Dosage Forms". However, this can be turned into a commercial opportunity for some companies which have developed patent-protected delivery systems to extend the product life cycle of their CFC pMDI products.

LESSONS LEARNT AND THE WAY FORWARD

To achieve the best chance of a fast and efficient development programme to bring a candidate drug to market, several important messages can be gleaned from projects which have gone well and from companies with consistently good track records.

There are benefits for pharmaceutical development to get involved early with preclinical research during the candidate drug selection phase. This is to move away from an "over-the-wall" hand-over approach of the candidate drug to be developed from "research" to "development". The drug selection criteria will be primarily based on pharmacological properties such as potency, selectivity, duration of action and safety/toxicology assessments. However, if all these factors are satisfactory and similar, there may be an important difference between the pharmaceutical properties of candidate drugs. A candidate drug with preferred pharmaceutical properties, for example, good aqueous solubility, crystalline, nonhygroscopic and good stability, should be selected to minimise the challenges involved in developing a suitable formulation. This is discussed further in Chapter 2.

Another important factor is good long-term planning, ideally from candidate drug nomination to launch, with consideration for the safety, clinical, pharmaceutical development, manufacturing operations and regulatory strategies involved to develop the product. There is a need for one central, integrated, company project plan that has been agreed on by all parties with a vested interest in the project. Needless to say, the plan should contain details of activities, timings, responsibilities, milestones, reviews and decision points. Reviews and decision points are required at the end of a distinct activity to ensure that the project is still meeting its objectives and should progress to the next stage of development. However, these reviews should not cause any delays to the programme, rather, they should ratify what is already progressing. The traditional sequential phases of product development (see Chapter 2) must be overlapped to accelerate the product to market. In reality, plans will inevitably change with time; they should be "living" documents which are reviewed and updated at regular intervals and then communicated to all parties. There may be several more detailed, lower-level plans focusing on departmental activities, e.g., for pharmaceutical development, but these plans must be linked to the top level central project plan.

Forward planning should provide the opportunity for a well thought out and efficient approach to product development, identifying requirements up front so as to avoid too much deliberation and backtracking along the way. It also should provide a visible communication tool.

Good planning is supported by adopting a systematic and structured approach to product development. The development process can be broken down into several key defined stages—product design, process design, product optimisation, process optimisation, scale-up and so on. Each stage will have inputs and outputs as shown in Figure 1.3, a simplified framework for product development. The appropriate definition and requirements at each stage are described in Chapters 5 and 8 of this text.

As product development can take several years to complete, it is important to have an effective document management system in place to record the work. The primary reference source for recording experimental work will usually be a laboratory notebook. The work should be checked, dated and counter-signed to satisfy GLP and intellectual property requirements. Experimental protocols are sometimes useful for defining programmes of work,

Figure 1.3 Framework for product development.

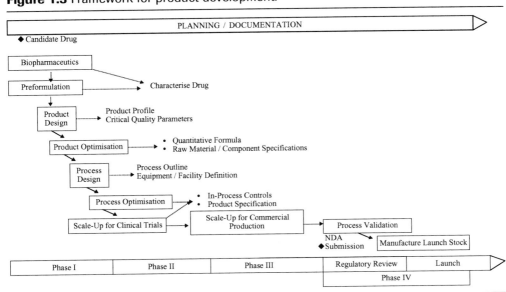

explaining the rationale for the studies and defining the acceptance criteria. When the studies are completed, the results can be reported with reference to the protocol and acceptance criteria. Laboratory notebooks are referenced in the protocols and reports so that the raw data can be retrieved in the event of an audit.

At the completion of key stages of the work, summary reports can be written, referencing all other protocols and reports relevant to that stage and highlighting the major recommendations and conclusions. In this way, a product development document file can be built up for transfer of information and technology, including the development history and rationale for progression. The file will also be vital for data retrieval in the event of a regulatory inspection.

Finally, successful product development is often associated with good teamwork. The process is multidisciplinary, relying on people with different specialist skills working together to make it happen. This is particularly important at the key interfaces such as preclinical research with pharmaceutical development and pharmaceutical development with manufacturing operations at the final production site. It is therefore useful to have representation on the project teams from all the key specialist functions to ensure buy-in to the plans, strategies and decisions and to have a good project management system in place.

SCOPE OF THE BOOK

This book is structured in a logical order to cover the various stages of drug development from candidate drug selection to development of the intended commercial dosage form.

In Chapter 2, the key stages of the R&D process are explained in some detail, with the outputs expected from each stage, to afford an appreciation of the entire process. The remainder of the book concentrates on candidate drug selection for development and development of the commercial dosage form where preformulation, biopharmaceutics and formulation play a vital role. Initial emphasis is on candidate drug selection and the importance of preformulation, formulation and biopharmaceutics input at this stage. Traditionally, not all pharmaceutical companies operate in this way, and the result from experience is often that pharmaceutical development has to accept whatever candidate drug comes out of research and address any unforeseen difficulties during development. The disadvantages of this approach, and the opportunities and benefits of pharmaceutical input to the candidate selection process, are clearly explained in the early chapters.

Available drug substance for preformulation and biopharmaceutics studies at the candidate drug selection stage can be a major challenge. Chapter 3 describes the preformulation studies that can be undertaken to maximise the information gained from small amounts of drug substance in order to select the preferred candidate drug for development. Various modern preformulation techniques which use minimal amounts of drug are described to evaluate the physicochemical properties of compounds, salts and polymorphs.

Chapter 4 describes the importance of drug delivery and biopharmaceutical factors in the candidate drug selection phase. Consideration is given to the intended route of administration and what predictions can be made and useful information gained from biopharmaceutical assessment of the candidate drug.

Following candidate selection, usually one candidate drug is nominated for development. The importance of establishing the product design attributes are discussed in Chapter 5. The value of this exercise is often underestimated in the rush to develop products quickly. However, the quality of the product design can often influence the success of developing a commercially viable product with a desired product profile in a timely manner to market.

Chapters 6 and 7 focus on preformulation and biopharmaceutics, respectively, as an aid to product design. The emphasis is on generating the appropriate data to characterise the candidate drug and aid product design and development. The objective at this stage is to determine the physicochemical properties of the candidate drug which are considered important in the development of a stable, effective and safe formulation. Limited availability of drug substance, speed and careful consideration of the programme of work depending on the intended dosage form and route are all considered here and illustrated with the aid of worked examples. Modern instrumental techniques and personal computer (PC)–based "expert systems" are discussed as useful tools.

To develop a product from inception to market, the product and process have to be optimised and the process scaled up and transferred to commercial production. Definitions and descriptions of the requirements for all these stages of development are discussed in Chapter 8, although the major discussion is on the preformulation/formulation input to product optimisation. The many factors which a formulator should consider in the selection of pharmaceutical excipients and packaging are discussed. Useful sources of information and techniques for selection such as expert systems and experimental design tools are included.

Drugs are generally administered via the mouth, eyes, nose, skin, or by inhalation or injection, and so these routes are covered in more detail in separate chapters of this book. Special considerations and issues for the formulation development of each route and type of dosage form are discussed, based on the considerable relevant experience of the various contributors.

REFERENCES

Anonymous. (1993). Global differences in registration requirements. *Pharmaceut. J.* 251:610–611.

Karia, R., Y. Lis, and S. R. Walker. 1992. The erosion of effective patent life—An international comparison. In *Medicines, regulation, research and risk* 2nd ed., edited by J. P. Griffin. Belfast: Queen's University Press, pp. 287–301.

Lis. Y., and S. R. Walker. 1988. Pharmaceutical patent term erosion—A comparison of the UK, USA and Federal Republic of Germany (FRG). *Pharmaceut. J.* 240:176–180.

McKinsey & Co. 1991. In *Managing product creation, a management overview*, edited by P. Burall. London: The Design Council for the UK Department of Trade and Industry.

Spence, C., ed. 1997. *The pharmaceutical R & D compendium: CMR International/SCRIP's guide to trends in R & D*. Richmond, Survey, UK: CMR International/SCRIP Publication.

Tucker, D. 1984. *The world health market, the future of the pharmaceutical industry*. Bücher, Germany: Euromonitor Publications Ltd.

Wells, J. I. 1988. *Pharmaceutical preformulation. The physicochemical properties of drug substances*. Chichester, UK: Ellis Horwood, and New York: Wiley.

Part I

AIDING CANDIDATE DRUG SELECTION

2

Aiding Candidate Drug Selection: Introduction and Objectives

Mark Gibson

AstraZeneca R&D Charnwood
Loughborough, United Kingdom

STAGES OF THE DRUG DISCOVERY AND DEVELOPMENT PROCESS

The development of a new medicinal product from a novel synthesised chemical compound, a chemical extracted from a natural source or a compound produced by biotechnological processes, is a long and complex process and involves many different disciplines working together. The drug discovery and development process for a typical research-based pharmaceutical company can be broken down into five distinct stages as described briefly below. At each stage, there will be several activities running in parallel, with the overall objective of discovering a candidate drug and developing it to market as efficiently as possible. It should be noted that different companies may use slightly different terminology and perform some activities sooner or later, but the overall process is essentially the same.

Strategic Research

Feasibility studies are conducted to demonstrate whether interfering in a particular biological mechanism has an effect that might be of therapeutic value.

The strategic research of a particular company is usually guided by factors such as its inherent research competence and expertise, therapeutic areas of unmet medical need and market potential/commercial viability. Companies often wish to develop a portfolio of products within a specific therapeutic area to capture a segment of the market. By focusing on a particular therapeutic area, a company can build on its existing expertise and competence in all of its functions with the aim of becoming a leading company in that field.

Exploratory Research

Investigation of the biological mechanism and identification of a "chemical lead" that interferes with it.

During the exploratory research stage, diverse compounds are screened for the desired biological activity. The aim is to find a chemical or molecular entity that interferes with the process and to provide a valuable probe of the underlying therapeutic problem. Traditionally, this has been achieved by the organic chemist synthesising compounds one at a time for the biologist to test in a linear fashion. Over the last decade, there has been a rapid development in the technologies for creating very large and diverse quantities of synthetic and biosynthetic molecules and for testing large numbers for activity in less time. These technologies have been labelled "combinatorial chemistry" and automated "high-throughput screening" (HTS), respectively. The key impact has been to accelerate the synthesis of new compounds from, say, 50 compounds per chemist year to many tens of thousands and to be able to test these against many biological targets (e.g., biological receptors or biochemical pathways) very quickly (Doyle et al. 1998).

The rate of technology development specifically associated with HTS for pharmaceutical drug discovery has increased markedly over recent years with automated techniques involving miniaturisation, to allow assays on very small samples (e.g., 1 µL volume), and the ability to analyse thousands of samples a day using well microplates (Burbaum 1998). In addition to the use of HTS for pharmacological activity, HTS tests have been developed for assessing metabolism and pharmacokinetic and toxicity factors to speed up the drug discovery process.

In simple terms, a biologically active compound can be considered to consist of a supportive framework with biofunctional groups attached that bind to a target to induce a biological response. Each compound is, in effect, a unique combination of numerous possible groups. Combinatorial techniques have replaced traditional synthetic approaches to generate many possible combinations rapidly for biological testing.

Approaches to lead generation during exploratory research often depend on how much is already known about the therapeutic target under consideration. For example, if the three-dimensional structure of the target (such as an enzyme-inhibitor complex) is known, chemical leads could be found and optimised through combinatorial chemistry and HTS. Alternatively, in some cases, the only available biochemical knowledge might be the structure of a ligand for the enzyme. If there were no information at all, then the only approach might be limited to HTS of batches of compounds from combinatorial libraries.

Even with combinatorial chemistry and HTS, lead generation can be extremely laborious because of the vast number of different molecules possible (framework and biofunctional group combinations). To ease this burden, some rational drug design and quantitative structure activity relationships (QSARs) are often introduced to direct the programme and utilise a company's finite screening resource as efficiently as possible.

"Representative" libraries of compounds, where each member is selected to give information about a larger cluster of compounds, are designed and used to reduce the amount of compounds that have to be made and tested.

Together with combinatorial chemistry and rational drug design, genomics is rapidly emerging as a useful technique to enable companies to significantly increase the number of drug targets and improve on candidate selection success. A number of companies have seen the potential in defining patient groups based on their genotypes and are now investing lots of money to gain a clearer understanding of the genes that are important to drug action.

Candidate Drug Selection

The chemical lead is used to generate specific chemical compounds with the optimal desired characteristics, for example, potency, specificity, duration, safety and pharmaceutical aspects. One or more candidate drugs are nominated for development.

During the candidate drug selection stage, the chemical lead is optimised by testing a range of selected compounds in *in vitro* and *in vivo* (animal) studies. The objective is to select one or more candidate drugs for development with the most desired characteristics. Pharmacological characteristics might include acceptable absorption, potency, duration of action and selectivity for the receptor or enzyme. Safety characteristics will normally include non-carcinogenicity, non-teratogenicity, non-mutagenicity, and general non-toxicity. The potential for these characteristics can be predicted from relatively short-term preclinical toxipharmacological animal studies and *in vitro* tests.

In the interests of rapid drug development, it is also important to select a compound with preferred pharmaceutical and chemical synthesis properties at this stage. A list of preferred characteristics for a compound intended for oral solid dosage form development is given in Table 2.1.

Higher priority in the selection process will, in most cases, be given to a compound's optimal pharmacological and safety characteristics. However, in the event of having a choice from a range of compounds all possessing similar pharmacological and safety properties, there may be a significant advantage for formulation development in selecting a compound with the most preferred pharmaceutical properties. It is useful to conduct preformulation studies and biopharmaceutics studies at the candidate drug selection stage to determine the

Table 2.1
Preferred drug synthesis and pharmaceutical properties for compounds intended for oral solid dosage form development.

Drug Synthesis Factors	Formulation/Drug Delivery Factors
• Least complex structure (none/few chiral centres)	• Exists as a stable polymorphic form
• Few synthesis steps as possible	• Non-hygroscopic
• High yields as possible	• Crystalline
• Non-explosive route or safety issues	• Acceptable solid-state stability of candidate drug
• Commercial availability of building blocks and contract manufacturers	• Acceptable oral bioavailability
• Low cost of goods compared to overall cost of product on market	• Not highly coloured or strong odour (to ensure batch reproducibility and reduce problems with blinding in clinical studies)
• No predicted problems in scale-up	• Compatible with key excipients

most relevant physicochemical and biopharmaceutical properties of potential candidate drugs to aid candidate selection.

Biopharmaceutics is the study of how the physicochemical properties of the candidate drugs, the formulation/delivery system and the route of administration affect the rate and extent of drug absorption. Appropriate biopharmaceutical information generated at this stage can also be very important in directing the candidate selection process and for future dosage form design during development.

The benefits of providing preformulation and biopharmaceutics input during the candidate drug selection stage, to characterise the candidate drug and provide useful information to support the selection of the optimal compound for pharmaceutical development, are emphasised in Chapters 3 and 4. Generally, any pharmaceutical issues can be discovered earlier, before the candidate drug reaches development, and any implications for product design and development considered in advance. Pharmaceutical development's involvement in the selection process and "buy-in" to the nomination decision can often enhance the team's working relationship with their research colleagues. The objective is to achieve a seamless transition from research to development, as opposed to the traditional "over-the-wall" approach that many pharmaceutical companies experience to their costs. Earlier involvement by the Pharmaceutical Development group at the preclinical stage should also result in better planning for full development.

In spite of all these potential advantages of early pharmaceutical involvement to candidate drug selection, there may be several barriers within a company which can hinder this way of working. Distance between the Research group and the Development group should not really be considered a barrier, although this can be the case for groups on different continents with different cultures and languages. The important factor for success seems to be the development of a formal mechanism for interaction, supported by senior management in the company. This often takes the form of a joint project team with regular meetings to review progress. However, there may still be a lack of appreciation of what input or expertise pharmaceutical development can offer at the candidate drug selection stage. Opportunities to demonstrate what can be done and to educate Research colleagues should be sought to try and overcome this attitude.

Another potential barrier is any overlapping expertise there may be in Research and Development groups. For example, overlap may occur between Preformulation in Pharmaceutical Development and Physical Chemistry in Research, or between Biopharmaceutics in Development and Drug Metabolism in Research. In these cases, it is important to clarify and agree which group does what activity.

A common perceived barrier to providing early preformulation and biopharmaceutics input can be the quantity of compound required for evaluation at this stage. The Research group may believe that significantly more compound is required; with modern instrumental techniques, however, this is often not the case.

Other potential barriers which can influence the success of the relationship with Research at the candidate drug selection stage are the Pharmaceutical Development response time not being fast enough to support Research and the lack of resources that Pharmaceutical Development can give to support the candidate drug selection programme. Several compounds may have to be evaluated simultaneously to generate comparative data to aid the selection process. Preformulation and Biopharmaceutics have to keep pace with the pharmacological and safety testing, otherwise there is no point in generating the data. One way of achieving this is to allocate dedicated resources to these projects using people trained to rapidly respond to the preformulation and biopharmaceutics requirements. Simple formulations can be used at this stage, and rank order information is often acceptable, rather than definitive quantitative information. Analytical methods should not require rigorous validation at this stage to provide these data. Excessive documentation and rigid standard operating procedures that can slow down the work are not usually necessary and should be avoided.

Exploratory Development

The aim of exploratory development is to gauge how the candidate drug is absorbed and metabolised in healthy human volunteers before studying its effect on those actually suffering from the disease for which it is intended. Occasionally, it is necessary to conduct further small-scale studies in patients in order to make a decision whether to progress the candidate drug into full development. This stage is often referred to as Phase I clinical studies or Concept Testing (Proof of Concept). Usually a small number of healthy volunteers (who do not have the condition under investigation or any other illness) receives the drug candidate provided as a simple formulation, which can be different from the intended commercial formulation. For example, a simple aqueous oral solution or suspension may be used, rather than a capsule or tablet, to minimise the formulation development work at this early stage.

If the candidate drug does not produce the expected effects in human studies, or produces unexpected and unwanted effects, the development programme is likely to be stopped at this stage. In the United Kingdom, there is no requirement, at the time of this writing, to make a submission to the local regulatory authorities for permission to conduct the trials in human volunteers. However, this is likely to change in the future to bring the United Kingdom in line with the rest of the world.

Full Development

Completion of longer-term safety and clinical studies (Phase II and Phase III) in patients suffering from the disease are accomplished at this stage. Phase II studies are dose ranging studies in a reasonable patient population (several hundred) to evaluate the effectiveness of the drug and common side-effects. During Phase II, the intended commercial formulation should be developed, and the product/process optimised and eventually scaled up to commercial production scale. The candidate drug should ideally be in the intended commercial formulation for the Phase III trials. After the satisfactory completion of Phase II trials, large patient populations (several hundred to thousands) are involved to statistically confirm efficacy and safety. Some patients will be given the drug, some a placebo product (required to be identical in appearance) and some may be given a known market leader (with all products appearing identical). The doctors and patients in the study will not know whether the patients are getting the test drug, placebo or market leader; by switching the medication in a controlled way (double-blind trials), objectivity and statistical assessment of the treatment under investigation are assured. Most regulatory authorities, including the U.S. Food and Drugs Administration (FDA), the Medicines Control Agency (MCA) in the United Kingdom and the European Agency for the Evaluation of Medicinal Products (EMEA), require three phases of clinical trials and sufficient data to demonstrate that the new product can be licensed as safe, effective and of acceptable quality. Once these clinical studies are complete, the company can decide whether it wishes to submit a marketing authorisation application to a regulatory authority for a medicinal drug product. Approval is usually followed by product launch to market.

SUMMARY

Pharmaceutical companies with the best track records for drug discovery and rapid development to market tend to have a seamless transfer from Research to Development. There are many opportunities and benefits to be gained by the involvement of Pharmaceutical Development groups, such as Preformulation and Biopharmaceutics, during the candidate drug selection stage: It may be surprising what valuable information can be obtained using modern preformulation instrumental techniques and biopharmaceutical techniques from relatively small quantities of compound. These topics are discussed further in Chapters 3 and 4 of this text.

REFERENCES

Burbaum, J. 1998. Engines of discovery. *Chemistry in Britain* (June): 38–41.

Doyle, P. M., E. Barker, C. J. Harris, and M. J. Slater. 1998. Combinatorial technologies—A revolution in pharmaceutical R&D. *Pharmaceutical Technology Europe* (April): 26–32.

3

Preformulation Predictions from Small Amounts of Compound as an Aid to Candidate Drug Selection

Gerry Steele

AstraZeneca R&D Charnwood
Loughborough, United Kingdom

Prior to nomination into full development, a candidate drug should undergo a phase traditionally called preformulation. Preformulation is the physicochemical characterization of the solid and solution properties of compounds and although now relatively old, the definition of preformulation proposed by Akers (1976) is particularly apt:

> Preformulation testing encompasses all studies enacted on a new drug compound in order to produce useful information for subsequent formulation of a stable and biopharmaceutically suitable drug dosage form.

Furthermore, Wells' book on the subject (1988) closes by exhorting pharmaceutical scientists:

> Do not neglect these foundations. Good preformulation will inevitably lead to simple and elegant formulations and successful commercial products.

The scope of preformulation studies to be carried out will depend not only on the expertise, equipment and drug substance available but also on any organizational preferences or restrictions. Some companies like to conduct detailed characterization studies, whilst others prefer to do the minimum amount of work required to progress compounds as quickly as possible into development. Both of these approaches have pros and cons. However, for the smooth progression of compounds through the preformulation phase, a close interaction between departments of Medicinal Chemistry in Research, Pharmaceutical Sciences, Analytical Chemistry and Drug Substance Process Development is essential.

Although preformulation typically begins in earnest during the lead optimization (LO) phase, there may be some involvement during lead identification (LI). In LI, support may be given to Medicinal Chemistry for solid-state screening to ensure that, e.g., batches of a compound are the same polymorph. LO normally takes around two years; during the last three to six months, the number of compounds being seriously considered for nomination will have been narrowed to around three. This phase is known as prenomination. During this period, there may be a number of compounds with sufficient activity to merit consideration, and so studies must be designed to select which compound to proceed with into development. Clear differences in *in vivo* activity may be sufficient to determine which of the candidates is selected. However, other factors that may be important from a pharmaceutical and drug synthesis point of view should also be considered if there is a choice. For example, physicochemical characteristics of the compound(s), ease of scale-up for compound supply, availability of analytical procedures and the nature of the anticipated dosage form should also be taken into consideration in the decision process.

Ideally, for an oral solid dosage form, a water-soluble, non-hygroscopic, stable and easily processed crystalline compound is preferred for development purposes; however, other formulation types will have their own specific requirements.

Table 3.1 summarizes the prenomination studies that could be carried out on a candidate drug. These are considered to be the minimum tests that should be undertaken, recognizing that during the prenomination phase only a limited quantity of compound, e.g., 50 mg, is typically available for characterization. However, it should be emphasized that this is a critical decision period that can profoundly affect the subsequent development of a candidate drug. Thus, the tests shown are considered to be those important for making a rational decision as to which compound, salt or polymorph to proceed with into development. A poor decision at this point could mean a substantial amount of revisionary work, such as a change of salt or polymorph being necessary, and a possible delay to the development of the drug to the market.

After nomination to full development, the increased quantity of candidate drug available will allow a more complete physicochemical characterization of the chosen compound(s) to be carried out, with particular emphasis on the dosage form. These tests should allow a rational, stable and bioavailable formulation to be progressed, which will be discussed in more detail in Chapter 6.

INITIAL PHYSICOCHEMICAL CHARACTERIZATION

Many of the tests carried out, for example, proof of structure, are normally performed out by discovery: nuclear magnetic resonance (NMR), mass spectra and elemental analysis. Although important from a physicochemical point of view, these will not be discussed in this chapter. Rather, we will focus on those tests carried out during prenomination that will have an important bearing in the selection of an optimal candidate drug.

Table 3.1
Suggested physicochemical tests carried out during prenomination.

Tier 1		
Test/Activity	Guidance to Amount	Timing/Comments
Elemental analysis	4 mg	LO
Initial HPLC methodology	2 mg	LO
NMR spectroscopy	5 mg	LO
Mass spectroscopy	5 mg	LO
General, e.g., MW, structural and empirical formulae	–	LO
IR/UV Visible Spectroscopy	5 mg	LO
Karl Fischer	20 mg	LO
pK_a	10 mg	LO
log P/log D	10 mg	LO
Initial solubility	10 mg	LO/Prenomination
Initial solution stability	Done on above samples	LO//Prenomination
Crystallinity investigations	20–30 mg	LO/Prenomination
Hygroscopicity	5–10 mg	LO/Prenomination
Initial solid stability	10 mg	Prenomination
Salt selection		
Decide/manufacture salts		Prenomination
Characterize salts—use DVS, X-ray, DSC, solubility/stability tests	10–50 mg each salt	Prenomination
Initial polymorphism studies, etc.—investigations of selected salt or neutral compound. Production— use different solvents, cooling rates, precipitation, evaporation techniques, etc	100 mg	Prenomination (also included is the propensity of the CD to form hydrates, solvates and amorphs)
Polymorphism, etc. investigations of selected salt or neutral compound. Characterization.		Prenomination
DSC/TGA/HSM	2 mg per technique/sample	Prenomination
X-ray powder diffraction, including temp and RH	10 mg per sample, zero background holder	Prenomination
FTIR/Raman	2 mg per sample	Prenomination
Crystal habit—microscopy, light and SEM	10 mg	Prenomination
Stability-stress wrt, temp/humidity	100 mg	Prenomination
Choose polymorph, amorph or hydrate		Prenomination

pK_a Determinations

Many potential candidate drugs are weak acids or bases, therefore, one of the most pertinent determinations carried out prior to development is the pK_a or ionization constant. Strong acids, e.g., HCl, are ionized at all pH values, whereas the ionization of weak acids is dependent on pH. It is useful to know the extent to which the molecule is ionized at a certain pH, since properties such as solubility, stability, drug absorption and activity are affected by this parameter. The basic theory of the ionization constant is covered by most physical chemistry textbooks, and a most useful text is that by Albert and Sargeant (1984). Fundamental to our appreciation of the determination of this parameter, however, is the Brønstead and Lowry theory of acids and bases. This states that an acid is a substance that can donate a hydrogen ion, and a base is one that can accept a proton.

For a weak acid, the following equilibrium holds:

$$HA \rightleftharpoons H^+ + A^-$$

For the sake of brevity, a detailed discussion and derivation of equations will be avoided; however, it is important that the well-known Henderson–Hasselbach equation is understood (equation 1). This equation relates the pK_a to the pH of the solution and the relative concentrations of the dissociated and undissociated parts of a weak acid:

$$pH = pK_a + \log\frac{[A^-]}{[HA]} \tag{1}$$

where $[A^-]$ is the concentration of the dissociated species, and $[HA]$ is the concentration of the undissociated species. This equation can be manipulated into the form given by equation 2 to yield the percentage of a compound that will be ionized at any particular pH.

$$\%\text{ionization} = \frac{100}{1+\left(pH - pK_a\right)} \tag{2}$$

One simple point to note about equation 1 is that at 50 percent dissociation (or ionization), pK_a = pH. It should also be noted that, usually, pK_a values are preferred for bases instead of pK_b values (pK_w = pK_a + pK_b).

Some methods used in the determination of ionization constants are shown in Table 3.2. Figure 3.1 shows the curve obtained from the titration of a hydrochloride salt with sodium hydroxide. The pK_a obtained from this experiment was 7.9.

If a compound is poorly soluble in water, the pK_a may be difficult to measure. One way around this problem is to measure the apparent pK_a of the compound in solvent and water mixtures and then extrapolate the data back to a purely aqueous medium using a Yasuda-Shedlovsky plot. The organic solvents most frequently used are methanol, ethanol, propanol, dimethylsulphoxide (DMSO), dimethyl formamide (DMFA), acetone and tetrahydrofuran (THF). However, methanol is by far the most popular because its properties are closest to water. A validation study in water-methanol mixtures has been reported by Takács-Novák et al. (1997) and the determination of the pK_as of ibuprofen and quinine in a range of organic solvent–water mixtures has been reported by Avdeef et al. (1999).

If the compound contains an ultraviolet (UV) chromophore that changes with the extent of ionization, then a method involving UV spectroscopy can be used. This method involves measuring the UV spectrum of the compound as a function of pH. Mathematical analysis of

Table 3.2
Some reported methods for the determination of pK_as.

Method	Reference
Potentiometric titration	Rosenberg and Wagenknecht (1986)
UV spectotroscopy	Asuero et al. (1986)
Solubility measurements	Zimmerman (1986a, 1986b)
HPLC techniques	Gustavo González (1993)
Capillary zone electrophoresis	Chauret et al. (1995)
Foaming activity	Alverez Núñez and Yalkowsky (1997)

the spectral shifts can then be used to determine the pK_a(s) of the compound. This method is most suitable for compounds in which the ionizing group is close to or actually within an aromatic ring, which usually results in large UV shifts upon ionization.

The pK_a of a compound may be estimated using ACDpKa software, which also contains a large database of measured pK_a data. The use of the computer program SPARC (scalable processor architecture) for estimating the pK_a of pharmaceuticals has been described by Hilal et al. (1996).

The UV method requires only 1 mg of compound, and the potentiometric method requires 3 mg of compound. The compound is equilibrated with an octanol/aqueous buffer

Figure 3.1 Titration curve obtained by titration of a hydrochloride salt of a weak base with NaOH.

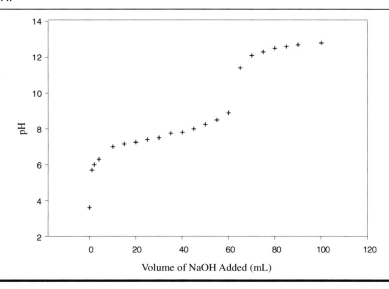

Volume of NaOH Added (mL)

mixture for 30 min, and the resulting emulsion is centrifuged to separate the two constituent phases. Once separated, the concentration of each layer is determined by high performance liquid chromatography (HPLC) and log D/log P is calculated. Bearing in mind the drive to determine the maximum amount of information from the minimum quantity of compound, Morgan et al. (1998) have developed microscale titrimetric and spectrophotometric methods for determination of the pK_a and log Ps of candidate drugs (see next section).

The Partition and Distribution Coefficients

The relationship between chemical structure, lipophilicity and its disposition *in vivo* has been reviewed by a number of authors (e.g., Koehler et al. 1988). It has been shown that many biological phenomena can be correlated with this parameter, such that "quantitative structure activity relationships" (QSARs) may be deduced. These include solubility, absorption potential, membrane permeability, plasma protein binding, volume of distribution and renal and hepatic clearance.

The lipophilicity of an organic compound is usually described in terms of a partition coefficient, log P, which can be defined as the ratio of the concentration of the unionized compound, at equilibrium, between organic and aqueous phases:

$$\log P = \frac{[\text{unionized compound}]_{org}}{[\text{unionized compound}]_{aq}} \qquad (3)$$

It is worth noting that this is a logarithmic scale, therefore, a log P = 0 means that the compound is equally soluble in water and in the partitioning solvent. If the compound has a log P = 5, then the compound is 100,000 times more soluble in the partitioning solvent. A log P = –2 means that the compound is 100 times more soluble in water, i.e., it is quite hydrophilic.

Log P values have been studied in approximately 100 organic liquid–water systems. Since it is virtually impossible to determine log P in a realistic biological medium, the octanol-water system has been widely adopted as a model of the lipid phase (Leo et al. 1971). Whilst there has been much debate about the suitability of this system (see, e.g., Dearden and Bresnen 1988), it is the most widely used in pharmaceutical studies. Octanol and water are immiscible, but some water does dissolve in octanol in a hydrated state. This hydrated state contains 16 octanol aggregates, with the hydroxyl head groups surrounded by trapped aqueous solution. Lipophilic (unionized) species dissolve in the aliphatic regions of the octanol, whilst ionized species (see below) are drawn to the polar regions (Franks et al. 1993). The partitioning of solutes in different solvent systems has been reported by El-Tayar et al. (1991).

The most common method for determining partition and distribution coefficients is the shake flask method. In this technique, the candidate drug is shaken between octanol (previously shaken together to presaturate each phase with the other) and water layers, from which an aliquot is taken and analyzed using UV absorption, HPLC or titration. In terms of experimental conditions, the value of the partition coefficient obtained from this type of experiment is affected by such factors as temperature, insufficient mutual phase saturation, pH and buffer ions and their concentration, as well as the nature of the solvents used and solute examined (Dearden and Bresnen 1988).

The role of log P in absorption processes occurring after oral administration has been discussed by Navia and Chaturvedi (1996). Generally, compounds with log P values between

1 and 3 show good absorption, whereas those with log Ps greater than 6 or less than 3 often have poor transport characteristics. Highly non-polar molecules have a preference to reside in the lipophilic regions of membranes, and very polar compounds show poor bioavailability because of their inability to penetrate membrane barriers. Thus, there is a parabolic relationship between log P and transport, i.e., candidate drugs that exhibit a balance between these two properties will probably show the best oral bioavailability.

The partition coefficient refers to the intrinsic lipophilicity of the drug, in the context of the equilibrium of unionized drug between the aqueous and organic phases. As we noted in the last section, if the drug has more than one ionization centre, the distribution of species present will depend on the pH. The concentration of the ionized drug in the aqueous phase will therefore have an effect on the overall observed partition coefficient. This leads to the definition of the distribution coefficient (log D) of a compound, which takes into account the dissociation of weak acids and bases. For a weak acid this is defined by

$$D = \frac{[\text{HA}]_{org}}{[\text{HA}]_{aq} + [\text{A}^-]_{aq}} \tag{4}$$

It can be seen that combining this equation with equation 1 gives an equation relating the distribution to the intrinsic lipophilicity (log P), the pK_a of the molecule and the pH of the aqueous phase:

$$\log\left(\frac{P}{D-1}\right) = pH - pK_a$$
$$\log\left(\frac{P}{D-1}\right) = pK_a - pH \tag{5}$$

Figure 3.2 shows the effect of ionization on the partitioning of a proton pump inhibitor compound. This compound has a log P of 3.82 and three pK_as, i.e., ≤1, 5.26 and 8.63. At low pH, both the benzimidazole and diethylamine nitrogens are protonated, and hence the tendency of the compound is to reside in the aqueous phase. As the pH increases, deprotonation of the protonated nitrogen of the benzimidazole takes place; as the compound is less ionized, the compound resides more in the octanol phase. At neutral pH, deprotonation of the diethylamine nitrogen renders the molecule neutral, and hence its lipophilicity is at a maximum. A further increase in the pH results in deprotonation of the second nitrogen to form an anion which, being ionized, is more hydrophilic, resulting in a decrease in log D.

HPLC techniques have also been used in the determination of log P values. Lambert et al. (1990), for example, have described the development of a preformulation lipophilicity screen utilizing a C_{18} derivatized HPLC column. They appeared to prefer this column to the traditional reverse-phase HPLC columns, which may yield a poor correlation between log P and the capacity factor (k'). A potential problem with the use of HPLC retention data is that it is not a direct method and thus requires calibration. Futhermore, there may be problems with performing experiments above pH 8.

Barnett et al. (1992) have described a method for estimating partition coefficients from data collected using a filter probe extractor. They developed the method to analyze data from two component mixtures (e.g., in the presence of an impurity) for which there existed no suitable method. The technique is based on model fitting and may also be used for pure compounds.

Figure 3.2 Ionization and partitioning scheme for a proton pump inhibitor.

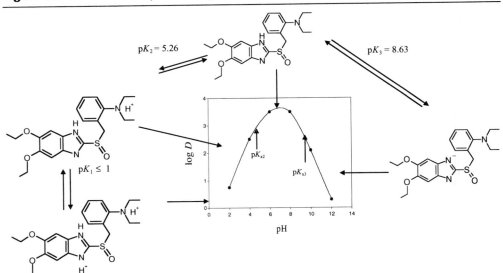

Log D membrane, or log D_{mem}, is another way of measuring the lipophilicity of a compound (e.g., Austin et al. 1995). However, it is fair to say that it is much less frequently used than the octanol/water partition system. Log D_{mem} utilizes liposomes prepared from the synthetic phospholipid dimyristoylphosphatidylcholine (DMPC), and although the system is more physiologically relevant than octanol, it suffers from a lack of predictability. This method requires 1 mg of compound, whereby a solution of the compound is equilibrated with a solution of DMPC liposomes at 37°C for 2 h. The free and liposome-bound compounds are then separated by centrifugation, and the solutions are analyzed by HPLC. Log D_{mem} is then calculated as the log of the ratio of the concentration of compound in the liposome phase to that of the compound in the aqueous phase.

More recently, computer methods have been devised to calculate these values. The molecule is broken down into fragments of known lipophilicity, and the log P is calculated using various computer routines. Alternatively, there are atom-based methods, and lipophilicity is calculated by summing the atom-type values. Although discrepancies do occur between measured and calculated log Ps (clog Ps), agreement is reasonably good. Programs and methods for calculating log P values have been reviewed by van de Waterbeemd and Mannhold (1996). Clearly this requires no compound and can be a useful starting place for these types of measurements.

INITIAL SOLUBILITY

The solubility of a candidate drug may be the critical factor determining its usefulness, since aqueous solubility dictates the amount of compound that will dissolve and, therefore, the amount available for absorption. If a compound has a low aqueous solubility, it may be subject to dissolution rate-limited absorption within the gastro-intestinal (GI) residence time.

Recently, the importance of solubility, in biopharmaceutical terms, has been highlighted by its use in the biopharmaceutics classification system (BCS) described by Amidon et al. (1995). In this system, compounds are defined in terms of combinations of their solubility and permeability, e.g., high solubility, high permeability or low solubility, high permeability. High solubility is defined as the highest dose strength that is soluble in 250 mL or less of aqueous media across the physiological pH range. Poorly soluble drugs can be defined as those with an aqueous solubility of less than 100 µg/mL. If a drug is poorly soluble, then it will only slowly dissolve, perhaps leading to incomplete absorption (Hörter and Dressman 1997). The importance of solubility (and permeability) in drug discovery and development arenas has also been discussed by Lipinski et al. (1997).

James (1986) has provided some general rules regarding solubility:

- Electrolytes dissolve in conducting solvents.

- Solutes containing hydrogen capable of forming hydrogen bonds dissolve in solvents capable of accepting hydrogen bonds and vice versa.

- Solutes having significant dipole moments dissolve in solvents having significant dipole moments.

- Solutes with low or zero dipole moments dissolve in solvents with low or zero dipole moments.

There will be some exceptions to these rules, but a good rule of thumb is "like dissolves like". In this respect, solvents fall into three classes: (a) protic solvents such as methanol and formamide which are hydrogen bond donors, (b) dipolar aprotic solvents (e.g., acetonitrile, nitrobenzene) with dielectric constants greater than 15 but which cannot form hydrogen bonds with the solute and (c) aprotic solvents in which the dielectric constant is weak and the solvent is non-polar, e.g., pentane or benzene.

If solubility of a compound is accompanied by degradation, the quotation of a solubility figure is problematic. In this case, it is preferable to quote a solubility figure but with the caveat that a specified amount of degradation was found. Obviously, large amounts of degradation will render the solubility value meaningless. A technique to estimate the water solubility of a number of water unstable prodrugs of 5-fluorouracil has been reported by Beall et al. (1993).

The U.S. Pharmacopeia (USP) gives the following definitions of solubility:

Descriptive Term	Parts of Solvent Required for 1 Part of Solute
Very soluble	Less than 1
Freely soluble	From 1 to 10
Soluble	From 10 to 30
Sparingly soluble	From 30 to 100
Slightly soluble	From 100 to 1,000
Very slightly soluble	From 1,000 to 10,000
Practically insoluble or insoluble	10,000 and over

Many candidate drugs are ionizable organic compounds, and thus there are a number of parameters that will determine the solubility of a compound. These parameters include, e.g., molecular size and substituent groups on the molecule, degree of ionization, ionic strength, salt form, temperature, crystal properties and complexation.

Molecular Size

Large organic molecules have a smaller aqueous solubility than smaller molecules, this being due to interactions between the non-polar groups and water, i.e., solubility is dependent on the number of solvent molecules that can pack around the solute molecule (James 1986). Figure 3.3 shows the effect of molecular weight on the solubility of some amino acids in water (data from James 1986).

Effect of Ionization on Solubility

The solubility of a compound, at a given pH, is a function of the solubility of the ionized form and the limiting solubility of the neutral molecule. This gives rise to equations 6 and 7, which describe the relationship between the intrinsic solubility of the free acid or base S_O, the pK_a and the pH.

$$S = [HA] + [A^-] \qquad \text{for acids} \qquad (6)$$

$$S = [B] + [BH^+] \qquad \text{for bases} \qquad (7)$$

Figure 3.3 Solubility of amino acids in water as a function of molecular weight.

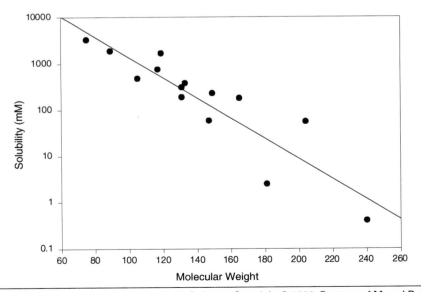

Data from *Solubility and related phenomena*, by K. C. James, Copyright © 1986. Courtesy of Marcel Dekker, Inc.

By setting $S_O = [HA]$ for acids or $[B]$ for bases and recalling our definition of the ionization constant, it follows that for weak acids with only one ionization centre, the change in solubility with respect to pH is given by

$$S = S_O\{1 + 10^{pH - pKa}\} \qquad (8)$$

Thus, it is possible to calculate the solubility of a compound at any pH if the intrinsic solubility and pK_a of the free acid or base are known.

A weak acid with two ionizable acid groups shows a more dramatic increase in solubility with respect to pH as described by equation 9 (Zimmerman 1986a).

$$S = S_O\left\{1 + \frac{K_{a1}}{[H^+]} + \frac{K_{a1}K_{a2}}{[H^+]^2}\right\} \text{ or } S = S_O\left\{1 + 10^{pH - pK_{a1}} + 10^{2pH - pK_{a1} + pK_{a2}}\right\} \qquad (9)$$

Figure 3.4 shows the pH-solubility profile of the disodium salt of a weak acid, demonstrating that the solubility reaches a plateau around pH 5. This is the limiting solubility (S^*) of the dianion under these experimental conditions. The experimentally determined pH-solubility curve for an amine hydrochloride salt is shown in Figure 3.5. The observed behaviour can be attributed to a number of physico-chemical phenomena (Serrajuden and Mufson 1985). For example, at a low pH, the solubility is suppressed due to the common ion effect. However, the rise in solubility at pH values > 5 is more difficult to explain. In this case, supersaturation due to self-association appears to be the most likely explanation (Ledwidge and Corrigan 1998).

Using conventional techniques, it is unlikely that a complete solubility profile can be generated in the prenomination phase due to a lack of compound. However, if the intrinsic solubility of the free base or acid is known, then the solubility can be calculated at any pH.

In the case of amphoteric compounds, equation 10 is relevant at a pH below the isoelectric point, and equation 11 above the isoelectric point.

$$pH - pK_a = \log\left(\frac{S - S_O}{S_O}\right) \qquad (10)$$

$$pH - pK_a = \log\left(\frac{S_O}{S_O - S}\right) \qquad (11)$$

Recently, an instrument for determining intrinsic solubility and pH-solubility profiles has been introduced. Known as pSOL™, it claims that with as little as 0.1 mg a complete solubility profile can be derived (Avdeef et al. 2000).

Additives

Additives may increase or decrease the solubility of a solute in a given solvent. In the case of salts, those that increase the solubility are said to "salt in" the solute, and those that decrease the solubility to "salt out" the solute. The effect of the additive depends very much on the influence it has on the structure of the water or its ability to compete with solvent water molecules. Both effects are described by the empirically derived Setschenow equation

$$\log\frac{S_O}{S} = kM \qquad (12)$$

Figure 3.4 pH–solubility curve of a disodium salt of a weak acid.

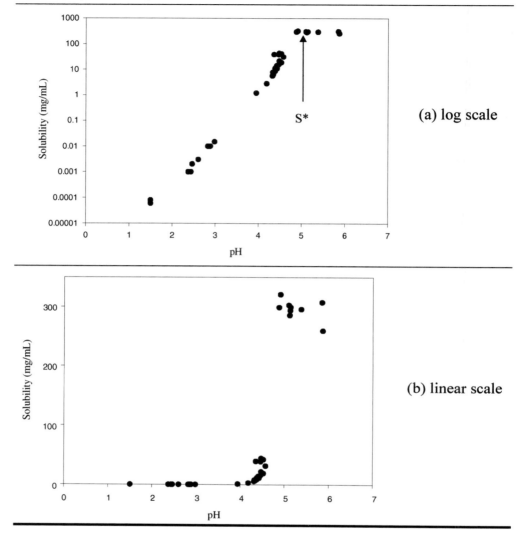

(a) log scale

(b) linear scale

where S_O = the solubility of the non-electrolyte in pure water, S = the solubility of the non-electrolyte in the salt solution, M = concentration of the salt and k = the salting out constant which is equal to $0.217/S_O$ at low concentrations of added salt.

Another aspect of the effect of electrolytes on the solubility of a salt is the concept of the solubility product for poorly soluble substances. The experimental consequences of this phenomenon are that if the concentration of a common ion is high, then the other ion must become low in a saturated solution of the substance, i.e., precipitation will occur. Conversely, the effect of foreign ions on the solubility of sparingly soluble salts is just the opposite, and the solubility increases. This is the so-called salt effect.

Figure 3.5 pH–solubility profile of an amine hydrochloride salt.

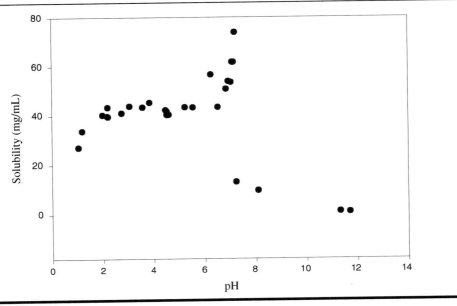

Setschenow (salting out) constants have been determined for eight hydrochloride salts of some α-adrenergic agonists and β-adrenergic agonist/blocker drugs (Thomas and Rubino 1996). The constants were calculated by determining the solubility of the salts in sodium chloride water, and the results showed that they were greatest for those with the lowest aqueous solubility and highest melting point. In addition, the number of aromatic rings and aromatic ring substituents appeared to contribute to the values of the salting out constants.

Temperature

Since dissolution is usually an endothermic process, increasing solubility of solids with a rise in temperature is the general rule. Therefore, most graphs of solubility plotted against temperature show a continuous rise, but there are exceptions, e.g., the solubility of sodium chloride is almost invarient, whilst that for calcium hydroxide falls slightly from a solubility of 0.185 g/mL at 0°C to 0.077 g/mL at 100°C. Figure 3.6 shows the exponential increase in solubility ($n = 5$) with increasing temperature of a hydrochloride salt in methanol/HCl.

Initial Investigations

Since compound supply is likely to be limited, then only a few solvent systems can be investigated during initial solubility studies. Typically, the solubility of the compounds in water, 0.9 percent w/v saline, 0.1 M HCl and 0.1 M NaOH will be determined. If there is sufficient compound, then the solubility in other systems may be considered (e.g., co-solvents such as

Figure 3.6 Temperature-solubility curve for a hydrochloride salt in methanol/HCl.

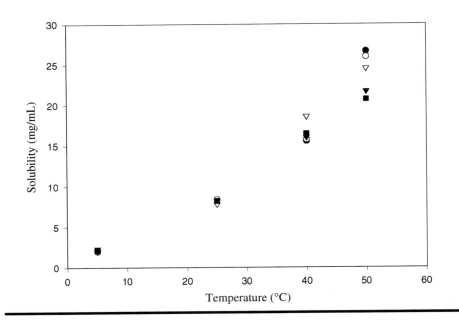

PEG400 and propylene glycol). In addition, the solubility in oils and surfactant systems (e.g., Tween 80) may be considered. For reasonably soluble compounds, it may well be that only a "greater than" figure can be quoted.

INITIAL STABILITY INVESTIGATIONS

Knowledge about the chemical and physical stability of a candidate drug in the solid and liquid state is extremely important in drug development for a number of reasons. In the longer term, the stability of the formulation will dictate the shelf life of the marketed product, however, to achieve this formulation, careful preformulation work will have characterized the compound such that a rational choice of conditions and excipients is available to the formulation team.

Candidate drugs being evaluated for development are often one of a series of related compounds that may have similar chemical properties, i.e., similar paths of degradation may be deduced. However, this rarely tells us the *rate* at which they will decompose, which is of more importance in pharmaceutical development terms. To elucidate their stability with respect to temperature, pH, light and oxygen, a number of experiments need to be performed. The major objectives of the preformulation team are, therefore, to identify conditions to which the compound is sensitive and to identify degradation profiles under these conditions.

The major routes of drug degradation in solution are via hydrolysis, oxidation or photochemical means. Conners et al. (1986) have dealt very well with the physical chemistry involved in the kinetic analysis of degradation of pharmaceuticals, and the reader is referred there for a detailed discussion.

Solution Stability

Hydrolysis

Mechanistically, hydrolysis takes place in two stages. In the first instance, a nucleophile, such as water or the OH^- ion, adds to, for example, an acyl carbon, to form an intermediate from which the leaving group then breaks away. The structure of the compound will affect the rate at which this reaction takes place, and the stronger the leaving conjugate acid, the faster the degradation reaction will take place (Loudon 1991).

Degradation by hydrolysis is affected by a number of factors, of which solution pH, buffer salts and ionic strength are the most important. In addition, the presence of co-solvents, complexing agents and surfactant can also affect this type of degradation.

As noted, solution pH is one of the major determinants of the stability of a compound. Hydroxyl ions are stronger nucleophiles than water; thus degradation reactions are usually faster in alkaline solutions than in water, i.e., OH^- ions catalyze the reaction. In solutions of low pH, H^+ can also catalyze hydrolysis reactions: catalysis by H^+ and OH^- is termed specific acid-base catalysis. Of course, H^+ and OH^- ions are not the only ions that may be present during an experiment or in a formulation. It is well known that buffer ions such as acetate or citric acid can catalyze degradation, and in this case the effect is known as general acid-base degradation. Therefore, although it is prudent to adjust the pH to the desired value to optimize stability, this should always be done with the minimum concentration necessary. Stewart and Tucker (1985) provide a useful, simple guide to hydrolysis and discuss the mechanism of hydrolysis. Table 3.3 shows some examples of the functional groups that undergo hydrolysis.

Oxidation

The second most common way a compound can decompose in solution is via oxidation. Reduction/oxidation (redox) reactions involve either the transfer of oxygen or hydrogen atoms

---

Table 3.3
Examples of classes of drugs that are subject to hydrolysis.

Class	Example
Ester	Aspirin
Thiol ester	Spirolactone
Amide	Chloramphenicol
Sulphonamide	Sulphapyrazine
Imide	Phenobarbitone
Lactam	Methicillin
Lactone	Spironolactone
Halogenated aliphatic	Chlorambucil

Reprinted with permission from Prediction of drug stability—Part 2: Hydrolysis, by P. J. Stewart and I. G. Tucker, in *Aust. J. Hosp. Pharm.*, 1985, Vol. 15, pages 11–16.

or the transfer of electrons. Oxidation is promoted by the presence of oxygen, and the reaction can be initiated by the action of heat, light or trace metal ions that produce organic free radicals. These radicals propagate the oxidation reaction, which proceeds until inhibitors destroy the radicals or until side reactions eventually break the chain. A typical oxidation sequence is that shown by dopamine (Myers and Jenke 1993). To test whether a compound is sensitive to oxygen, simply bubble air through the solution, or add hydrogen peroxide, and assess the amount of degradation that takes place.

Racemization

Although hydrolysis and oxidation constitute the main mechanisms by which drugs can decompose, racemization is another way in which the compound can change in solution. For example, Fyhr and Högström (1988) investigated the racemization of ropivacaine hydrochloride. They found that although ropivacaine showed a high stability against hydrolysis, it underwent racemization from the S-form to the R-form via pseudo-first-order, reversible kinetics with respect to the S-form.

Kinetics of Degradation

Essentially, we must determine the amount of the compound remaining with respect to time under the conditions of interest. Alternatively, the appearance of degradation product could also be used to monitor the reaction kinetics. Thus, the rate of a reaction can be defined as the rate of change of concentration of one of the reactants or products.

For a simple drug decomposition, therefore, the following situation holds:

$$\text{Drug} \rightarrow \text{Product(s)}$$

Since the concentration of the compound will decrease with time, the equation relating these quantities is given by

$$-\frac{d[D]}{dt} = k[D]^n \tag{13}$$

where k is the rate constant for the reaction at that particular temperature and n is the reaction order, which is the dependence of the rate on the reactant concentrations.

Zero-Order Reactions

For zero-order reactions, the rate of reaction is independent of concentration and does not change (with time) until the reactant has been consumed.

$$\text{Rate} = -\frac{d[D]}{dt} = k_O \tag{14}$$

The final form of the zero-order equation is given by

$$[D]_t = [D]_O - k_O t \tag{15}$$

Therefore, if we plot the concentration ($[D]_O$ = initial and $[D]_t$ = at time t) directly as a function of time, the slope is equal to the rate constant, k_O, for this reaction. Moreover, the time required for any specific amount of reactant to disappear is proportional to the initial amount present. Many reactions in the solid state or in suspensions undergo decomposition by zero-order kinetics.

First-Order Reactions

In first-order reactions, the rate of reaction decreases with time as the concentration of the reactant decreases according to

$$\text{Rate} = -\frac{d[D]}{dt} = k_1[D] \tag{16}$$

The final form of the first-order equation is given by

$$\log_{10}[D] = \log_{10}[D_O] - \frac{k_1}{2.303} \tag{17}$$

Therefore, if the logarithm of the concentration of the compound (for convenience, percent log remaining is often used) is plotted against time, a line with slope equal to $-k_1/2.303$ is obtained, where k is known as the rate constant. Further manipulation of the rate equation yields the expression for the half-life (time taken for the concentration to fall to half its initial value and halve in concentration thereafter; see equation 18). The unit of the rate constant is time^{-1}.

$$t_{1/2} = \frac{0.693}{k_1} \tag{18}$$

It should be noted that the half-life of the reaction is independent of the initial concentration.

Many hydrolysis reactions technically follow second-order kinetics, but since water is present in such an excess, its concentration negligibly changes with time. Thus, the rate is dependent only on the rate of decomposition of the drug in solution; this type of reaction is termed a *pseudo*-first-order reaction. Most compounds that degrade in solution follow this order. Second-order kinetics are observed when a reactant reacts with itself or when the reaction rate depends on the concentration of more than one reactant.

Temperature can affect reactions, and, in general, an increase in temperature will increase the rate of reaction. The effect of temperature on reaction is described by the Arrhenius relationship

$$\log k = \log A - \frac{E_a}{2.303RT} \tag{19}$$

where k is the observed pseudo-first-order rate constant for the reaction, A is a constant and E_a is the observed energy of activation of the reaction. R is the gas constant and T is the temperature in Kelvin (8.314 J/mol K).

Due to insufficient drug quantity, a complete degradation profile will probably not be possible during prenomination studies, but it should be possible to assess the stability of the candidate drug at a few pH values (acid, alkali and neutral) to establish the approximate stability of the compound with respect to hydrolysis. To accelerate the reaction, temperature elevation will probably be necessary to generate the data. Although it is difficult to assign a definite temperature for these studies, 50–90°C in the first instance is a reasonable compromise. This should be followed by extrapolation via the Arrhenius equation to 25°C. Hydrolytic stability of >100 days at 25°C should be taken as a goal of these studies. In terms of candidate drug selection, if all other factors are equal, the compound that is most stable should be the one taken forward into development.

Normally, the stability of solutions is assessed using HPLC to determine the amount of decomposition of a compound with time. However, a recent paper by Willson et al. (1996) has indicated that microcalorimetry can determine decomposition reactions with an annual degradation rate of 0.03 percent, i.e., a half-life of 2200 years! However, the nature and form of the reaction and the calorimetric output need to be assessed extremely carefully, and this can require careful work-up of the technique to bring it into routine use.

Initial Solid–State Stability

The solid-state degradation of candidate drugs, particularly in the candidate selection phase, is an important consideration, since degradation rates as slow as 0.5 percent per year at 25°C may affect the development of the compound. Monkhouse and van Campen (1984) have reviewed solid-state reactions and make the point that decomposition in the solid state will be different from that in a liquid insofar as the concepts of concentration and order of reaction are less applicable. Moreover, solid-state degradation reactions can be complex and can involve both oxidation and hydrolysis together. As with solutions, solids can also exhibit instability due to the effects of light. This is further complicated by the fact that in solids these reactions usually only occur on the surface. Figure 3.7 shows how a solid drug might decompose.

Three phases have been identified: the lag, acceleration and deceleration phases. Depending on the conditions of temperature and the humidity to which the solid is exposed, the acceleration phase may follow zero, first or higher orders. A general equation has been proposed to describe the process.

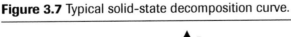

Figure 3.7 Typical solid-state decomposition curve.

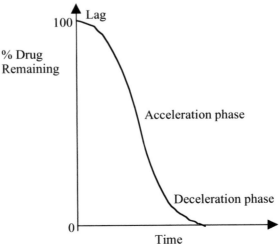

$$\frac{d\alpha}{dt} = k\alpha^{1-x}(1-\alpha)^{1-y} \qquad (20)$$

where α is the fraction of the reaction which has occurred at time t, such that $\alpha = 0$ when $t = 0$, and $a = 1$ at $t = \infty$; k is the rate constant; and x and y are constants characteristic of the reaction rate law, i.e., when $x = y = 1$, the reaction is zero order. If, however, $x = 1$ and $y = 0$, the reaction is first order. If x and y have fractional values, the reaction will be autocatalytic.

To accelerate the degradation so that the amount degraded becomes quantifiable in a shorter period of time, elevated temperatures are used, and the amount of degradation is typically calculated using the Arrhenius equation. The assumption made during these studies is that the degradation mechanism at higher temperatures is the same as that at 25°C. However, this need not be the case, and a non-linear Arrhenius plot may be an indication of change of mechanism as the temperature is increased. Furthermore, many compounds are hydrates that dehydrate at higher temperatures, which can change the degradation mechanism in the solid state.

In terms of the chemical stability of compounds with respect to moisture uptake, the following descriptions have been used to describe classes of surface moisture (Cartensen and Li Wan Po 1992):

- *Limited water:* Water is used up during the degradation reaction, and there is not enough present to degrade the compound completely.

- *Adequate water:* Sufficient water is present to decompose the compound completely.

- *Excess water:* This is an amount of water equal to or greater than the amount of moisture necessary to dissolve the drug. As such, this may develop as the mass of intact drug decomposes with time.

With regard to crystallinity, it should be noted that amorphous materials are generally less stable than the corresponding crystalline phase. In amorphous solids, the net effect of water sorption is to lower the glass transition temperature, T_g, and hence plasticize the material. In turn, this increases molecular mobility and therefore increases chemical reactivity (Ahlneck and Zografi 1990). Often, amorphous phases crystallize with exposure to moisture.

In prenomination studies, a useful protocol to assess the effects of these factors is as follows. The compound is accurately weighed into each of six open glass vials. These are then placed (in duplicate if possible) under the following conditions: light stress (5000 lx, 25°C), 40°C/75 percent relative humidity (RH) and 30°C/60 percent RH. Typically, the sample would be sampled as necessary up to three months to determine its stability. After each time point, all samples are assessed visually and with a suitable HPLC (or liquid chromatography–mass spectrometry (LC–MS) method that can detect degradation products. In addition, differential scanning calorimetry (DSC) and X-ray powder diffraction (XRPD) can be used to detect phase changes.

Photostability

As illustrated in the book *Drugs Photochemistry and Photostability,* edited by Albini and Fasani (1998), a wide range of drug types can undergo photochemical degradation. Theoretically, candidate drugs with absorption maxima greater than 280 nm may decompose in sunlight. However, instability due to light will probably only be a problem if the drug significantly absorbs light with a wavelength greater than 330 nm and, even then, only if the reaction proceeds at a significant rate (Albini and Fasani 1998). Light instability is a problem in both the solid and solution state, and formulations therefore need to be designed to protect the compound from its deleterious effects.

The number of compounds showing photoinstability is large, e.g., Tønneson (1991) has stated that more than 100 of the most commonly used drugs are unstable with respect to light. There are a number of chemical groups that might be expected to give rise to decomposition. These include the carbonyl group, the nitroaromatic group, the *N*-oxide group, the C=C bond, the aryl chloride group, groups with a weak C–H bond, sulphides, alkenes, polyenes and phenols (Albini and Fasani 1998).

It is therefore important to establish the propensity of a candidate drug to decompose due to light as soon as possible in preformulation studies, since this can have ramifications for its formulation and packaging (Merrifield et al. 1996). The first evidence that compounds are light sensitive is usually discovered during LO studies. Thus, candidate drugs should be assessed in the prenomination phase with respect to light stability to alert the formulation team whether special measures are needed to protect the drug from light. Indeed, this could be used as a selection criterion in many cases to reject unsuitable candidate drugs.

An International Conference on Harmonisation (ICH) guideline for the photostability testing of new drug substances and products has been recently been published in e.g. the European Pharmacopoeia (1996). This states that photostability testing should consist of forced degradation and confirmatory testing. The forced degradation experiments can involve the candidate drug alone, in solution or in suspension using exposure conditions that reflect the nature of the compound and the intensity of the light sources used. The samples are then analyzed at various time-points using appropriate techniques (e.g., HPLC). In addition, changes in physical properties such as appearance and clarity or colour should be noted. Confirmatory studies involve exposing the compound to light whose total output is not less than 1.2 million lx · h and has a near UV energy of not less than 200 watt hours/m^2. Light sources for testing photostability include artificial daylight tubes, xenon lamps, tungsten-mercury lamps, laboratory light and natural light (Anderson et al. 1991). A novel microcalorimetric technique for measuring the photoreactivity of solids and solutions has been described by Lehto et al. (1999).

In terms of the kinetics, light degradation in dilute solution is first order, however, in more concentrated solutions, decomposition approaches pseudo-zero order (Conners et al. 1986). The reason for this is that as the solution becomes more concentrated, degradation becomes limited due to the limited number of incident quanta and quenching reactions between the molecules. It should be noted that ionizable compounds, e.g., ciprofloxacin, can show large differences in photostability between the ionized and unionized forms (Torniainen et al. 1996).

Solids can undergo photolysis and oxidation. For example, de Villiers et al. (1992) showed that Form II of furosemide was less stable to light than Form I, particularly in the presence of oxygen. The decomposition showed more complex behaviour with the reaction consisting of a number of steps. The first step occurred on the surface, which was followed by a gas phase mass transfer step. After this, the reaction proceeded by diffusion via a porous reacted zone and chemical reaction at the boundary.

Under the constant intense light source of the Hanau suntest, degradation is measured using 10 μM of the candidate drug in pH 7.4 at room temperature. Under these conditions, if the compound shows a half-life of greater than 5 h, it is classified as stable. If the compound has a half-life of less than 5 min, it is classfied as very photolytically unstable.

CRYSTALLINITY

Polymorphism and Related Phenomena

Haleblain and McCrone (1969) have defined polymorphism as "a solid crystalline phase of a given compound resulting from the possibility of at least two different arrangements of that compound in the solid state". This definition encompasses conformational polymorphism, i.e., the existence of different conformers of the same molecule in different polymorphic modifications.

In general, polymorphs of a given compound have different physicochemical properties, such as melting point, solubility and density, so that the occurrence of polymorphism has important formulation, biopharmaceutical and chemical process implications. In addition to polymorphs, solvates (inclusion of the solvent of crystallization), hydrates (inclusion of water of crystallization) and amorphous forms (where no long-range order exists) may also exist. Figure 3.8 shows an example of the polymorphism of estrone (Busetta et al. 1973).

It is thus necessary that the preformulation protocol investigates and characterizes these phenomena (Smith 1986) so that:

Figure 3.8 Structures of the polymorphs of estrone.

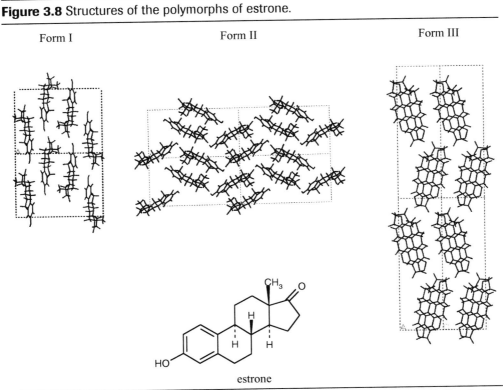

| Form I | Form II | Form III |

estrone

3D Search and Research Using the Cambridge Structural Database, Allen, F. H. and Kennard, O. *Chemical Design Automation News*, 8 (1), pp. 1 & 31–37, 1993.

- the desired forms can be consistently manufactured;

- the effects of pharmaceutical manipulations are understood, e.g., granulation, milling and compression; and

- the effect of storage conditions on the dosage form can be evaluated and predicted, e.g., crystal growth in suspensions, creams and metered dose inhalers (MDIs).

In general, true polymorphs can be classified into two different types (Table 3.4; Giron 1995):

1.   enantiotropic—one polymorph can be reversibly changed into another one by varying the temperature or pressure.

2.   monotropic—the change between the two forms is irreversible

There are a number of ways to screen for polymorphism and related phenomena. However, as Kuhnert-Brandstatter and Gasser (1971) have stated,

> Investigations of polymorphism can never be considered to be completely exhaustive in that there is always the possibility that with a specific seeding a heretofore unknown crystal modification may appear . . . and . . . there is always the possibility of finding a new modification from some unique solvent and condition.

Although Gavezotti and Filippini (1995) agreed that polymorphism of organic crystals was very frequent at room temperature, they felt that the appearance of polymorphs was not as common as it sometimes appeared to be.

Table 3.4
Thermodynamic rules for polymorphic transitions.

Enantiotropy	Monotropy
transition < melting I	transition > melting I
I stable > transition	I always stable
II stable < transition	–
transition reversible	transition irreversible
solubility I higher < transition	solubility I always lower
solubility I lower > transition	–
transition II → I endothermic	transition II→I exothermic
$\Delta H_f^I < \Delta H_f^{II}$	$\Delta H_f^I > \Delta H_f^{II}$
IR peak I before II	IR peak I after II
density I < II	density I > density II

Reprinted from *Thermochimica Acta*, Vol. 248, D. Giron, Thermal analysis and calorimetric methods in the characterization of polymorphs and solvates, Pages 1–59, Copyright 1995, with permission from Elsevier Science.

Bearing this in mind, the choice of conditions to screen for polymorphism can be summarized as follows (Führer 1986):

- Crystallization from different solvents at different speeds and temperatures
- Precipitation
- Concentration or evaporation
- Crystallization from the melt
- Grinding and compression
- Lyophilization
- Spray drying

In addition, newer techniques based on supercritical fluids to crystallize compounds have been reported (Subramaniam et al. 1997).

In the prenomination phase, the polymorphism screen will be limited due to the amount of compound available, and strategies must therefore be employed to reflect this situation. Initially, the Medicinal Chemistry batches should be analyzed to gain preliminary evidence for the propensity of the compound to show variations in the solid-state form of the compound. It is possible that the Process Research and Development department will also be working on the synthesis and crystallization of the compound. Therefore, a useful starting place for searching for polymorphs is to screen the material produced by the process chemists as they attempt to optimize the crystallization conditions. Work can also be undertaken by the Pharmaceutical and Analytical departments, in parallel, to use some of the above methods to generate polymorphs. However, these initial studies will probably have to be carried out on a micro- or semi-microscale.

One way of assessing whether the solid is a metastable form of the compound is to slurry the compound in a range of solvents. In this way, a solvent-mediated phase transformation may be detected using the usual techniques (Davey et al. 1986).

Solvates

The phenomenon whereby solvent or water is incorporated in the crystal lattice or in interstitial voids, for example, has been termed pseudopolymorphism. When incorporated into a crystal lattice, the solvent usually has a space-filling role, especially where solvent molecules do not show strong interactions. If the crystal has large empty channels or holes, their nature will determine which solvent will be included and the structure of the resulting solvate. Although solvates can show higher solubilities and dissolution rates compared to non-solvated species (e.g., Stoltz et al. 1988; Suleiman and Najib 1989), solvates cannot normally be used in the pharmaceutical arena. Residual solvents have been classified the ICH into three classes:

1. *Class I solvents:* Solvents to be avoided. These include known human carcinogens, strongly suspected human carcinogens and environmental hazards, e.g., benzene, carbon tetrachloride and 1,2 dichloroethane.

2. *Class II solvents:* Solvents to be limited. These include non-genotoxic animal carcinogens or possible causative agents (e.g., acetonitrile, cyclohexane, toluene, methanol and N,N-dimethylacetamide) of irreversible toxicity such as neurotoxicity

or teratogenicity. Also included are solvents suspected of other significant but re-versible toxicities.

3. *Class III solvents:* Solvents with low toxic potential, e.g., acetic acid, acetone, ethanol ethyl acetate and ethyl ether. Also included are solvents with low toxic potential to man are also included here; no health-based exposure limit is needed. Class III solvents have permissible daily exposures (PDEs) of 50 mg or more a day.

Usually solvates arise in the manufacturing process and have been identified as such and, where appropriate, characterized. It is important that solvates are desolvated before use. Usually vacuum drying is used; however, it has been noted for several compounds that solvated alcohol can be removed more quickly by exposure of the solvate to water vapour (Pikal et al. 1983).

Whilst the use of solvates is not a usual practice, because of toxicity, it is interesting to note that according to Glaxo's British patent 1,429,184, the crystal form of beclomethasone dipropionate used in the MDI is the trichlorofluoromethane solvate. By using the solvate, it was found that crystal growth due to solvation of the propellant chlorofluorocarbon (CFC) was prevented.

Hydrates

The most common case of solvation is for the incorporation of water molecules, which are almost always involved in hydrogen bonding. Indeed, it is the hydrogen bonding network that contributes to the coherence of the crystal, such that they usually show slower dissolution rates compared to the corresponding anhydrates. Byrn (1982) has illustrated the importance of this topic by stating that there are more than 90 hydrates listed in the USP.

Three types of hydrates have been identified:

1. *Isolated lattice site water.* In this situation, the water molecules are not in contact with each other, i.e., they are separated by the drug molecules.

2. *Lattice channel water.* Here the water molecules lie in channels, are hydrogen bonded and perform a space-filling role.

3. *Metal ion co-ordinated water.* This arises in the salts of weak acids, e.g., calcium salts where the metal ion co-ordinates with the water molecules, and is included in the growing lattice structure.

In some structures, both (2) and (3) can occur together. Nedocromil sodium trihydrate, for example, shows both metal co-ordinated water and channel water.

Hydrates can be polymorphic; amiloride hydrochloride, for example, is available in two polymorphic dihydrate forms, each of which can be dehydrated to an anhydrous crystalline form. By milling or compressing both forms, it was shown that Form A was more stable than Form B. Moreover, it was shown that the anhydrate rapidly rehydrated to Form A dihydrate on exposure to atmospheric relative humidity (Jozwiakowski et al. 1993).

In terms of the selection of the best form to take forward into development, Bray et al. (1999) have described a number of experiments undertaken to characterize the properties of a number of hydrates of the fibrinogen antagonist L-738,167. Four solid-state forms of the compound were identified using XRPD, DSC and moisture uptake studies. The four forms were a pentahydrate, a trihydrate and two others where the stoichiometry was determined to be 2.41 and 0.59. The trihydrate was shown to convert to the pentahydrate above 50 percent RH and hence was rejected as a candidate. From suspension studies, it was found that the 0.59 hydrate converted to the pentahydrate; however, the 2.41 hydrate did not. Thus, the pentahydrate and 2.41 hydrate were recommended with the caveat that additional formulation and processing experiments should be carried out to choose which of these hydrates should be used in a solid dosage form.

Amorphous Forms

Amorphous forms are, by definition, non-crystalline materials, i.e., they possess no long-range order. Their structure can be thought of as being similar to that of a frozen liquid with the thermal fluctuations present in a liquid frozen out, leaving only "static" structural disorder (Elliot et al. 1986). According to the USP, the degree of crystallinity depends on the fraction of crystalline material in the mixture, which is termed the two-state model. Another way of viewing this situation is that the crystallinity has a range from 100 percent for perfect crystals (zero entropy) to 0 percent (non-crystalline or amorphous); this is known as the one-state model. The characteristics and significance of the amorphous state with regard to pharmaceuticals have been reviewed by Hancock and Zografi (1997), who schematically illustrated the most common ways in which the amorphous state is formed, e.g., vapour condensation, supercooling of a melt, precipitation from solution and milling and compaction of crystals.

One consequence of a disordered structure is that amorphous forms are thermodynamically unstable; therefore, they are the most energetic form. The tendency of amorphous forms is thus to revert to a more stable form—this is particularly true when the formulation is in an aqueous suspension (Haleblain 1975). Another consequence for some compounds with a low degree of crystallinity can be a decrease in chemical stability.

Because of these problems with physical and chemical stability, it is not usual to proceed into development with a candidate drug in such a state. Attempts to crystallize the amorphous phase should always be undertaken, however, it should be borne in mind that amorphous phases, if chemically and physically stable, can have some advantages over the crystalline phase. For example, a stabilized amorphous form of novobiocin was found to be 10 times more soluble and therapeutically active compared to the crystalline form.

Ab initio Crystal Structure Solution from XRPD Patterns and Polymorph Prediction

It is now becoming possible to use molecular modelling techniques to solve crystal structures and predict solid properties. For example, *Powdersolve*, part of the CERIUS^2 software package, which solves crystal structures from XRPD, will soon be commercially available from Molecular Simulations Incorporated (Engel et al. 1999). In brief, this technique uses a simulated annealing and a rigid-body Reitveld refinement procedure, whereby the calculated and measured XRPD patterns are compared; when they agree sufficiently, the structure is deemed to be solved. Other programs also exist. Kariuki et al. (1999), for example, used a genetic algorithm technique to solve the structure of fluticasone propionate using data from a laboratory XRPD. The determination of crystal structures from powder diffraction data was also the subject of a paper by David et al. (1998). Using a simulated annealing technique, the structures of capsaicin, promazine hydrochloride and thiothixene were solved.

There are also now computer programs available for the *ab initio* prediction of polymorphs (e.g., Verwer and Leusen 1998). Polymorph Predictor, another module of CERIUS^2, is based on a potential energy function program and a search program to locate potential minima of that potential function. It does have limitations, for example, by neglecting polarization effects, the results are less accurate for molecules such as salts that are common in the pharmaceutical industry. Moreover, atoms such as fluorine and divalent sulphur are not optimally parameterized. The molecules need to be rigid; however, a few successes for flexible molecules have been reported. A number of polymorphs of 4-amidinoindanone guanylhydrazone (AIGH) were correctly predicted (Karfunkel et al. 1996). More recently, Payne et al. (1999) have successfully predicted the polymorphs of primidone and progesterone.

CRYSTAL MORPHOLOGY

The external shape of a crystal is termed the habit, and a variety of shapes have been defined in Table 3.5. The habit of a crystal arises due to the way in which the solutes orientate themselves when growing; therefore, the general shape of a crystal is the result of the way individual faces grow. During growth, the fastest growing faces are usually eliminated.

Since solvents can preferentially adsorb to crystal faces during the growth process, crystals of a substance produced under different crystallization conditions may exhibit an entirely different physical appearance, even though they still belong to the same crystal system.

Crystal morphology or habit is important, since it can influence many properties of the compound. For example, powder flow properties, compaction and stability have all been found to be dependent on crystal morphology. It has been shown that tolbutamide B (platelike)

Table 3.5
Examples of crystal habits.

Habit	Description
Acicular	Elongated prism, needlelike
Angular	Sharp edged, roughly polyhedral
Bladed	Flattened acicular
Crystalline	Geometric shape fully developed in fluid
Dendritic	Branched crystalline
Fibrous	Regular or irregular threadlike
Flaky/Platy	Plate or saltlike
Granular	Equidimensional irregular shape
Irregular	Lacking any symmetry
Nodular	Rounded irregular shape
Prismatic	Columnar prism
Spherical	Global shape
Tabular	Rectangular with a pair of parallel faces

caused powder bridging in the hopper and a capping problem when tableted. Form A, on the other hand, was tableted without problems (Simmons et al. 1972). Danjo et al. (1989) have investigated the compaction and flow properties of powders and found that with increasing shape factor the flowability of the particles increased. Moreover, it was found that the porosity of a powder bed decreased as the sphericity increased. Hong-guang and Ru-hua (1995) investigated the tableting properties of needle-, cube- and plate-shaped paracetamol crystals. They found that the needle-shaped powder had the worst compression properties, showing greater capping and lamination, than the plate- or cube-shaped crystals. Compounds with different crystal habits can also exhibit differences in dissolution rate. For example, Wanatabe et al. (1982) have shown the effect of the different habits of aspirin on the dissolution of the compound. Finally, Wadsten et al. (1990) have reported that crystal habit was responsible for an observed change in the bioavailablity of pentetrazole.

If a compound exhibits a particular morphology that may cause formulation problems, it may be worthwhile investigating ways in which to change the habit via crystallization from different solvents. Additionally, the effect of impurities on the crystal habit should not be overlooked, as these can act as crystal poisons or promote growth in a particular crystallographic direction. Figure 3.9 shows scanning electron micrographs of a variety of crystal habits found for some candidate drugs. In general, those habits that are bound by plane faces are termed euhedral, whilst irregularly shaped crystals are described as anhedral. The most accurate way

Figure 3.9 SEM micrographs of some crystal morphologies.

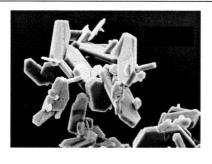
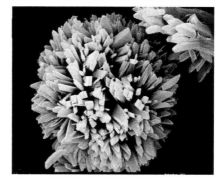
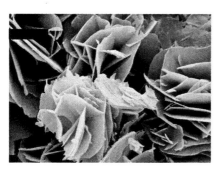
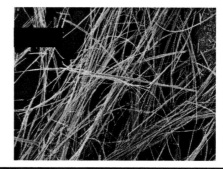

of determining the symmetry of a crystal is to use an optical goniometer to measure the angles between the crystal faces. However, this technique requires a good quality crystal of adequate size, >0.05 mm in each direction.

The CERIUS^2 software can be used to model the morphology of crystals as well as the effect of additives on morphology. Both the BFDH (Bravais, Friedel, Donnay and Harker) model and the attachment energy model, in conjunction with force field methods, are used in morphology prediction. The attachment energy approach gives the growth morphology of the crystal studied, but it is also possible to calculate the shape of a small particle in equilibrium with its growth environment by computing the surface energy of each relevant face.

Surface interactions between solvent molecules and growing faces can also be modelled. It is well known that the stronger the solvent binds to a particular face, the more it will inhibit the growth of that face so that morphology will be affected. This can be simulated by computer; the interaction of paracetamol with ethanol, for example, has been reported (Green and Meenan 1996). The ability to predict crystal morphology, i.e., to identify key growth faces, combined with the ability to analyze the surface chemistry of each of the faces in detail (including interactions with solvent molecules, excipients and impurities), enables rational control of morphology and crystal growth. For example, an undesirable morphology (a plate) can be transformed into a more isometrical shape.

In addition to morphological assessments of crystals, optical microscopy can be used to measure their refractive indices. Wanantabe et al. (1980) have shown that to identify the crystal, it is not necessary to measure the principal refractive indices: simply measuring two that are unique and reproducible is sufficient. These were termed the *key refractive indices* that, according to these researchers, are all that are needed to identify any particular compound.

HYGROSCOPICITY

Many compounds and salts are sensitive to the presence of water vapour or moisture. When compounds interact with moisture, they retain the water by either bulk or surface adsorption, capillary condensation, chemical reaction and, in extreme cases, a solution (deliquescence). Deliquescence is where a solid dissolves and saturates a thin film of water on its surface. It has been shown that when moisture is absorbed to the extent that deliquescence takes place at a certain critical relative humidity, the liquid film surrounding the solid is saturated. This process is dictated by vapour diffusion and heat transport rates (Kontny et al. 1987).

The opposite of deliquescence is efflorescence, which occurs when the crystal loses water of crystallization below a critical water vapour pressure. For example, Griesser and Burger (1995) found that caffeine hydrate lost its water of crystallization even at 61 percent RH. It has also been observed that the three known polymorphs of oxytetracycline have different hygroscopicity profiles (Burger et al. 1985).

Moisture is also an important factor that can affect the stability of candidate drugs and their formulations. Sorption of water molecules onto a candidate drug (or excipient) can often induce hydrolysis (see, e.g., Yoshioka and Cartensen 1990). In this situation, by sorbing onto the drug-excipient mixture, the water molecules may ionize either or both of them and induce a reaction. For example, we have found that a primary amine, when mixed with lactose, was apparently stable even when stored at 90°C for 12 weeks. However, when the experiment was carried out in the presence of moisture, extensive degradation by way of the well-known Mailliard reaction took place. Other properties such as crystal structure, powder flow, compaction, lubricity, dissolution rate and polymer film permeability may also be affected by moisture adsorption (Ahlneck and Zografi 1990).

The influence that moisture has on stability depends on how strongly it is bound, i.e., it depends on whether the moisture is in a free or bound state. Generally, degradation arises as a function of free water, which may be due to its ability to change the pH of the surfaces of candidate drug and excipient (Monkhouse 1984). On the other hand, bound water is not available if it is (1) a crystal hydrate, (2) hydrogen bonded or (3) sorbed or trapped in an amorphous structure.

Callaghan et al. (1982) have classified the degree of hygroscopicity into four classes (Table 3.6). More recently, the European Pharmacopoeia Technical Guide (1999, p. 86) has defined hygroscopicity, based on the static method, after storage at 25°C for 24 h at 80 percent RH:

- *Slightly hygroscopic:* Increase in mass is less than 2 percent m/m and equal to or greater than 0.2 percent m/m.

- *Hygroscopic:* Increase in mass is less than 15 percent m/m and equal to or greater than 0.2 percent m/m.

- *Very hygroscopic:* Increase in mass is equal to or greater than 15 percent m/m.

- *Deliquescent:* Sufficient water is absorbed to form a liquid.

If a compound is very hygroscopic, it would normally be rejected. However, the decision to proceed with a compound that takes up less water should be taken on a case-by-case basis. For example, although a compound may take up 5 percent moisture, it may not be accompanied by any serious effects, that is, it may remain stable and free flowing despite a high level of surface moisture. Moreover, there may be phase change to a hydrate, which may be beneficial in some circumstances.

SALT SELECTION

If a compound possesses an ionization centre, then the possibility of forming a salt exists. Salt evaluation should be an integral part of the prenomination phase and is usually carried out to alter the physicochemical properties of the free acid or base. Factors that can be changed by

---

Table 3.6
Hygroscopicity classification.

Class 1: Non-hygroscopic	Essentially no moisture increases occur at relative humidities below 90%.
Class 2: Slightly hygroscopic	Essentially no moisture increases occur at relative humidities below 80%.
Class 3: Moderately hygroscopic	Moisture content does not increase more than 5% after storage for 1 week at relative humidities below 60%.
Class 4: Very hygroscopic	Moisture content increase may occur at relative humidities as low as 40 to 50%.

Reprinted from Equilibrium moisture content of pharmaceutical excipients, by J. C. Callaghan et al., in *Drug Dev. Ind. Pharm.*, Vol. 8, pp. 355–369. Courtesy of Marcel Dekker, Inc.

salt formation include solubility, dissolution hygroscopicity, taste, physical and chemical stability or polymorphism.

Gould (1986) has identified a number of pivotal issues with respect to salt selection for basic drugs. The uses of salts to control a number of properties are illustrated in Table 3.7. The range of salts used in drug products is shown in Table 3.8 (Berge et al. 1977), and Table 3.9 shows the pK_as of some weak acids used in salt formation.

Morris et al. (1994) have extended the scope of Gould's review and described an integrated approach to the selection of the optimal salt form for new drug candidates. In the first tier of their decision-making process, the salts are evaluated in terms of their hygroscopicity. Those salts that show a great propensity to sorb moisture are eliminated from consideration. The rationale behind using moisture sorption as the criterion for selection is that excessive moisture sorption by a salt may cause handling, stability (chemical and physical) and manufacturing problems. Furthermore, if the moisture content changes on a batch-to-batch basis, this can lead to variation in potency of the prepared dosage forms. Those salts that survive this primary screen proceed to the second tier, whereby any crystal structure changes induced by high levels of moisture are elucidated. In addition, the aqueous solubility of the remaining salts is determined to ascertain whether there may be dissolution or bioavailability problems. In the final tier, the stability of the final candidate salts is then investigated under accelerated conditions (temperature, humidity and presence of excipients). If desired, compatibility testing with excipients may be conducted at this stage. Consideration of ease of synthesis, analysis, potential impurities and so on must also be taken into account.

Intimately related to the salt selection procedure is the phenomenon of polymorphism. This is where the compound can crystallize in different crystal forms which, in turn, can produce different physicochemical properties as well as different bioavailabilities. If a salt has the propensity to form many polymorphs, then, unless production of the desired form can be easily controlled, it should be rejected in favour of one that shows less polymorphic behaviour.

To comply with the concept that in preformulation studies minimal amounts of compound are used, an *in situ* salt screening technique for basic compounds has been developed by Tong and Whitesell (1998). The steps involved in this process are listed below:

1. Only acids with a pK_a that is at least two pH units should be considered.

2. Solubility studies on the base in solutions of the chosen acids should then be carried out. The concentration of the acid should be at a concentration such that, after the formation of the salt, it is in excess. It was recommended that the amount of base added should be accurately recorded since it affects the amount of acid consumed in preparing the salt. Solubility measurements during the experiment should also be carried out and the pH of the final solution recorded.

3. The solids formed (both wet and dry) should then be carried out using the usual techniques (e.g., DSC, thermogravimetric analysis [TGA] and XRPD).

Good agreement between the solubilities of salts prepared by conventional means and the solubility of the base in the *in situ* technique was found, except for the succinate. This was probably due to the fact that, as prepared, it was a hydrate—a potential drawback of the technique. Indeed, it was stated (Tong and Whitesell 1998) that the *in situ* technique should not replace traditional salt selection techniques. Rather, it should be used as a salt screening tool to rule out those salts that have poor solubility characteristics, thus obviating the need for their synthesis.

Table 3.7

Strategies for altering the physicochemical properties of weak bases via salt formation.

Action	Decrease Change and Reason	Property	Increase Change and Reason	Action
Use more flexible aliphatic acids with aromatic bases. Move to more highly substituted acids that destroy crystal symmetry.	DECREASE Increase solubility Form oil	←Melting Point→	INCREASE Process problems Reduce solubility	Use small counter-ions, e.g., Cl⁻, Br⁻. Use aromatic conjugate anions if aromatic base. Use small hydroxy acids if drug has good hydrogen bonding potential.
Increase melting point. Increase hydrophobicity of conjugate anion.	DECREASE Suspensions Controlled release	←Solubility→ (Dissolution rate)	INCREASE Bioavailability Liquid formulation	Decrease pK_a and increase solubility of conjugate acid. Decrease melting point. Increase hydroxylation of conjugate acid. If common ion dependence, move small organic acid.
	DECREASE		←Stability→	INCREASE	Reduce hygroscopicity by increasing hydrophobicity of acid. Also move to carboxylic rather than sulphonic or mineral acid. Use acid of higher pK_a to raise pH of solution. Decrease solubility and increase crystallinity by increase of melting point.
Increase hydrophobicity of conjugate anion.	DECREASE To control hygroscopicity	←Wettability→	INCREASE Dissolution/ bioavailability	Increase polarity of conjugate anion. Lower pK_a of conjugate acid. Attempt recrystallization from different solvents to alter crystal habit. Move to acid with high degree of hydroxylation.

Reprinted from *International Journal of Pharmaceutics*, Vol. 33, P. L. Gould, Salt selection for basic drugs, Pages 201–217, Copyright 1986, with permission from Elsevier Science.

Table 3.8
FDA-approved commercially marketed salts.

Anion	Percentage	Anion	Percentage
Acetate	1.26	Iodide	2.02
Benzenesulphonate	0.25	Isothionate	0.88
Benzoate	0.51	Lactate	0.76
Bicarbonate	0.13	Lactobionate	0.13
Bitartrate	0.63	Malate	0.13
Bromide	4.68	Maleate	3.03
Calcium edetate	0.25	Mandelate	0.38
Camsylate	0.25	Mesylate	2.02
Carbonate	0.38	Methylbromide	0.76
Chloride	4.17	Methylnitrate	0.38
Citrate	3.03	Methylsulphate	0.88
Dihydrochloride	0.51	Mucate	0.13
Edatate	0.25	Napsylate	0.25
Edisylate	0.38	Nitrate	0.64
Estolate	0.13	Pamoate	1.01
Esylate	0.13	Pantothenate	0.25
Fumarate	0.25	(Di)Phosphate	3.16
Gluceptate	0.18	Polygalactoronate	0.13
Gluconate	0.51	Salicylate	0.88
Glutamate	0.25	Stearate	0.25
Glycollylarsinate	0.13	Subacetate	0.38
Hexylresorcinate	0.13	Succinate	0.38
Hydrabamine	0.25	Sulphate	7.46
Hydrobromide	1.90	Teoclate	0.13
Hydrochloride	42.98	Triethiodide	0.13
Hydroxynaphthoate	0.25		

Cation	Percentage	Cation	Percentage
Organic		*Metallic*	
Benzathine	0.66	Aluminium	0.66
Chloroprocaine	0.33	Calcium	10.49
Choline	0.33	Lithium	1.64
Diethanolamine	0.98	Magnesium	1.31
Ethyldiamine	0.66	Potassium	10.82
Meglumine	2.29	Sodium	61.97
Procaine	0.66	Zinc	2.95

Table 3.9
pK_as of weak acids used in salt formation.

Name	pK_a
Acetate	4.76
Benzoate	4.20
Oleate	~4.0
Fumarate	3.0, 4.4
Succinate	4.2, 5.6
Ascorbate	4.21
Malate	3.5, 5.1
Gluconate	3.60
Tartrate	3.0, 4.3
Citrate	3.13
Besylate	2.54
Napsylate	0.17
Phosphate	2.15, 7.20, 12.38
Mesylate	1.92
Tosylate	−0.51
Sulphate	−3.0
Hydrochloride	−6.1
Hydrobromide	−8.0

Salts of Weak Acids

There are fewer salt-forming species for weak acids than there are for weak bases, and the available information suggests that, in general, alkali metal salts exhibit greater solubility than the corresponding alkaline earth salts. However, as shown by Chowan (1978), no specific conclusions can be drawn about which cation will produce the greater solubility. In that paper, he attempted to predict solubilities on the basis of lattice and hydration energies and the ionic radii of the cation. He was, however, unable to show an agreement between theory and experiment, except in general terms. In the case of amine salts, Anderson and Conradi (1985) were also unable to correlate hydrophilicity of the amine with the observed solubility order. On the other hand, the solubility did show a good correlation with the melting point of the salts. This information points to interactions within the crystal dominating properties when considering amine salts. Therefore, attempts to increase solubility through increased hydrophilicity of the amine counterion may not be successful.

As an example of using a salt of a weak acid to overcome a processing problem, Hirsch et al. (1978) used the calcium salt of fenoprofen to overcome the low melting point of the free acid (40°C). By increasing the melting point, problems with frictional heat due to mechanical handling were overcome.

Rubino (1989) has investigated the solid-state properties of the sodium salts of drugs (e.g., barbiturates, sulphonamides and hydantoins). When the logarithm of their aqueous solubilities was plotted against their melting points, a reciprocal relationship was found to hold. It was found that in many cases hydrate formation occurred, and the stoichiometry was found to be different before and after equilibration. It was concluded that the solubility of the salts was primarily controlled by the properties of the solid phase which is in equilibrium with the solution phase. Rubino and Thomas (1990) followed up this work and examined the influence of solvent composition on the solubilities and solid-state properties of these sodium salts. In many cases, it was found that the solubilities of the salts in the mixed solvent (propylene glycol/water) were lower than those found in water alone. On the other hand, several salts showed an increase in solubility in the solvent mixes. This was not related to the intrinsic lipophilicity of the acidic form of the drug but was related to hydrate formation. Moreover, it was found that those compounds with a low dehydration temperature showed increased solubility in propylene glycol–water and vice versa. Thus it would appear that crystal hydrate formation plays a significant role in determining whether a co-solvent can be used to enhance the solubility of sodium salts. In terms of hygroscopicity, it is not possible, again, to be specific with regard to the cation.

In another study by Cotton et al. (1994), a salt selection procedure was carried out because the free acid of L-649,923, an orally active leukotriene D_4 antagonist, was inherently unstable because it rapidly hydrolyzed to a less active form of the compound. Therefore, to ensure that this did not occur, the compound had to be isolated as a salt. The physical and chemical properties of the sodium, calcium, ethylene diamine and benzathine salts were evaluated, and the calcium salt was selected as the most pharmaceutically acceptable form of the compound.

Usually companies do not investigate other salt-forming species other than those shown in Table 3.8. However, Gu and Strickley (1987) have described the physical properties of the tris-(hydroxymethyl)aminomethane (THAM) salts of four analgesic/antiinflammatory agents with sodium salts and free acids. They concluded that the THAM salts had superior hygroscopicity properties compared to the sodium salts and did not show any loss in aqueous solubility or intrinsic dissolution rate. The one exception to this was the THAM salt of naproxen. Ketoralac is now marketed as the tromethamine or THAM salt.

Fini et al. (1991) have investigated the N-(2-hydroxyethyl)-pyrrolidine (epolamine) salt of diclofenac and found that it was more soluble and dissolved more rapidly than diclofenac sodium. Furthermore, studies showed that this salt gave faster plasma levels when administered orally; this salt has been marketed for both systemic and topical use (Giachetti et al. 1996).

Salts of Weak Bases

As shown in Table 3.8, there are many more acids that can be used to form salts with weak bases. However, in terms of usage, the hydrochloride is by far the most frequently used; hence, this salt should be used as a benchmark to compare other salts. According to Gould (1986), to be able to form a salt of a basic compound, the pK_a of the of the salt-forming acid has to be less than or equal to the pK_a of the basic centre of the compound. Thus, very weakly basic compounds having a pK_a of around 2 will only form salts with strong acids such as hydrochloric, sulphuric and toluenesulphonic. Bases with higher pK_as have a greater range of possibilities for salt formation, as shown by the range of weaker acids in Table 3.8.

Increasing and decreasing the solubility of a compound are two of the most important reasons for salt selection. One of the major factors determining the solubility of a salt is the pH of the resultant solution. That is, the salts of the stronger acids will produce slurries with a lower pH which will promote dissolution of the base. For example, the pK_a of HCl is –6.1; therefore, on dissolution of a hydrochloride salt, the resultant low solution pH will promote a high solubility of the basic drug. However, other factors may also play a part in solubility enhancement through salt formation. For example, reduction in the melting point of the salt, or improved hydrogen bonding, may also contribute to the process. In this respect, the use of hydroxyl groups in the conjugate acid to increase hydrogen bonding capacity of the salt can be of use, and it is best to avoid conjugate acids with hydrophobic groups or those that contain long alkyl chains (Gould 1986).

Salt formation is not always a successful strategy for increasing the solubility of compounds. For example, Miyazaki et al. (1981) have shown that the formation of hydrochloride salts does not always enhance solubility and bioavailability due to the common ion effect in gastric fluid that is rich in chloride ions.

Salts can also affect the dissolution properties of a compound even though solubility characteristics may be similar. This was illustrated by Shah and Maniar (1993) who examined these properties for bupivacaine and its hydrochloride salt. The difference in the intrinsic dissolution behaviour was explained as being due to the pH of the diffusion layer; that is, when a solid dissolves, there is a stagnant film where the pH is different compared to the bulk dissolution medium. Thus when the base dissolved in an acidic medium, e.g., pH 1–5, the pH increased to 6–7 due to self-buffering. In alkaline solutions, however, the pH did not change because ionization was suppressed due to the pK_a of the drug being 8.2. In the case of the salt, however, the opposite occurred: in acid, the pH remained unchanged and alkaline pH values were reduced to about 5–7. The reduction in pH arose due to the release of HCl as the salt dissolved.

Usually salt formation is carried out to increase the solubility of the base, however, salts with lower solubilities are sometimes prepared to, e.g., mask taste, provide slower dissolution and increase chemical stability. An example of salt formation to decrease dissolution rate is described by Benjamin and Lin (1985), who prepared a range of salts of an experimental antihypertensive as shown in Table 3.10. The solubilities and intrinsic dissolution rates (IDR) of the prepared salts of this compound are also shown in Table 3.10. These *in vitro* tests showed that there were significant differences in the dissolution rate when the experiments were performed in water and buffer. However, the difference in the IDRs of the salts was similar in 0.1 M HCl. Hence, it was recommended that ebonate, 3-hydroxynaphthoate or napsylate salts should be formulated as enteric-coated dosage forms. This would avoid dissolution in the stomach acid, which could cause local GI irritation, and would still provide release of the compound.

We have investigated the effect of salt formation on the solubility of a development compound in water and saline (Table 3.11). Although there was the expected range of solubilities of the free base and the salts in water, solubilities were reduced when the experiment was conducted in isotonic saline. There was a relationship between the pH of the suspensions and the resulting solubility, as shown in Figure 3.10. However, the scatter of results indicated that the solubility was not simply due to pH but was also influenced by the nature of the conjugate base. In saline, the mechanism of the reduction in solubility is less clear. The decrease observed for the hydrochloride salt is probably due to the common ion effect as noted above.

The possibility of producing slowly dissolving salbutamol salts for delivery to the lung was investigated by preparing its adipic and stearic acid salts (Jashnani et al. 1996). The aqueous solubilities of the adipate and stearate salts were 353 and 0.6 mg/mL, respectively, compared to the free base and sulphate, which had solubilities of 15.7 and 250 mg mL, respectively. In terms of the IDR, the stearate dissolved much more slowly than the other salts and the free base. This was explained as due to the deposition of a stearate-rich layer on the dissolving surface of the compacted salt surface.

In another study, Walkling et al. (1983) found that xilobam, as the free base, was sensitive to high humidity and temperature. In an effort to overcome this problem, the tosylate, 1-napsylate, 2-napsylate and saccarinate salts were prepared and assessed with respect to their

Table 3.10
Solubilities and intrinsic dissolution rates
of the salts of an experimental antihypertensive.

Salts	Solubility in Water (mg free base/mL)	Intrinsic Dissolution Rate* (mg free base/min/cm^2)		
		0.1 M HCl	0.05 M (pH 7.5) Phosphate Buffer	Water
Acetate	24.20	20.36	15.69	18.60
Hydrochloride	31.70	3.43	7.64	6.32
Tartrate	26.61	13.21	3.65	4.39
Sulphate	10.81	6.25	3.04	2.56
p-Hydroxybenzoate	5.04	12.41	0.83	0.64
Eudragit-L	0.08	0.15	0.27	—
Eudragit-S	0.08	0.17	0.14	—
Free base	0.32	14.97	0.15	—
Napsylate	0.62	0.13	0.11	—
Ebonate	0.24	0.20	0.06	—
3-Hydroxy-2-naphthoate	0.35	0.13	0.04	—

*The intrinsic dissolution rates were determined using the rotating disc method, which normally needs around 100 mg of compound.

Reprinted from Preparation and in vitro evaluation of salts of an antihypertensive agent to obtain slow release, by E. J. Benjamin and L. H. Liu, in *Drug Dev. Ind. Pharm.*, Vol. 11, pp. 771–790. Courtesy of Marcel Dekker, Inc.

Table 3.11
Solubility of a free base and selected salts in water and isotonic saline.

Salt	Solubility (mM)		Mp/°C	pH*
	Water	Saline		
Free base	—	0.46		
Hydrochloride	10.9	0.74	201	4.52
		0.66		
Tartrate	23.2	1.34	160	2.95
		1.07		
p-Toluenesulphonate (tosylate)	1.39	1.77	170	5.39
1-Hydroxy-2-naphthoate (xinafoate)	0.11	0.14	176	6.00
Hemisuccinate	1.36	2.15	182	5.96
Hexanoate	2.97	3.85	131	5.87

*pH = saturated suspension of compound.

Figure 3.10 Solubility as a function of suspension pH of the salts shown in Table 3.8.

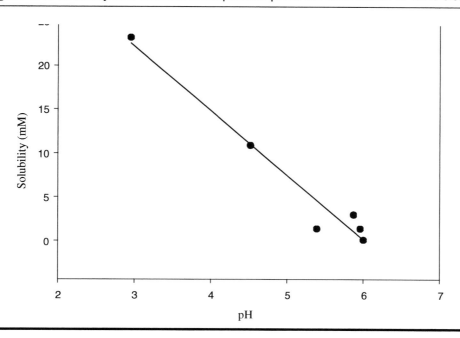

solid-state stability by storing samples at 74 percent RH and 70°C for up to 7 days. In addition to the stability studies, the dissolution of tablets made from the salts was investigated. The results obtained from the stability study are shown in Table 3.12. These data and data from the dissolution studies showed that not only was 1-napsylate the most stable, it also dissolved the most rapidly.

Saesmaa and Halmekoski (1987) have reviewed the slightly water-soluble salts of the β-lactam antibiotics, and their paper consists of much information on the early literature of these compounds. As examples, they describe the use of the benzathine salts of penicillin G and V for depot injections. The benzathine salt of penicillin V has also been used to mask the

Table 3.12
Amount of xilobam remaining after storage at 70°C and 74% RH for 7 days.

Salt	Free Base	Tosylate	Saccharinate	2-Napsylate	1-Napsylate
% Xilobam remaining	18.0	82.5	81.1	77.4	99.6

taste of the antibiotic for pediatric use. In another example, they quoted a comparison of the napsylate and hydrochloride salts of talampicillin. Because of its lower water solubility, the napsylate had more acceptable organoleptic properties (when formulated as a syrup) compared to the hydrochloride salt; it had blood levels comparable to a tablet formulation of the hydrochloride.

It is worth adding a note of caution with regard to salt formation. In a series of benzathine and emboate salts of the β-lactam antibiotics—ampicillin, amoxicillin, cephalexin and talampicillin—studied by XRPD (Saesmaa et al. 1990), the results showed that the emboate salts of ampicillin, amoxicillin and cephalexin were nearly identical in structure to that of the stoichiometric physical mixture of the two starting materials. Furthermore, the XRPD of benzathine amoxicillin and amoxicillin trihydrate were identical. In contrast, the benzathine salts of ampicillin and cephalexin were formed, illustrating that formation of the salt should always be confimed by solid-state characterization tehniques.

Stability of the salt could also be an important issue. For example, Nakanishi et al. (1998) found that the hydrochloride of the anticancer drug, NK109, was less stable than the sulphate salt. This was thought be due to the low pK_a (5.3) and the volatility of HCl. When NK109 was stressed (at 70°C under reduced pressure), it was found that the chloride changed colour from orange to amber and was accompanied by decrease in purity (99.45 to 98.78) compared to the sulphate, which showed no change.

Hydrolysis of a salt back to the free base may also take place if the pK_a of the base is sufficiently weak. As an example, a hydrochloride salt of an investigational compound was prepared from a weak base containing a pyridine moiety with a pK_a of 5.4. When this salt was slurried in water or subjected to high humidity, hydrolysis back to the free base was induced. Figure 3.11 shows the DSC thermograms of the hydrochloride and the free base and a sample of the hydrochloride slurried in water. A DSC thermogram of a physical mix of the base and the hydrochloride is also included. Hydrochloride salts may also have disadvantages compared to other salts in terms of tablet production. For example, Nururkar et al. (1985) reported that a hydrochloride salt of an investigational compound caused the rusting of tablet punches and dies.

METHODS FOR EVALUATING PHYSICOCHEMICAL PROPERTIES

There are many techniques available to characterize compounds. Indeed, in polymorphism studies it is advisable to identify the modifications present by more than one technique. In 1985, the U.S. Food and Drug Administration (FDA) indicated (The Gold Sheet) that the principal physicochemical techniques (in their approximate order of usefulness) that could be used to characterize polymorphs should be (Poulson 1985)

- melting point (hot stage microscopy);

- infrared spectroscopy;

- XRPD;

- thermal analytical techniques (e.g., DSC, differential thermal analysis [DTA], TGA, etc.);

- solid-state Raman spectroscopy;

- crystalline index of refraction;

Figure 3.11 DSC Thermograms of a free base, its hydrochloride salt (plus physical mix) and the effect of slurrying in water.

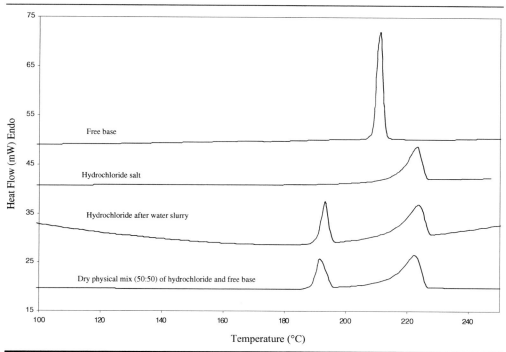

- phase solubility analysis;

- solution-pH profile determination;

- solution calorimetry; and

- comparative intrinsic dissolution rates.

More recently, Byrn et al. (1995) have proposed a strategic conceptual approach to the regulatory considerations regarding the characterization of pharmaceutical solids. This is based on flowcharts for polymorphs, hydrates, desolvated solvates and amorphous forms. The main techniques listed above are included, as well as cross-polarisation/magic angle spinning (CP/MAS) solid-state NMR. In addition to these techniques, hygroscopicity measurements can also be used to characterize the various salts of candidate drugs.

For reference, Threlfall (1995) has produced an excellent review of the analysis of organic polymorphs. Spectral methods (IR, Raman and solid-state NMR) for the characterization of polymorphs and solvates have been reviewed by Brittain (1997). The basis of some of the techniques used in solid-state characterization has been discussed earlier in this chapter in the section on salt selection. A few examples are given here to show the utilization of these techniques. Characterization of pharmaceutical solvates by combined TGA and infrared anaylsis has been described by Rodriguez and Bugey (1997).

Hygroscopicity

Dynamic Vapour Sorption (DVS)

Measurement of the hygroscopic properties of a compound can be conveniently carried out on small quantities of compound using a DVS-1 water sorption analyzer (Scientific and Medical Ltd., Manchester, UK). The relative humidity is generated by bubbling nitrogen through a water reservoir where it is saturated with moisture. Using a mixing chamber, the moist nitrogen is mixed with dry nitrogen in a fixed ratio, thus producing the required relative humidity. The moist nitrogen is then passed over the sample, and the instrument is programmed such that the increase in weight due to moisture is monitored with time using an ultrasensitive microbalance. The compound takes up moisture and reaches equilibrium, at which point the next relative humidity stage is programmed to start. The adsorption and desorption of moisture can be studied using this instrument, and the effect of temperature can be investigated as well. Using this technique, a quantity as small as 1 mg can be assessed.

Normally, the moisture sorption-desorption profile of the compound is investigated. This can reveal a range of phenomena associated with the solid. For example, on reducing the relative humidity from a high level, hysteresis (separation of the sorption-desorption curves) may be observed. As reported by Umprayn and Mendes (1987), there are two types of hysteresis loops. The first is an open hysteresis loop, where the final moisture content is higher than the starting moisture content. This is due to so-called ink-bottle pores, where condensed moisture is trapped in pores with a narrow neck. On the other hand, the hysteresis loop may be closed, and this is presumed to be due to compounds having capillary pore sizes. Figure 3.12 shows two batches of magnesium stearate exhibiting these types of moisture sorption-desorption phenomena.

Alternatively, there may be a larger uptake of moisture, which can indicate a phase change. In this case, the desorption phase is characterized by only small decreases in the moisture content (depending on the stability of the hydrate formed) until at a low RH the moisture is lost. In some cases, hydrated amorphous forms are formed on desorption of the hydrate formed on the sorption phase. Figure 3.13 shows the uptake of moisture of an amorphous phase with increasing relative humidity. In this case, the sorption of moisture caused the sample to crystallize as a hydrate, which at higher RHs crystallized into a higher hydrate. The higher hydrate was found to be stable to decreasing RHs, until RHs less than 10 percent resulted in the loss of all the sorbed moisture to regenerate the amorphous phase.

In terms of salt selection procedures, the critical relative humidity (CRH) of each salt should be identified. This is defined as the point at which the compound starts to sorb moisture (Cartensen et al. 1987). Clearly, compounds or salts that exhibit excessive moisture uptake should be rejected. The level of this uptake is debatable, but those exhibiting deliquesence (where the sample dissolves in the moisture that has been sorbed) should be automatically excluded from further consideration.

The automation of moisture sorption measurements is a relatively recent innovation (Marshall et al. 1994). Prior to this advance, moisture sorption of compounds (~ 10 mg) was determined by exposing weighed amounts of compound in dishes placed in sealed desiccators containing saturated salt solutions. Saturated solutions of salts that give defined relative humidities (as a function of temperature) have been reported by Nyqvist (1983). A typical range at 25°C is given in Table 3.13. The samples are then stored at a selected temperature and analyzed at various time points for moisture and stability, usually by TGA and HPLC, respectively.

When conducting these experiments, it is wise to analyze the solid phase during or after the experiments to ascertain the effect of the moisture sorption. For example, scanning electron microscopy (SEM), DSC or XRPD can be used to examine whether a sample has changed

Figure 3.12 DVS isotherm of magnesium stearate showing two types of sorption-desorption behaviour.

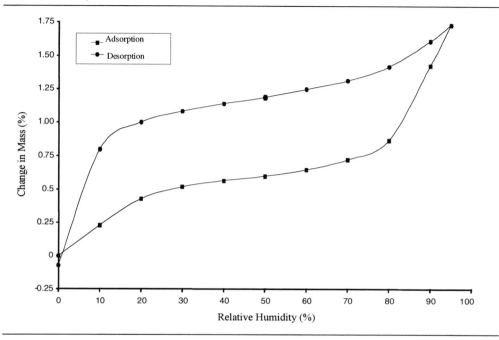

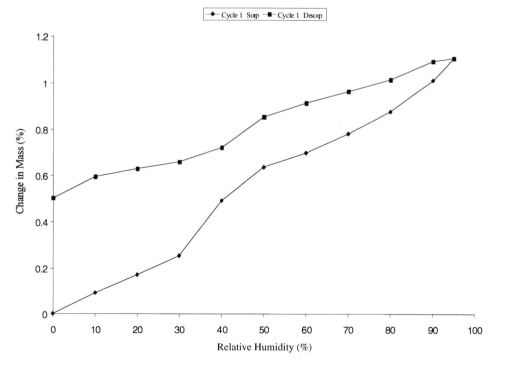

Figure 3.13 DVS isotherm for hydrate showing phase changes.

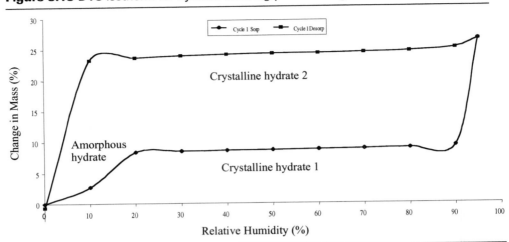

Table 3.13
Relative humidities generated by various saturated salt solutions.

Salt Solution	% Relative Humidity at 25°C
Silica gel	0
Potassium acetate	20
Calcium chloride	32
Sodium bromide	58
Potassium bromide	84
Dipotassium hydrogen phosphate	92
Water	100

Adapted from Nyqvist (1983).

after hygroscopicity experiments. It is also now possible to examine the effect of moisture of compounds *in situ* using environmental SEM (Clarke et al. 1998).

Isothermal Microcalorimetry

Isothermal microcalorimetry can also be used be to determine, amongst other things, the hygroscopicity of substances (Pudipeddi et al. 1996; Jakobsen et al. 1997). In the ramp mode, this technique can be used, like DVS, to examine milligram quantities of compound. This instrument utilizes a perfusion attachment with a precision flow switching valve. The moist gas is pumped into a reaction ampoule through two inlets, one that delivers dry nitrogen at 0 percent RH and one that delivers nitrogen that has been saturated by passing it through two humidifier chambers maintained at 100 percent RH. The required RH is then achieved by the switching valve which varies the proportion of dry to saturated gas. The RH can then be increased or decreased to determine the effect of moisture on the physicochemical properties of the compound.

It is probably more popular to perform microcalorimetry in the static mode. In the so-called internal hygrostat method described by Briggner et al. (1994), the compound under investigation is sealed into a vial with a sealed pipette tip containing the saturated salt solution chosen to give the required RH. This is shown in Figure 3.14.

Figure 3.15 shows the heat output recorded when using an 84 percent RH internal hygrostat for the sample whose DVS isotherm is shown in Figure 3.13. In this example, there is a transformation of one crystalline hydrate to a higher hydrate.

Thermal Analysis

There a number of interrelated thermal analytical techniques that can be used to characterize the salts and polymorphs of candidate drugs. As noted in Table 3.8, the melting point of a salt can be manipulated to produce compounds with desirable physicochemical properties for specific formulation types. Giron (1995) has reviewed thermal analytical and calorimetric methods used in the characterization of polymorphs and solvates. Of the thermal methods available for investigating polymorphism and related phenomena, DSC, TGA and hot stage microscopy (HSM) are the most widely used.

Differential Scanning Calorimetry

There are two types of DSC. The first type is the heat flux type (e.g., Mettler and du Pont) where sample and reference cells are heated at a constant rate and thermocouples are used to

Figure 3.14 Internal hygrostat for microcalorimetry experiments.

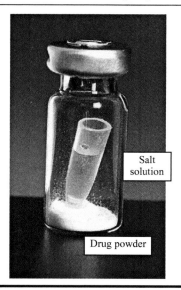

Salt
solution

Drug powder

Figure 3.15 Microcalorimetric output from an internal hygrostat experiment (corresponds to crystalline hydrate 1 to crystalline hydrate 2 transformation illustrated in Figure 3.13).

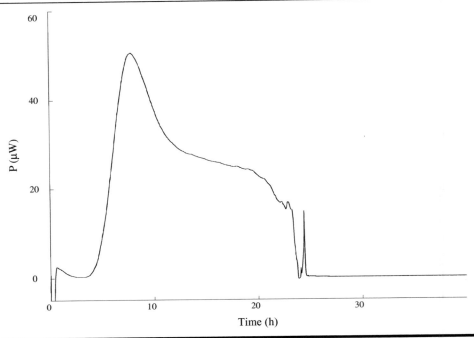

detect the extent of the differential heat transfer between the two pans. The other DSC system is the power compensated type (e.g., Perkin-Elmer). With this type of calorimeter, if an exothermic or endothermic event occurs when a sample is heated, the power added or subtracted to one or both of the furnaces to compensate for the energy change occurring in the sample is measured. Thus, the system is maintained in a thermally neutral position at all times, and the amount of power required to maintain the system at equilibrium is directly proportional to the energy changes that are occurring in the sample. In both instruments, a few milligrams of the compound under study are weighed into an aluminium pan that can be open, hermetically sealed, or pierced to allow the escape of water, solvent or decomposition products from pyrolysis reactions.

There are a number of variables that can affect DSC results (see, e.g., van Dooren 1982). These include the type of pan, heating rate, the nature and mass of the compound, the particle size distribution, packing and porosity, pre-treatment and dilution of the sample. Normally the experiments are carried out under a nitrogen atmosphere. Phenomena that can be detected using this technique include melting (endothermic), solid-state transitions (endothermic), glass transitions, crystallization (endothermic), decomposition (exothermic) and dehydration or desolvation (endothermic). DSC can also be used for purity analysis (see Giron and Goldbronn 1995). However, this is restricted to those compounds that are >98 percent pure. It may be appropriate, if no HPLC methods are available, to use DSC to estimate purity, but it should be emphasized that DSC is much less reliable than HPLC.

A heating rate of 10°C/min is a useful compromise between speed of analysis and detecting any heating-rate dependent phenomena. Should any heating-rate dependent phenomena be evident, experiments should be repeated varying the heating rate to attempt to identify the nature of the transition(s). These may be related to polymorphism, discussed earlier in this chapter, or to particle size. Figure 3.16 shows the effect of particle size and heating rate on the polymorphic transition of a development compound. At 10°C/min, the sample showed a single endotherm; however, when the sample was milled, it gave a thermogram that showed a melt–recrystallization–melt transformation. By reducing the heating rate it can be seen that, rather than being due to a polymorphic transformation induced by the milling process, the transformation was due to a reduction in particle size.

A number of parameters can be measured from the various thermal events detected by DSC. For example, for a melting endotherm the onset, peak temperatures and enthalpy of fusion can be derived. The onset temperature is obtained by extrapolation from the leading edge of the endotherm to the baseline. The peak temperature is the temperature corresponding to the maximum of the endotherm, and enthalpy of fusion is derived from the area of the thermogram. It is the accepted custom that the extrapolated onset temperature is taken as the melting point; however, some users report the peak temperature in this respect. We tend to report both for completeness.

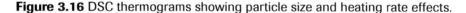

Figure 3.16 DSC thermograms showing particle size and heating rate effects.

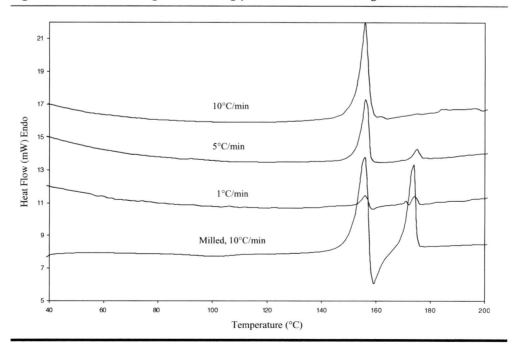

Recycling experiments can also be conducted whereby a sample is heated and then cooled. The thermogram may show a crystallization exotherm for the sample, which on subsequent reheating may show a melting point different from the first run. In a similar way, amorphous forms can be produced by cooling the molten sample to form a glass.

Figure 3.17 shows the DSC behaviour of the methanolate, the desolvated solvate and two polymorphs of the hydrochloride salt of a development compound. These thermograms are

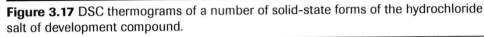

Figure 3.17 DSC thermograms of a number of solid-state forms of the hydrochloride salt of development compound.

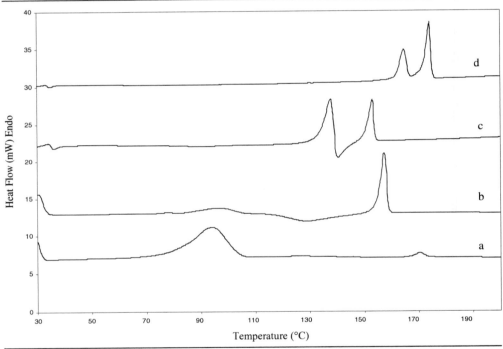

(a) This is the methanol solvate, which showed a desolvation endotherm between 75 and 100°C: TGA recorded a weight loss of 4.5 percent. A second much smaller endotherm was detected at ~170°C; however, no thermal events at this temperature were noted using HSM.

(b) This thermogram was obtained after the methanol solvate was desolvated in an oven. As can be seen, the thermogram contained a number of thermal events. The first, at ~100°C, corresponded to small weight loss (residual solvent) detected by TGA. An exotherm corresponding to crystallization was noted at ~125°C, which indicated that desolvation produced an amorphous form which, on heating, crystallized. The non-crystalline nature of this phase was confirmed by XRPD. The crystalline material produced by this heating process melted at ~160°C.

(c) This is the DSC thermogram of the first polymorph of the compound, which consisted of an endotherm corresponding to the melting followed by an exotherm due to immediate recrystallization to form a higher melting form of the compound.

(d) The second polymorphic form of the compound consisted of two thermal events, the first of which was a solid-state transition, i.e., a transformation without a melt. The second was confirmed by HSM to be the melting endotherm.

quite complicated and would be difficult to interpret in the absence of other measurements and observations such as TGA, HSM and XRPD.

Because of the polymorphism of the compound shown in Figure 3.17, a number of alternative salts were prepared in an attempt to overcome a problem in production. Figure 3.18 shows the range of thermograms obtained from these salts. This clearly shows that DSC can be an extremely informative technique, but it should not be used in isolation. Additional information from other techniques is almost always required for complete interpretation of the results.

The calibration of a DSC employs the use of standards, and Giron-Forest et al. (1989) has listed a number materials that can be used (Table 3.14). In this respect ultra-pure indium and lead traceable standards are probably the most convenient for a two-point calibration. The relevant data are as follows:

- Indium: onset temperature = 156.61 ± 0.25°C, ΔH = 28.45 ± 0.50 J/g

- Lead: onset temperature = 327.47 ± 0.50°C, ΔH = 23.01 ± 1.0 J/g

Modulated Differential Scanning Calorimetry

In modulated DSC (MDSC) experiments, the heating programme is applied sinusoidally such that any thermal events are resolved into reversing and non-reversing components. This allows complex and even overlapping processes to be deconvoluted (Coleman and Craig 1996). The heat flow signal in conventional DSC is a combination of "kinetic" and heat capacity responses, and Fourier transform (FT) techniques are used to separate the heat flow component from the underlying heat flow signal. The cyclic heat flow part of the signal (heat capacity,

Figure 3.18 DSC of the salts of the compound shown in Figure 3.16.

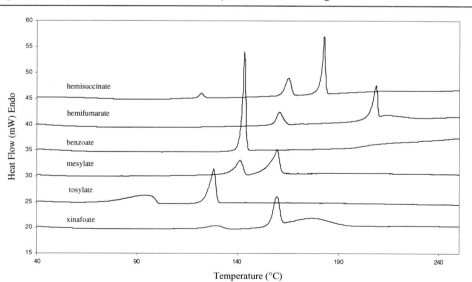

Table 3.14
Standards for thermal analysis.

Temperature (°C)	Substance
0	Water
26.87	Phenoxybenzene
114.2	Acetanilide
151.4	Adipic acid
156.6	Indium
229	Tin
232	Caffeine
327.5	Lead
419.6	Zinc

Reprinted from *J. Pharm. Biomed. Anal.*, Vol. 7, D. Giron-Forest et al., Thermal analysis methods for pharmacopeial materials, Pages 1421–1433, 1989, with permission from Elsevier Science.

$C_p \times$ heating rate) is termed the reversing heat flow component. The non-reversing part is obtained by subtracting this value from the total heat flow curve. It is important to note that all of the noise appears in the non-reversing signal.

In MDSC experiments the following experimental conditions need to be optimized:

- Samples should be small, thin and completely encapsulated in the DSC pan. This minimizes temperature gradients and maximizes conductivity during the heating and cooling cycles. Good thermal contact must also be ensured between the pans and the DSC head.

- The heat capacity heat flow contribution during the heating and cooling cycles is completely reversible.

The limitations of MDSC have been described as follows (Craig and Royall 1998):

- The sample does not follow the heating signal.

- There needs to be a sufficient number of cycles to cover the thermal event under investigation.

- Some samples may fluctuate in temperature during the sinusoidal ramp.

Royall et al. (1998) have described its use in the characterization of amorphous saquinavir. Using this technique, the glass transition could be separated from a relaxation endotherm that appeared as part of the transition. Although it is useful in this respect, the measurements can be affected by such instrumental parameters as temperature cycling and modulation period.

Rabel et al. (1999) have investigated the use of MDSC in preformulation studies. Its use in investigating glass transitions was discussed; however, this was extended to consider its use with regard to desolvation and degradation. For example, they showed that MDSC could deconvolute concomitant melting and degradation thermal events. The events were separated as melt (endothermic), which was reversible, and as decomposition, which was non-reversible. Polymorphic transformations were also investigated. The solid-state transformation of losartan was subjected to the MDSC programme and in this case the transition was seen in the non-reversible heat flow, and almost no reversible transition was detected.

Hot Stage Microscopy

HSM is a thermal analytical technique whereby a few milligrams of material is spread on a microscope slide which is then placed in the hot stage and heated. Figure 3.19 shows a simplified schematic diagram of a typical HSM set-up. It consists of a sample chamber with windows which allow the light from the microscope to pass through the sample. The sample can be heated at different rates in the sample chamber, and the atmosphere can be controlled. Sub-ambient work can also be carried out using liquid nitrogen as a coolent. The use of videotaping is highly recommended, as this allows the experiment to be left unattended and other work to be performed. Also, portions of particular interest can be slowed down or speeded up to ascertain the exact nature of the thermal events under observation. It is strongly recommended that HSM be carried out in conjuction with DSC and TGA. Indeed, direct observation by HSM can sometimes reveal subtle changes not readily detected by the other instrumental thermal analytical techniques. Although now quite old, McCrone's (1957) book on the subject is a useful introduction to this technique. In addition, the recent paper by Vitez et al. (1998) is recommended.

The DSC thermogram for carbamazepine (Figure 3.20) shows a number of thermal events; without the aid of HSM these events would be difficult to ascribe to any particular thermal event.

Figure 3.21 shows the sequence of events recorded on heating a sample of carbamazepine. On heating, the sample melted, which corresponded to the first endotherm recorded in the DSC thermogram. As the sample was heated further, a second form of the compound recrystallized from the melt as acicular crystals; however, this event was not detected by DSC

Figure 3.19 Hot stage microscopy (HSM) unit.

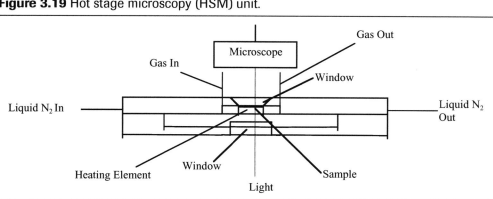

Figure 3.20 DSC thermogram of carbamzepine.

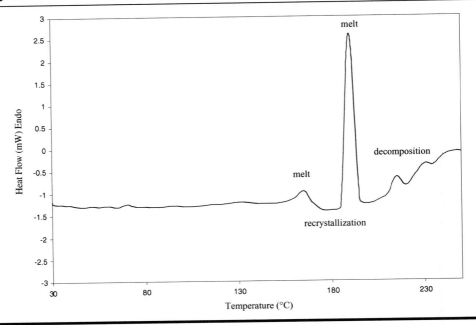

analysis. The acicular crystals continued to grow until the second crystal form of the compound melted, corresponding to the second, large endotherm on the DSC thermogram.

Thermogravimetric Analysis

TGA is a related thermal analytical technique that can be used to detect the amount of weight lost on heating a sample (Komatsu et al. 1994). It is based on a sensitive balance that records the weight of the sample as it is heated. Normally, 5 to 10 mg of compound is examined, and like DSC, the experiments are normally conducted under flowing nitrogen. An example of the weight loss profile on heating a hydrate is shown in Figure 3.22.

As illustrated in Figure 3.22, the TGA experiment can detect the presence of water or solvent in different locations in the crystal lattice. In this example, a trihydrate, two-thirds of the water is hydrogen-bonded channel water easily removed by heating, i.e., "loosely bound". The remaining third is more tightly bound and associated with a sodium ion in the crystal lattice. Thus, this technique has the advantage over a Karl Fischer titration or a loss on drying experiment that can only detect the total amount of moisture present. In addition, TGA requires less compound than the other two techniques. It is good practice not to use too small a sample weight in the analysis, as this may give rise to inaccuracies due to buoyancy and convection current effects.

The total amount of moisture lost in TGA experiments is not affected by the heating rate, however, the temperature at which it occurs may vary (Figure 3.23). In addition, the dehydration mechanism and activation of the reaction may be dependent on the particle size and sample weight (Agbada and York 1994). The TGA is calibrated using magnetic standards.

Figure 3.21 HSM photographs of carbamazepine.

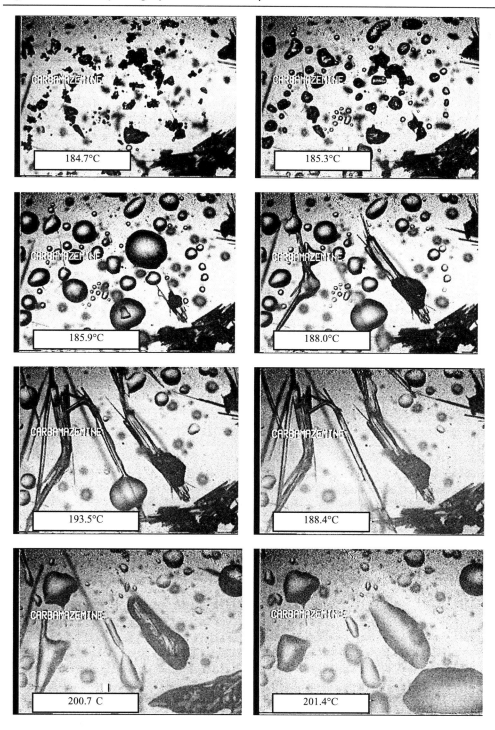

Figure 3.22 Thermogravimetric analysis (TGA) of a hydrate showing two weight losses.

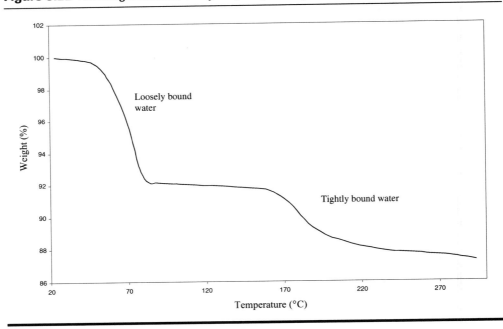

Infrared (IR) Spectroscopy

In addition to being a chemical identification technique, IR spectroscopy is also able to distinguish different solid-state structures of compounds. Since different arrangements of atoms in solid-state will lead to different molecular environments, this leads to different stretching frequencies that can be used to distinguish polymorphic forms of a compound. In addition, the inclusion of solvent or water can be detected using this technique; for example, the broad –OH stretch associated with water will be seen. IR spectroscopy has been used effectively to characterize the various forms of carbamazepine, and four ranges appear to be important in their differentiation (Krahn and Mielck 1987):

- **3490–3460 cm^{-1} (N–H valence stretch)**
Form I	3489 cm^{-1}
Form II	3473 cm^{-1}
Form III	3468 cm^{-1}

- **1700–1680 cm^{-1} (–C–O–R vibration)**
Form I	1695 cm^{-1}
Form II	1688 cm^{-1}
Form II	1680 cm^{-1}

- **Circa 1600 cm^{-1} (vibration of the –C = C– and –C = O bonds –NH deformation)**
  Forms I and III exhibited two bands with differing intensity while Form II showed a single band.

Figure 3.23 Effect of TGA heating rate on moisture loss.

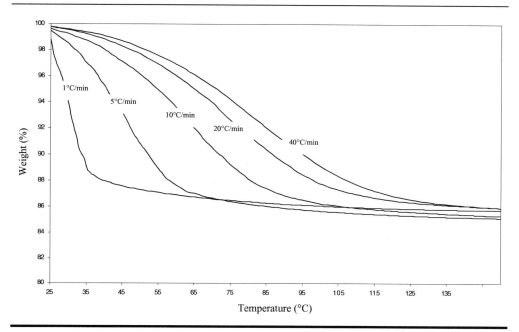

- **830–770 cm^{-1} (out of plane vibration –C–H)**

  Form I   811, 800 and 783 cm^{-1}
  Form II   815, 783 and 770 cm^{-1}
  Form III   810 and 775 cm^{-1}

Takla and Dakas (1989) have also shown that IR spectroscopy can be used to detect polymorphism due to the keto-enol tautomerism of acetohexamide.

Experimentally, IR spectroscopy can be accomplished in a number of ways: by Nujol mull, KBr disc or the diffuse reflectance technique. In the KBr disc technique, the compound is mixed with KBr and compressed into a disc using a press and die. This can be a disadvantage if the compound undergoes a polymorphic transformation under pressure (see Chan and Doelker, 1985). One way to overcome this problem is to use the diffuse reflectance Fourier transform (DRIFT) technique, whereby a few milligrams of compound is dispersed in approximately 250 mg of KBr and the spectrum obtained by reflection from the surface.

The Fourier transform–infrared (FT-IR) spectra of two polymorphs, an amorphous form and a methanol solvate of a hydrochloride salt, are shown in Figure 3.24 (see Figure 3.17 for the corresponding DSC thermograms). The spectra can be used to give information on how the molecule is packed in the solid state and which groups of the molecule are in a different environment. As can be seen, the spectrum of the amorphous form of the compound is less well defined and reflects the multitude of molecular environments present in this form of the compound.

Figure 3.24 Infrared spectra of a number of solid-state forms of a compound.

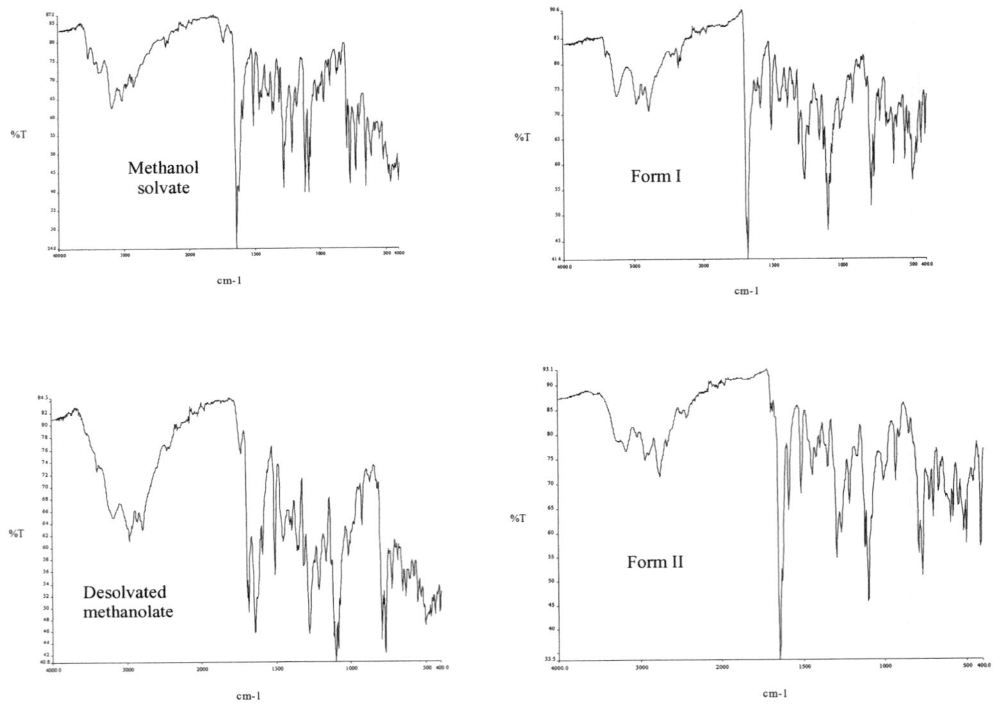

In all figures, abscissa is 4000–400 cm^{-1} and ordinate is % transmittance.

Heating experiments are also possible using IR spectroscopy. Bartolomei et al. (1997) used variable temperature IR spectroscopy to confirm that a solid-solid transition took place on heating two forms of flucinolone acetonide. The spectrum at 230°C showed frequency shifts characteristic of Form A transforming into Form B. However, these did not match the frequencies of Form B. The analytical potential of FT-IR thermomicroscopy of sulphaproxyline and difluprednate has been studied by Ghetti et al. (1994). Spectra were recorded for every 2°C increase of temperature and, in the case of sulphaproxyline, between 184 and 186°C the NH bands at 3140 and 2870 cm^{-1} disappeared and a broad band at 3280 cm^{-1} appeared. This is characteristic of the melt phase of this polymorph. At 190°C this band was replaced by a strong band at 3300 cm^{-1} that was distinctive of Form I of the compound. Other changes were also noted.

X-Ray Powder Diffraction

The book by Jenkins and Snyder (1996) is particularly recommended as an excellent introduction to the science of XRPD. Some of the salient points made in this book and in other sources are presented below.

X rays are part of the electromagnetic spectrum lying between ultraviolet and gamma rays, and they are expressed in angstrom units (Å). Diffraction is a scattering phenomenon, and when X rays are incident on crystalline solids, they are scattered in all directions. Scattering occurs due to the radiation wavelength being in the same order of magnitude as the interatomic distances within the crystal structure.

Bragg's law describes the conditions under which diffraction will occur. Diffraction will occur if a perfectly parallel and monochromatic X-ray beam, of wavelength λ, is incident on a crystalline sample at an angle θ that satisfies the Bragg equation:

$$n\lambda = \frac{2d}{\sin \theta} \qquad (21)$$

where n = order of reflection (an integer, usually 1); λ = wavelength of X ray; d = distance between planes in crystal (d-spacings); and θ = angle of incidence/reflection.

An X-ray diffractometer is made up of an X-ray tube generating X rays from, e.g., Cu K_α or Co source and a detector. The most common arrangement in pharmaceutical powder studies is the Bragg-Brentano θ-θ configuration. In this arrangement, the X-ray tube is moved through angle θ, and the detector is moved through angle θ. The sample is fixed between the detector and X-ray source as shown in Figure 3.25.

The powder pattern consists of a series of peaks that have been collected at various scattering angles, which are related to d-spacings, so that unit cell dimensions can be determined. In most cases, measurement of the d-spacings will suffice to positively identify a crystalline material. If the sample does not show long-range order, i.e., it is amorphous, the X rays are not coherently scattered, and no peaks will be observed. Figure 3.26 shows an example of a crystalline and an amorphous phase.

Although XRPD analysis is a relatively straightforward technique for the identification of solid-phase structures, there are sources of error, including the following:

Figure 3.25 Bragg-Bentano geometry used in XRPD experiments.

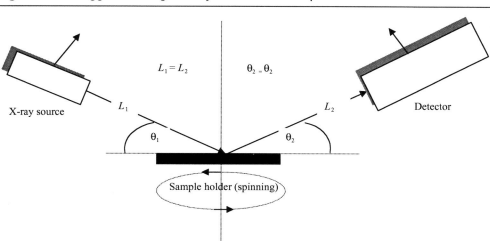

Figure 3.26 XRPD patterns of a compound with a crystalline and an amorphous phase.

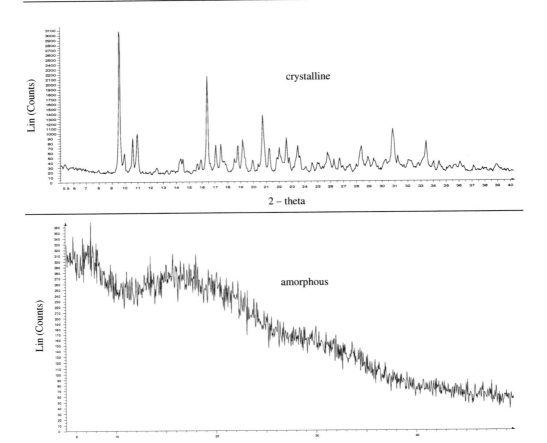

- *Variations in particle size.* Large particle sizes can lead to non-random orientation, and so particles <10 μm should be used, i.e., the sample should be *carefully* ground. However, if the size is too small, e.g., 1 μm, this leads to broadening of the diffraction peaks. Indeed, if the crystal sizes are too small, then the sample may appear to be amorphous.

- *Preferred orientation.* If a powder consists of, e.g., needle- or plate-shaped particles, these tend to become aligned parallel to the specimen axis, and thus certain planes have a greater chance of reflecting the X rays. To reduce the errors due to this source, the sample is usually rotated. Alternatively, the sample can be packed into a capillary. Figure 3.27 shows some examples of preferred orientation.

- *Statistical errors.* The magnitude of statistical errors depends on the number of photons counted. To keep this number small, scanning should be carried out at an appropriately slow speed.

Figure 3.27 Examples of preferred orientation.

a) One peak dominates the diffraction pattern.

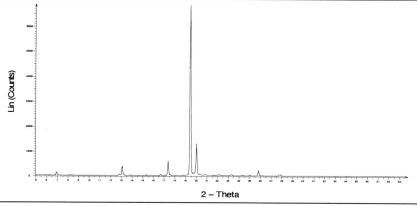

(b) Two batches have apparently different XRPD patterns.

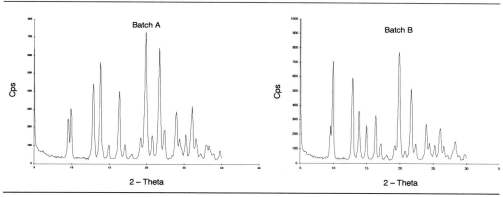

(c) Effect of grinding samples shown in (b).

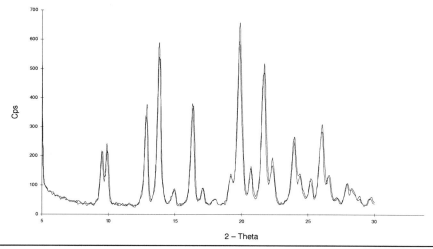

In all figures, abscissa is degress 2 – theta, and ordinate is intensity.

- *Sample height.* The sample should be level with the top of the holder. If the sample height is too low, the pattern shifts down the 2θ scale, and if it is too high, it moves up the 2θ scale.

Sample preparation procedures for XRPD have been reported (JCPDS Data Collection and Analysis Sub-committee (Jenkins et al. 1986). Possible causes for compositional variations between as-received and samples prepared (by grinding) for X-ray analysis are given in Table 3.15. The greatest potential source of problems is due to grinding, which can introduce strain, amorphism and polymorphic changes. Furthermore, the atmosphere surrounding the sample can create problems due to loss or gain of moisture or carbon dioxide. This is particularly true if a heating stage is used.

As already mentioned, the limited amount of compound available can be problematic. However, modern diffractometers can use so-called zero-background holders (ZBH). These are made from a single crystal of silicon that has been cut along a non-diffracting plane and then polished to an optically flat finish (Misture et al. 1994). Thus, X rays incident on this surface will be negated by Bragg extinction. In this technique, a thin layer of grease is placed on the ZBH surface, and the sample of ground compound is placed on the surface. The excess is removed such that only a monolayer is examined. The total thickness of the sample and grease should be of the order of a few microns. According to Misture et al. (1994), it is important that the sample is deagglomerated so that the monolayer condition is met. Using this technique, the diffraction pattern of approximately 10 mg of compound can be obtained. One disadvantage of the ZBH is that weak reflections may not be readily detectable because of the small sample size used.

The powder X-ray diffractometer can be calibrated using a variety of standards. These are available from the Laboratory of the Government Chemist (LGC) in the United Kingdom or the National Institute of Standards and Technology (NIST) in the United States. The types of standards used in XRPD are shown in Table 3.16 (Jenkins and Snyder 1996). Analyzing one or two peaks of LaB_6, at least weekly, should give confidence in the diffractometer performance and alert the user to any problems that may be developing.

Table 3.15
Possible causes for compositional variations
between "as received" and ground samples.

Induced by Grinding Problems	Induced by Irradiation	Special
Amorphism	Polymerisation	Hydration
Carbonisation Strain	Decomposition	Loss of water in vacuum
Decomposition		Decomposition at high temperature
Polymorphic change		
Solid-state reactions		
Contamination by the mortar		

Reprinted with permission from Jenkins, R., T. G. Fawcett, D. K. Smith, J. W. Visser, M. C. Morris, and L. K. Frevel. JCPDS–International centre for diffraction data sample preparation methods in X-ray powder diffraction. *Powder Diff.* 1:51–63. Copyright, JCPDS–International Centre for Diffraction Data, 1986.

Table 3.16
Standards used in X-ray diffraction studies.

Type	Use	Standard
External 2θ standards		Silicon
		α-Quartz
		Gold
Internal *d*-spacing standards	Primary	Silicon (SRM 640b)
	Primary	Fluorophlogopite (SRM 675)
	Secondary	Tungsten, silver, quartz and diamond
Internal intensity standards	Quantitative	Al_2O_3 (SRM 676)
		α- and β-Silicon nitride (SRM 656)
	Intensity	Oxides of Al, Ce, Cr, Ti and Zn (SRM 674a)
	Respirable	α-Silicon dioxide (SRM 1878a)
	Quartz	Cristobalite (SRM 1879a)
External sensitivity standards		Al_2O_3 (SRM 1976)
Line profile standards	Broadening calibration	LaB_6 (SRM 660)

Source: Jenkins and Snyder (1996).

A heating stage may also be of value for investigating thermal events detected during DSC experiments. For example, if a compound undergoes a solid-state transition from a low melting form to a high melting form, this can be detected by a change in the diffraction pattern. Using the Anton Parr TTK-450 temperature attachment, the compound can be investigated between subambient temperatures and several hundred degrees. Figure 3.28 shows the diffraction patterns obtained on heating a sample. Prior to the start of the XRPD experiment, the compound was partially amorphous due to desolvation and micronization. However, as the sample was heated, the XRPD peaks became sharper and stronger, indicating an increase in crystallinity. This corresponds to the annealing exotherm observed in the DSC thermogram. This DSC experiment showed a melt–recrystallization–melt polymorphic transformation, which is also shown by the XRPD, whereby a change in crystal structure was evident as the sample was heated, followed by a diffuse pattern from the final melt. In a similar way, the sample can be exposed to varying degrees of humidity *in situ* and the diffraction pattern determined.

Phase Solubility Analysis

Methods used for the estimation of the aqueous solubility of organic compounds have been presented by in a book by Yalkowsky and Banerjee (1992). Solubilities can also be estimated by visual observation as follows. The solubility of a compound is initially determined by weighing out 10 mg (or other suitable amount) of the compound. To this is added 10 μL of the solvent of interest. If the compound does not dissolve, a further 40 μL of solvent is added

Figure 3.28 Temperature-XRPD pattern of a compound undergoing a polymorphic change.

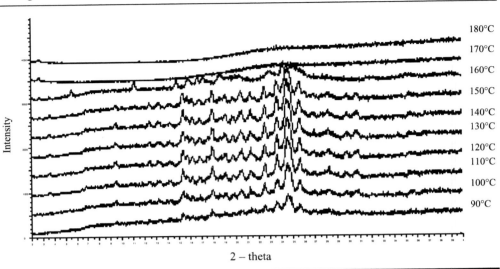

and its effect noted. Successive amounts of the solvent are then added until the compound is observed to dissolve. This procedure should give an approximate value of the solubility.

It should be noted that this is a crude method of solubility determination and takes no account of the kinetic aspects of the dissolution processes involved in solubility measurements. To more accurately determine the concentration of a saturated solution of a compound, the following procedure can be used. A known volume of the solvent, water or buffer is pipetted into a scintillation vial, and the compound of interest is added until saturation is observed to occur. The solution is then stirred or shaken for approximately 1 h at the desired temperature. If the compound dissolves, then more compound is added and the experiment restarted. It is recommended that the experiment be conducted at least overnight, but longer time periods may be required if the compound has a very low solubility: for example, saturation of morphine in water at 35°C was obtained only after approximately 48 h (Roy and Flynn 1989).

Depending on the amount of compound available, replicate experiments should be carried out. After stirring or shaking, the solvent should be separated from the suspension by centrifugation or by filtration using polytetrafluoroethylene (PTFE) filters. The filtrate is then assayed preferably by HPLC; however, UV-visible spectroscopy can also be used to determine the solubility, if compound stability or impurities are not an issue. This is termed the thermodynamic solubility. It is also useful to measure the pH of the filtrate and to analyze any undissolved material by DSC to detect any phase changes that may have occurred.

For high-throughput screening of solubilities, where the amount of compound may be severely restricted, reporting kinetic solubilities may be adequate. In this respect, Quarterman et al. (1998) have described a technique based on a 96-well microtitre technique with an integral nephelometer. The process of determining kinetic solubilities by this method was summarized as follows. Aliquots of the aqueous solution are placed in the microtitre wells, to which are added 1 μL of the compounds in DMSO, and the plate is shaken. The turbidity of the solutions is then measured using the nephelometer; this process is repeated up to 10 times. If turbidity is detected in a cell the experiment is terminated, i.e., solution additions are stopped and the solutions ranked in terms of number of additions that caused turbidity. The authors emphasized, however, that the purpose of this experiment is to rank the compounds in terms of their solubility but will not give a precise measure of a compound's solubility.

Due to the differences in melting point and other characteristics of polymorphs, solubility differences are often observed. Usually the most stable form of the compound has the lowest solubility in any solvent. It has already been noted that solids can undergo phase changes by way of the solution phase (Davey et al. 1986). When the solvent is in contact with the metastable phase, it dissolves, and the stable phase nucleates and grows from solution. So it is always worth slurrying a compound and assessing the solid phase to determine whether a solution mediated phase transformation to the stable phase has taken place.

Figure 3.29 shows the dissolution profile obtained during a solubility experiment for the amorphous form of a development compound. The initial dissolution of the compound is high but falls as the compound crystallizes and the equilibrium reaches that of a crystalline form of the compound. By measuring the solubility of polymorphs, the thermodynamic quantities involved in the transition from a metastable to a stable polymorph can be calculated. Experimentally, the solubilities of the polymorphs are determined at various temperatures, and then the log of the solubility is plotted against the reciprocal of the temperature (the van't Hoff method). A straight line results (the problem of non-linearity has been dealt with by

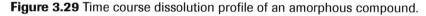

Figure 3.29 Time course dissolution profile of an amorphous compound.

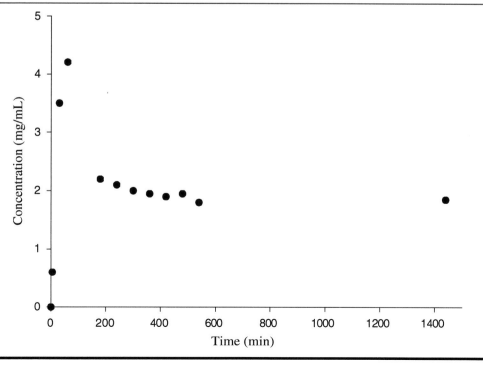

Grant et al. 1984), from which the enthalpy of solution can be calculated from the slope. If the lines intersect, it is known as the transition temperature, and one consequence of this is that there may be a transition from one polymorph to another, depending on the storage conditions. For example, the formation of the monohydrate of metronidazole benzoate from a suspension of the anhydrate was predicted from such data (Holgaard and Møller 1983).

Solution Calorimetry

Solution calorimetry involves the measurement of heat flow when a compound dissolves into a solvent. There are two types of solution calorimeters, i.e., isoperibol and isothermal. In the isoperibol technique, the heat change caused by dissolution of the solute gives rise to a change in the temperature of the solution. This results in a temperature-time plot from which the heat of solution is calculated. By contrast, in isothermal solution calorimetry (where, by definition, the temperature is maintained constant), any heat change is compensated by an equal, but opposite, energy change, which is then the heat of solution (Grant 1999). The newest microsolution calorimeter can be used with 3–5 mg of compound. Experimentally, the sample is introduced into the equilibrated solvent system and the heat flow is measured by a heat conduction calorimeter.

Dissolution of a solute involves several thermal events, such as heat associated with wetting, breakage of lattice bonds and solvation energy. The peak can be integrated directly to give an enthalpy of dissolution. The relative stabilities of polymorphs can be investigated in this way by the magnitude and sign (endothermic/exothermic) of the enthalpy of dissolution. A more endothermic (or less exothermic) response indicates that the energy of solvation of the solute does not compensate for the breaking of lattice bonds, and it is therefore the more stable solid (polymorph) (Goa and Rytting 1997).

Solution calorimetry was used by Pikal et al. (1978) to determine the heats of solution of different forms of some β-lactam antibiotics. It has also been used to quantitate binary mixtures of three crystalline forms of sulphamethoxazole (Guillory and Erb 1985). Solution calorimetry, in conjunction with thermal analysis, was used by Wu et al. (1993) to examine the two polymorphs of losartan. The heats of solution for polymorphs I and II were measured in water and *N,N*-dimethylformamide, however, the heats of transition were insignificant (ΔH_T = 1.72 kcal/mol).

Solution calorimetry can also been used to evaluate amorphous/crystalline content in a binary mixture. For example, Table 3.17 shows the enthalpy of solution of the amorphous and crystalline forms of a compound (Figure 3.30). The enthalpy of solution for the amorphous compound is an exothermic event, whilst that of the crystalline hydrate is endothermic. Enthalpy of solution is a sum of several thermal events, i.e., heat of wetting (incorporating sorption processes such as surface sorption and complexing), disruption of the crystal lattice and solvation. The order of magnitude of $\Delta_{sol}H^{\infty}$ for the crystalline compound suggests that the disruption of the crystal lattice predominates over the heat of solvation. In addition, the ready solubility of the compound in aqueous media is probably governed by entropy considerations.

Solution calorimeters are calibrated using KCl in water (for endothermic processes) and tris HCl in 0.01 M HCl (for exothermic processes) standards. For example, the heat of solution ΔH_s) of KCl at 25°C (298.15 K) is 235.86 ± 0.23 J/g. Similarly, the ΔH_s for tris HCl at 25°C is −29.80 kJ/mol (Kilday 1980).

Table 3.17
Heat of solution for an amorphous and a crystalline substance.

Determination	Amorphous [$\Delta_{sol}H^{\infty}$(kJ/mol)]	Crystalline [$\Delta_{sol}H^{\infty}$(kJ/mol)]
1	−9.92	37.59
2	−11.60	37.89
3	−10.42	37.47
4	−11.53	37.32
Mean	−10.87	37.57
SD	0.72	0.21
C of V/%	6.60	0.56

Figure 3.30 Isothermal solution calorimetry of an amorphous and a crystalline phase.

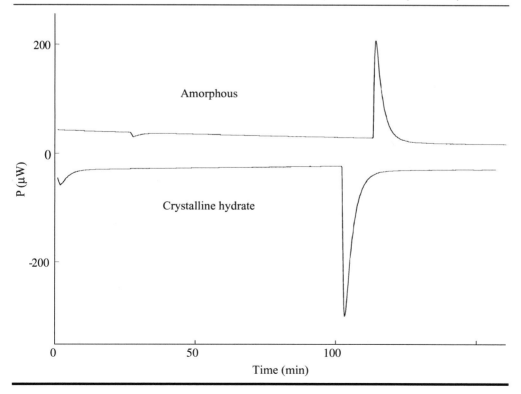

Intrinsic Dissolution

During the preformulation stage, an understanding of the dissolution rate of a drug candidate is necessary, since this property of the compound is recognized as a significant factor involved in drug bioavailability. Dissolution of a solid usually takes place in two stages: solvation of the solute molecules by the solvent molecules followed by transport of these molecules from the interface into the bulk medium by convection or diffusion. The major factor that determines the dissolution rate is the aqueous solubility of the compound, however, other factors such as particle size, crystalline state (polymorphs, hydrates), pH and buffer concentration can affect the rate. Moreover, physical properties such as viscosity and wettability can also influence the dissolution process.

Ideally, dissolution should simulate *in vivo* conditions. To do this, it should be carried out in a large volume of dissolution medium, *or* there must be some mechanism whereby the dissolution medium is constantly replenished by fresh solvent. Provided this condition is met, the dissolution testing is defined as taking place under sink conditions. Conversely, if there is a concentration increase during dissolution testing, such that the dissolution is retarded by a concentration gradient, the dissolution is said to be non-sink. Whilst the use of the USP paddle dissolution apparatus is mandatory when developing a tablet, the rotating disc method has great utility with regard to preformulation studies. The intrinsic dissolution rate is the dissolution rate of the compound under the condition of constant surface area. The rationale for the use of a compressed disc of pure material is that the intrinsic tendency of the test material to dissolve can be evaluated without formulation excipients.

Intrinsic dissolution rates of compounds obtained from rotating discs have been theoretically determined by Levich (1962). Under hydrodynamic conditions, the intrinsic dissolution rate is usually proportional to the solubility of the solid. However, as predicted by Levich, the dissolution rate obtained will be dependent on the rotation speed. Jashnani et al. (1993) have reported the validation of an improved rotating disc apparatus after finding that the original apparatus gave non-zero intercepts when experiments of albuterol discs were conducted at various rotation speeds.

In the experimental procedure, a disc is prepared by compression of ~200 mg of the candidate drug in a hydraulic press—an IR press is ideal and gives a disc with a diameter of 1.3 cm. It should be noted that some compounds do not compress well and may exhibit elastic compression properties; that is, the disc may be very weak, rendering the experiment impossible. In addition to poor compression properties, another complication is that some compounds can undergo polymorphic transformations due to the application of pressure. This should therefore be borne in mind if there is insufficient compound to perform, e.g., XRPD post-compaction.

If the disc has reasonable compression properties, it is then attached to a holder and set in motion in the dissolution medium (water, buffer or simulated gastric fluid): we use a rotation speed of 100 rpm. A number of analytical techniques can be used to follow the dissolution process, however, UV-visible spectrophotometry and HPLC with fixed or variable wavelength detectors (or diode array) appear to be the most common. The UV system employs a flowthrough system and does not require much attention, however, if HPLC is used, then any aliquot taken should be replaced by an equal amount of solvent. The IDR is given by the slope of the linear portion of the concentration versus time curve divided by the area of the disc and has the units of $mg/min \cdot cm^2$.

Figure 3.31 shows the increase in absorbance due to dissolution of approximately 200 mg of a sodium and a calcium salt of a weak acid. The sodium salt, which was soluble to approximately 300 mg/mL, dissolved much more rapidly than the calcium salt, whose solubility was only 1.4 mg/mL.

Figure 3.31 Plot of increase in absorbance versus time for a sodium and calcium salt of a compound undergoing intrinsic dissolution into water.

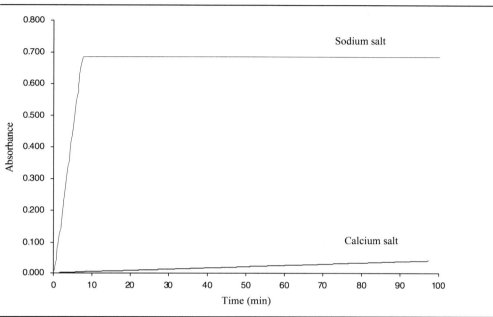

Crystalline Index of Refraction

Because different polymorphs have different internal structures, they will belong to different crystal systems; therefore, polymorphs can be distinguished using polarised light and a microscope. The crystals can be either isotropic or anisotropic. In isotropic crystals, the velocity of light is the same in all directions, while anisotropic crystals have two or three different light velocities or refractive indices. In terms of crystal systems, only the cubic system is isotropic; the other six are anisotropic.

The refractive indices, along with some other optical properties, of Form I and II of paracetamol have been reported (Nichols 1998). These are shown in Table 3.18. From these data, it was concluded that Form I of paracetamol could be optically distinguished from Form II because of its lower birefringence and strongly dispersed extinction. Its morphology was also different.

High Performance Liquid Chromatography

HPLC is now considered to be an established standard technique in most Preformulation and Formulation laboratories. We use HPLC to assess the degradation of the compound in the solid or solution state. From our measurements, we should be able to determine, e.g., the kinetics of degradation. Furthermore, if we can identify the degradation products of the reaction by combining this technique with mass spectroscopy, then it may also be possible to elucidate the degradation mechanism. The advantages of HPLC lie in the combination of sensitivity, efficiency, reliability and speed of analysis of the technique. Only brief guidance is

Table 3.18
Optical data for paracetamol Forms I and II.

Optical Data	Form I	Form II
Refractive index ($n_D{}^{25}$)		
nα	1.580 ($\pm$ 0.001)	1.491 ($\pm$ 0.001)
nβ	1.643 ($\pm$ 0.001)	1.667 ($\pm$ 0.001)
nγ	1.704 ($\pm$ 0.001)	1.840 ($\pm$ 0.001)
nγ when lying on {101}	1.683 ($\pm$ 0.001)	
Birefringence	0.124	0.349
Optic sign	(–)	(–)
Optic axial angle	86° (calculated)	81° (calculated)
Dispersion of optic axes	v > r (strong, crossed)	v > r (weak)
Acute bisectrix (Bx$_a$)	α	α
Extinction	Straight for sections perpendicular to the *b*-axis. Inclined and dispersed when viewed along the *b*-axis; γ^ {101} = 36.2° in white light 34.0° (656 nm, red) 38.2° (488 nm, blue)	Straight for prisms and symmetrical in rhomboid-shaped 002 cleavage fragments
Optical orientation	X = a = b	X = α = c Y = β = b Z = γ = a

From the *Microscope,* 46(3), 117–122 (1998) with permission.

presented here—a more detailed discussion of HPLC methodology and applications is beyond the scope of this book.

Prior to developing an HPLC method, its intended use must be carefully considered. For example, if the analysis is required to obtain an approximate value for the amount of candidate drug, such as for a solubility experiment, a "crude" method may be acceptable. Alternatively, if the HPLC method is to separate and determine related substances, i.e., synthesis intermediates and degradation products, from the compound of interest, a more robust method will have to be developed. Other considerations will include the amount of compound to be determined, from what type of matrix (e.g., formulation, reaction mixture, drug substance) and the number of and how quickly analyses are to be performed.

For most assays, where the compound is easily detected and there are relatively high concentrations in a simple matrix, then isocratic elution is usually preferred, since it is simple and no post-equilibration phase is required prior to the next analysis. However, with degradation products, excipients or synthetic intermediates, products of side reactions of differing lipophilicites are likely to be encountered, and then gradient elution may be used.

Gradient elution offers the advantage of sharper peaks, increased sensitivity, greater peak capacity and selectivity (increased resolving power). On the other hand, gradient elution may lead to an extended analysis time due to post-run equilibration. In addition, the system dwell times of different HPLC configurations may result in major differences in retention times and selectivity.

The type of detector to be used is usually dictated by the chemical structure of the compound under investigation. Since most compounds of pharmaceutical interest contain aromatic rings, UV detection is the most common detection method. When using this technique, the most appropriate wavelength is selected from the UV spectrum of the pure compound and that of the system suitability sample. Usually, the λ_{max} is chosen, however, in order to remove unwanted interference, it may be necessary to move away from this value. Where possible, the use of wavelengths <250 nm should be avoided due to the high level of background interference and solvent adsorption. In practical terms, this requires the use of far-UV grade solvents and the avoidance of organic buffers.

Other types of detection include refractive index, fluorescence or mass selective detectors. The use of other types of detectors, such as those based on fluorescence, may be used for assaying compounds that can be specifically detected at low concentrations in the presence of non-fluorescent species. However, since few compounds are naturally fluorescent, they require chemical modification, assuming they have a suitable reactive group, to give a fluorescent derivative.

During the early stages of development, the amount of method validation carried out is likely to be limited due to compound availability. At the very least, a calibration curve should be obtained using either an internal standard or external standard procedure. The latter procedure is commonly employed by injecting a fixed volume of standard samples containing a range of known concentrations of the compound of interest. Plots of peak height and/or area versus concentration are checked for linearity by subjecting the data to linear regression analysis. Other tests may be carried out, such as the limit of detection, precision of the detector response, accuracy, reproducibility, specificity and ruggedness, if more extensive validation is required.

CONCLUDING REMARKS

The preformulation phase is a critical learning time about candidate drugs. Typically, it begins during the LO phase and continues through prenomination and into the early phases of development. Decisions made on the information generated during this phase can have a profound effect on the subsequent development of those compounds. Therefore, it is imperative that preformulation should be performed as carefully as possible to enable rational decisions to be made. The quantity and quality of the drugs can affect the data generated; so can the equipment available and the expertise of the personnel conducting the investigations.

In some companies, there are specialized preformulation teams, but in others the information is generated by a number of other teams. Whichever way a company chooses to organize its preformulation information gathering, one of the most important facets is the close communication between its various departments.

Preformulation studies should not be conducted on a checklist basis. Rather, they should form the basis of a controlled investigation into the physicochemical characteristics of candidate drugs.

ACKNOWLEDGEMENTS

I would like to recognize the contributions of David O'Sullivan, Phil Plumb, Clare Westwood, Tal Austin and Steve Cosgrove made to the science of preformulation at AstraZeneca R&D Charnwood. Special thanks also go the students from Loughborough University who have contributed to our work—Arvind Varsani, Alan Tatham, Will Barton, Gavin Gunn and Dee Patel.

REFERENCES

Agbada, C. O., and P. York. 1994. Dehydration of theophylline monohydrate powder-effects of particle size and sample weight. *Int. J. Pharm.* 106:33–40.

Ahlneck, C., and G. Zografi. 1990. The molecular basis of moisture effects on the physical and chemical stability of drugs in the solid state. *Int. J. Pharm.* 62:87–95.

Akers, M. J. 1976. Preformulation testing of solid oral dosage forms. Methodology, management and evaluation. *Can. J. Pharm. Sci.* 11:1–10.

Albert, A., and E. P. Sargeant. 1984. *The determination of ionisation constants: A laboratory manual*, 3rd ed. London: Chapman Hall.

Albini, A., and E. Fashini, eds. 1998. *Drugs: Photochemistry and photostability.* Cambridge, UK: The Royal Society of Chemistry.

Alverez Núñez, F. A., and S. H. Yalkowsky. 1997. Foaming activity and pKa of some surface active compounds. *Int. J. Pharm.* 151:193–199.

Amidon, G. L., H. Lennernäs, V. P. Shah, and J. R. Crison. 1995. A theoretical basis for a biopharmaceutic drug classification: The correlation of in vitro drug product dissolution and in vivo bioavailability. *Pharm. Res.* 12:413–420.

Anderson, B. D., and R. A. Conradi. 1985. Predictive relationships in the water solubility of salts of a nonsteroidal anti-inflammatory drug. *J. Pharm. Sci.* 74:815–820.

Anderson, N. H., D. Johnston, M. A. McLelland, and P. Munden. 1991. Photostability testing of drug substances and drug products in UK pharmaceutical laboratories. *J. Pharm. Biomed. Anal.* 9:443–449.

Asuero, A. G., M. J. Navas, M. A. Herrador, and A. F. Recamales. 1986. Spectrophotometric evaluation of acidity constants of isonicotinic acid. *Int. J. Pharm.* 34:81–92

Austin, R. P., A. M. Davis, and C. N. Manners. 1995. Partitioning of ionizing molecules between aqueous buffers and phospholipid Vesicles. *J. Pharm Sci.* 84:1180–1183.

Avdeef, A., C. M. Berger, and C. Brownell. 2000. pH-metric solubility. 2. Correlation between the acid-base titration and the saturation shake-flask solubility-pH methods. *Pharm. Res.* 17:85–89.

Avdeef, A., K. J. Box, J. E. A. Comer, M. Gilges, M. Hadley, C. Hibbert, W. Patterson, and K. Y. Tam. 1999. pH-metric log P 11. Pka determination of water-insoluble drugs in organic-solvent mixtures. *J. Pharm. Biomed. Anal.* 20:631–641.

Barnett, S. P., A. P. Hill, D. J. Livingstone, and J. Wood. 1992. A new method for the calculation of partition coefficients from experimental data for both mixtures and pure compounds. *Quant. Struct.-Act. Relat.* 11:505–509.

Bartolomei, M., M. C. Ramusino, and P. Ghetti. 1997. Solid state investigation of flucinolone acetonide. *J. Pharm. Biomed. Anal.* 15:1813–1820.

Beall, H. D., J. J. Getz, and K. B. Sloan. 1993. The estimation of relative water solubility for prodrugs that are unstable in water. *Int. J. Pharm.* 93:37–47.

Benjamin, E. J., and L. H. Lin. 1985. Preparation and in vitro evaluation of salts of an antihypertensive agent to obtain slow release. *Drug Dev. Ind. Pharm.* 11:771–790.

Berge, S. M., L. D. Bighley, and D. C. Monkhouse. 1977. Pharmaceutical salts. *J. Pharm. Sci.* 66:1–18.

Bray, M. L., H. Jahansouz, and M. J. Kaufman. 1999. Selection of optimal hydrate/solvate forms of a fibrinogen receptor antagonist for solid dosage development. *Pharm. Dev. and Tech.* 4:81–87.

Briggner, L.-E., G. Buckton, K. Bystrom, and P. Darcy. 1994. Use of isothermal microcalorimetry in the study of changes in crystallinity induced during the processing of powders. *Int. J. Pharm.* 105:125–135.

Brittain, H. G. 1997. Spectral methods for the characterization of polymorphs and solvates. *J. Pharm. Sci.* 86:405–412.

Burger, A., W. Brox, and A. W. Ratz. 1985. Polymorphie und pseudopolymorphie von celiprololhydrochlorid. *Acta Pharm. Technol.* 31:230–235.

Busetta, B., C. Courseille, and M. Hospital. 1973. Crystal and molecular structure of three polymorphous forms of estrone. *Acta Cryst.* B29:298–313.

Byrn, S. R. 1982. *Solid state chemistry of drugs.* New York: Academic Press.

Byrn, S. R., R. Pfeiffer, M. Ganey, C. Hoiberg, and G. Poochikian. 1995. Pharmaceutical solids: A strategic approach to regulatory considerations. *Pharm. Res.* 12:945–954.

Callaghan, J. C., G. W. Clearly, M. Elefant, G. Kaplan, T. Kensler, and R. A. Nash. 1982. Equilibrium moisture content of pharmaceutical excipients. *Drug Dev. Ind. Pharm.* 8:355–369.

Cartensen, J. T., K. Danjo, S. Yoshioka, and M. Uchiyama. 1987. Limits to the concept of solid-state stability. *J. Pharm. Sci.* 76:548–550.

Cartensen, J. T., and A. Li Wan Po. 1992. The state of water in drug decomposition in the moist solid state. Description and modelling. *Int. J. Pharm.* 83:87–94.

Chan, H. K., and E. Doelker. 1985. Polymorphic transformation of some drugs under compression. *Drug Dev. Ind. Pharm.* 11:315–332.

Chauret, N., D. K. Lloyd, D. Levorse, and D. A. Nicoll-Griffith. 1995. Automated pK_a determination of soluble and sparingly soluble drugs by capillary zone electrophoresis. *Pharm. Sci.* 1:59–62.

Chowan, Z. T. 1978. pH solubility profiles of organic carboxylic acids and their salts. *J. Pharm. Sci.* 67:1257–1260.

Clarke, M. J., U. J. Potter, C. Gilpin, M. J. Tobyn, and J. N. Staniforth. 1998. Imaging of hygroscopic ultrafine pharmaceutical powders using low temperature and environmental scanning electron microscopy. *Pharm. Pharmacol. Commun.* 4:419–425.

Coleman, N. J., and D. Q. M. Craig. 1996. Modulated temperature differential scanning calorimetry: A novel approach to pharmaceutical thermal analysis. *Int. J. Pharm.* 135:13–29.

Connors, K. A., G. L. Amidon, and V. J. Stella. 1986. *Chemical stability of pharmaceuticals. A handbook for pharmacists,* 2nd ed. New York: John Wiley and Sons.

Cotton, M. L., P. Lamarche, S. Motola, and E. B. Vadas. 1994. L-649,923—The selection of an appropriate salt form and preparation of a stable oral formulation. *Int. J. Pharm.* 109:237–249.

Craig, D. Q. M., and P. G. Royall. 1998. The use of modulated temperature DSC for the study of pharmaceutical systems: Potential uses and limitations *Pharm. Res.* 15:1152–1153.

Danjo, K., K. Kinoshita, K. Kitagawa, K. Iida, H. Sunada, and A. Otsuka. 1989. Effect of particle shape on the compaction and flow properties of powders. *Chem. Pharm. Bull.* 37:3070–3073.

David, W. I. F., K. Shankland, and N. Shankland. 1998. Routine determination of molecular crystal structures from powder diffraction data. *Chem. Commun.* 931–932.

Davey, R. J., P. T. Cardew, D. McEwan, and D. E. Sadler. 1986. Rate processes in solvent-mediated phase transformations. *J. Cryst. Growth* 79:648–653.

Dearden, J. C., and G. M. Bresnen. 1988. The measurement of partition coefficients. *Quant. Struct.-Act. Relat.* 7:133–144.

De Villiers, M. M., J. G. van der Watt, and A. P. Lötter. 1992. Kinetic study of the solid-state photolytic degradation of two polymorphic forms of furosemide. *Int. J. Pharm.* 88:275–283.

El-Tayar, N., R. S. Tsai, B. Testa, P. A. Carrupt, and A. Leo. 1991. Partitioning of solutes in different solvent systems: Contribution of hydrogen-bonding capacity and polarity. *J. Pharm. Sci.* 80:590–598.

Elliot, S. R., C. N. R. Rao, and J. M. Thomas. 1986. The chemistry of the non-crystalline state. *Agnew. Chem. Int. Ed. Engl.* 25:31–46.

Engel, G. E., S. Wilke, O. König, K. D. M. Harris, and F. J. J. Leussen. 1999. *PowderSolve*—A complete package for crystal structure solution from powder diffraction patterns. *J. Appl. Cryst.* 32: 1169–1179.

Fini, A., G. Fazio, I. Orienti, V. Zecchi, and I. Rapaport. 1991. Chemical properties-dissolution relationship. Part 4. Behaviour in solution of the diclofenac N-(2-hydroxyethyl) pyrrolidine salt (DHEP). *Pharm. Acta Helv.* 66:201–203.

Franks, N. P., M. H. Abraham, and W. R. Lieb. 1993. Molecular organization of liquid *n*-octanol: An x-ray diffraction analysis. *J. Pharm. Sci.* 82:466–470.

Führer, C. 1986. Crystal engineering. *Acta Pharm. Technol.* 32:161–163.

Fyhr, P., and C. Högström. 1988. A preformulation study on the kinetics of the racemization of ropivacaine hydrochloride. *Acta Pharm. Suec.* 25:121–132.

Gavezotti, A., and G. Filppini. 1995. Polymorphic forms of organic crystals at room conditions—thermodynamic and structural implications. *J. Am. Chem. Soc.* 117:12,299–12,305.

Ghetti, P., A. Ghedini, and R. Stradi. 1994. Analytical potential of FT-IR microscopy. I. Applications to the drug polymorphism study. *Boll. Chim. Farm.* 133:689–697.

Giachetti, C., A. Assandri, G. Mautone, E. Tajana, B. Palumbo, and R. Palumbo. 1996. Pharmacokinetics and metabolism of N-(2-hydroxyethyl)-2,5-[^{14}C]-pyrolidine (HEP, epolamine) in male healthy volunteers. *Eur. J. Drug Met. Pharmcokinet.* 21:261–268.

Guillory, J. K., and D. M. Erb. 1985. Using solution calorimetry to quantitate binary mixtures of three crystalline forms of sulfamethoxazole. *Pharm. Manuf.* (Sept.): 28–33.

Giron, D. 1995. Thermal analysis and calorimetric methods in the characterization of polymorphs and solvates. *Thermochim. Acta* 248:1–59.

Giron, D., and C. Goldbronn. 1995. Place of DSC purity analysis in pharmaceutical development. *J. Thermal Anal.* 44:217–251.

Giron-Forest, D. Ch. Goldbronn, and P. Piechon. 1989. Thermal analysis methods for pharmacopeial materials. *J. Pharm. Biomed. Anal.* 7:1421–1433.

Goa, D., and J. H. Rytting. 1997. Use of solution calorimetry to determine the extent of crystallinity of drugs and excipients. *Int. J. Pharm.* 151:183–192.

Gould, P. L. 1986. Salt selection for basic drugs. *Int. J. Pharm.* 33:201–217.

Grant, D. J. W. 1999. Report and recommendation of the USP advisory panel on physical test methods: crysrallinity determination by solution calorimetry. *Pharmacop. Forum.* 25:9266–9268.

Grant, D. J. W., M. Mehdizadeh, A. H. L. Chow, and J. E. Fairbrother. 1984. Nonlinear van't Hoff solubility–temperature plots and their pharmaceutical interpretation. *Int. J. Pharm.* 18:25–38.

Green, D. A., and P. Meenan. 1996. Acetaminophen crystal habit: Solvent effects. In *Crystal growth of organic materials*, edited by A. S. Myerson, D. A. Green, and P. Meenan. ACS Conference Proceedings, pp. 78–84.

Griesser, U. J., and A. Burger. 1995. The effect of water vapor pressure on desolvation kinetics of caffeine 4/5-hydrate. *Int. J. Pharm.* 120:83–93.

Gu, L., and R. G. Strickley. 1987. Preformulation salt selection—physical property comparisons of the tris(hydroxymethyl)aminomethane (THAM) salts of four analgesic/anti-inflammatory agents with the sodium salts and the free acids. *Pharm. Res.* 4:255–257.

Gustavo González, A. 1993. Practical digest for the evaluation of acidity constants of drugs by reversed phase high performance liquid chromatography. *Int. J. Pharm.* 91:R1–R5.

Haleblian, J. K. 1975. Characterization of habits and crystalline modification of solids and their pharmaceutical applications. *J. Pharm. Sci.* 64:1269–1288.

Haleblian, J., and W. McCrone. 1969. Pharmaceutical applications of polymorphism. *J. Pharm. Sci.* 58:911–929.

Hancock, B. C., and G. Zografi. 1997. Characteristics and significance of the amorphous state in pharmaceutical systems. *J. Pharm. Sci.* 86:1–12.

Hilal, S. H., Y. El-Shabrawy, L. A. Carreira, S. W. Karickhoff, S. S. Toubar, and M. Rizk. 1996. Estimation of the ionization pK_a of pharmaceutical substances using the computer program SPARC. *Talanta* 43:607–619.

Hirsch, C. A., R. J. Messenger, and J. L. Brannon. 1978. Fenoprofen: Drug form selection and preformulation stability studies. *J. Pharm. Sci.* 67:231–236.

Holgaard, A., and N. Møller. 1983. Hydrate formation of metronidazole benzoate in aqueous suspensions. *Int. J. Pharm.* 15:213–221.

Hong-guang, W., and Z. Ru-hua. 1995. Compaction behaviour of paracetamol powders of different crystal shapes. *Drug Dev. Ind. Pharm.* 21:863–868.

Hörter, D., and J. B. Dressman. 1997. Influence of physicochemical properties on dissolution of drugs in the gastrointestinal tract. *Adv. Drug Del. Rev.* 25:3–14.

Jakobsen, D. F., S. Frokjaer, C. Larsen, H. Niemann, and A. Buur. 1997. Application of isothermal microcalorimetry in preformulation. I. Hygroscopicity of drug substances. *Int. J. Pharm.* 156:67–77.

James, K. C. 1986. *Solubility and related phenomena.* New York: Marcel Dekker.

Jashnani, R. K., P. R. Byron, and R. N. Dalby. 1993. Validation of an improved Wood's rotating disk dissolution apparatus. *J. Pharm. Sci.* 82:670–671.

Jashnani, R. K., and P. R. Byron. 1996. Dry powder aerosol generation in different environments: Performance comparisons of albuterol, albuterol sulphate, albuterol adipate and albuterol stearate. *Int. J. Pharm.* 130:13–24.

Jenkins, R., and R. L. Snyder. 1996. *Introduction to x-Ray powder diffractometry.* New York: John Wiley & Sons.

Jenkins, R., T. G. Fawcett, D. K. Smith, J. W. Visser, M. C. Morris, and L. K. Frevel. 1986. JCPDS—International centre for diffraction data sample preparation methods in X-ray powder diffraction. *Powder Diff.* 1:51–63.

Jozwiakowski, M. J., S. O. Williams, and R. D. Hathaway. 1993. Relative physical stability of the solid forms of amiloride hydrochloride. *Int. J. Pharm.* 91:195–207.

Karfunkel, H. R., Z. J. Wu, A. Burkhard, G. Rihs, D. Sinnreich, H. M. Buerger, and J. Stanek. 1996. Crystal packing calculations and Rietveld refinement in elucidating the crystal structures of two modifications of 4-amidoindanone guanylhydrazone. *Acta Cryst.* B52:555–561.

Kariuki, B. M., K. Psallidas, K. D. M. Harris, R. L. Johnston, R. W. Lancaster, S. E. Staniforth, and S. M. Cooper. 1999. Structure determination of a steroid directly from powder diffraction data. *Chem. Commun.* 1677–1678.

Kilday, M. V. 1980. Systematic errors in an isoperibol solution calorimeter measured with standard reference reactions. *J. Res. Natl. Bur. Stand.* 85:449–465.

Koehler, M. G., S. Grigoras, and W. J. Dunn III. 1988. The relationship between chemical structure and the logarithm of the partition coefficient. *Quant. Struct.-Act. Relat.* 7:150–159.

Komatsu, H., K. Yoshii, and S. Okada. 1994. Application of thermogravimetry to water-content determinations of drugs. *Chem. Pharm. Bull.* 42:1631–1635.

Kontny, M. J., G. P. Grandolfi, and G. Zografi. 1987. Water vapor sorption of water-soluble substances: Studies of crystalline solids below their critical relative humidities. *Pharm. Res.* 4:104–112.

Krahn, F. U., and J. B. Mielck. 1987. Relations between several polymorphic forms and the dihydrate of carbamazepine. *Pharm. Acta Helv.* 62:247–254.

Kuhnert-Brandstätter, M., and P. Gasser. 1971. Solvates and polymorphic modifications of steroid hormones. I. *Microchem. J.* 16:419–428.

Lambert, W. J., L. A. Wright, and J. C. Stevens. 1990. Development of a preformulation screen utilizing a C-18-derivitized polystyrene-divinylbenzene high-performance liquid chromatographic (HPLC) column. *Pharm. Res.* 7:577–586.

Ledwidge, M. T., and O. I. Corrigan. 1998. Effects of surface active characteristics and solid state forms on the pH solubility profiles of drug–salt systems. *Int. J. Pharm.* 174:187–200.

Lehto, V.-P., J. Salonen, and E. Laine. 1999. Real time detection of photoreactivity in pharmaceutical solids and solutions with isothermal microcalorimetry. *Pharm. Res.* 16:368–373.

Leo, A., C. Hansch, and D. Elkins. 1971. Partition coefficients and their uses. *Chem. Rev.* 71:525–616.

Levich, V. G. 1962. *Physicochemical hydrodynamics.* Englewood Cliffs, N. J., USA: Prentice Hall.

Lipinski, C. A., F. Lombardo, B. W. Dominy, and P. J. Feeney. 1997. Experimental and computational approaches to estimate solubility and permeability in drug discovery and development settings. *Adv. Drug Del. Rev.* 23:2–25.

Loudon, G. C. 1991. Mechanistic interpretation of pH-rate profiles. *J. Chem. Ed.* 68:973–984.

Marshall, P. V., P. A. Cook, and D. R. Williams. 1994. A new analytical technique for characterising the water vapour sorption properties of powders. *Int. Symp. Solid Dosage Forms*, Stockholm.

Mayers, C. L., and D. R. Jenke. 1993. Stabilization of oxygen-sensitive formulations via a secondary oxygen scavenger. *Pharm. Res.* 10:445–448.

McCrone, W. C. 1957. *Fusion methods in chemical microscopy.* New York: Interscience Publishers Inc.

Mehta, A. C. 1995. Analytical issues in the chemical stability testing of drugs in solution. *Anal. Proc.* 32:67–69 (1995).

Merrifield, D. R., P. L. Carter, D. Clapham, and F. D. Sanderson. 1996. *Addressing the problem of light instability during formulation development. Photostab. Drugs Drug Formulations*, edited by H. H. Tønnesen, London: Taylor and Francis, pp. 141–154.

Misture, S. T., L. Chatfield, and R. L. Snyder. 1994. Accurate powder patterns using zero background holders. *Powder Diff.* 9:172–179.

Miyazaki, S., M. Oshiba, and T. Nadai. 1981. Precaution on the use of HCl salts in pharmaceutical formulation. *J. Pharm. Sci.* 70:594–596.

Monkhouse, D. C. 1984. Stability aspects of preformulation and formulation of solid pharmaceuticals. *Drug Dev. Ind. Pharm.* 10:1373–1412.

Monkhouse, D. C., and L. van Campen. 1984. Solid State reactions—theoretical and experimental aspects. *Drug Dev. Ind. Pharm.* 10:1175–1276.

Morgan, M. E., K. Liu, and B. D. Anderson. 1998. Microscale titrimetric and spectrophotometric methods for determination of ionization constants and partition coefficients of new drug candidates. *J. Pharm. Sci.* 87:238–245.

Morris, K. R., M. G. Fakes, A. B. Thakur, A. W. Newman, A. K. Singh, J. J. Venit, C. J. Spagnuolo, and A. T. M. Serajuddin. 1994. An integrated approach to the selection of optimal salt form for a new drug candidate. *Int. J. Pharm.* 105:209–217.

Nakanishi, T., M. Suzuki, A. Mashiba, K. Ishikawa, and T. Yokotsuka. 1998. Synthesis of NK109, an anticancer benzo[*c*]phenanthridine alkaloid. *J. Org. Chem.* 63:4235–4239.

Navia, M. A., and P. R. Chaturvedi. 1996. Design principles for orally bioavailable drugs. *DDT* 1:179–189.

Nichols, G. 1998. Optical properties of polymorphic forms I and II of paracetamol. *Microscope* 46:117–122.

Nururkar, A. N., A. R. Purkaystha, and P. C. Sheen. 1985. Effect of various factors on the corrosion and rusting of tooling material used in tablet manufacturing. *Drug Dev. Ind. Pharm.* 11:1487–1495.

Nyqvist, H. 1983. Saturated salt solutions for maintaining specified relative humidities. *Int. J. Pharm. Tech. & Prod. Mfr.* 4:47–48.

Paulson, B., ed. 1985. Polymorph changes important to FDA. *The Gold Sheet* 19:1–20.

Payne, R. S., R. J. Roberts, R. C. Rowe, and R. Docherty. 1999. Examples of successful crystal structure prediction: Polymorphs of primidone and progesterone. *Int. J. Pharm.* 177:231–245.

Pikal, M. J., J. E. Lang, and S. Shah. 1983. Desolvation kinetics of cefamandole sodium methanolate: Effect of water vapour. *Int. J. Pharm.* 17:237–262.

Pikal, M. J., A. L. Lukes, J. E. Lang, and K. Gaines. 1978. Quantitative crystallinity determinations for β-lactam antibiotics by solution calorimetry: Correlations with stability. *J. Pharm. Sci.* 67:767–772.

Pudipeddi, M., T. D. Sokoloski, S. P. Duddu, and J. T. Carstensen. 1996. Quantitative characterization of adsorption isotherms using isothermal microcalorimetry. *J. Pharm. Sci.* 85:381–386.

Quarterman, C. P., N. M. Banham, and A. K. Irwan. 1998. Improving the odds—high throughput techniques in new drug selection. *Eur. Pharm. Rev.* 3:27–31.

Rabel, S. R., J. A. Jona, and M. B. Maurin. 1999. Applications of modulated differential scanning calorimetry in preformulation studies. *J. Pharm. Biomed. Anal.* 21:339–345.

Roderiguez, C., and D. E. Bugey. 1997. Characterization of pharmaceutical solvates by combined thermogravimetric and infrared analysis. *J. Pharm. Sci.* 86:263–266.

Rosenberg, L. S., and D. M. Wagenknecht. 1986. pKa determination of sparingly soluble compounds by difference potentiometry. *Drug Dev. Ind. Pharm.* 12:1449–1467.

Roy, S. D., and G. L. Flynn. 1989. Solubility behaviour of narcotic analgesics in aqueous media: Solubilities and dissociation constants of morphine, fentanyl and sufentanil. *Pharm. Res.* 6:147–151.

Royall, P. G., D. Q. M. Craig, and C. Doherty. 1998. Characterization of the glass transition of an amorphous drug using modulated DSC. *Pharm. Res.* 15:1117–1130.

Rubino, J. T. 1989. Solubilities and solid state properties of the sodium salts of drugs. *J. Pharm. Sci.* 78:485–489.

Rubino, J. T., and E. Thomas. 1990. Influence of solvent composition on the solubilities and solid state properties of the sodium salts of some drugs. *Int. J. Pharm.* 65:141–145.

Saesmaa, T., and J. Halmekoski. 1987. Slightly water-soluble salts of β-lactam antibiotics. *Acta Pharm. Fenn.* 96:65–78.

Saesmaa, T., T. Makela, and V. P. Tannienen. 1990. Physical studies on the benzathine and embonate salts of some β-lactam antibiotics. Part 1. X-ray powder diffractometric study. *Acta Pharm. Fenn.* 99:157–162.

Serrajudin, A. T. M, and D. Mufson. 1985. pH-solubility profiles of organic bases and their hydrochloride salts. *Pharm. Res.* 2:65–68.

Shah, J. C., and M. Maniar. 1993. pH-dependent solubility and dissolution of bupivacaine and its relevance to the formulation of a controlled release system. *J. Controlled Rel.* 23:261–270.

Simmons, D. L., R. J. Ranz, N. D. Gyannchandani, and P. Picotte. 1972. Polymorphism in pharmaceuticals. II. Tolbutamide. *Can. J. Pharm. Sci.* 7:1436–1442.

Smith, A. 1986. Pharmaceutical and biological applications of thermal analysis studies in polymorphism and hydration. *Anal. Proc.* 23:388–389.

Stewart, P. J., and I. G. Tucker. 1985. Prediction of drug stability—Part 2: Hydrolysis. *Aust. J. Hosp. Pharm.* 15:11–16.

Stoltz, M., A. P. Lötter, and J. G. van der Watt. 1988. Physical characterization of two oxyphenbutazone pseudopolymorphs. *J. Pharm. Sci.* 77:1047–1049.

Subramaniam, B., R. A. Rajewski, and K. Snavely. 1997. Pharameutical processing with supercritical carbon dioxide. *J. Pharm. Sci.* 86:885–890.

Suleiman, M. S., and N. M. Najib. 1989. Isolation and physicochemical characterization of solid forms of glibenclamide. *Int. J. Pharm.* 50:103–109.

Takács-Novák, K., K. J. Box, and A. Avdeef. 1997. Potentiometric pKa determination of water-insoluble compounds: Validation study in methanol/water mixtures. *Int. J. Pharm.* 151:235–248.

Takla, P. G., and C. J. Dakas. 1989. Infrared study of tautomerism in acetohexamide polymorphs. *J. Pharm. Pharmacol.* 41:227–230.

Thomas, E., and J. Rubino. 1996. Solubility, melting point and salting-out relationships in a group of secondary amine hydrochloride salts. *Int. J. Pharm.* 130:179–185.

Threlfall, T. L. 1995. The analysis of organic polymorphs. *Analyst* 120:2435–2460.

Tong, W.-Q., and G. Whitesell. 1998. In situ salt screening—A useful technique for discovery support and preformulation studies. *Pharm. Dev. Tech.* 3:215–223.

Tønneson, H. H. 1991. Photochemical degradation of components in drug formulations. Part 1: An approach to the standardization of degradation studies. *Pharmazie* 46:263–265.

Torniainen, K., and S. Tammilehto, and V. Ulvi. 1996. The effect of pH, buffer type and drug concentration on the photodegradation of ciprofloxacin. *Int. J. Pharm.* 132:53–61.

Umprayn, K., and R. W. Mendes. 1987. Hygroscopicity and moisture adsorption kinetics of pharmaceutical solids: A review. *Drug Dev. Ind. Pharm.* 13:653–693.

Van Dooren, A. A. 1982. Effects of heating rates and particle sizes on DSC peaks. *Anal. Proc.* 554–555.

Van de Waterbeemd, H., and R. Mannhold. 1996. Programs and methods for calculation of log P values. *Quant. Struct.-Act. Relat.* 15:410–412.

Verwer, P., and F. J. J. Leusen. 1998. Computer simulation to predict possible crystal polymorphs. *Rev. Comput. Chem.* 12:327–365.

Vitez, I. M., A. C. Newman, M. Davidovich, and C. Kiesnowski. 1998. The evolution of hot-stage microscopy to aid solid-state characterizations of pharmaceutical solids *Thermochim. Acta* 324:187–196.

Walkling, W. D., B. E. Reynolds, B. J. Fegely, and C. A. Janicki. 1983. Xilobam: Effect of salt form on pharmaceutical properties. *Drug Dev. Ind. Pharm.* 9:809–819.

Wadsten, T., L. Simon, and G. S. Talpas. 1990. Crystal habit as the basis of the change in bioactivity of pentetrazole. *Pharmazie* 45:66–67.

Watanabe, A., Y. Yamaoka, and K. Kuroda. 1980. Study of crystalline drugs by means of polarizing microscope. III. Key refractive indices of some crystalline drugs and their measurement using an improved immersion method. *Chem. Pharm. Bull.* 28:372–378.

Watanabe, A., Y. Yamaoka, and K. Takada. 1982. Crystal habits and dissolution behaviours of aspirin. *Chem. Pharm. Bull.* 30:2958–2963.

Wells, J. I. 1988. *Pharmaceutical preformulation. The physicochemical properties of drug substances.* Chichester, UK: Ellis Horwood Ltd. p. 219.

Willson, R. J., A. E. Beezer, and J. C. Mitchell. 1996. Determination of thermodynamic and kinetic parameters from isothermal heat conduction microcalorimetry: Applications to long term reaction studies. *J. Phys. Chem.* 99:7108–7113.

Wu, L.-E., C. Gerard, and M. A. Hussain. 1993. Thermal analysis and solution calorimetry studies on losartan polymorphs. *Pharm. Res.* 10:1793–1795.

Yalkowsky, S. H., and S. Banerjee. 1992. *Aqueous solubility. Methods for estimation for organic compounds.* New York: Marcel Dekker Inc.

Yoshioka, S., and J. L. Cartensen. 1990. Nonlinear estimation of kinetic parameters for solid-state hydrolysis of water-soluble drugs. Part 2. Rational presentation mode below the critical moisture content. *J. Pharm. Sci.* 79:799–801.

Zimmerman, I. 1986a. Determination of pK$_a$ values from solubility data. *Int. J. Pharm.* 13:57–65.

Zimmerman, I. 1986b. Determination of overlapping pK$_a$ values from solubility data. *Int. J. Pharm.* 31:69–74.

4

Biopharmaceutical Support in Candidate Drug Selection

Anna-Lena Ungell
Bertil Abrahamsson

AstraZeneca
Mölndal, Sweden

Adminstration via the oral route has been, and still is, the most popular and convenient route for patient therapeutics. However, even though it is the most convenient route, it is not the simplest route, as the barriers of the gastro-intestinal (GI) tract are in many cases difficult to circumvent. The main barriers of the GI tract to systemic delivery are the environment in the stomach and intestinal lumen, the presence of different enzymes, the physical barrier of the epithelium and the liver extraction. These barriers are of functional importance for the organism in controlling intake of water, electrolytes and food constituents and still remain a complete barrier to harmful organisms such as bacteria, viruses and toxic compounds.

Generally, drug absorption from the GI tract requires that the drug is brought into solution in the GI fluids and that it is capable of crossing the intestinal membrane into the systemic circulation. It has therefore been suggested that the drug must be in its molecular form before it can be absorbed. Therefore, the rate of dissolution of the drug in the GI lumen can be a rate-limiting step in the absorption of drugs given orally. Particles of drugs, e.g., insoluble crystalline forms or specific delivery systems such as liposomes, are generally found to be absorbed to a very small extent. The cascade of events from release of the drug from its dosage form, i.e. *dissolution* of the drug in the gut lumen, *interactions* and/or degradation within the lumen and the *uptake* of its molecular form across the intestinal membrane into the systemic circulation, is schematically shown in Figure 4.1. For rapid and effective design and development of new drug products, methods for drug absorption are required that describe the different steps involved before and during the absorption process. The need for such specific

Figure 4.1 Drawing showing the different steps in the absorption process including the dissolution of the compound from the solid dosage form, interactions with the dissolved material in the gastro-intestinal lumen and the uptake of the compound through the epithelial membrane.

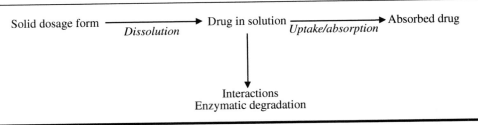

methods is determined by the information on the rate-limiting step in the cascade of events (e.g., solubility, permeability or metabolic instability limited). The results from these methods act as a guide to a more efficient discovery process in which resources are given to optimising structures that lead to the selection of a good drug candidate with well-defined pharmacokinetic and physicochemical properties. A method now available is multivariate analysis for analysing large data sets. Screening and optimisation of several parameters in parallel, e.g., permeability, metabolic stability, solubility, potency, duration and toxicity, represent a growing area for rationalising drug discovery using multivariate statistical models (Eriksson et al. 1999). The importance of this is obvious: There is no point in using resources to increase the potency of an oral drug candidate if the drug is not predicted to be orally bioavailable. The consideration of biopharmaceutical properties in the selection of candidate drugs has also been shown in a recent survey, based on statistics published by the Pharmaceutical and Research Manufacturers of America (PhRMA), to be the most common reason for terminating drug development projects in the clinical phase.

The dissolution rate and/or the aqueous solubility of the drug will also affect the outcome of studies using biological methods, in very early phases of screening. If not dissolved in the test system, low solubility drugs will not appear on the receiver side/blood side of a membrane or will show incomplete absorption *in vivo*. Consequently, the drug will be considered a low permeability drug and be discarded as being of no potential use as a systemically active drug. The situation is even more complex, since there are also mechanistic membrane processes that can give the same result. Such processes include drug efflux systems that transport the drug from inside the epithelial cell to the lumen of the intestine [e.g., efflux proteins (Hunter and Hirst 1997)] or metabolism during transport and adhesion to plastics in the test system (Table 4.1). The evaluation of the reason for low transport is therefore crucial for the design of proper screening procedures.

In the drug discovery process, the selection of a suitable candidate drug is the milestone for continuing into a costly development and clinical phase. Some *optimal absorption criteria* from a biopharmaceutical point of view are shown below:

- High permeability coefficient (determined using in vitro assays such as Caco-2 cell monolayers, Ussing chambers, intestinal perfusions, etc.; see below) throughout the GI tract [Extended Release (ER) formulation]

Table 4.1
Suggested reasons for low permeability values
during transport studies with *in vitro* models.

Adhesions to plastics

Low solubility

Complexation with ions in the buffer

Metabolism in the lumen or in the intestinal segment

Low activity/viability of the tissue (active transport)

Analytical problems (analytical response limited)

Large UWL (unstirred water layer) or mucus layer (unstirred models)

True low permeability

- Passive diffusion–directed transport or known mechanism for carrier-mediated transport or interaction

- High solubility in aqueous media and over a wide pH range (e.g., pH 1–7).

- No degradation/metabolism in intestinal luminal fluids, intestinal homogenates and/or microsomal preparations from the intestine and liver (i.e., low first-pass metabolism)

- Complete absorption in the GI tract in vivo in several animal species

These criteria are usually difficult to achieve, and the relationship between the *in vitro effect of the drug* (potency/concentration needed), *therapeutic effect and index* (acceptable variation in plasma concentration from safety and efficacy point of view) and the *rate and extent of absorption* must therefore be evaluated carefully for each project and drug. Furthermore, the physicochemical characteristics (e.g., the ability of the drug to be formulated into a relevant delivery system) of the drug as determined in preformulation studies also guide the selection of a potential drug candidate.

The biopharmaceutical information gathered in the candidate drug selection process regarding the characteristics of the drug molecule (e.g., dissolution, solubility, stability in fluids at the site of administration, enzymatic stability, membrane transport and bioavailability) is also very useful as input to the subsequent formulation development. This information is important, for example,

- to determine suitable formulation types and technologies,

- to set biopharmaceutical targets for formulation development,

- to define initial biopharmaceutical test methods and studies needed to reach the targets and

- as background data for interpretation of different studies used in the development of a formulation.

Thus, a well-performed drug substance characterisation minimises the risk of a suboptimal final formulation as a result of neglecting important biopharmaceutical prerequisites for a certain drug substance. Furthermore, such information also allows an efficient development process based on science, while trial and error approaches are avoided.

The ideal model for the biopharmaceutical assessment of drug transport, metabolism and dissolution should have certain characteristics, i.e., should represent the main physiological or physicochemical barrier as relevantly as possible to the human *in vivo* situation. No single method can represent all barriers and at the same time give information about the mechanisms underlying the absorption process. Furthermore, no single method can provide all the information needed, from the synthesis of a series of compounds in the screening phase (discovery) to the development of the specific formulation intended for human use. Many different methods have been developed over the last 20 years for use in different phases of drug discovery and development. This chapter will deal with some of these techniques to gain a basic knowledge of drug absorption. Also, it will give a description of related methods, and the functional use of the information provided by these methods, to aid in the selection of a candidate drug and the development of formulations intended for use in humans.

DRUG DISSOLUTION AND SOLUBILITY

Drug dissolution is a prerequisite for oral absorption. Thus, a drug that is not fully dissolved cannot be completely absorbed through the GI epithelium. It is thus extremely important to understand drug dissolution and solubility in aqueous media, both in early drug discovery studies and as a prerequisite for the subsequent formulation development. More specifically, drug dissolution/solubility data give important information that provides answers to the following biopharmaceutical questions during the discovery phase:

- Will the drug absorption be limited by the drug dissolution/solubility?

- Will the drug dissolution/solubility limit the bioavailability to an extent that endangers the clinical usefulness of the drug?

- Which types of vehicles are needed in preclinical studies to provide the desired drug exposure?

- Should the substance form be changed to improve dissolution (e.g., salt, polymorph, particle size)?

After the choice of a candidate drug, solubility and dissolution data are used for guidance in the following:

- Should dissolution rate-enhancing principles be applied in the formulation development (e.g., wetting agents, micronisation, solubilising agents, solid solutions, emulsions and nanoparticles)?

- In the case of modified release formulations, which formulation principles are suitable and which release mechanisms can be expected?

- Which test conditions should be used for *in vitro* dissolution testing of solid formulations?

It should be emphasised that *dissolution* is the dynamic process by which a material is dissolved in a solvent and is characterised by a rate (amount dissolved per time unit), while *solubility* is the amount of material dissolved per volume unit of a certain solvent. Solubility is often used as a short form for "saturation solubility", which is the maximum amount of drug that can be dissolved at equilibrium conditions. Finally, the term *intrinsic solubility* is sometimes used as well, which is the solubility of the neutral form of a proteolytic drug.

Theoretically, the dissolution rate is most often described by the Noyes-Whitney equation (equation 1):

$$\frac{dm}{dt} = \left(\frac{D \times A}{h}\right) \times (Cs - Ct) \tag{1}$$

where D is the diffusion coefficient of the drug substance in a stagnant water layer around each drug particle with a thickness h, A is the drug particle surface area, Cs is the saturation solubility and Ct is the drug concentration in the bulk solution. If the drug concentration in the bulk (Ct) in equation 1 is negligible as compared to the saturation solubility (Cs), the dissolution rate is not affected by Ct. This state is denoted a "sink condition" and is often assumed to be the case *in vivo*, owing to the continuous removal of a drug from the intestine due to the absorption over the intestinal wall. A, Ct and h in equation 1 will be time dependent, whereas the other variables are constants at a certain test condition. The surface area (A) of a dissolving particle will be constantly reduced by time (provided that no precipitation occurs); the thickness of the diffusion layer (h) is dependent on the radius of the particle size; and the bulk solution will increase toward its maximum when the total amount has been dissolved. In addition, no solid drug powder is monodisperse, i.e., the starting material will consist of a dispersion of different particle sizes with different surface areas (A). Extensions of equation 1 have therefore been derived that take into account some or all of these factors. A full review of such equations and underlying assumptions, and a presentation of some other less used theories for dissolution, can be found elsewhere (Abdou 1989). A modification of equation 1 was recently presented that takes into account all time-dependent factors that can be useful for predictions of the dissolution rate (Hintz and Johnson 1989).

Basic theoretic considerations and experimental methods regarding solubility are reviewed in more detail in Chapter 3.

The present chapter focuses on aspects of drug solubility/dissolution of specific relevance for biopharmaceutical support in candidate drug selection and preformulation. These aspects include solubility in candidate drug screening, physiological aspects of test media, solubility of amphiphilic drugs and substance characterisation prior to solubility/dissolution tests.

Aspects of Solubility in Candidate Drug Screening

Although drug solubility is an important factor in drug absorption in the GI tract, it has not been extensively screened for as a barrier to absorption. Drug solubility should, however, be complementary to models predicting drug permeability through the lipid membrane. Solubility as a high-throughput screening (HTS) parameter has therefore been discussed rather intensively. The importance of solubility as a selective tool during early screening of hundreds of compounds, to choose a drug with a potential to be absorbed *in vivo* in humans, has not been fully evaluated, however. Several drugs that are very useful in the clinical situation have very low water solubility. For example, candesartan cilexetil, an effective and well-tolerated antihypertensive drug, has a water solubility of about 0.1 μg/mL. On the other hand, more soluble drugs will minimise the risk of failure during the subsequent development phase and may avoid delays, increased costs or discontinuation of the project.

Another aspect of solubility is seen during screening for good pharmacokinetic properties of candidate drugs. The HTS systems or *in vitro* assays are the critical point for most drugs insoluble in water. This means that if the drug is not soluble in the buffer solution used in the *in vitro* system, it cannot be properly experimentally evaluated. The most common negative effect of this is that the concentration needed to induce transport across the epithelial membrane in the *in vitro* model is too low to be detected on the receiver side (see Table 4.1). For this reason, vehicles known to increase the solubility of sparingly soluble compounds are used (see section "Vehicles for Absorption Studies"). However, since these vehicles are based on surfactant systems, toxic effects may be seen on the membrane (Oberle et al. 1995), and the permeability values obtained may be overestimated. New methods are now available for screening large numbers of compounds in small volumes (e.g., the Nephelometer [BMG labtechnologies GmbH]). This method is based on turbidimetric determinations and is therefore not an exact tool. It can, however, contribute substantially as a first estimate of solubility of sparingly soluble compounds and make it possible to understand the results of the screening methods and to design specific experiments using vehicles.

Determinations of Drug Dissolution Rate

The dissolution rate, rather than the saturation solubility, is most often the primary determinant in the absorption process of a sparingly soluble drug. Experimental determinations of the dissolution rate are therefore of great importance. The main area for dissolution rate studies is evaluation of different solid forms of a drug (e.g., salts, solvates, polymorphs, amorphous, stereoisomers) or effects of particle size. The dissolution rate can either be determined for a constant surface area of the drug in a rotating disc apparatus or as a dispersed powder in a beaker with agitation.

The *rotating disc method* is in most cases the technique of choice for determining the drug dissolution rate of drug substances. Compressed discs of the pure drug without any excipients are placed in a holder (see Figure 4.2a, b). The disc is immersed in a dissolution medium and rotated at a high speed (e.g., 300–1000 rpm). The disc may be centrally or excentrally mounted to the stirring rod. The dissolution process is preferably monitored by on-line measurements of the dissolved drug. A more detailed description of the application of the rotating disc method in a preformulation programme can be found elsewhere (Niklasson et al. 1985).

The dissolution rate is determined by linear regression from the slope of the initial linear part of the dissolution time curve. It is often expressed as amount of drug dissolved per time and surface area unit (G), e.g., mg/cm^2·s, by dividing the rate by the surface area of the disc. This dissolution rate is specific for the rotational speed (ω) of the disc and is linearly related to the square root of the rotational speed of the disc according to hydrodynamic theories that have been experimentally verified (Levich 1962). Thus, if experiments are performed at several rotational speeds, and the dissolution rate at each speed is plotted versus the square root of the rotational speed, a linear relationship should be obtained. It should be noted that this determination of dissolution rate is still dependent on other experimental hydrodynamic conditions, such as positioning of the disc, shape of the vessel and viscosity. An equation has therefore been derived that allows for determination of an "intrinsic dissolution rate" (k_1) that is independent of the drug diffusion in the boundary layer (Niklasson and Magnusson 1985);

$$\frac{1}{G} = \frac{1}{k_1} + \frac{k'}{R \times \omega^{0.5}} \tag{2}$$

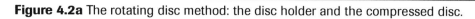

Figure 4.2a The rotating disc method: the disc holder and the compressed disc.

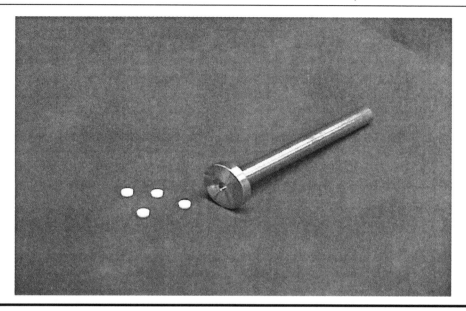

Figure 4.2b The rotating disc method: experimental set-up for the rotating disc.

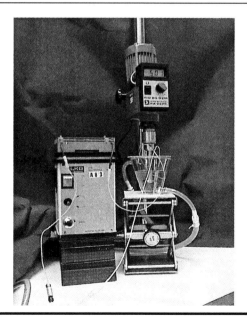

where k' is a proportionality constant. The rotating disc must be mounted eccentrically at a certain distance (R) from the center of the stirring rod to perform this evaluation. A plot is made between $1/G$ and $1/(R \times \omega^{0.5})$ at different agitation rates, which should yield a straight line. The reciprocal of the "intrinsic dissolution rate" ($1/k_1$) is determined by extrapolating the line to the y axis. If G is determined at different speeds, and laminar flow along the disc can be assumed, other theoretical evaluations can be made of the data, such as determination of the diffusion coefficient of the drug in the boundary layer around the solid particles and the thickness of the diffusion boundary layer (Levich 1962).

The main merits of the rotating disc apparatus are the well-defined hydrodynamic conditions and constant surface area. These reduce the risk of artefacts in dissolution rate determinations caused by non-ideal test conditions. Furthermore, it is possible to determine an intrinsic dissolution rate and to perform other mechanistic evaluations of the dissolution process. The main limitation of the method is that it is not suitable for drugs that form fragile or porous discs, since it is not possible to maintain a constant surface area.

The drug dissolution rate of powder may be determined by methods such as in a beaker with appropriate agitation, as described in the pharmacopoeial methods. The dissolution rate determined by such approaches will be method dependent, and it will not be possible to derive an intrinsic value of the dissolution rate. The main reason for using this type of experimental approach can be understood when the effect of the drug particle size must be considered. Experimental errors and uncontrollable variations may occur for hydrophobic drugs due to agglomeration in the test medium or due to floating. The use of a wetting agent in the test medium (such as a surfactant in concentrations well below the critical micelle concentration [CMC]), may be needed to avoid such undesired effects.

Biopharmaceutical Interpretation of Dissolution/Solubility Data

It is desirable to predict the influence of drug dissolution on oral absorption based on measurements of dissolution or solubility, both before the selection of a candidate drug, in order to obtain a drug molecule with acceptable properties, and in the preformulation phase, to determine the need for solubility-enhancing formulation principles. The primary variable for judgements of *in vivo* absorption is the dissolution rate rather than the solubility. Drug dissolution will limit the bioavailability when the dissolution rate is too slow to provide complete dissolution in the part of the intestine where it can be absorbed. In addition, the drug concentration in the intestinal fluids will be far below the saturation solubility, under the assumption that "sink conditions" in the GI tract will be obtained due to absorption of the drug. However, most often, solubility data are more readily available than dissolution rates for a drug candidate, especially in early phases when the amount of drug available does not allow for accurate dissolution rate determinations. Predictions of *in vivo* effects on absorption caused by poor dissolution must thus often be made on the basis of solubility data rather than dissolution rate. This can theoretically be justified by the direct proportionality between dissolution rate and solubility under "sink conditions" according to equation 1. A list of proposed criteria to be used to avoid a reduction in absorption caused by poor dissolution is given in Table 4.2. These criteria are discussed in further detail in this chapter. A solubility in water of ≥ 10 mg/mL in pH range 1–7 has been proposed as an acceptable limit to avoid absorption problems, while another suggestion is that drugs with water solubilities <0.1 mg/mL often lead to dissolution limitations to absorption (Kaplan 1972; Hörter and Dressman 1997). It should be noted that these limits may be conservative, especially in the context of screening and selection for candidate drugs. For example, a drug with much lower solubility, such as

Table 4.2
Proposed limits of drug dissolution on solubility to avoid absorption problems.

Factor	Limit	Reference
Solubility in pH 1–7	>10 mg/mL at all pH	Kaplan (1972)
Solubility in pH 1–8 and dose	Complete dose dissolved in 250 mL at all pH	Amidon et al. (1995)
Water solubility	>0.1 mg/mL	Hörter and Dressman (1997)
Dissolution rate in pH 1–7	>1 mg/min/cm^2 (0.1–1 mg/nm/cm^2 borderline) at all pH	Kaplan (1972)

felodipine (0.001 mg/mL), provides complete absorption when administered in an appropriate solid dosage form (Wingstrand et al. 1990). This may be explained both by successful application of dissolution-enhancing formulation principles and by more favourable drug solubility *in vivo* owing to the presence of solubilising agents such as bile acids.

Another model for biopharmaceutical interpretation based on solubility data is found in the biopharmaceutical classification system (BCS) (Amidon et al. 1995). Four different classes of drugs have been identified, based on drug solubility and permeability as outlined in Table 4.3. If the administered dose is completely dissolved in the fluids in the stomach, which is assumed to be 250 mL (50 mL basal level in stomach plus administration of the solid dose with 200 mL of water), the drug is classified as a "high solubility drug". Such good solubility should be obtained within a range of pH 1–8 to cover all possible conditions in a patient and exclude the risk of precipitation in the small intestine due to the generally higher pH there than in the stomach. Drug absorption is expected to be independent of drug dissolution for drugs that fulfil this requirement, since the total amount of the drug will be in solution before entering the major absorptive area in the small intestine, and the rate of absorption will be determined by the gastric emptying of fluids. Thus, this model also provides a very conservative approach for judgements of dissolution-limited absorption. However, "highly soluble drugs" are advantageous in pharmaceutical development since no dissolution-enhancing principles are

Table 4.3
Biopharmaceutical classification system.

Class	Solubility	Permeability
I	High	High
II	Low	High
III	High	Low
IV	Low	Low

needed, and process parameters that could affect drug particle form and size are generally not critical formulation factors. Furthermore, if certain other criteria are met, in addition to favourable solubility, regulatory advantages can be gained. Bioequivalence studies for bridging between different versions of clinical trial material and/or of a marketed product can be replaced by much more rapid and cheaper *in vitro* dissolution testing (*Guidance for Industry*, FDA 1999; *Note for Guidance on Investigation*, EMEA 1998).

The assumption of "sink condition" *in vivo* is valid in most cases when the permeability of the drug over the intestinal wall is fast, which is a common characteristic of lipophilic, poorly soluble compounds. However, if such a drug is given at a high dose in relation to the solubility, Ct (see equation 1) may become significant even if the permeation rate through the gut wall is high. If the drug concentration is close to Cs (see equation 1) in the intestine, the primary substance-related determinants for absorption are the administered dose and Cs rather than the dissolution rate. It is important to identify such a situation, since it can be expected that the dissolution rate-enhancing formulation principle will not provide any benefits and that higher doses will provide only a small increase in the amount of absorbed drug. As a rough estimate for a high permeability drug, it has been proposed that this situation can occur when the relationship between the dose (mg) and the solubility (mg/mL) exceeds a factor of 5,000 if a dissolution volume of 250 mL is assumed (Amidon 1996). For example, if the solubility is 0.01 mg/mL, this situation will be approached if doses of about 50 mg or more are administered. It should, however, be realised that this diagnostic tool is based on theoretical simulations rather than *in vivo* data. For example, physiological factors that might affect the saturation solubility are neglected (described in more detail below).

In order to predict the fraction absorbed (F_a) in a more quantitative manner, factors other than dissolution, solubility or dose must be taken into account, such as regional permeability, degradation in the GI lumen and transit times. Several algorithms with varying degrees of sophistication have been developed that integrate the dissolution or solubility with other factors. A more detailed description is beyond the scope of this chapter, but a comprehensive review has been published by Yu et al. (1996). Computer programmes based on such algorithms are also commercially available and permit simulations to identify whether the absorption is limited by dissolution or solubility (Gastroplus™, Simulations Plus Inc, Lancaster, Calif., USA). As an example, Figure 4.3 shows simulations performed to investigate the dependence of dose, solubility and particle radius on the F_a for an aprotic, high-permeability drug.

Physiological Aspects of Dissolution and Solubility Test Conditions

The dissolution of a drug in the gut lumen will depend on luminal conditions, e.g., pH of the luminal fluid, volume available, lipids and bile acids and the hydrodynamic conditions produced from the GI peristaltic movements of the luminal content toward the lower bowel. Such physiological factors influence drug dissolution by controlling the different variables in equation 1 that describe the dissolution rate. This is summarised in Table 4.4 adapted from Dressman et al. (1998).

The test media used for determining solubility and dissolution should therefore ideally reflect the *in vivo* situation. The most relevant factors to be considered from an *in vivo* perspective are

- pH (for proteolytic drugs),
- ionic strength and composition,

Figure 4.3 Simulations of fraction of drug absorbed after oral administration for a high-permeability drug ($P_{eff} = 4.5 \times 10^{-4}$ cm/s) for doses 1–100 mg, water solubilities 0.1–10 g/mL and radius of drug particles 0.6–60 μm. During variations of one variable, the others are held constant at the midpoint level (dose 10 mg, solubility 1 μg/mL and particle radius 6 μm).

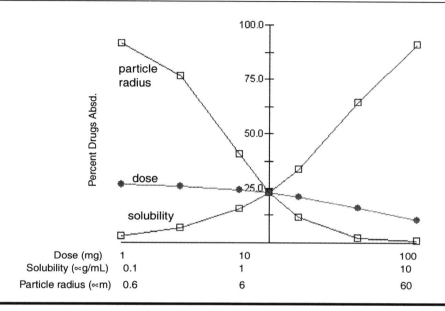

Dose (mg)	1	10	100
Solubility ($\propto$g/mL)	0.1	1	10
Particle radius ($\propto$m)	0.6	6	60

Table 4.4
Physicochemical and physiological parameters important to drug dissolution in the gastro-intestinal tract.

Factor	Physicochemical Parameter	Physiological Parameter
Surface area of drug (A)	Particle size, wettability	Surfactants in gastric juice and bile
Diffusivity of drug (D)	Molecular size	Viscosity of lumenal contents
Boundary layer thickness (h)		Motility patterns and flow rate
Solubility (Cs)	Hydrophilicity, crystal structure, solubilisation	pH, buffer capacity, bile, food components
Amount of drug already dissolved (Ct)		Permeability
Volume of solvent available (Ct)		Secretions, co-administered fluids

Pharmaceutical Research, vol. 15, 1998, pages 11–22, Dissolution testing as a prognostic tool for oral drug absorption: Immediate release dosage forms, J. B. Dressman et al., Table 2, with kind permission from Kluwer Academic Publishers.

- surface active agents and

- temperature.

The pH varies in the GI tract from 1 to 8 (see Table 4.5), and so the dissolution properties should therefore be known over this pH range for orally administered drugs. A more thorough review of intestinal pH conditions can be found elsewhere (Charman et al. 1997).

It may be argued that, for immediate release formulations intended to quickly dissolve in the stomach, only the more acidic pH levels are of relevance. However, dissolution may occur at higher pH levels for several reasons, e.g., concomitant food intake, co-medication, diseases or instant tablet emptying to the small intestine. In addition, since drug absorption over the gastric wall is negligible, the drug will always enter the more neutral conditions in the intestine.

Dissolution studies at pH 1 are generally performed in HCl, which is also present in the stomach. However, to perform studies over the entire pH interval, different buffers are needed to control the pH. In the intestine, pH is controlled by bicarbonate, which is not practical to use *in vitro* because of the need for continuous bubbling with CO_2. Non-physiologic buffer systems, such as phosphates, acetates or citrates, are therefore often used. It is important to note that the solubility may vary for different buffers at the same pH, due to different "salting in" and "salting out" effects or differences in solubility products (see Chapter 3) when the drug and buffer component are of opposite charge. If such effects occur, the solubility parameters will also be dependent on the concentration of the buffer system, and the influence of the buffer will increase at higher concentrations. Excessive buffer concentrations beyond what is needed to control the pH should therefore be avoided.

The dominant ions in the GI tract are sodium, chloride and bicarbonate (see Table 4.5), and their concentrations vary between luminal sites along the GI tract (Lindahl et al. 1997). The total concentration of these ions, expressed as ionic strength, has been determined to be 0.10–0.16 and 0.12–0.19 in the stomach and small intestine, respectively. The presence of such ions may affect solubility, especially by the common ion effect (see Chapter 3).

The presence of physiological surface-active agents in the stomach and small intestine will influence the solubility and the dissolution of sparingly soluble drugs by improved wetting of solid particle surface areas and by micellar solubilisation. This has been reviewed in more detail by Gibaldi and Feldman (1970) and Charman et al. (1997).

Table 4.5

The pH and concentration of most dominant ions in different parts of the GI tract in humans (based on Lindahl et al. 1997; Charman 1997).

	pH		Ionic Concentrations (nM)		
	Fasting	Fed	Na+	HCO−3	Cl−
Stomach	1–2	2–5[1]	70	<20	100
Upper small intestine	5.5–6.5		140	50–110	130
Lower small intestine	6.5–8				
Colon	5.5–7				

[1]Dependent on volume, pH and buffer capacity of the food.

The main endogenous surfactants are the bile acids, which are excreted into the upper jejunum by the bile flow. The bile acids—cholic acid, chenodeoxycholic acid and deoxycholic acid—are present as conjugates with glycine and taurine as the sodium salts. The total concentrations of bile acids in the upper small intestinal transit are 4–6 mM in the fasting state and 10–40 mM after ingestion of a meal. The bile acids are reabsorbed in the terminal small intestine by active uptake. During normal physiological conditions, micelle formation and solubilisation may already occur at the lower bile acid concentrations in the fasting state. The micelles formed not only contain bile acids but are a mixture with endogenous phospholipids excreted by the bile (lecithin) and products from the digestion of dietary fat, such as monoglycerides. The saturation solubility of a sparingly soluble drug has, in some cases, been increased by several orders of magnitude by the addition of physiological amounts of lecithin to a bile salt solution, whereas no solubility improvements are obtained by the formation of mixed micelles for others. It should also be noted that, while the solubility of a very sparingly water-soluble drug is increased by the formation of a mixed micelle, the rate of dissolution might be decreased. This is exemplified in Figure 4.4a and b showing the saturation solubility and the dissolution rate at different concentrations of lecithin in a bile acid solution for a compound that has a water solubility of <1 μg/mL.

Bile acids not only affect the solubility by solubilisation of sparingly soluble compounds, they may also decrease the solubility by forming sparingly soluble salts or complexes with drugs. Indications of such phenomena have been shown for a variety of drugs such as pafenolol, tubocurarine, neomycine, kanamycine, nadolol, atenolol and propranolol (Yamaguchi et al. 1986a,b,c; Grosvenor and Löfroth 1995).

Solubility or dissolution studies in the presence of physiological surfactants may provide important information with respect to the *in vivo* absorption process of sparingly soluble compounds, although it is hardly possible to reconstitute the full complexity and dynamics

Figure 4.4a The solubility of a poorly soluble compound (water solubility <1 μg/mL) at different concentrations of sodium taurocholate (NaTC) mixed with lecithin in two different ratios, 2.5:1 and 50:1.

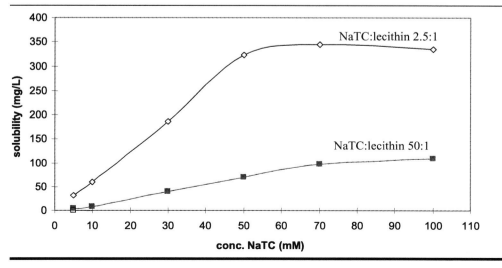

Figure 4.4b The dissolution rate of a poorly soluble compound (water solubility <1 μg/mL) versus the saturation solubility obtained by testing in different concentrations of NaTC mixed with lecithin at two different ratios, 2.5:1 and 50:1.

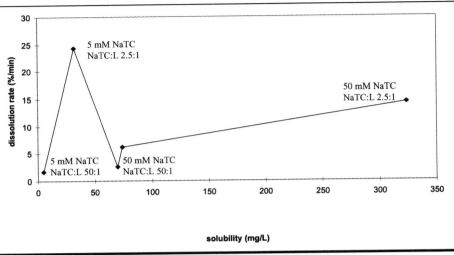

of the *in vivo* situation in an *in vitro* model. While bile acids and lecithin are available in purified forms, their use is somewhat limited by their high price. Much less well-defined ox bile preparations are also available, which contain a mixture of conjugated bile acids and other bile components.

The temperature in dissolution and solubility tests should preferably be identical to the *in vivo* temperature at the site of administration, since the solubility is dependent on the temperature. The most suitable temperature depends on the intended administration route. For oral administration, testing at 37°C is the obvious choice.

Special Considerations for Surface-Active Drugs

Many drugs consist of both hydrophobic and hydrophilic structural groups, since these are often needed to optimise oral absorption. It is therefore not surprising that surface-active properties have been identified for a large number of drugs. Such drugs may provide unexpected dissolution and solubility properties, owing to the formation of micelles or other forms of self-aggregation. This is exemplified in Figure 4.5 which shows the solubility of an amphiphilic drug at different temperatures in a phosphate buffer solution. The saturation solubility is drastically increased at about 37°C due to the formation of micelles. The temperature at which micelles are formed in a certain test medium is called the critical micelle temperature (CMT).

If the drug substance is suspected to be surface active, which will be indicated by the molecular structure, the surface-active properties should be further investigated during the biopharmaceutical preformulation phase. The potential for micelle formation should be investigated and, if relevant, the CMC and the CMT should be determined. CMC is determined by measuring a colligative property such as conductivity, surface tension or osmotic pressure

Figure 4.5 Solubility of an amphilic drug at different temperatures in a phosphate buffer, illustrating the effect on solubility at the micelle formation at the critical micelle temperature (CMT).

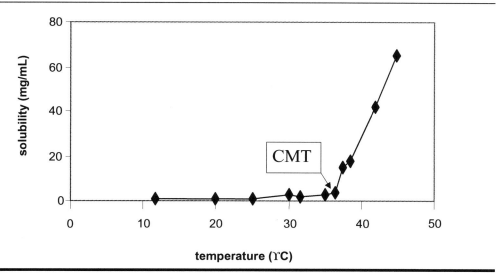

in water solutions of the drug in different concentrations. Typically, for all methods, an increase or decrease is seen in the measured variable at increasing drug concentrations, which is followed by a plateau level. The inflection point between the two phases is the CMC. It should be noted that CMC and CMT are dependent on the composition of the test medium. For example, salts, buffers and the presence of other amphiphilic compounds affect the micelle formation and thereby the solubility of an amphiphilic compound.

Substance Characterisation Prior to Biopharmaceutical Solubility/Dissolution Tests

Several substance properties can affect dissolution and/or solubility, such as purity; particle size and distribution; surface area; and the presence of polymorphs, hydrates or other solvates or amorphous forms. To avoid misleading or inconclusive results in extensive solubility or dissolution studies, it is important to characterise the drug substance form with respect to such properties, especially in the later biopharmaceutical preformulation phase. Methods for such characterisation are described in more detail in Chapters 3 and 7.

LUMINAL INTERACTIONS

The rate and extent of drug absorption can be affected by degradation, metabolism and complex binding in the GI lumen. There is a general change in the composition of the luminal fluid along the GI tract (Hörter and Dressman 1997; Dressman and Yamada 1991). The differences are mainly in the concentration and nature of ions, bile, proteins, osmolality, surface tension and lipids. The interaction of a drug with the luminal content can induce precipitation of the drug with ions to form insoluble salts (Dakas and Takla 1991; Hörter and Dressman 1997), or binding to enzymes or proteins (Sjöström et al. 1999), or simply a partition of the drug into luminal compartments (micelles, cell debris). This will result in a reduction of the effective concentration of the drug at the absorption site and will thus lower the flux of the drug across the membrane. For instance, pH in lumen changes along the GI tract and is different before and after a meal (Table 4.5), starting at pH 1–2 during fasting conditions in the stomach, rising to 5–6.5 in the duodenum and going slowly up to 7–8 in the ileum region. It then decreases to 6–7 in the proximal colon and approaches 7–8 in the rectum. This luminal pH is especially important for the release of the drug from the dosage form or the dissolution in the luminal media. The predicted absorption, based on pH partition hypothesis, of some ionisable drugs was originally based on this luminal pH, and actual values of absorption obtained from *in vivo* animal studies differed markedly. The reason for this pH shift has been explained in different ways over the years but has been accepted to be caused by an acidic "microclimate region" adjacent to the mucosal membrane (McEwan and Lucas 1990). The pH during the actual transport of a drug through the epithelial membrane in the intestinal mucosa is therefore approximately one pH unit lower. This microclimate pH favours absorption of weak acids and weak bases (Figure 4.6). This means that, for an ionisable drug, the luminal pH is the most important pH for the release of the drug from the dosage form and for dissolution/solubility. However, the pH at the surface of the membrane (i.e., microclimate) will determine the rate of absorption of this drug through the membrane. Both of these pH values vary along the GI tract.

Figure 4.6 Surface pH hypothesis for weak acids and bases. A model for the influence of the microclimate pH in rat proximal jejunum on weak electrolyte permeation. The weak acid A^- is converted to neutral by the presence of H^+ in the microclimate. The undissociated form can easily be absorbed through the mucosa. In contrast, the weak base B is protonated by the H^+ to BH^+ which is less absorbed through the membrane.

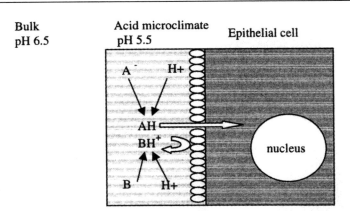

From G. T. A. McEwan and M. L. Lucas (1990), The effect of *E. coli* Sta enteroxine on the absorption of weakly dissociable drugs from the rat proximal jejunum in vivo, *Br. J. Pharmacol,* vol. 101: pp. 937–943.

A common phenomenon for drugs is decomposition at acidic pH. The drug stability should therefore be investigated along the entire physiological range (pH 1–8) if such degradation can be expected. Typically, the percentage of drug that remains is determined at different times, and a first-order rate constant or half-life is determined for the degradation process. This is exemplified in Figure 4.7 for omeprazole in a range of different pH values (Pilbrant and Cederberg 1985).

Complexation

Complexation of drugs in the GI tract can occur with the luminal content. Any non-metallic atom, whether free or contained in a neutral molecule, or an ionic compound that can donate an electron pair, may serve as a donor. The acceptor is frequently a metal ion. In general, complexes can be divided into two classes, depending on whether the acceptor component is a metal ion or an organic molecule (Dakas and Takla 1991, Hörter and Dressman 1997). Complex formation with components of food, such as milk, can give precipitation of the drug compound and reduce the bioavailability and fraction of the dose absorbed. Complex formation of peptide-like compounds and enzymes in the GI tract lumen has also recently been reported (Sjöström et al. 1999) and a reduced bioavailability was observed.

The complex formation of a coumarin derivative with magnesium ions present in antacid formulations has also been reported (Ambre and Fuher 1973). The formation of a more absorbable species of the coumarin derivative was found, i.e., magnesium-bis-hydroxy-coumarin (Dakas and Takla 1991). Complex formation is therefore not just negative for drug

Figure 4.7 Omeprazol stability as a function of pH. Logarithm of the observed rate constant (k_{obs}, 1/h) for the intial, pseudo-first-order degradation of omeprazole in water solution at constant pH plotted as a function of pH.

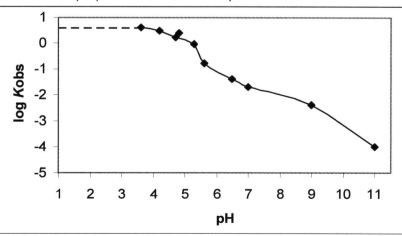

Reprinted from Development of an oral formulation of omeprazol by Å. Pilbrant and C. Cederberg from *Scand. J. Gastroenterol.,* 1985, Suppl. 120, Vol. 108, pp. 113–120.

absorption but can be used positively in formulation development for increasing the solubility of a drug, e.g., the use of cyclodextrins.

The composition and concentration of bile acids is different in different species and also varies along the GI tract (Lindahl et al. 1997, Dressman and Yamada 1991). The composition will affect the wetting ability of the bile and may also give variations in interactions. Drug interactions with bile have been reported (e.g., beta-blockers) (Yamaguchi et al. 1986a,b,c; Grosvenor and Löfroth 1995) and involve binding to the bile acid dimers or micelles or precipitation, which causes an unexpectedly low absorption in the GI tract.

Degradation and Metabolism

The gastric and intestinal fluids contain a multitude of different enzymes that can potentially metabolise different drugs (see Table 4.6). In addition, the microflora, being most significant in the colon, also have a significant metabolising capacity. A list of such metabolic reactions is shown in Table 4.7.

Interaction with the luminal content may be a *chemical or enzymatic/microbial degradation*. The chemical degradation is usually related to pH changes in the gut lumen but can also be a result of the reductive environment (redox potential negative) produced by the presence of anaerobic bacteria (Shamat 1993).

Enzymes are present throughout the GI tract, both within the brush-border membrane and in the lumen. The general gradient is decreased luminal degradation aborally to the small intestine and increased brush-border and intracellular degradation. The main enzymes include proteases, peptidases, esterases, cytochrome P450 enzymes and conjugating enzymes (see Table 4.6). Some enzymes, such as cytochrome P450 isoforms, are especially involved in the biotransformation of lipophilic compounds of both endogenous and exogenous origin, such as steroids, bile acids, fatty acids and prostaglandins (Arlotto et al. 1991). Cytochrome P450 3A4 is present mainly in the upper GI tract and is concentrated primarily to the villus tips (Paine et al. 1997; Pascoe et al. 1983). CYP 3A is the most abundant isoform in the human intestine (Paine et al. 1997) and, among the CYP 3A, CYP 3A4 is often found in co-existence with the MDR1 gene product, the efflux protein, P-glycoprotein, and shares a significant substrate specificity overlap (Wacher et al. 1998). The main CYP 450 isoforms in the intestine vary with animal species and the intestinal region.

Techniques for studying enzymatic degradation of compounds include

- homogenised intestinal segments, sometimes centrifuged into different subcellular fractions after high-speed centrifugation [crude homogenates, S9 (supernatant fraction constituting the cell plasma content), microsomal fraction (ER and other membrane fractions)];

- degradation in luminal perfusates or fluids (chyme) and identification of metabolites after transport across the intestinal membrane, as in the Ussing chamber model (Ungell et al. 1992); and

- cell monolayers such as Caco-2 cells (Delie and Rubas 1997).

Caco-2 cells express the main enzymes involved in drug metabolism (Delie and Rubas 1997; Artursson and Borchardt 1997) in quantities similar to those in the human small intestine rather than as is present in colonocytes. However, the very important cytochrome P450 3A family, which is the main CYP 450 in the human intestine, is absent in the Caco-2 cell

Table 4.6
Enzymes found in the GI tract.

Source	Enzyme	Substrate
Salivary glands	Amylase	Starch
Stomach	Pepsinogens/pepsins	Proteins and polypeptides
Exocrine pancreas	Trypsin	Proteins and polypeptides
	Chymotrypsin	Proteins and polypeptides
	Elastase	Elastin and other proteins
	Carboxypeptidase A,B	Proteins and polypeptides
	Pancreatic lipase	Triglycerides
	Pancreatic amylase	Starch
	Ribonuclease	RNA
	Deoxyribonuclease	DNA
	Phospholipase A	Lecithin
Intestinal mucosa	Enterokinase	Trypsinogen
	Aminopeptidases	Polypeptides
	Dipeptidases	Dipeptides
	Maltase	Maltose, maltotriose
	Lactase	Lactose
	Sucrase	Sucrose
	Isomaltase	Alpha-limit dextrins
	Nuclease and related enzymes	Nucleic acids
	Intestinal lipase	Monoglycerides
	Cytochrome P450	Steroids
	Esterases	Esters of prodrugs

Adapted from Ganong (1975).

monolayers, a fact that can explain differences in permeability between this model and intestinal tissues for drugs that are substrates to this enzyme family. The existence of metabolism can also be evaluated by incubation of the drug using pure enzyme preparations.

The *bacterial* content in the lumen of the GI tract varies with the region, starting with approximately 10^2 organisms in the mouth and increasing to as much as 10^{12} in the colon. Microbial degradation therefore increases aborally to the stomach and largely takes place in the colon (Shamat 1993). Illing (1981) and Coates et al. (1988) reviewed the techniques employed for studying the role of the gut flora in drug metabolism. In general, incubations are made with the drug and the gut content of an animal, or man, in a suitable medium, under anaerobic conditions. The degradation pathways are mainly reductive (of nitro compounds, sulphoxides, corticoids, doubles bonds and azo bonds), hydrolysis (of esters, amides, glucoronides and

Table 4.7
Some metabolic reactions of the intestinal microflora.

Reactions	Example
Reductions	
Nitro compounds	Clonazepam
Sulphoxides	Sulinac
21-Hydroxycorticoids	Aldosterone
Double bonds	Digoxin
Azo compounds	Prontosil
Hydrolysis	
Nitrate esters	Glyceryl trinitrate
Sulphate esters	Sodium picosulphate
Succinate esters	Carbenoxolone
Amides	Methotrexate
Glucuronides	Morphine glucuronide
Glucosides	Sennosides
Removal of functional groups	
N-dealkylation	Methamphetamine
Deamination	Flucytosine
Other reactions	
Heterocyclic ring fission	Levamisole
Side-chain cleavage	Steroids

Reprinted from *International Journal of Pharmaceutics,* Vol. 97, M. A. Shamat, The role of the gastrointestinal microflora in the metabolism of drugs, Pages 1–13, 1993, with permission from Elsevier Science.

glucosides), *N*-dealkylations and deamination (Shamat 1993). Anaerobic metabolism can also affect the formulation components, giving false release rates of the drug. This mechanism has been used for targeting drugs to the colon using azopolymer bonds (Saffran et al. 1986; van den Mooter et al. 1997). The degradation of compounds by the gut flora *in vitro* seems not always to be correlated to the *in vivo* situation, and so *in vivo* measurements must be performed (Shamat 1993).

Enzymatic *degradation of prodrugs* to the active drug can occur in the intestinal lumen (by the gut flora or by luminal or brush-border enzymes) or during transport across the intestinal membrane (intracellular enzymes). Where the prodrug is degraded depends on the nature of the prodrug bond, and the *in vitro* assay is very important for establishing optimal biotransformation rates and regional absorption/degradation. In general, the most commonly used *in vitro* models for the biotransformation of prodrugs are incubation with intestinal fluids, liver or intestinal microsomal incubations, and plasma/blood incubations. It is also very important to consider species differences in metabolic activity for prodrug activation. Permeability models, such as Caco-2 cell monolayers, have also been used to evaluate the importance of ester hydrolysis of prodrugs in parallel with transport (Narawane et al. 1993; Augustijns et al. 1998).

ABSORPTION/UPTAKE OVER THE GI MEMBRANES

Mechanisms of Drug Absorption

Several factors originating from the chemical structure and property of the drug molecule, and from the physiology within the environment in the GI tract, affect the flow of molecules across the intestinal membrane. These factors include solubility, partition coefficient, pK_a, molecular weight, molecular volume, aggregate, particle size, pH in the lumen and at the surface of the membrane, GI secretions, absorptive surface area, blood flow, membrane permeability and enzymes (for more factors, see Ungell 1997, and Table 4.8). Complete absorption occurs when the drug has a maximum permeability coefficient and maximum solubility at the site of absorption (Pade and Stavchansky 1998).

The uptake of drugs across the intestinal membrane can occur transcellularly across the lipid membrane or paracellularly between the epithelial cells in the tight junctional gap (see Figure 4.8) (Ungell 1997). The transcellular route is generally via carrier proteins or by passive diffusion. In addition, the transport across the cell membrane can be via endocytotic processes. Efflux proteins carrying the drug from the inside back into the lumen (e.g., P-glycoprotein, MRP1–6, etc.) have recently been proposed to be important for the overall absorption of drugs in the GI tract (Saitoh and Aungst 1995; Hunter and Hirst 1997; Makhey et al. 1998; Döppenschmitt et al. 1998; Anderle et al. 1998). Models have now been developed for specific studies of the mechanism behind low permeability or active transport via carrier systems, such as oligopeptide transporters, dipeptide transporters, amino acid transporters and monocarboxylic transporters (Tsuji and Tamai 1996).

Table 4.8
Physicochemical and physiological factors that influence drug bioavailability after oral administration (from Ungell 1997, with permission).

Physicochemical	Physiological
Hydrophobicity	Surface area at the site of administration
Molecular size	Transit time and motility
Molecular conformation	pH in the lumen and at surface
pK_a	Intestinal secretions
Chemical stability	Enzymes
Solubility	Membrane permeability
Complexation	Food and food composition
Particle size	Disease state
Crystal form	Pharmacological effect
Aggregation	Mucus and UWL
Hydrogen bonding	Water fluxes
Polar surface area	Blood flow
	Bacteria
	Liver uptake and bile excretion

Figure 4.8 Schematic drawing of the mechanisms and routes of drug absorption across intestinal epithelia. Drugs can be absorbed transcellularly (**1**) and paracellularly (**2**) by passive diffusion or transcellularly via carrier-mediated transport (**3**) or endocytosis (**4**). Enzymes in the brush-border region or intracellular enzymes and the efflux proteins, e.g., P-glycoprotein (**5**) contribute to the elimination of harmful compounds.

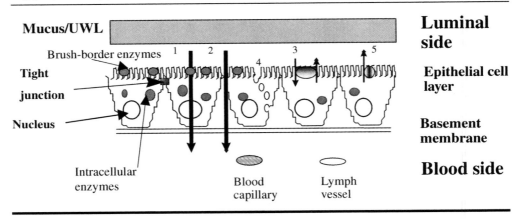

Apart from permeability of the intestine to molecules, the time the molecule spends in the region of absorption, i.e., transit time, becomes important. Generally, transit times in humans are seconds in the oesophagus, 0.5 to 1.5 h in the stomach, 3–4 h in the small intestine and 8–72 h in the colon.

Regionally, the different physiological factors will change and, thereby, also the potential impact on the drug molecule (Dressman and Yamada 1991; Hörter and Dressman 1997; Ungell et al. 1997). For developing extended oral drug release dosage forms, knowledge of the regional differences in the absorption pattern becomes very important in evaluation and success (Thomson et al. 1986; Ungell et al. 1997; Kararli 1995; Pantzar et al. 1993; Narawane et al. 1993). In addition, these mechanisms are also species different (Kararli 1995) and must be correlated to the human situation. If the regional difference in absorption probability of the drug is known (regional permeability and interactions), increased absorption can be achieved by the use of an absorption window, e.g., targeting the drug to a specific region to avoid critical regions of enzymes or low permeability.

MODELS FOR STUDYING THE ABSORPTION POTENTIAL OF DRUGS

Models for studying drug absorption that are available in industry and at universities and contract organisations are mainly (see Hillgren et al. 1995; Ungell 1997; Borchardt et al. 1996; Stewart et al. 1995)

- computational methods,

- partitioning between water and oil,

- cell cultures,

- membrane vesicles,

- intestinal rings or sacs,

- excised segments from animals in the Ussing chamber,

- *in vitro* and *in situ* intestinal perfusions,

- *in vivo* cannulated or fistulated animals and

- *in vivo* gavaged animals.

All of these models have values that must be correlated to human data, mainly F_a (fraction absorbed) (Ungell 1997; Lennernäs et al. 1997; Artursson et al. 1993; Lennernäs et al. 1996; Artursson and Karlsson 1991) (see Figure 4.9). Correlations have been made in different laboratories using different models (Ussing, Perfusion, and Caco-2) (Matthes et al. 1992; Rubas et al. 1993; Tanaka et al. 1995; Lennernäs et al. 1997; Fagerholm et al. 1996) and in different laboratories using the same model (Caco-2) (Artursson et al. 1996).

Methods to describe the process of transport over the GI membrane must describe different mechanisms of absorption for a wide variety of molecules and must be predictive of the absorption process in man. If a New Chemical Entity (NCE) cannot penetrate the intestinal epithelium, it will not be successfully developed as a pharmaceutical product. This also means that, if the rate-limiting step in the absorption process of the drug molecule is not described in the model, the result will be a false positive.

Figure 4.9 Schematic drawing of a screen ladder. The screen ladder can be used for understanding different complexities in the results, using different screening models (from Ungell 1997, with permission).

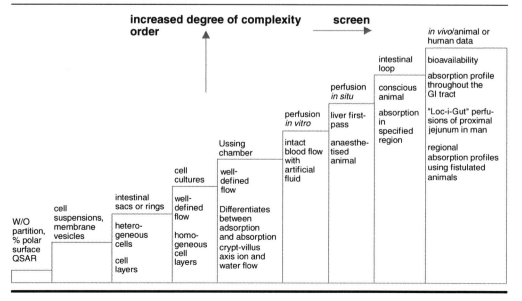

The literature mentions numerous non-biological (biophysical and computational) and biological *in vitro* and *in vivo* methods for screening barriers of absorption (for more information see: Borchardt et al. 1996; Kararli 1989; Ungell 1997; Hillgren et al. 1995; Lipinski et al. 1996; Lundahl and Beigi 1997; Yang et al. 1997; Hjort-Krarup et al. 1998; Quilianova et al. 1999; Stewart et al. 1997; Lee et al. 1997; Altomare et al. 1997; van der Waterbeemd et al. 1996; Winiwarter et al. 1998). Each method describes a part of the absorption process, mainly the transport through the lipid membrane. However, it is clear that, for drug discovery and rational drug development, there is no single ultimate method, but instead there is a need for more than one of these screening methods. It is also evident from the literature that we need more information regarding the absorption mechanisms of the particular drug entity and its analogues, to be able to obtain structure/absorption relationships and to design the most proper method for screening, e.g., HTS. Below is a short review of the different methods available for studying drug absorption.

Non-biological Methods for the Prediction of Oral Drug Absorption

Passive diffusion through the lipid membrane of the GI tract is the main drug absorption mechanism. This is a process generally thought to be governed by physicochemical factors of the drug molecule, such as lipophilicity, surface charges, molecular volume/molecular weight and conformational flexibility (Navia and Chaturvedi 1996). The size of the molecule and the charge will also govern whether the molecule can passively pass across the epithelium via the paracellular pathway and between the cells via the tight junctional complex. However, it has been argued that the paracellular route is almost non-existent and seems to be important only for drugs with molecular weights below 200 g/mol and for non-ionic or cationic molecules (Karlsson et al. 1994, 1999; Lennernäs 1997).

The non-biological models describing the transmembrane process are very rapid and involve no use of animals. Computer-based models of structure/absorption relationships belong to this group. They have recently become increasingly popular due to the use of chemical libraries and possibilities for testing large sets of biological data, with multivariate analysis models such as partial least squares (PLS) and principal component analysis (PCA) (Eriksson et al. 1999). In fact, the non-biological methods can, in many cases, replace the biological methods, and can be used in an HTS manner. The most challenging ideas for industry today involve trying to avoid time and resource consuming synthesis of structural analogues with no potential of being developed as pharmaceutical products; they therefore focus more on the analogues that have such potential.

The most widely accepted parameter for predicting drug absorption is the *partition coefficient* reflecting partitioning of the drug only into a lipid phase (e.g., octanol/water), the log *P* (or log *D*) value (see Chapter 3), and general rule-of-thumb models such as the Lipinski Rule (Lipinski et al. 1996). This rule states that molecules with a molecular weight of less than 500 g/mol, with a clog *P* of less than 5, with hydrogen donors fewer than 5 and acceptors fewer than 10 will have greater possibilities for being orally available. This rule is based on historical data (up to 1997) from a vast number of drugs entering the Investigational New Drug Application (IND) phase, including drugs that fulfilled the criteria of pharmacological activity. The rule is also based on several other assumptions: that the transcellular transport is molecular weight dependent, the drug is *only* absorbed through passive diffusion, the four parameters describe the molecular structure correctly and the drug is not solubility restricted. Only the high value of the limit is set; the lower limit of, for instance, clog *P* is not within the rule. In addition, the parameters in the Lipinski Rule describe the two-dimensional structure of the molecule, but do not take into account the three-dimensional structure and the true conformation of the molecule. However, regardless of the restrictions of the rule, it can be used as a rule of thumb in the same way as log *P* or log *D* is being used, but is a better predictor than lipophilicity alone.

The optimal range in *lipophilicity* that would reflect a good absorption potential has been suggested to be a log *P* value between 0 and 3 (Navia and Chaturvedi 1996) or above 3 (Wils et al. 1994a), depending on the method used. This is a general rule of thumb because it means that very hydrophilic drugs (log *P* < −3) and very lipophilic drugs (log *P* > 6) are often associated with incomplete absorption *in vivo* (Navia and Chaturvedi 1996; Wils et al. 1994a). Drugs with log *P* values between −3 and 0 and a log *P* between 3 and 6 often give varying results (Navia and Chaturvedi 1996). However, the prediction of incomplete absorption for hydrophilic and very lipophilic drugs has been argued. Hydrophilic drugs, such as atenolol and sotalol, are absorbed from the GI tract although their partition coefficients are low, and very lipophilic drugs, such as Fluvastatin, are completely absorbed (Lindahl et al. 1996). The lack of correlation and the varying results obtained by this method are understandable, since lipophilicity is far from being the only determinant of drug absorption.

Today, however, there is a more complex view of the factors governing the partitioning into a lipid phase, e.g., multiple molecular structure descriptors, including number of hydrogen bonds (acceptors and donors) (Burton et al. 1992), polar surface area (Palm et al. 1996), polarity, integy moments, polarisability, distances between functional groups of importance, etc. (Zamora and Ungell 2001; Norinder et al. 1996; Palm et al. 1997; Cruciani et al. 2000; Goodford 1985). Future quantitative structure activity relationship (QSAR) models will therefore be based more on multivariate analysis, analysing a complex set of molecular descriptors.

Below is a short description of some of the non-biological methods that can be used to predict drug absorption. For more detailed information, see, e.g., Ungell (1997), Lipinski et al. (1996), Palm et al. (1997), Burton et al. (1992), Norinder et al. (1996), van der Waterbeemd et al. (1996), Cruciani et al. (2000).

Computer-Based Prediction Models

A good relationship has been established between the number of *hydrogen bonds* of small model peptides and their permeability coefficients, determined using Caco-2 cell monolayers (Burton et al. 1992). The method reflects the ability of the molecule to form hydrogen bonds with the surrounding solvent. The more bonds the molecule forms with water (luminal fluid), the less potential it has to diffuse into a lipid phase of a membrane.

The total number of hydrogen bonds in the molecule can easily be calculated, including the bonds the molecule can form internally. This may be one of the reasons for the lack of correlation seen for the drug Fluvastatin, a very lipophilic drug (log *P* 3.8) that has a total of 8 hydrogen bonds (Lindahl et al. 1996). The total number of hydrogen bonds that should be the limit is 5, according to the Lipinsky Rule (Lipinsky et al. 1996), if the drug is to be completely absorbed in the GI tract in man (Lindahl et al. 1996).

Polar surface area is another important determinant of drug absorption, as first proposed by Palm et al. (1996). The method was described as dynamic molecular surface properties. These were calculated with consideration of all low energy conformations of some beta-blockers, and the water-accessible surface areas, which were calculated and averaged according to a Bolzmann distribution. They found a linear relationship between permeability coefficients, measured both with Caco-2 cells and with excised segments from the rat intestine, and percentage polar surface area of beta-blockers with different lipophilicity. According to calculated values of log D_{oct} at pH 7.4, there was not as good a relationship, with some additional impaired ranking order between the substances (calculated according to the method of Hansch and co-workers, for references, see Palm et al. 1996). Polar surface area has also recently been proposed to explain why drugs with very high log D values are not absorbed (Artursson et al. 1996). The authors suggest that these very lipophilic drugs instead show a high degree of polar surface area towards the environment, which will reduce their ability to diffuse through a lipid phase. This was shown by a bell-shaped correlation between permeability coefficients determined in HT-29 (18-C) monolayers and log D and, in contrast, a linear relationship between permeability coefficients and calculated polar surface area (Artursson et al. 1996). A good correlation between the fraction absorbed of a variety of drugs and the polar surface, as well as for hydrogen acceptors and donors, has been proposed to exist (Palm et al. 1997).

QSAR Models

Several theoretical models attempting to predict the absorption properties from molecular descriptors have been published in the last few years (Palm et al. 1996; Zamora and Ungell 2001; Norinder et al. 1997; Hjort-Krarup et al. 1998; Winiwarter et al. 1998). These theoretical models can be based on several different experimental data sets from various absorption models, such as Caco-2 cells, Ussing chambers, *in vivo* fraction absorbed and permeability in humans (Palm et al. 1996; Palm et al. 1997; Artursson et al. 1996; Norinder et al. 1997; Winiwarter et al. 1998). There are several new, recently published approaches in this area for creating predictive models for drug absorption properties, the MOLSURF™ methodology (Norinder et al. 1997) being one. Another approach is to use the GRID™ methodology, a strategy designed by Goodford (1985) to study interaction fields of a molecule, the target, with a small chemical group, the probe. The GRID™ methodology has been successfully applied in the receptor-substrate interaction analysis. The VOLSURF™ program analyses these interaction fields and obtains different surface properties and volumes to describe the interaction. In recent work by Zamora and Ungell (2001), Caco-2 data and data from Ussing chamber experiments were used for predicting permeability properties of a set of beta-blockers using the VOLSURF™ program. Until recently, it was believed that computer-based methods were only to be used for passive transcellular diffusion. Data have been presented that also indicate the use of these methods for active transport and efflux via carrier systems (Neuhoff et al. 1999). The average time for the calculation of each compound is, at the least, seconds, but this differs between models. The more complex and flexible the structure becomes, the more time is required for the calculation. All of the methods described above are computer-based models and do not require any synthesis of compounds. This means that if they can be used in the early screening of thousands of compounds, the time required for evaluating these compounds will be reduced enormously, compared with the synthesis and determination of absorption by biological methods and difficult analytical procedures.

Extraction into a Lipid Phase

Measurement of log P (or log D) usually uses a determination of a drug molecule extracted into the lipid phase of an octanol/water or octanol/buffer extraction system (for references, see Palm et al. 1996; Leahy et al. 1989; Manhold et al. 1990; Leo et al. 1975). The predictive value of log P or log D has been questioned. First, octanol is not the ideal lipid phase because of its own hydrogen bonding capacity. A delta log P, determined between two lipid phases, has instead been suggested, e.g., between octanol/water and iso-octane/water (Kim et al. 1993). Second, Leahy et al. (1989) showed that there is no simple relationship between log P and drug absorption. The curve is represented by a sigmoidal shape with a plateau (or even reported as a bell shaped form) (Wils et al. 1994a; Yodoya et al. 1994). The reason for this is not known, but it is suggested to be a consequence of decreased aqueous solubility (Navia and Chaturvedi 1996), uncertainty in the evaluation of the value of log P (Palm et al. 1996) or a high degree of polar surface area (Artursson et al. 1996).

Measurements of partitioning of drugs into *lipid vesicles, liposomes or cell membranes* as predictive models for drug absorption are also described in the literature (Hillgren et al. 1995; Balon et al. 1999; Stewart et al. 1997). This may be due to the similarity of these systems to biological membranes and the wish for a "pure membrane system" with the correct lipid and protein composition, but without enzymes and carrier proteins.

Chromatography

Retention time measurements, k', through different types of *chromatographic systems* have recently become very popular, e.g., immobilised artificial membrane (IAM) columns, reversed-phase C18 columns and liposome columns. IAM columns show a good correlation to the determined log D values and drug absorption *in vivo* in mice for a group of cephalosporins. IAMs also predicted drug permeability through Caco-2 cells. The method is based on the retention of molecules on a column consisting of a solid phase of immobilised phospholipids tethered to a hydrocarbon string onto a silica column. In between the phospholipid strings, C_{10} and C_3 alkyl groups are bound to the column. The mobile phase is 100 percent aqueous. The substance is thought to be retained on the column mainly in the ranking order of lipophilicity. As the molecule faces the more polar head groups of the phospholipids, this reflects the biological membrane, more than would separation on a HPLC column (Pidgeon et al. 1995; Yang et al. 1997).

The method is reported to be very simple and may be used for fast screening of a large quantity of compounds. A good correlation has been reported between IAM chromatography and the membrane partition coefficient for structurally related hydrophobic drugs, but not for nonrelated compounds (Pidgeon et al. 1995).

The IAM method is similar to a separation on a HPLC column, which has been used for screening substances for drug absorption (Pidgeon et al. 1995; Merino et al. 1995). The method of Merino et al. (1995) is based on a fluorimetric reversed-phase HPLC method for quantification of quinolones in absorption and partition samples. The retention times of two of the quinolones correlated well with data obtained *in vivo*. The results of this type of separation also reflect the membrane partition coefficient of drugs and can therefore be used when the ranking order of related compounds is evaluated. However, drugs with a very large gap between their lipophilicity will require a gradient system for elution, which can mislead the interpretation. Non-related compounds will give different correlation lines with membrane permeability and partitioning coefficients because of the different mobile phase polarity and differences in the chemical structure (Rathbone and Tucker 1991).

The chromatographic systems (as for log D or log P calculations or measurements) must be correlated to a biological parameter, e.g., permeability over Caco-2 cells or intestinal segments in the Ussing chamber, for a better correlation to the absorption process. However, if this can be done with a wide range of molecules, as was reported for IAM chromatography (Pidgeon et al. 1995), before starting a large synthesis strategy, it might improve, in terms of time and effectiveness, the finding of a drug with good absorption potential.

Liposome chromatography has also recently been used as a tool for predicting permeability (Lundahl and Beigi 1997; Beigi et al. 1998). For most drugs tested, the method does not predict drug absorption better than other chromatographic methods, such as reversed-phase columns, but some additional knowledge can nevertheless be gathered. The interaction between the drug and the lipophilic phase can be studied with this method, which may play an important role in the determination of the retention factor. This was especially evident when ionisable drugs were studied. Further evaluation is needed to understand whether this information can also contribute to the overall understanding of the process of drug transport across the lipid membrane.

Another method that should be mentioned here is capillary electrophoresis, which has recently been reported as a new tool for predicting drug absorption using beta-blockers (Örnskov et al. 2001). This method can very easily be used as an HTS instrument if it can also be proved useful for other types of drug structures.

In Vitro Biological Methods

Many drugs will not perform only according to physicochemical rules, and their absorption cannot be predicted properly using biophysical methods. These are the drugs that are susceptible to any of the carrier-mediated processes (both in absorptive and secretory directions) or the molecules that are degraded during transport. The transport processes used by these drugs must be studied by biological methods, and information is also needed regarding cofactors and scaling factors to the fraction absorbed in humans.

Biological methods are therefore used when the mechanisms of absorption (paracellular, transcellular or carrier-mediated) and the enzymatic degradation or regional difference in permeability are to be evaluated. A short description of the best-known biological *in vitro* methods follows, and more detailed information on each of the methods can be found in, e.g., Ungell (1997), Stewart et al. (1997), Hillgren et al. (1995), Borchardt et al. (1996), and Kararli (1989, 1995).

Methods Describing Drug Uptake

Membrane Vesicles and Intestinal Rings

As a group of methods membrane vesicles and intestinal rings are technically quick and easy to use, even for persons not very skilled in using biological material. They represent the uptake of a drug into the enterocytes.

The use of brush-border *membrane vesicles* (BBMV) in the discovery or development of drugs is usually restricted to mechanistic studies of enzyme interactions or ion transport–coupled processes. The method is based on a homogenisation of an inverted frozen intestine to give a purified fraction of the apical cell membranes from a chosen part of the GI tract (Kararli 1989; Kessler et al. 1978) (see Figure 4.10). The method can frequently be used for isolated studies of the brush-border membrane transport characteristics without any basolateral membrane influence. It has been used for studies concerning the intestinal peptide carrier system (Yuasa et al. 1993) to clarify the mechanism of absorption of fosfomycin (Ishizawa et al. 1992), glucose, amino acids and salicylate uptake (Osiecka et al. 1985). Membrane vesicles have been isolated from numerous animals, including man (Hillgren et al. 1995). The functionality of the preparation (i.e., whether the membrane is closed) is assessed by using substrates to specific carriers, such as glucose, phosphate or amino acids, and the orientation of the membrane, i.e., right side or inside out, is assessed by enzyme markers. Recently, BBMV was tested as a screening model for a large number of compounds using 96-well Multiscreeen Filtration plates (Quilianova et al. 1999). After correction for unspecific binding to the tissue,

Figure 4.10 Technique for purification of BBMV. Flowchart for purification of BBMW from intestinal tissue (from Kararli 1989).

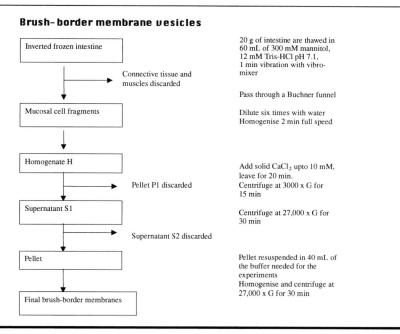

Brush-border membrane vesicles

Inverted frozen intestine

Connective tissue and muscles discarded

20 g of intestine are thawed in 60 mL of 300 mM mannitol, 12 mM Tris-HCl pH 7.1, 1 min vibration with vibro-mixer

Pass through a Buchner funnel

Mucosal cell fragments

Dilute six times with water
Homogenise 2 min full speed

Homogenate H

Pellet P1 discarded

Add solid CaCl$_2$ upto 10 mM, leave for 20 min.
Centrifuge at 3000 x G for 15 min

Supernatant S1

Centrifuge at 27,000 x G for 30 min

Supernatant S2 discarded

Pellet

Pellet resuspended in 40 mL of the buffer needed for the experiments
Homogenise and centrifuge at 27,000 x G for 30 min

Final brush-border membranes

the permeability values were found to show a good correlation to the *in vivo* human fraction absorbed.

This represents a method of lipid membrane extraction and can be used in drug absorption studies for evaluation of a biological log *D* value (see the above section on non-biological methods). This was actually first used for measurements of the lipid composition (Hillgren et al. 1995). Different regions of the GI tract can be used, evaluating the influence of regional differences in lipid composition on the permeability of drugs, as has been suggested by Thomson et al. (1986); Ungell et al. (1997) and Kim et al. (1994). The major disadvantage of the method is that these processes represent only a fraction of the complete absorption process, i.e., into the cell. No paracellular process can be studied, nor can processes that need the basolateral membrane and its function for absorption, e.g., processes linked to the active transport of Na$^+$ by the basolateral Na$^+$/K$^+$ adenosine triphosphatase (ATP-ase) (Kararli 1989). There may be a day-to-day variation in vesicle preparation and a leakage of drugs from the vesicles during washing and filtration, which can affect the drug concentration (Osiecka et al. 1985). However, despite these drawbacks, it can be used for mechanistic studies of the drug absorption process, although there are only data on a direct correlation to human *in vivo* absorption values.

The second method in this group is the *intestinal rings or slices*. This method for studying drug absorption has been used extensively for kinetic analysis of carrier-mediated transport of glucose, amino acids and peptides (Kararli 1989; Osiecka et al. 1985; Porter et al. 1985; Kim et al. 1994; Leppert and Fix 1994). The method is easy to use; the intestine of the animal is cut into rings or slices of approximately 30–50 mg (2 to 5 mm in width) which are put into an incubation medium for a short period of time (often up to 1 min) with agitation and oxygenation. Samples of the incubation medium and rings are analysed for drug content after the incubation. The intestine is sometimes everted on a glass rod before cutting, and different regions of the intestinal tract can be used (see Figure 4.11).

The main advantage of this method is its ease of preparation. As in the BBMV, this method can also frequently be used for testing many different drugs simultaneously. The intestinal rings have several disadvantages, however. Diffusion into the tissue slices takes place on the side of the tissue (not only through the lipid membrane), as the connective tissue and muscle layers are exposed to the incubation solution. Correction is not always made for the adsorption of a drug on the surface of the tissue, and the slices do not maintain their integrity for more than 20–30 min (Osiecka et al. 1985; Levine et al. 1970). The method is also restricted by the limits of the analytical methods. Nevertheless, good mechanistic correlation to *in vivo* measurements has been achieved with the method in kinetic studies of carrier-mediated mechanisms of peptides (Kim et al. 1994). The method was evaluated for the prediction of *in vivo* absorption potential (Leppert and Fix 1994), and it was shown that, under appropriate conditions, uptake into everted intestinal rings closely paralleled known *in vivo*

Figure 4.11 Schematic drawing of intestinal sacs and rings. After preparation, the intestinal sacs or rings are put into a beaker with incubation buffer of the pH of interest. After incubation for 10–20 min at 37°C, the rings/sacs are taken up, dried and analysed for compound content. In some cases, correction for unspecific binding to the tissues (muscles, lamina propria, etc.) is made. For the everted sac model, a catheter can be inserted for withdrawal of sample solution and oxygenation on the serosal side.

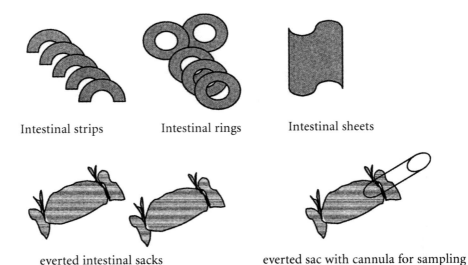

Intestinal strips   Intestinal rings   Intestinal sheets

everted intestinal sacks   everted sac with cannula for sampling bioavailability. The method has also recently been experimentally improved for better hydro-dynamics and a requirement for lower volumes during the incubation period (Uch and Dressman 1997; Uch et al. 1999).

Methods with Well-Defined Transport Direction

Cell Cultures

The Caco-2 cell monolayers and other cell cultures (HT-29, IEC-18) from human carcinoma have become increasingly popular as permeability methods in the past few years (Artursson 1990; Hidalgo et al. 1989; Ma et al. 1992; Wils et al. 1994b). Recently, cell lines such as MDCK (Madin-Darby canine kidney) have also received attention, especially for screening large numbers of compounds. The cell monolayers consist of polarised cells grown onto a filter support. When fully differentiated, the cells express the transport characteristics of mature cells (see Figure 4.12). Caco-2 cells (Artursson 1990) and HT-29 (18-C1) (Wils et al. 1994b) grow into tight epithelia extremely useful for the measurement of permeability coefficients of various molecules.

The Caco-2 cell monolayer shows an epithelium membrane barrier function similar to the colon of man (Artursson et al. 1993; Lennernäs 1997) but has carrier-mediated systems similar to the small intestine (e.g., bile acid transporter, dipeptide carrier, glucose carriers and vitamin B_{12}) (for references, see Borchardt 1991; Walter et al. 1995). The transport of pharmaceutical drugs is studied using both 6-, 12- and 25-well systems and side-by-side diffusion cells as in the Ussing chamber. The cells have also been used for culturing cocultures with lymphocytes for studying the transport of particles through lymphoid tissues (M-cells) (Kerneis et al. 1997; Delie and Rubas 1996) and have recently also been grown upside down in order to study transport in the opposite direction (Garberg et al. 1999).

Much is known about the performance of this method in predicting the absorption of drugs in humans. A good correlation is seen especially for lipophilic high permeability drugs

Figure 4.12 Schematic drawing of a cell culture model, Caco-2 cells. Cells are seeded on filter support and are left to differentiate for 1–3 weeks before the transport experiments. Experiments are started by adding the compound to the donor side and taking out samples from the receiver side at times up to 2 h. The incubation with the compound is done with good stirring and at 37°C.

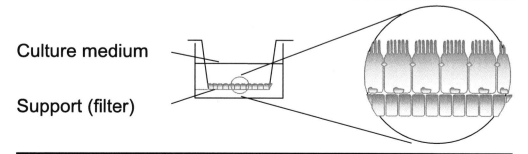

Culture medium

Support (filter)

using the transcellular pathway and the *in vivo* permeability coefficients measured by perfused human jejunum (Loc-i-Gut® technique, Lennernäs et al. 1996). Apart from studies of passive transcellular transport (Artursson 1990; Artursson and Karlsson 1991), the Caco-2 cell method has also been used for studying mechanisms of passive paracellular transport (Artursson et al. 1993), carrier-mediated (peptidomimetics and antibiotics) (Walter et al. 1995), oligopeptide transporter (Hidalgo et al.1995), monocarboxylic acid transporters (Tsuji and Tamai 1996), efflux systems (p-glycoprotein and other efflux systems) (Kuo et al. 1994; Delie and Rubas 1996; Döppenschmitt et al. 1998; Anderle et al. 1998), the effect of enhancers (Surendran et al. 1995; Lindmark et al. 1997; Anderberg and Artursson, 1994) and recently also cloned Caco-2 cells with specific carrier systems (Wenzel et al. 1996; Artursson and Borchardt 1997). The importance of the unstirred water layer for the transport of very lipophilic drugs has also been studied (Karlsson and Artursson 1991), and the HT-29 cell lines have been used for predicting drug absorption and investigating the mechanisms of mucus as a barrier to absorption (Wikman et al. 1993; Wils et al. 1994b; Matthes et al. 1992; MacAdam, 1993). There are also numerous studies of the metabolic capacity of the Caco-2 cells and possible induction of enzyme expression and carrier proteins (Delie and Rubas 1997; Artursson and Borchardt 1997).

The advantages of the cell culture method are many, i.e., good performance on frequent use, both for the prediction of drug absorption in humans and mechanistic studies, and probably the best potential for use in HTS strategies. The monolayers are extremely useful in automated systems and, to speed up this automation, very young cells, three days old, have been evaluated for drug absorption studies (BIOCOAT system, BD VIasante™; Chong et al. 1997). The experiments are rapid, have good precision, are less time-consuming and are less controversial than, for instance, *in vivo* animal studies. In addition, cell culture allows evaluation of drug transport under very controlled conditions and offers the major advantage that the cells are derived from humans. The MDCK cell line is, however, an easy cell line to cultivate, although it is derived from dogs instead of humans, which may give species different results. The disadvantages of cell lines in culture are the tightness of the epithelium (although this can probably be regulated), showing a more colon-like system and giving extremely low permeability coefficients for hydrophilic drugs. Further disadvantages include the unknown quantity and predictive value of the different carrier-mediated systems (Lennernäs et al. 1996; Lennernäs 1997), and the unknown composition of the lipid membrane and its lack of crypt-villus axis, which is important for fluid and ion transport *in vivo*. There are also differences in results from laboratories using this method for establishing a relationship between the permeability coefficients of compounds and the values of the F_a, as reported in the literature. The reason for the differences has not been fully evaluated but may have to do with the cultivation procedure, which can affect enzyme and carrier expressions, cell density and passage number, and may have to do with differences in the experimental set-up (e.g., stirred or unstirred, concentration of compounds tested, etc.) (Delie and Rubas 1997; Anderle et al. 1998).

Excised Intestinal Segments

The *everted sac* (everted intestine) method is based on the preparation of a 2–3 cm long tube of the gut which is tied off at the ends after evertion on a glass rod (Kararli 1989) (see Figure 4.11). The serosa becomes the inside of the sac and the mucosa faces the outer buffer solution. As a modification of this procedure, the serosal layer and muscular layers can also be stripped off before evertion on the glass rod (Hillgren et al. 1995). The presence or absence of the serosal layer may give different transport rates of compounds, e.g., salicylic acid (Hillgren et al. 1995). This has also been found for the Ussing chamber technique (see section below). An oxygenated buffer solution is injected into the sac, which is put into a flask containing the drug of interest. Samples of fluid are taken from the buffer solution in the flask. The sac is weighed before and after the experiments to compensate for fluid movement. In one modification of the method, one end of the tissue is cannulated with a polyethylene tubing (Kararli 1989), also making it easier to withdraw samples from the serosal side of the intestine.

An advantage of this method is that it is rapid and many drugs can be tested simultaneously, especially low permeability drugs, owing to the low volume of the serosal compartment. There is good performance as regards stirring conditions on the mucosal side, although the oxygenation of the tissue is poor, as a result of the unstirred and unoxygenated serosal layer inside the uncannulated sac. Another advantage of this method is that it needs no specialised equipment, in contrast to the Ussing chamber and cell culture models.

Disadvantages are mainly the viability issue and the diffusion through the lamina propria. Histological studies have shown that structural changes start as early as 5 min after the start of incubation, and a total disruption of the epithelial tissue can be seen after 1 h (Levine et al. 1970). As for intestinal rings, there is no correction for the binding of drug substance onto the surface of the mucosa (when uncannulated sacs are used).

Ussing Chamber

The Ussing chamber technique is an old technique for studying transport across an epithelium, developed by Ussing and Zerhan in 1951. It has been used extensively in physiological studies concerning the pharmacology and physiology of ion and water fluxes across the intestinal wall. It has also recently been used for drug absorption studies using excised intestinal tissues from different animals—rabbits, dogs, rats or monkeys (Palm et al. 1996; Ungell et al. 1997; Artursson et al. 1993; Jezyk et al. 1992; Rubas et al. 1993; Polentarutti et al. 1999)—and for human biopsies (Biljsma et al. 1995; Söderholm et al. 1998). The method is generally based on excision of intestinal segments from the animal. These segments may be stripped of the serosa and the muscle layers and mounted between two-diffusion half-cells (Grass and Sweetana 1988) (see Figure 4.13). The permeability coefficients

$$P_{\text{app}} = \frac{dq}{dt} \times \frac{1}{AC_o}$$

of the compounds are calculated from the measurement of the rate of transport, dQ/dt, of molecules from one side of the segment to the other (either mucosa to serosa or serosa to mucosa), divided by the exposed area of the segment (A) and the donor concentration of the drug (Co).

Stirring of the solutions on both sides of the membrane is very important, especially for lipophilic drugs (Karlsson and Artursson 1991). This can be achieved either by a gas lift system, as originally proposed by Ussing and Zerhan (1951), by a more refined gas lift system, as shown by Grass and Sweetana (1988) or by stirring with rotors (Polentarutti et al. 1999). The viability of the tissues is verified with the measurement of potential difference (*PD*), short circuit current and calculation of the transepithelial electrical resistance by Ohm's law (Polentarutti et al. 1999; Söderholm et al. 1998; Ungell et al. 1992; Biljsma et al. 1995; Sutton et al. 1992). The values that set the limits of viability should be in the range of what has been measured *in vivo*, e.g., for rat jejunum and ileum, 5 and 6 mV, respectively. Extracellular marker molecules such as mannitol, inulin, Na-fluorescein and PEG 4000 have been used to verify a tight epithelium (for references, see Pantzar et al. 1994) and for testing effects of enhancers

Figure 4.13 Schematic drawing of an Ussing chamber. Excised tissues from the animal intestine are stripped of the serosal and muscle layers and are mounted in between the two chamber halves. The experiment is run by adding the compound to one side and taking out samples from the other side for up to several hours after excision at 37°C. Oxygenation of the tissue can be performed separately from the stirring of the solutions. The viability of the tissue can be monitored simultaneously using a voltmeter and connected current generator.

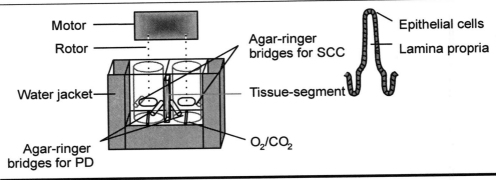

and increased fluid absorption (Borchardt et al. 1996; Karlsson et al. 1994, 1999). It has also become very popular to verify a viable and intact epithelium using biochemical markers such as lactate dehydrogenase (LDH) release (Oberle et al. 1995) and morphology evaluations (Polentarutti et al. 1999; Söderholm et al. 1998). The more viable the segment, the better the interpretation of the results. Extreme values of permeability values can be discarded from the data set giving better and more reliable results and a better overall understanding of drug transport (Polentarutti et al. 1999). The model has also been used for identifying metabolites formed during transport (Ungell et al. 1992) and evaluation of carrier-mediated transport and prodrugs (Schwaan et al. 1995), although not as extensively as the Caco-2.

This method has several advantages for predicting *in vivo* drug absorption in humans. First, there is a good correlation with the permeability coefficients of human jejunum *in vivo* (Lennernäs et al. 1997) for both passively transported and low- and high-permeability compounds. Second, the technique can be used for different regions of the GI tract, evaluating the regional absorption characteristics of drugs (Ungell et al. 1997; Polentarutti et al. 1999; Jezyk et al. 1992; Narawane et al. 1993; Pantzar et al. 1993). Furthermore, mucosal types (buccal, nasal, oesophageal, stomach, rectal, skin) other than the intestine can be used, making it possible to evaluate other administration sites with the same model. The method using diffusion cells can also be employed for cultured monolayers using a modified insert for the monolayer membrane. The method is very useful for evaluating mechanisms of absorption. It can shed light on the importance of ionic transport processes on the transport of drug molecules due to the physiological presence of a crypt-villus axis and a heterogeneous population of cells (mature and immature as well as cells with different functions). The method also has the advantage of being available for human tissues, slices or biopsies from surgically removed tissues (Biljsma et al. 1995; Söderholm et al. 1998), which represents one of the most challenging developments of this method for future screening of drugs, especially for mechanistic studies and enzymatic evaluation of drugs and prodrugs for which experiments with human tissue are needed.

The major disadvantage of this absorption method is the diffusion pathways for the molecules, which are unphysiological, i.e., the lack of vascular supply forces the molecules to diffuse through the lamina propria, and, in the case that unstripped tissues also are used, through the serosal layer. It was recently proposed that the presence of the serosal and muscular layers might have different impacts on the transport of molecules with different physicochemical characteristics, which are both size and lipophilicity dependent (Breitholtz et al. 1999). The lamina propria, muscle layers and serosal layer can also be different in the different animals and regional segments. Some reports have also proposed that there may be difficulties with the unstirred water layers and that there is concern regarding the stirring conditions, especially of the solution in the donor compartment. Segments from animals are often used (as for most of the absorption models), which must then be verified for human tissue. This is especially important metabolically and for carrier-mediated transport processes. The integrity and viability of the tissue must be verified simultaneously because it will strongly impair the transport of the drug molecules (see above). The model is probably not designated as an HTS tool. However, correctly used as a mechanistic secondary screening tool, data from the Ussing chamber technique are more closely related to the human situation than many of the other biological methods available.

Intestinal Perfusion Method

There are reports in the literature on the isolated perfused intestine as a technique for absorption studies and *in situ* perfusions (Blanchard et al. 1990; Oeschsenfahrt and Winne 1974; Chiou 1995; Krugliak et al. 1994; Fagerholm et al. 1996). A segment of 10–30 cm of the intestine is cannulated on both ends and perfused with a buffer solution at a flow rate of 0.2 mL/min (Fagerholm et al. 1996) (see Figure 4.14). The blood side can also be cannulated through the mesenteric vein and artery. The difference between *in situ* and *in vitro* is the use of the rat circulation *in vivo* (which is a vascular perfusion in the *in vitro* situation) (Windmueller et al. 1970; Fagerholm et al. 1996). This then gives the opportunity of evaluating the influence of hepatic clearance on the absorption of drugs.

Both perfusion methods can use different evaluation systems for testing drug absorption, using the difference between "in" and "out" concentrations in the perfusion solutions, and/or disappearance and appearance on both sides of the membrane, and also by analysing the drug concentration on the blood side. The permeability, usually called the P_{eff}, is calculated from the following equation,

$$P_{eff} = -Q_{in} \times \frac{\ln\left(\dfrac{C_{out}}{C_{in}}\right)}{2\pi rL} \quad \text{(parallel tube model)}$$

where Q is the flow rate, C_{in} and C_{out} are the inlet and outlet concentrations of each drug, respectively, and $2\pi rL$ is the mass transfer surface area within the intestinal segment. Different lengths are used between 10 and 30 cm, but the best flow characteristics are achieved with 10 cm (Fagerholm et al. 1996). PEG 4000 is used for corrections of fluid flow and to verify the absence of leakage in the model. In addition, as for the Ussing chamber using excised segments and Caco-2 cells, many use mannitol as a permeability marker molecule (Krugliak et al. 1994). This is more sensitive to changes in the intestinal barrier function, compared to PEG 4000

Figure 4.14 Schematic drawing of the intestinal perfusion technique. The intestine of the animal is catheterised in both ends and a flow of buffer solution of 37°C is perfused using a pump. For *in vitro* studies in which only the absorption over the intestine is to be measured, the vascular support can be cannulated, and a separate buffer solution can be perfused through the intestine. If the influence of the liver on drug absorption is to be studied, an *in situ* system with an intact anaesthetised animal can be used by only perfusion of the intestine, keeping the blood flow of the vascular support intact.

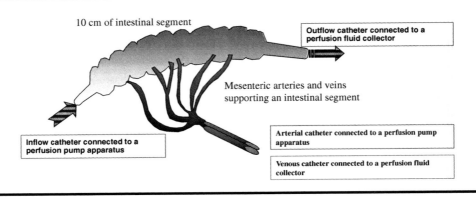

alone. *In situ* perfusions have recently been extensively used for mechanistic studies of efflux of drugs (Lindahl et al. 1999).

The major advantage of this type of absorption method is the presence of a blood supply giving the tissue oxygen and the correct flow characteristics on the serosal side of the membrane, e.g., less diffusion through the lamina propria. Secondly, different parts of the GI tract can be used as in the Ussing chamber technique. Good stirring, i.e., flow characteristics, of the mucosal/luminal solution has been reported (Fagerholm et al. 1996). A very good correlation with perfusions has been found to the human fraction absorbed and human permeability of different types of drugs (Fagerholm et al. 1996, Amidon et al. 1988).

The disadvantage of the method is the use of anaesthesia, which has been reported to affect drug absorption (Uhing and Kimura 1995a,b). PEG 4000 is used to verify the integrity of the barrier, which can lead to misinterpretation of the integrity of the tissue due to the high molecular weight of the marker. An additional disadvantage, although less important for mechanistic studies, is that the method is time and animal consuming, which makes it less useful for screening purposes. Some discrepancies between the disappearance rates of drugs and their appearance on the blood side have also been reported, indicating a loss of the drug in the system either by enzymatic degradation or by adhesion to the plastic catheters.

In Vivo *Biological Methods*

Methods primarily used are *in situ* perfusions of the rat gut, regionally cannulated/fistulated rats and dogs, bioavailability models in different animals, intestinal perfusions in man (Loc-i-Gut®, Lennernäs et al. 1992) (Figure 4.15) and triple-lumen perfusions (Gramatte et al. 1994) and bioavailability studies in man.

Figure 4.15 The multichannel tube system with double balloons allowing for segmental jejunal perfusion. The balloons are filled with air when the proximal balloon has passed the ligament of Treitz. Gastric suction is obtained by a separate tube (Lennernäs et al. 1992).

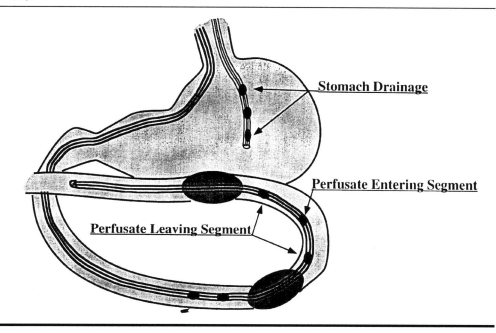

For regional absorption assessments in small animals like the rat, the drug substance is usually administered via a cannula situated in the region to be tested, intraduodenal, intrajejunal, intraileum or intracolonic. Blood samples are withdrawn from an arteric/venous cannula inserted in the carotid artery/jugular vein (Borchardt et al. 1996; Sjöström et al. 1999). For regional absorption assessment in the dog, a chronic fistula is surgically inserted in the region of interest and blood samples are taken from superficial veins in the forelegs (Borchardt et al. 1996). Regional absorption differences can be seen for a compound as regards permeability coefficients (Ungell et al. 1997) and metabolism in the intestinal lumen, in the brush-border region or within the cells of the epithelium. The importance of good regional absorption performance (e.g., high and similar absorption throughout the GI tract) of a selected compound may be crucial for the development of extended release formulations and should therefore be evaluated early in the screening phase for optimal drug candidate selection.

These complex studies are usually very time-consuming and cost-ineffective and are too complex for detailed evaluation of the mechanisms of absorption. Furthermore, only drugs that have been approved as non-toxic can be used for studies in man, and these methods are thus not used early in development studies. However, for the completeness of the understanding of the absorption of a certain drug, for correct information to support the pharmaceutical dosage form program and for correlation of the performance of the more simple animal models, some experiments must be performed *in vivo* in animals and in humans early in the clinical phase. Such experiments include membrane permeability coefficient assessment; absorption, distribution, metabolism, and excretion (ADME) studies; dose and concentration dependency; food interactions; regional absorption performance; and evaluation of enhancer systems. All *in vitro* methods used, regardless of what mechanism or part of the absorption process they represent, must be correlated to the *in vivo* situation and, if possible, also to absorption in humans. This is not a simple evaluation since different methods represent different parts of the total process and the main barrier will affect the main part of the results. Values for *in vivo* absorption in man are not easy to obtain, and the values are often a result of a recalculation of data obtained for other purposes. The values of Fa for drugs in the literature are therefore most uncertain. Published, compiled data on bioavailability can be found in Benet et al. (1996).

More mechanistic studies in humans during Phase I must be performed for better feedback to discovery and pharmaceutical development, and thereby for faster performance through the clinical phases. It was recently suggested that a biopharmaceutical classification of drug permeability coefficients and dissolution issues must be determined early in the development program for rational drug design (Amidon 1996).

PERMEABILITY COEFFICIENTS VERSUS F_a

Using the HT-29–18-C1 cell line, permeabilities of various molecules have been compared with *in vivo* oral data (Wils et al. 1994b). This report found a threshold value of 2×10^{-6} cm/s. Over this value, the drugs showed more than 80 percent absorption *in vivo*, and were poorly absorbed below this value. A similar threshold value can be seen for Caco-2 cells (1×10^{-6} cm/s) (Artursson and Karlsson 1991) and, according to a recent paper by Yazdanian et al. (1997) (0.5×10^{-6} cm/s), for excised jejunal segments of the rat in the Ussing chamber (10×10^{-6} cm/s) (Lennernäs et al. 1997), for perfusion of the rat jejunum and for the perfused human jejunum *in vivo* (0.5×10^{-4} cm/s) (Fagerholm et al. 1996). These threshold values indicate a parallel shift for different methods concerning the predictive permeability versus F_a *in vivo*, which was recently suggested for the methods *in situ* rat perfusion, Ussing chamber with rat jejunal segments and the perfusion of the human jejunum (Lennernäs et al. 1997) and at different laboratories using the same Caco-2 cell model (Artursson et al. 1996). The parallel shift for permeability coefficients between different methods and animals is expected since the lipid membrane composition can vary with both species and diet (Thomson et al. 1986; Ungell et al. 1997). This is no cause for concern if the ranking order is the same between the methods used.

The values of the permeability coefficients also indicate experimental windows of different sizes. The Caco-2 cells seem to operate roughly between 0.1 and 200×10^{-6} cm/s (Artursson and Karlsson 1991), the excised segments in the Ussing chamber between 1 and 200×10^{-6} cm/s and the perfused rat intestine and perfused human jejunum between 0.1 and 10×10^{-4} cm/s. A difference in the operating window can also be seen for the same model at different laboratories. Yazdanian and co-workers recently published permeability values for a vast number of compounds using the Caco-2 cell model (Yazdanian et al. 1997). In spite of the large data set in this paper, the values are difficult to interpret since they form an "all-or-none" shape of the correlation curve to Fa in humans, and the steep part of the curve shows a very narrow range in permeability values. For instance, there is a 100-fold change in Fa that shows a minor change in the permeability value, e.g., 0.38×10^{-6} cm/s for ganciclovir to 0.51×10^{-6} cm/s for acebutalol (Yazdanian et al. 1997). The reason for this phenomenon is not known. Owing to differences in the handling of animals, age, species, food, tissues, tissue media, clones of cultured cells or different passages, laboratories will have different prediction factors for absorption when they use the different methods available (Artursson et al. 1996; Thomson et al. 1986; Ungell et al. 1997; Ungell 1997).

The ranking order between the different drugs might also be different between laboratories because of the different levels of viability and integrity of the biological systems used (Ungell 1997). The integrity of the tissue change is time related, which means that there is a limit in time for use of the different systems (Levine et al. 1970; Polentarutti et al. 1999). It may also be related to buffer solutions, oxygenation of the solutions, stirring conditions, preparation of the tissues and other physical handling, and temperature (Ungell 1997). The surface exposed to the drug is different in different models and for high and low permeability drugs, as suggested by Artursson et al. (1996) and Strocchi and Levitt (1993). The "true" exposed surface area is the same as the serosal surface area for cultured monolayers (Artursson et al. 1996) but is very variable for excised segments for the Ussing chamber or perfusions, depending on which region of the GI tract is used. As a result of different handling during preparation of the tissues, the effective surface area for absorption may also be different, and a time-dependent change in surface area during the course of the experiments has been reported (Polentarutti et al. 1999). The change in area by time will affect high and low permeability drugs differently (Strocchi and Levitt 1993). For a full understanding of the differences in results between laboratories and between species, these parameters may perhaps be useful as a complement to other valuable information regarding the performance of the experiments and the technique used.

The variability between experiments and laboratories presents difficulties when comparing values from different laboratories. Each laboratory should therefore be careful in standardising and correlating their own models to human absorption values before using them as predictive tools. Indeed, the guidelines from FDA regarding the use of a compound data set for classification of their candidate drugs using the BCS could be helpful in standardising *in vitro* techniques (Amidon 1996).

IN VIVO TECHNIQUES FOR STUDIES IN MAN

The physicochemical tests, *in vitro* methods and animal experiments used in the biopharmaceutical preformulation phase can never fully reflect the conditions in man, and studies of the drug absorption prerequisites can therefore be very valuable. This is especially relevant if (a) contradictory results have been obtained in model experiments, (b) the substance has complicated absorption properties (e.g., active transport) or (c) a modified release formulation will be developed. The most important information that can be obtained in such human studies is

- intestinal drug permeability/absorption and

- bioavailability after administration at different regions in the GI tract.

This type of study is not only useful for drug substance characterisation prior to formulation development but may also be performed to elucidate absorption effects of certain formulation components.

Intestinal Permeability Measurements

The extent of absorption is determined by several drug properties such as dissolution, degradation/metabolism in the GI lumen and permeability over the GI wall. Human intestinal permeability can be quantified *in vivo* by use of an intubation technique called Loc-i-Gut® (Lennernäs et al. 1996) (see Figure 4.15). This is a multichannel tube with two balloons, which is positioned in the proximal jejunum. A closed segment is created in the jejunum by inflating the two balloons. Thereafter, an isotonic drug solution is continuously perfused through the intestine, and sampling from the segment for assessment of drug concentrations is performed in parallel. The intestinal permeability (P_{eff}) is calculated by the following equation:

$$P_{eff} = \frac{\left(C_{in} - C_{out}\right)}{\left(C_{out}\right)} \times \frac{Q_{in}}{2\pi rL}$$

where C_{in} and C_{out} are the drug concentrations in the inlet solution and in the perfusate leaving the tube, respectively, and Q_{in} is the flow rate of the inlet solution. The surface of the closed segment is described by $2\pi rL$, where L is the length (10 cm) and r is the intestinal radius (1.75 cm). The recovery of a non-absorbable marker is used to check that no fluid is leaking out of the closed segment.

The intestinal permeability has been determined by this technique for a large number of substances (Tamamatsu et al. 1997). A relationship between P_{eff} and the extent of absorption has also been established (see Figure 4.16), which has clearly shown that permeability can be the limiting step in the absorption process and that a certain permeability (about 4×10^{-4} cm/s) is needed to obtain complete absorption.

It is also possible to study the influence of active carriers on the transport over the intestinal mucosa by this technique. This can be done by comparing the P_{eff} with and without an

Figure 4.16 The relationship between fraction absorbed (Fa) drug in humans after oral administration and jejunal gut wall permeability is determined in humans for different drugs.

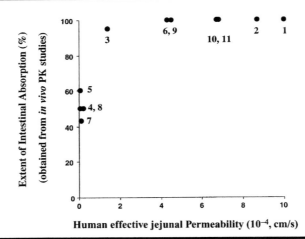

inhibitor of the carrier system in the perfusion solution or by comparing the P_{eff} for different drug concentrations in the perfusion solution. For example, the P_{eff} of verapamil was increased at higher drug concentrations in the perfusion solution (Sandström et al. 1998). An active efflux of the drug into the lumen by P-glycoprotein membrane transporters could explain this, since verapamil is known to be a substrate for this carrier.

Regional Bioavailability Assessment

The bioavailability of a drug after administration to different regions in the GI tract can be determined either by remote control capsules or by intubation techniques. The two most frequently used remote control devices, the "high frequency capsule" and Intellisite, are shown in Figure 4.17a and b (Parr et al. 1999). The drug must be dissolved or suspended in a small

Figure 4.17a The high-frequency (HF) capsule. When the capsule has reached the intended region, it is exposed to an HF field. This induces an increased temperature in a heating wire, which leads to melting of a nylon thread and release of a steel needle. The needle perforates a latex balloon which contains the drug solution, and the drug is released.

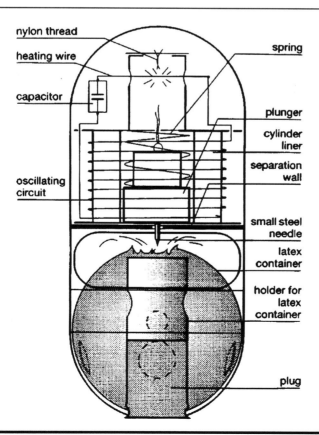

Figure 4.17b The InteliSite™ capsule. When the capsule has reached the desired location, it is exposed to a magnetic field, which increases the temperature in the capsule. This causes two memory alloys to straighten, which rotates the inner sleeve of the capsule. A series of slots in the sleeve surface are thereby aligned, and the drug solution is released through the openings.

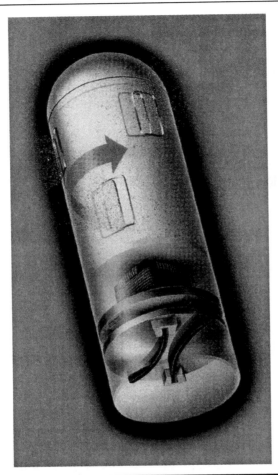

volume (1 mL) which is included in a chamber or balloon in the remote control device. The location of the device in the GI tract is determined by fluoroscopy or gamma scintigraphy. When the target location has been reached, "microwaves" externally trigger a drug release mechanism and the drug appears in the intestines as a bolus dose. Markers such as radionuclides can also be included in the device together with the drug solution to verify when drug release occurs (Bode et al. 1996).

Different intubation techniques have been used for regional absorption studies. The terminal ileum and colon can be reached either by an oral tube (Abrahamsson et al. 1997) or by colonoscopy (Gleiter et al. 1985; Parr et al. 1999). In the latter case, the tube is inserted "from the end of the colon". The position of the tube is determined by fluoroscopy before administering the drug, preferably as a solution, through the tube.

Both types of techniques have been shown to provide very valuable results, but certain pros and cons can be identified. For example, multiple doses are possible, and the rate of drug administration can be varied in the case of intubation, whereas this is presently not possible for remote control devices. The potential risk of not obtaining appropriate drug release at the desired site is lower for intubations, owing to its simplicity, as compared with the more highly technological remote control devices. On the other hand, the tube or the perfusion may disturb the normal physiological flow conditions in the intestine. Furthermore, in the case of colonoscopy, the colon content must be emptied before insertion of the colonoscope, which leads to unphysiological test conditions. For both types of techniques, it is crucial to investigate drug adhesion/partitioning to the device material and drug stability for relevant time periods before starting any *in vivo* experiments.

In these studies, standard bioavailability variables such as the extent of bioavailability determined from area under the curve (AUC), rate of bioavailability related to peak plasma drug levels (C_{max}) and time to peak (t_{max}) are determined. A more detailed presentation of the assumptions and interpretations of bioavailability data is given in Chapter 7. The bioavailability after administration in more distal parts of the intestine, such as the terminal ileum and different parts of the colon, is compared with a reference administration either as an oral solution or as a regional delivery to the upper small intestine. This is exemplified in Figure 4.18, which shows the plasma drug concentrations of metoprolol after administration to jejunum, terminal ileum and colon ascendens or transversum.

VEHICLES FOR ABSORPTION STUDIES

Early preformulation studies are often performed to obtain initial information regarding drug absorption but may be restricted by solubility problems of the active drug. During early

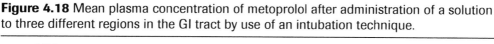

Figure 4.18 Mean plasma concentration of metoprolol after administration of a solution to three different regions in the GI tract by use of an intubation technique.

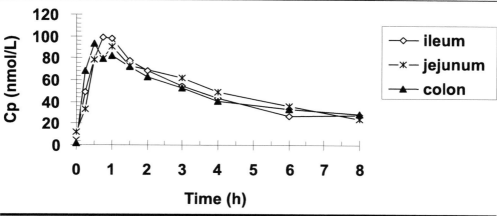

studies, such as *in vitro* methods and in *in vivo* methods using animals, *vehicles to solubilise* the molecule are used. However, as many of these vehicles are surfactants or lipid systems, they may also act as "membrane breakers" and are therefore classified as enhancers of absorption (Oberle et al. 1995; van Hoogdalem et al. 1989; Swenson et al. 1994; Anderberg and Artursson 1994). The absorption enhancers/vehicles may act differently on the permeability of low and high permeability drugs and may also affect carrier-mediated transport or metabolism, e.g., chremophore and Tween-80, which are known to inhibit P-glycoprotein (Hunter and Hirst 1997). The membrane integrity may be impaired, and whether it is the lipid fluidity or the tight junctions that are affected depends on the concentration and on the vehicle system used. The outcome of the use of the vehicle system will thereby depend on the physicochemical nature of the drug and on the metabolic pathway or transport mechanism or route it uses. There are very few reports showing the effects of vehicle systems on the integrity of the mucosal membrane. Excised intestinal segments in the Ussing chamber have been used to verify the change in permeability to mannitol and propranolol using different vehicles, both surfactant and lipid based systems (Hanisch et al. 1998). Effects of surfactants on the viability of mucosal tissues have been reported using LDH release (Oberle et al. 1995), change in teansepithelial electrical resistance (TEER) over Caco-2 cells (Anderberg and Artursson 1994) and lipid vehicles such as monoglycerides (Borchardt et al. 1996; Yeh et al. 1994).

At present, no inert vehicle system is available that in general will solubilise all sparingly soluble compounds during *in vitro* screening or that is specifically intended for *in vivo* administration in animals. This is, of course, impossible, since the molecules have different structural backbones and behaviour in aqueous solutions, and thus, have different physicochemical properties. Instead, it is advisable to use a vehicle with as few side-effects as possible and, in addition, to standardize screening and to test the particular vehicle *in vitro* and *in vivo* using marker molecules (Hanisch et al. 1998, 1999).

Many vehicles also give analytical problems when liquid chromatography-mass spectrometry (LC-MS) is used, e.g., PEG 400, ChremophorEL and solutol. The vehicle may, of course, impair the pharmacological effect and activity of the active drug or receptor. This must be taken into account when choosing the right vehicle for discovery screening tests and early preformulation studies.

Systems that *enhance drug absorption* do not always contain ingredients that act on the epithelial membrane (increased membrane permeability) but act by other mechanisms, such as by increasing the solubility, changing pH at the absorption site or decreasing the binding to luminal material. The result of the enhancement is then an increased force in the absorption process, i.e., the effective concentration at the absorption site. Some examples in the literature of enhancers can be seen in Table 4.9.

We must very often consider an enhancer system to be able to develop a dosage form for a drug with low bioavailability because of the difficulty in performing any more structural changes without loss of potency. The Caco-2 cells, Ussing chambers and perfused intestinal segments methods are often used for enhancer studies or evaluation of the toxicity of the enhancers (Anderberg and Artursson 1994; van Hoogdalem et al. 1989; LeCluyse and Sutton 1997). It has been found that the effects of enhancers on the biological system are both species and method related. For instance, it has been found that Caco-2 cell monolayers are very sensitive to surfactants, and the rat intestinal tract seems to be more sensitive than that of the rabbit (Anderberg and Artursson 1994). Some enhancers have also been used in delivery systems for humans. Best known are the salts of the fatty acids caprate and caprylate (C8 and C10), which have been used for rectal administration of antibiotic drugs such as cefoxitin (Lindmark et al. 1997). The toxic or sensory feeling experienced with the use of the enhancers in humans has not been fully evaluated. Enhancer systems using mixtures of monoglycerides (C8

Table 4.9
Most commonly used classes of enhancers to drug absorption from the GI tract.

Non-steroidal anti-inflammatory drugs (NSAIDs) and derivatives	**Mixed micelles**
	Glyceryl monooleate + sodium taurocholate
Sodium salicylate	Linoleic acid + HCO60
Sodium 5-methoxysalicylate	**Calcium binding agents**
Indomethacin	EDTA (ethylenediaminetetraacetic acid)
Diclofenac	**Phenothiazines**
Surfactants	Chlorpromazine
Nonionic: polyoxyethylene ethers	**Liposomes**
Anionic: sodium laurylsulfate	**Azone**
Cationic: quaternary ammonium compounds	**Fatty acid derivatives of carnitine and peptides**
Bile salts	Palmitoyl-DL-carnitine
Dihydroxy bile salts: sodium deoxycholate	N-Myristoyl-L-propyl-L-propyl-glycinate
Trihydroxy bile slats: sodium cholate	**Saponins**
Derivative: sodium tauro-24,25-dihydrofusidate (STDHF)	**Concanavalin A**
	Phosphate and phosphonate derivatives
Medium chain fatty acids	DL-alpha-glycerophosphate
Octanoic acid	3-amino-1-hydroxypropylidene-1.1-diphosphonate (APD)
Decanoic acid	
Medium chain glycerides	**Polyacrylic acid**
Glyceryl-1-monooctanoate	Diethyl maleate (DEM) and diethylethoxy-methylene malonate
Glyceryl-1-monooctanoate	
Enamines	
DL-Phenylalanine ethylacetoacetate enamine	

Reprinted from *Pharmacology and Therapeutics*, Vol. 44, E. J. van Hoogdalem et al., Intestinal drug absorption enhancement, Pages 407–443, 1989, with permission from Elsevier Science.

and C10), intented to increase the oral absorption in humans of a large number of different types of poorly absorbable drugs, have recently been patented, and studies on the mechanisms behind the enhancer effect have also been published (Le Cluyse and Sutton 1997; Sekine et al. 1985; van Hoogdalem et al. 1989; Constantinides 1993; Yeh et al. 1994; Borchardt et al. 1996).

FUNCTIONAL USE OF ABSORPTION MODELS

There are different strategies for the use of these absorption models in the industry, e.g., screening of structural analogues, mechanistic studies and problem solving, as well as in early formulation perspectives and correlation to *in vivo* data. This means that there is no ultimate method for both the discovery and development of pharmaceutical drugs, but rather a battery of models to be used in different phases of the projects. The functional use of the different models available could be to use computational methods for the large majority of compounds, both to select drugs of interest for synthesis and to gather information on what important factors will govern the molecule through the membrane via the different transport routes (see section on absorption mechanisms). When analogues have been synthesised, a selected group of compounds should be run in HTS screens for solubility, permeability and metabolic stability. The information is entered in the computational models to gather additional data, and simultaneously, also put into more complex models of absorption and used for correlation to *in vivo* values found in animals (Figure 4.19). The more complex secondary screening models should also address the biopharmaceutical aspects, i.e., solubility, interactions in the gut lumen, regional permeability/absorption differences and degradation by bacteria.

HTS is the initial phase in the discovery process, where chemical entities are tested for biological activity in specific target assays. The technology and the high-throughput standardisation have also lately been discussed for the structure/absorption relationship using

Figure 4.19 Scheme expressing the functional use of the screening tools in an HTS manner for the prediction of oral drug absorption. Compound groups from the HTS of potency are fed into the QSAR models for selection of good candidates to be synthesised and run through the more complex biological models. After data have been received from the biological screening, the compound information can be fed back into the computer-based model compound analogues and fed at the same time into more complex biological models for elucidating mechanisms of absorption or formulation development.

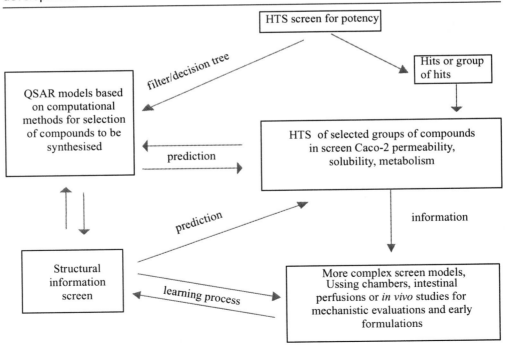

Caco-2 cell monolayers or other cell lines as well as intrinsic clearance determination (half-lives) for structure/stability evaluation. The overall strategy for the industry is to use this screening tool as efficiently as possible, and not necessarily for all compounds in the chemical library. The standardised systems have a high throughput where thousands of chemical compounds can be tested in a short period of time and where the time for feedback into the projects is the most important success factor. Because of the importance of the measured values resulting from such assays for a forthcoming candidate drug selection, the importance of the assay for correct prediction of the human situation becomes evident.

As concerns the absorption of drugs in the GI tract, HTS in the industry has focused on Caco-2 cell monolayer permeability assays. Other cell lines have been and are also currently being used, such as MDCK, T84 cells, CHO cells, LDCK, HT29, other clones of Caco-2, etc. The purpose of using cell lines at this stage is to proceed quickly to the next step of the evaluation of a potentially available oral drug, which requires only a representative value for acceptable or non-acceptable permeability. The cell lines differ in the presence of carrier-mediated transport systems and metabolic activity, and thus the outcome differs. For the design of more specific screening tools, e.g., transporters, specific cells of a certain age and differentiation are used (Döppenschmitt et al. 1998; Anderle et al. 1998; Delie and Rubas 1997) as are cloned human transporters in cells (Artursson and Borchardt 1997).

REFERENCES

Abdou, H., ed. 1989. Theory of dissolution. In *Dissolution, bioavailability & bioequivalence*, Easton, Penn., USA: MACK Publishing Company, pp. 11–36.

Abrahamsson, B., K. Lindström, L. Nyberg, A. Pettersson, M. Sunzel, A-L. Ungell, and W. Månsson. 1997. Regional absorption of metoprolol in humans determined by a new method suitable for studies in the whole gastro-intestinal (GI) tract. *Proceedings of the controlled Release Society*. 24:359–360.

Altomare, C., A. Carotti, G. Trapani, and G. Liso. 1997. Estimation of partitioning parameters of non-ionic surfactants using calculated descriptors of molecular size, polarity, and hydrogen bonding. *J. Pharm. Sci.* 86:1417–1425.

Ambre, J. J. and L. T. Fuher. 1973. Effect of coadministration of aluminium and magnesium hydroxides on absorption of anticoagulants in man. *Clin. Pharmacokinet. Ther.* 14:231.

Amidon, G. L. 1996. A Biopharmaceutic Classification System: Update May 1996. In *Biopharmaceutics drug classification and international drug regulation*. Bornem, Belgium: Capsugel Symposium Services, pp. 11–30.

Amidon, G. L., P. J. Sinko, and D. Fleisher. 1988. Estimating human oral fraction dose absorbed: A correlation using rat intestinal membrane permeability for passive and carrier-mediated compounds. *Pharm. Res.* 5:651–654.

Amidon, G. L., H. Lennernäs, V. P. Shah, and J. R. Crison. 1995. Theoretical considerations in the correlation of in vitro drug product dissolution and in vivo bioavailability: A basis for biopharmaceutical drug classification. *Pharm. Res.* 12:413–420.

Anderberg, E. K., and P. Artursson. 1994. Cell cultures to access drug absorption enhancement. In *Drug absorption enhancement*, edited by A. G. de Boer. Reading, UK: Harwood Academic Publishers, pp. 101–118.

Anderle, P., E. Niederer, W. Rubas, C. Hilgendorf, H. Spahn-Langguth, H. Wunderli-Allenspach, H. P. Merkle, and P. Langguth. 1998. P-glycoprotein (P-gp) mediated efflux in Caco-2 cell monolayers:

The influence of culturing conditions and drug exposure on P-gp expression levels. *J. Pharm. Sci.* 87:757–762.

Arlotto, M. P., J. M. Trant, and R. W. Estabrook. 1991. Measurement of steroid hydroxylation reactions by high performance liquid chromatography as indicator of P450 identity and function. *Methods Enzymol.* 206:454–462.

Artursson, P. 1990. Epithelial transport of drugs in cell culture I: A model for studying the passive diffusion of drugs over intestinal epithelia. *J. Pharm. Sci.* 79:476–482.

Artursson, P., and R. Borchardt. 1997. Intestinal drug absorption and metabolism in cell cultures: Caco-2 and beyond. *Pharm. Res.* 14:1655–1658.

Artursson, P., and J. Karlsson. 1991. Correlation between oral drug absorption in humans and apparent drug permeability coefficients in human intestinal epithelial (Caco-2) cells. *Biochem. Biophys. Res. Commun.* 175:880–885.

Artursson, P., A.-L. Ungell, and J.-E. Löfroth. 1993. Selective paracellular permeability in two models of intestinal absorption: Cultured monolayers of human intestinal epithelial cells and rat intestinal segments. *Pharm. Res.* 10:1123–1129.

Artursson, P., K. Palm, and K. Luthman. 1996. Caco-2 monolayers in experimental andtheoretical predictions of drug transport. *Adv. Drug Delivery Rev.* 22:67–84.

Augustijns, P., P. Annaert, P. Heylen, G. van den Mooter, and R. Kinget. 1998. Drug absorption studies of prodrugs esters using the Caco-2 model: Evaluation of ester hydrolysis and transepithelial transport. *Int. J. Pharm.* 166:45–53.

Balon, K., B. U. Riebesehl, and B. W. Müller. 1999. Drug liposome partitioning as a tool for the prediction of human passive intestinal absorption. *Pharm. Res.* 16:882–888.

Beigi, F., I. Gottschalk, Lagerqvist, C. Hägglund, L. Haneskog, E. Brekkan, Y. Zhang, T. Österberg, and P. Lundahl. 1998. Immobilized liposome and biomembrane partitioning chromatography of drugs for prediction of drug transport. *Int. J. Pharm.* 164:129–137.

Benet, L. Z., S. Oie, and J. B. Schwartz. 1996. Design and optimization of dosage forms regimens: Pharmacokinetic data. In *Goodman and Gilman's: Pharmacological basis of Therapy,* 9th ed., edited by J. G. Hardman, L. E. Limbird, P. B. Molinoff, R. W. Ruddan, and A. G. Gilman. New York: McGraw-Hill, pp. 1707–1792.

Bijlsma, P. B., R. A. Peeters, J. A. Groot, P. R. Dekker, J. A. Taminiau, and R. Van der Meer. 1995. Differential in vivo and in vitro intestinal permeability to lactulose and mannitol in animals and humans: a hypothesis. *Gastroenterology* 108:687–696.

Blanchard, J., L. M. Tang, and M. E. Earle. 1990. Reevaluation of the absorption of carbenoxolone using an in situ rat intestinal technique. *J. Pharm. Sci.* 79:411–414

Bode, H., E. Brendel, G. Ahr, U. Fuhr, S. Harder, and A. H. Staib. 1996. Investigation of nifedipine absorption in different regions of the human gastrointestinal (GI) tract after simultaneous administration of ^{13}C and ^{12}C nifedipine. *Eur. J. Clin. Pharmacol.* 50:195–201.

Borchardt, R. T., P. L. Smith, and G. Wilson. 1996. *Models for assessing drug absorption and metabolism.* New York: Plenum Press.

Borchardt, R. 1991. Rational delivery strategies to circumvent physical and metabolic barriers to the oral absorption of peptides. In *Peptides. Theoretical and practical approaches to their delivery.* Bornem, Belgium: Capsugel Library, p. 9.

Breitholz, K., U. Hägg, L. Utter, K. Wiklander, and A.-L. Ungell. 1999. The influence of the serosal layer on viability and permeability of rat intestinal segments in the Ussing chamber. *AAPS Pharm. Sci. Suppl.* 1:S653.

Burton, P. S., R. A. Conradi, A. R. Hilgers, N. F. H. Ho, and L. L. Maggiora. 1992. The relationship between peptide structure and transport across epithelial cell monolayers. *J. Contr. Rel.* 19:87–97.

Charman, W. N., C. J. H. Porter, S. Mithani, and J. B. Dressman. 1997. Physico-chemical and physiological mechanisms for the effects of food on drug absorption: The role of lipids and pH. *J. Pharm. Sci.* 86:269–282.

Chiou, W. L. 1995. The validation of the intestinal permeability approach to predict oral fraction of dose absorbed in humans and rats. *Biopharmaceut. Drug Disposition* 16:71–75.

Chong, S., S. A. Dando, and R. A. Morrison. 1997. Evaluation of BIOCOAT® intestinal epithelium differentiation environment (3-day cultured Caco-2 cells) as an absorption screening model with improved productivity. *Pharm. Res.* 14:1835–1837.

Coates, M. E., B. S. Drasar, A. K. Mallett, and I. R. Rowland. 1988. Methodological considerations for the study of bacterial metabolism. In *Role of the gut flora in toxicity and cancer*, edited by I. R. Rowland. London: Academic Press, pp. 1–21.

Constantinides, P. P. 1993. Lipid microemulsions for improving drug dissolution and oral absorption: Physical and biopharmaceutical aspects. *Pharm. Res.* 12:1561–1572.

Cruciani, G., P. Crivori, P. A. Carrupt, and B. Testa. 2000. Molecular fields in quantitative structure-permeation relationships: The Volsurf approach. *J. Mol. Structure (Theochemistry)* 503:17–30.

Dakas, C. J., and P. G. Takla. 1991. Physicochemical interactions affecting drug in the gastrointestinal tract: A review. *Epitheo. Klin. Farmakol. Farmakokinet. Int.* 5 (3):124–142.

Delie, F., and W. Rubas. 1996. Caco-2 monolayers as a tool to examine intestinal uptake of particulates. *Proc. Contr. Rel. Soc.* 23:149–150.

Delie, F., and W. Rubas. 1997. A human colonic cell line sharing similarities with enterocytes as a model to examine oral absorption: Advantages and limitations of the Caco-2 model. *Crit. Rev. Ther. Drug Carrier Systems* 14:221–286.

Döppenschmitt, S., H. Spahn-Langguth, C-G. Regårdh, and P. Langguth. 1998. Radioligand binding assay employing P-glycoprotein-overexpressing cells: Testing drug affinities to the secretory intestinal multidrug transporter. *Pharm. Res.* 15:1001–1006.

Dressman, J. B., G. L. Amidon, C. Reppas, and V. P. Shah. 1998. Dissolution testing as a prognostic tool for oral drug absorption: Immediate release dosage forms. *Pharm. Res.* 15:11–22.

Dressman, J. B., and K. Yamada. 1991. Animal models for oral drug absorption. In *Pharmaceutical bioeqvivalence*, edited by Welling and Tse. New York: Dekker, pp. 235–266.

EMEA. 1998. *Note for guidance on the investigation of bioavailability and bioequivalence.* Geneva, Switzerland: European Agency for the Evaluation of Medicinal Products.

Eriksson, L., E. Johansson, N. Kettaneh-Wold, and S. Wold. 1999. Multi- and megavariate data analysis using projection methods (PCA & PLS), Umeå, Sweden: Umetrics Ed.

Fagerholm, U., M. Johansson, and H. Lennernäs. 1996. The correlation between rat and human small intestinal permeability to drugs with different physico-chemical properties. *Pharm. Res.* 13:1335.

FDA. 2000. *Guidance for industry—Waiver of in vivo bioavailability and bioequivalence studies for immediate release solid dosage forms based on a biopharmaceutics classification system.* Rockville, Md., USA: Food and Drug Administration.

Ganong, W. F. 1975. Gastrointestinal function. Digestion and Absorption. In *Review of Medical Physiology*, 7th ed., edited by W. F. Ganong. Los Altos, Calif., USA: Lange Medical Publications.

Garberg, P., P. Eriksson, N. Schipper, and B. Sjöström. 1999. Automated absorption assessment using Caco-2 cells cultivated on both sides of polycarbonate membranes. *Pharm. Res.* 16:441–445.

Gibaldi, M., and S. Feldman. 1970. Mechanisms of surfactant effects on drug absorption. *J. Pharm. Sci.* 59:579–588.

Gleiter, C. H., K-H. Antonin, and P. Bieck. 1985. Colonoscopy in the investigation of drug absorption in healthy volunteers. *Gastrointestinal Endoscopy* 31:71–73.

Godbillon, J., D. Evard, and N. Vidon. 1985. Investigation of drug absorption from the gastrointestinal tract of man. III. Metoprolol in the colon. *Brit. J. Clin. Pharmacol.* 19:113s–118s.

Goodford, P. J. 1985. A computational method procedure for determining energetically favourable binding sites on biologically important macromolecules. *J. Med. Chem.* 28:849–857.

Gramatté, T., E. E. Desoky, and U. Klotz. 1994. Site-dependent small intestinal absorption of ranitidin. *Eur. J. Clin. Pharmacol.* 46:253–259.

Grass, G. M., and S. A. Sweetana. 1988. In vitro measurement of gastrointestinal tissue permeability using a new diffusion cell. *Pharm. Res.* 5:372–376.

Grosvenor, M. P., and J. E. Löfroth. 1995. Interaction between bile salts and beta-adrenoceptor antagonists. *Pharm. Res.* 12:682–686.

Hanisch, G., M. Kjerling, A. Pålsson, B. Abrahamsson, and A.-L. Ungell. 1999. Effects of vehicles for sparingly soluble compounds on the drug absorption *in vivo*. Abstract from conference: *Elderly people & medicines*, Stockholm conference center Älvsjö, 11–13 October.

Hanisch, G., C. von Corswant, K. Breitholtz, S. Bergstrand, and A.-L. Ungell. 1998. Can mucosal damage be minimised during permeability measurements of sparingly soluble compounds? *Fourth International Conf. on Drug Absorption: Towards prediction and enhancement of drug absorption*, Edinburgh.

Hidalgo, I. J., T. J. Raub, and R. T. Borchardt. 1989. Characterization of the human colon carcinoma cell line (Caco-2) as a model for intestinal epithelial permeability. *Gastroenterology* 96:736–749.

Hidalgo, I. J., P. Bhatnagar, C.-P. Lee, J. Miller, G. Cucullino, and P. L. Smith. 1995. Structural requirements for interaction with the oligopeptide transporter in Caco-2 cells. *Pharm. Res.* 12:317–319.

Hillgren, K. M., A. Kato, and R. T. Borchardt. 1995. *In vitro* systems for studying intestinal drug absorption. *Medicinal Res. Rev.* 15:83–109.

Hintz, R. J., and K. C. Johnson. 1989. The effect of particle size istribution on dissolution rate and oral absorption. *Int. J. Pharm.* 51:9–17.

Hjort-Krarup, L., I. T. Christensen, L. Hovgaard, and S. Frökjaer. 1998. Predicting drug absorption from molecular surface properties based on molecular dynamics simulations. *Pharm. Res.* 15:972–978.

Hunter, J., and B. H. Hirst. 1997. Intestinal secretion of drugs: The role of P-glycoprotein and related drug efflux systems in limiting oral drug absorption. *Adv. Drug Delivery Rev.* 25:129–157.

Hörter, D., and J. B. Dressman. 1997. Influence of physicochemical properties on dissolution of drugs in the gastrointestinal tract. *Adv. Drug Delivery Rev.* 25:3–14.

Illing, H. P. A. 1981. Techniques for microfloral and associated metabolic studies in relation to the absorption and enterohepatic circulation of drugs. *Xenobiotica* 11:815–830.

Ishizawa, T., S. Sadahiro, K. Hosoi, I. Tamai, T. Terasaki, and A. Tsuji. 1992. Mechanisms of intestinal absorption of the antibiotic, fosfomycin, in brush-border membrane vesicles in rabbits and humans. *J. Pharmacobio-Dynamics* 15:481–489.

Jezyk, N., W. Rubas, and G. M. Grass. 1992. Permeability characteristics of various intestinal regions of rabbit, dog and monkey. *Pharm. Res.* 9:1580–1586.

Kaplan, S. A. 1972. Biopharmaceutical considerations in drug formulation design and evaluation. *Drug Metab. Rev.* 1:15–34.

Kararli, T. T. 1989. Gastrointestinal absorption of drugs. *Crit. Rev. Ther. Drug Carrier Systems* 6:39–86.

Kararli, T. T. 1995. Comparison of the gastrointestinal anatomy, physiology, and biochemistry of humans and commonly used laboratory animals. *Biopharmaceut. Drug Disposition* 16:351.

Karlsson, J., and P. Artursson. 1991. A method for the determination of cellular permeability coefficients and aqueous boundary layer thickness in monolayers of intestinal epithelial (Caco-2) cells grown in permeable filter chambers. *Int. J. Pharm.* 71:51–64.

Karlsson, J., A.-L. Ungell, J. Gråsjö, and P. Artursson. 1999. Paracellular drug transport across intestinal epithelia: Influence of charge and induced water flux. *Eur. J. Pharm. Sci.* 9:47–56.

Karlsson, J., A.-L. Ungell, and P. Artursson. 1994. Effect of an oral rehydration solution on paracellular drug transport in intestinal epithelial cells and tissues: Assessment of charge and tissues selectivity. *Pharm. Res.* 11:S248.

Kerneis, S., A. Bogdanova, J.-P. Kraehenbuhl, and E. Pringault. 1997. Conversion by Peyer's patch lymphocytes of human enterocytes into M cells that transport bacteria. *Science* 277:949–952.

Kessler, M., O. Acuto, C. Storelli, H. Murer, M. Muller, and G. Semenza. 1978. A modified procedure for the rapid preparation of efficiently transporting vesicles from small intestinal brush border membranes. *Biochim. Biophys. Acta* 506:136–154.

Kim, D. C., P. S. Burton, and R. T. Borchardt. 1993. A correlation between the permeability characteristics of a series of peptides using an in vitro cell culture model (Caco-2) and those using an in situ perfused rat ileum model of the intestinal mucosa. *Pharm. Res.* 10:1710–1714.

Kim, J. S., R. L. Oberle, D. A. Krummel, J. B. Dressman, and D. Fleischer. 1994. Absorption of ACE inhibitors from small intestine and colon. *J. Pharm. Sci.* 83:1350–1356.

Krugliak, P., D. Hollander, C. C. Schlaepfer, H. Nguyen, and T. Y. Ma. 1994. Mechanisms and sites of mannitol permeability of small and large intestine in the rat. *Digestive dis. Sci.* 39:796–801.

Kuo, S.-M., B. Whitby, P. Artursson, and A. Ziemniak. 1994. Carrier-mediated transport of celiprolol in rat intestine. *Pharm. Res.* 11:648–653.

Leahy, D. H., J. Lynch, and D. C. Taylor. 1989. Mechanisms of absorption of small molecules. In *Novel drug delivery*, edited by L. F. Prescott and W. S. Nimmo. New York: Wiley and Sons, pp. 33–40.

LeCluyse, E. L., and S. C. Sutton. 1997. In vitro models for selection of development candidates. Permeability studies to define mechanisms of absorption enhancement. *Adv. Drug Delivery Rev.* 23:163–183.

Lee, C.-P., R. L. A. de Vrueh, and P. L. Smith. 1997. Selection of development candidates based on in vitro permeability measurements. *Adv. Drug Delivery Rev.* 23:47–62.

Lennernäs, H. 1997. Human jejunal effective permeability and its correlation with preclinical drug absorption models. *J. Pharm. Pharmcol.* 49:627–638.

Lennernäs, H., Ö. Ahrenstedt, R. Hallgren, L. Knutson, M. Ryde, and L. K. Paalzow. 1992. Regional jejunal perfusion: A new in vivo approach to study oral drug absorption in man. *Pharm. Res.* 9:1243–1251.

Lennernäs, H., S. Nylander, and A.-L. Ungell. 1997. Jejunal permeability: A comparison between the Ussing chamber technique and the single-pass perfusion in humans. *Pharm. Res.* 14 (5):667–671.

Lennernäs, H., K. Palm, and P. Artursson. 1996. Comparison between active and passive drug transport in human intestinal epithelial (Caco-2) cells in vitro and human jejunum in vivo. *Int. J. Pharm.* 127:103–107.

Leo, A., P. Y. C. Jow, C. Silipo, and C. Hansch. 1975. Calculation of hydrophobic constant (log *P*) from pi and f constants. *J. Med. Chem.* 18:865–868.

Leppert, P. S., and J. A. Fix. 1994. Use of everted intestinal rings for in vitro examination of oral absorption potential. *J. Pharm. Sci.* 83:976–981.

Levich, V. G. 1962. *Physicochemical hydrodynamics.* Englewood Cliffs, N.J., USA: Prentice Hall, pp. 1–80.

Levine, R. R., W. F. McNary, P. J. Kornguth, and R. LeBlanc. 1970. Histological reevaluation of everted gut technique for studying intestinal absorption. *Eur. J. Pharmacol.* 9:211–219.

Lindahl, A., B. Persson, A.-L. Ungell, and H. Lennernäs. 1999. Surface activity and concentration dependent intestinal permeability in the rat. *Pharm. Res.* 16:97–102.

Lindahl, A., R. Sandström, A.-L. Ungell, B. Abrahamsson, T. Knutson, L. Knutson, and H. Lennernäs. 1996. Jejunal permeability and hepatic extraction of fluvastatin in humans. *Clin. Pharmacol. Ther.* 60:1.

Lindahl, A., A.-L. Ungell, L. Knutson, and H. Lennernäs. 1997. Characterisation of fluids from the stomach and proximal jejunum in men and women. *Pharm. Res.* 14:497–502.

Lipinski, C. A., F. Lombardo, B. W. Dominy, and Feeney. 1996. Experimental and computational approaches to estimate solubility and permeability in drug discovery and development settings. *Adv. Drug Delivery Rev.* 23:3–25.

Lindmark, T., J. D. Söderholm, G. Olaisson, G. Alve'n, G. Ocklind, and P. Artursson. 1997. Mechanism of absorption enhancement in humans after rectal administration of ampicillin in suppositories containing sodium caprate. *Pharm. Res.* 14:930–935.

Lundahl, P., and F. Beigi. 1997. Immobilized liposome chromatography of drugs for model analysis of drug-membrane interactions. *Adv. Drug Delivery Rev.* 23:221–227.

Ma, T. Y., D. Hollander, D. Bhalla, H. Nguyen, and P. Krugliak. 1992. IEC-18, a nontransformed small intestinal cell line for studying epithelial permeability. *J. Lab. Clin. Med.* 120:329–341.

MacAdam, A. 1993. The effect of gastrointestinal mucus on drug absorption. *Adv. Drug Del. Rev.* 11:201–220.

Makhey, V. D., A. Guo, D. A. Norris, P. Hu, J. Yan, and P. J. Sinko. 1998. Characterization of the regional intestinal kinetics of drug efflux in rat and human intestine and in Caco-2 cells. *Pharm. Res.* 15:1160–1167.

Mannhold, R., K. P. Dross, and R. F. Rekker. 1990. Drug lipophilicity in QSAR practice: A comparison of experimental with calculated approaches. *Quantitative Structure-Activity Relationship* 9:21–28.

Matthes, I., F. Nimmerfall, J. Vonderscher, and H. Sucker. 1992. Mucus models for investigation of intestinal absorption. Part 4: Comparison of the *in vitro* mucus model with absorption models *in vivo* and *in situ* to predict intestinal absorption. *Pharmazie* 47:787–791.

McEwan, G. T. A., and M. L. Lucas. 1990. The effect of *E. coli* Sta enteroxine on the absorption of weakly dissociable drugs from the rat proximal jejunum in vivo. *Brit. J. Pharmacol.* 101:937–941.

Merino, V., J. Freixas, M. del Val Bermejo, T. M. Garrigues, J. Moreno, and J. M. Pla-Delfina. 1995. Biophysical models as an approach to study passive absorption in drug development: 6-fluoroquinolones. *J. Pharm. Sci.* 84 (6):777–782.

Narawane, M., S. K. Podder, H. Bundgaard, and V. H. L. Lee. 1993. Segmental differences in drug permeability, esterase activity and ketone reductase activity in the albino rabbit intestine. *J. Drug Targeting* 1:29–39.

Navia, M. A., and P. R. Chaturvedi. 1996. Drug discovery today. *Res. Focus Rev.* 1:179.

Neuhoff, S., H. Spahn-Langguth, C.-G. Regårdh, T. B. Andersson, U. Norinder, and P. Langguth. 1999. Computational approach to predict affinity of drugs to MDR1 encoded P-glycoprotein using Mol-Surf parametrization. *Arch. Pharm. Med. Chem.* 331 (suppl. 2):33.

Niklasson, M., A. Brodin, and L-O. Sundelöf. 1985. Studies of some characteristics of molecular dissolution kinetics from rotating discs. *Int. J. Pharm.* 23:97–108.

Niklasson, M., and A-B. Magnusson. 1985. Program for evaluating drug dissolution kinetics in preformulation. *Pharm. Res.* 253–320.

Norinder, U., T. Österberg, and P. Artursson. 1997. Theoretical calculation and prediction of Caco-2 cell permeability using MolSurf parametrization and PLS statistics. *Pharm. Res.* 14:1785–1791.

Oberle, R. L., T. J. Moore, and D. A. P. Krummel. 1995. Evolution of mucosal damage of surfactants in rat jejunum and colon. *J. Pharmacol. Toxicol. Methods* 33:75–81.

Oeschsenfahrt, H., and D. Winne. 1974. The contribution of solvent drag to the intestinal absorption of the basic drugs amidopyridine and antipyrine from the jejunum of the rat. *Naunyn-Schmiedeberg's Arch. Pharmacol.* 281:175–196.

Örnskov, E., J. Gottfries, and S. Folestad. 2001. Correlation of drug absorption with migration data from capillary electrophoresis using micellar electrolytes. *J. Pharm. Sci.*, in press.

Osiecka, I., P. A. Porter, R. T. Borchardt, J. A. Fix, and C. R. Gardner. 1985. *In vitro* drug absorption models. I. Brush border membrane vesicles, isolated mucosal cells and everted intestinal rings: Characterization and salicylate accumulation. *Pharm. Res.* 2:284–293.

Österberg, T., and U. Norinder. 2000. Theoretical calculation and prediction of P-glycoprotein-interacting drugs using MolSurf parametrization and PLS statistics. *Eur. J. Pharm. Sci.* 10:295–303.

Pade, V., and S. Stavchansky. 1998. Link between drug absorption solubility and permeability measurements in Caco-2 cells. *J. Pharm. Sci.* 87:1604–1607.

Paine, M. F., M. Khalighi, J. M. Fisher, D. Shen, K. L. Kunze, and C. L. Marsh. 1997. Characterization of interintestinal and intraintestinal variations in human CYP3A-dependent metabolism. *J. Pharmacol. Exp. Ther.* 288:1552–1562.

Palm, K., K. Luthman, A.-L. Ungell, G. Strandlund, and P. Artursson. 1996. Correlation of drug absorption with molecular surface properties. *J. Pharm. Sci.* 85:32.

Palm, K., L. P. Stenberg, K. Luthman, and P. Artursson. 1997. Polar molecular surface properties predict the intestinal absorption of drugs in humans. *Pharm. Res.* 14:568–571.

Pantzar, N., B. R. Weström, A. Luts, and S. Lundin. 1993. Regional small-intestinal permeability *in vitro* to different sized dextrans and proteins in the rat. *Scand. J. Gastroenterol.* 28:205–211.

Pantzar, N., S. Lundin, L. Wester, and B. R. Weström. 1994. Bidirectional small-intestinal permeability in the rat to common marker molecules in vitro. *Scand. J. Gastroenterol.* 29:703–709.

Parr, A. F., E. P. Sandefer, P. Wissel, M. McCartney, C. McClain, U. Y. Ryo, and G. A. Digenis. 1999. Evaluation of the feasibility and use of a prototype remote drug delivery capsule (RDDC) for noninvasive regional drug absorption studies in the GI tract of man and beagle dog. *Pharm. Res.* 16:266–271.

Pascoe, G. A., J. Sakai-Wong, E. Soliven, and M. A. Correia. 1983. Regulation of intestinal cytochrome P450 and heme by dietary nutrients. *Biochem. Pharmacol.* 32:3027–3035.

Perez-Buendia, M. D., B. Gomez-Perez, and J. M. Pla-Delfina. 1993. Permeation mechanisms through artificial lipoidal membranes and effects of synthetic surfactants on xenobiotic permeability. *Arzneim Forsch* 43:789–794.

Pidgeon, C., S. Ong, H. Liu, X. Qiu, M. Pidgeon, A. H. Dantzig, J. Munroe, W. J. Hornback, J. S. Kasher, L. Glunz, and T. Szczerba. 1995. IAM chromatography: An in vitro screen for predicting drug membrane permeability. *J. Med. Chem.* 38:590–594.

Pilbrant, Å., and C. Cederberg. 1985. Development of an oral formulation of omeprazol. *Scand. J. Gastroenterol.* Suppl 20, 108:113–120.

Polentarutti, B., A. Peterson, Å. Sjöberg, E.-K. Anderberg, L. Utter, and A.-L. Ungell. 1999. Evaluation of viability of excised rat intestinal segments in the Ussing chamber: Investigation of morphology, electrical parameters and permeability characteristics. *Pharm. Res.* 16:446–454.

Porter, P. A., I. Osiecka, R. T. Borchardt, J. A. Fix, L. Frost, and C. R. Gardner. 1985. *In vitro* drug absorption models. II: Salicylate, cefoxitin, alphamethyl dopa and theophylline uptake in cells and rings: Correlation with in vivo bioavailability. *Pharm. Res.* 2:293–298.

Quilianova, N., Y. Chen, A. Richard, and Z. Hu. 1999. Drug absorption screening model using rabbit intestinal brush border membrane vesicles (BBMV). Abstract from *AAPS meeting in Washington on membrane transporters*. April 1999, Washington.

Rathbone, M. J., and I. G. Tucker. 1991. Mechanisms, barriers and pathways of oral mucosal drug permeation. *Adv. Drug Delivery Rev.* 12:41–60.

Rubas, W., N. Jezyk, and G. M. Grass. 1993. Comparison of the permeability characteristics of a human colonic epithelial (Caco-2) cell line to colon of rabbit, monkey and dog intestine and human drug absorption. *Pharm. Res.* 10:113–118.

Saffran, M., G. S. Kumar, C. Savariar, J. C. Burnheim, F. Williams, and D. C. Neckers. 1986. A new approach to the oral administration of insulin and other peptide drugs. *Science* 233:1081–1084.

Sandström, R., A. Karlsson, L. Knutsson, and H. Lennernäs. 1998. Jejunal absorption and metabolism of R/S-verapamil in humans. *Pharm. Res.* 15:856–562.

Saitoh, H., and B. J. Aungst. 1995. Possible involvement of multiple P-glycoprotein mediated efflux systems in the transport of verapamil and other organic cations across rat intestine. *Pharm. Res.* 12:1304–1310.

Schwaan, P. W., R. C. Stehouwer, and J. J. Tukker. 1995. Molecular mechanism for the relative binding affinity to the intestinal peptide carrier. Comparison of three ACE inhibitors: Enalapril, enalaprilat and lisinopril. *Biochim. Biophys. Acta-Biomembranes* 1236:31–38.

Sekine, M., H. Terashima, K. Sasahara, K. Nishimura, R. Okada, and S. Awazu. 1985. Improvement of bioavailability of poorly absorbed II. Effect of medium-chain glyceride base on the intestinal absorption of cefmetazole sodium in rats and dogs. *J. Pharmacobio. Dyn.* 8:286–295.

Shamat, M. A. 1993. The role of the gastrointestinal microflora in the metabolism of drugs. *Int. J. Pharmaceut.* 97:1–13.

Sjöström, M., L. Lindfors, and A.-L. Ungell. 1999. Inhibition of binding of an enzymatically stable thrombin inhibitor to luminal proteases as an additional mechanism of intestinal absorption enhancement. *Pharm. Res.* 16:74–79.

Söderholm, J. D., L. Hedamn, P. Artursson, L. Franzen, J. Larsson, N. Pantzar, J. Permert, and G. Olaison. 1998. Integrity and metabolism of human ileal mucosa in vitro in the Ussing chamber. *Acta Physiol. Scand.* 162:47–56.

Stewart, B. H., O. H. Chan, R. H. Lu, E. L. Reyner, H. L. Schmid, H. W. Hamilton, B. A. Steinbaugh, and M. D. Taylor. 1995. Comparison of intestinal permeabilities determined in multiple *in vitro* and *in situ* models: Relationship to absorption in humans. *Pharm. Res.* 12 (5):693–699.

Stewart, B. H., O. H. Chan, N. Jezyk, and D. Fleischer. 1997. Discrimination between drug candidates using models for evaluation of intestinal absorption. *Adv. Drug Delivery Rev.* 23:27–45.

Strocchi, A., and M. D. Levitt. 1993. Role of villus surface area in absorption. *Dig. Dis. Sci.* 38:385.

Surendran, N., S. O. Ugwu, L. D. Nguyen, E. J. Sterling, R. T. Dorr, and J. Blanchard. 1995. Absorption enhancement of melanotan—1: Comparison of the Caco-2 and rat in situ models. *Drug Delivery: J. Delivery Target Ther. Agents* 2:49–55.

Sutton, S. C., A. E. Forbes, R. Cargyll, J. H. Hochman, and E. L. Le Cluyse. 1992. Simultaneous in vitro measurement of intestinal tissue permeability and transepithelial electrical resistance (TEER) using Sweetana-Grass diffusion cells. *Pharm. Res.* 9:316–319.

Swenson, E. S., W. B. Milisen, and W. Curatolo. 1994. Intestinal permeability enhancement: Efficacy, acute toxicity and reversibility. *Pharm. Res.* 11:1132–1142.

Tamamatsu, N., L. S. Welage, N. M. Idkaldek, D.-Y. Liu, P. I.-D. Lee, Y. Hayashi, J. K. Rhie, H. Lennernäs, J. L. Barnett, V. Shah, L. Lesko, and G. L. Amidon. 1997. Human intestinal permeability of piroxicam, propranolol, phenylalanine, and PEG 400 determined by jejunal perfusion. *Pharm. Res.* 14:1127–1132.

Tanaka, Y., Y. Taki, T. Sakane, T. Nadai, H. Sezaki, and S. Yamashita. 1995. Characterization of drug transport through tight-junctional pathway in Caco-2 monolayer: Comparison with isolated rat jejunum and colon. *Pharm. Res.* 12:523–528.

Thomson, A. B. R., M. Keelan, M. T. Clandinin, and K. Walker. 1986. Dietary fat selectively alters transport properties of rat jejunum. *J. Clin. Invest.* 77:279–288.

Tsuji, A., and I. Tamai. 1996. Carrier-mediated intestinal transport of drugs. *Pharm. Res.* 13:963–977.

Uch, A. S., and J. Dressman. 1997. Improved methodology for uptake studies in intestinal rings. *Pharm. Res.* 14 (11):S-29.

Uch, A. S., U. Hesse, and J. B. Dressman. 1999. Use of 1-methyl-pyrrolidone as a solubilising agent for determining the uptake of poorly soluble drugs. *Pharm. Res.* 16 (6):968–971.

Uhing, M. R., and R. E. Kimura. 1995a. The effect of surgical bowel manipulation and anaesthesia on intestinal glucose absorption in rats. *J. Clin. Invest.* 95:2790–2798.

Uhing, M. R., and R. E. Kimura. 1995b. Active transport of 3-O-methyl-glucose by the small intestine in chronically catheterised rats. *J. Clin. Invest.* 95:2799–2805.

Ungell, A.-L. 1997. *In vitro* absorption studies and their relevance to absorption from the GI tract. *Drug Dev. Indust. Pharm.* 23 (9):879–892.

Ungell, A.-L., A. Andreasson, K. Lundin, and L. Utter. 1992. Effects of enzymatic inhibition and increased paracellular shunting on transport of vasopressin analogues in the rat. *J. Pharm. Sci.* 81:640.

Ungell, A.-L., S. Nylander, S. Bergstrand, Å. Sjöberg, and H. Lennernäs. 1997. Membrane transport of drugs in different regions of the intestinal tract of the rat. *J. Pharm. Sci.* 87:360–366.

Ussing, H. H., and K. Zerhan. 1951. Active transport of sodium as the source of electric current in the short-circuited isolated frog skin. *Acta Physiol. Scand.* 23:110–127.

van den Mooter, G., B. Maris, C. Samyn, P. Augustijns, and R. Kinget. 1997. Use of Azo polymers for colon-specific drug delivery. *J. Pharm. Sci.* 86:1321–1327.

van der Waterbeemd, H., G. Camenisch, G. Folkers, and O. Raevsky. 1996. Estimation of Caco-2 cell permeability using calculated molecular descriptors. *Quant. Struct. Act. Relat.* 15:480–490.

van Hoogdalem, E. J., A. G. de Boer, and D. D. Breimer. 1989. Intestinal drug absorption enhancement. *Pharm. Ther.* 44:407–443.

Wacher, V. J., C.-Y. Wu, and L. Z. Benet. 1995. Overlapping substrate specificities and tissue distribution of cytochrome P450 3A and P-glycoprotein: Implications for drug delivery and activity in cancer chemotherapy. *Mol. Carcinog.* 13:129–134.

Wacher, V. J., J. A. Silvermann, Y. Zhang, and L. Z. Benet. 1998. Role of p-glycoprotein and cytochrome P450 3A in limiting oral absorption of peptides and peptidomimetics. *J. Pharm. Sci.* 87:1322–1330.

Walter, E., T. Kissel, M. Reers, G. Dickneite, D. Hoffmann, and W. Stuber. 1995. Transepithelial transport properties of peptidomimetic thrombin inhibitors in monolayers of a human intestinal cell line (Caco-2) and their correlation to *in vivo data. Pharm. Res.* 12:360.

Wenzel, U., I. Gebert, H. Weintraut, W.-M. Weber, W. Clauss, and H. Daniel. 1996. Transport characteristics of differently charged cephalosporin antibiotics in oocytes expressing the cloned intestinal peptide transporter PepT1 and in human intestinal Caco-2 cells. *J. Pharmacol. Exp. Ther.* 277:831–839.

Wikman, A., J. Karlsson, I. Carlstedt, and P. Artursson. 1993. A drug absorption model based on the mucus layer producing human intestinal goblet cell line HT29-H. *Pharm. Res.* 10 (6):843–852.

Wils, P., A. A. Warnery, V. Phung-Ba, S. Llegrain, and D. Scherman. 1994a. High lipophilicity decreases drug transport across intestinal epithelial cells. *J. Pharmacol. Exp. Ther.* 269:654.

Wils, P., A. Warnery, V. Phung-Ba, and D. Scherman. 1994b. Differentiated intestinal epithelial cell lines as in vitro models for predicting the intestinal absorption of drugs. *Cell Biol. Toxicol.* 10 (5–6):393–397.

Windmueller, H. G., A. E. Spaeth, and C. E. Ganote. 1970. Vascular perfusion of isolated rat gut: Norepinephrine and glucocorticoid requirements. *Amer. J. Physiol.* 218:197–204.

Wingstrand, K., B. Abrahamsson, and B. Edgar. 1990. Bioavailability from felodipine extended-release tablets with different dissolution properties. Int. J. Pharm. 60:151–156.

Winiwarter, S., N. M. Bonham, F. Ax, A. Hallberg, L. Lennernäs, and A. Karle'n. 1998. Correlation of human jejunal permeability (*in vivo*) of drugs with experimentally and theoretically derived parameters. A multivariate data analysis approach. *J. Med. Chem.* 41:4939–4949.

Winne, D. 1979. Rat jejunum perfused in situ: Effect of perfusion rate and intraluminal radius on absorption rate and effective unstirred layer thickness. *Naunyn-Schmiedeberg's Arch. Pharmacol.* 307:265–274.

Yamaguchi, T., C. Ikeda, and Y. Sekine. 1986a. Intestinal absorption of a beta-adrenergic blocking agent nadolol. I: Comparison of absorption behaviour of nadolol with those of other beta-blocking agents in the rat. *Chem. Pharm. Bull.* 24:3362–3369.

Yamaguchi, T., C. Ikeda, and Y. Sekine. 1986b. Intestinal absorption of a beta-adrenergic blocking agent nadolol.II: Mechanism of the inhibitory effect on the intestinal absorption of nadolol by sodium cholate in rats. *Chem. Pharm. Bull.* 34:3836–3843.

Yamaguchi, T., T. Oida, and C. Ikeda. 1986c. Intestinal absorption of a beta-adrenergic blocking agent nadolol. III: Nuclear magnetic resonance spectroscopic study on nadolol-sodium cholate micellar complex and intestinal absorption of nadolol derivatives in rats. *Chem. Pharm. Bull.* 34:4259–4264.

Yang, C. Y., S. J. Cai, H. Liu, and C. Pidgeon. 1997. Immobilized artificial membranes—screens for drug membrane interactions. *Adv. Drug Delivery Rev.* 23:229–256.

Yazdanian, M., S. L. Glynn, J. L. Wright, and H. Hawi. 1997. Correlating partitioning and Caco-2 cell permeability of structurally diverse small molecular weight compounds. *Pharm. Res.* 15:1490–1494.

Yeh, P. Y., P. L. Smith, and H. Ellens. 1994. Effect of medium-chain glycerides on physiological properties of rabbit intestinal epithelium in vitro. *Pharm. Res.* 11:1148–1153.

Yodoya, E., K. Uemura, T. Tenma, T. Fujita, M. Murakami, A. Yamamoto, and S. Muranishi. 1994. Enhanced permeability of tetragastrin across the rat intestinal membrane and its reduced degradation by acylation with various fatty acids. *J. Pharmacol. Exp. Ther.* 27:1509.

Yu, L. X., E. Lipka, J. R. Crison, and G. L. Amidon. 1996. Transport approaches to the biopharmaceutical design of oral drug delivery systems: Prediction of intestinal absorption. *Adv. Drug Delivery Rev.* 19:359–376.

Yuasa, H., G. L. Amidon, and D. Fleischer. 1993. Peptide carrier–mediated transport in intestinal brush border membrane vesicles of rats and rabbits: Cephradine uptake and inhibition. *Pharm. Res.* 10:400–404.

Yuasa, H., D. Fleischer, and G. L. Amidon. 1994. Noncompetetive inhibition of cephradine uptake by enalapril in rabbit intestinal brush border membrane vesicles: An enalapril specific inhibitory binding site on the peptide carrier. *J. Pharmacol. Exp. Ther.* 269:1107–1111.

Zamora, I., and A.-L. Ungell. 2001. Comparison between different absorption models using QSAR. *Pharm. Sci.* (in press).

Part II

EARLY DRUG DEVELOPMENT

5

Early Drug Development: Product Design

Mark Gibson

AstraZeneca R&D Charnwood
Loughborough, United Kingdom

THE IMPORTANCE OF PRODUCT DESIGN

It may seem obvious to state that a new product should be adequately defined before any serious product development is undertaken. In many cases, the value of the design phase is often underestimated in the rush to start development and get products to the market quickly. This can result in much wasted time and valuable resources. It can also lead to reduced staff motivation if a product is developed that is not wanted or if the product definition is constantly changing during development. The quality of the design activities can strongly influence the success of development of the right product to the market and ultimate return on investment.

Several non-pharmaceutical industries have long realised the necessity of investing time and money in an initial product design phase. The automobile, aeroplane or shipbuilding industries, for example, would not think of gearing up for large-scale manufacture of a new model until they were satisfied with the design phase. Thorough market research will have been completed to ensure customer requirements are being met. The product definition and technical specifications will have been agreed on, and the cost of goods estimated, so that the company is satisfied that the venture will be commercially viable! Pharmaceutical companies are now realising the value of product design to achieve successful product development.

Studies have shown that the initial design phase actually requires a relatively small investment, which can greatly influence the nature of the product and its ultimate commercial success (Berliner and Brimson 1988). The return on investment (ROI) of the conceptual design phase was shown to be five times greater than the ROI of later development work to develop and optimise the product and manufacturing process.

A simple definition of "product design" is: "the initial stage of product development, where 'global' agreement is required about the nature of the product to be developed". Figure 1.3 in Chapter 1 illustrates where product design fits into the overall product development process. Effective product design is considered to have the following important benefits:

- To provide clear direction and objectives for the project team

- To gain buy-in and input from all the key functions at the start of development (such as Pharmaceutical Development, Safety, Clinical, Manufacturing Operations, Quality Assurance, Regulatory and Marketing)

- To assess the feasibility of the project in commercial and technical terms

- To identify any risks early and hence manage them

- To avoid wasting valuable resources on developing a product which is not needed or wanted

- To provide a good reference source for the development plan

PRODUCT DESIGN CONSIDERATIONS

A useful outcome of the initial product design phase is a Product Design Report. This should document the careful evaluation of the following key elements:

- Target product profile/minimum product profile

- Design specification and critical quality parameters

- Commercial and marketing considerations

- Technical issues and risk assessment

- Safety assessment considerations

- Environmental, health and safety considerations

- Intellectual property considerations

Each of these elements are discussed in more detail below.

Target Product Profile/Minimum Product Profile

A "target product profile" (TPP) which defines the product attributes should be established for the intended marketed product based on all "customer" and "end-user" needs. Customers and end users include anyone in the supply chain, including both internal and external customers, such as those in manufacturing and in sales and marketing, distributors, doctors, nurses, pharmacists and patients. Each customer wants the right product (meeting their quality expectations) at the right time and at the right price. Additionally, each customer will have his or her own specific requirements.

The TPP is often expressed primarily in clinical terms, but should also include the pharmaceutical, technical, regulatory and commercial/marketing attributes required of the product. The TPP is based on the ideal product characteristics which are considered to be desirable, whereas the minimum product profile is based on the minimum product requirements which must be met for the product to be viable and worth developing. For example, the TPP may stipulate an ideal dosing regimen of once daily. However, the minimum product profile may state that the dosing regimen must be no more than twice daily for the product to be competitive.

The ideal attributes for a fictitious product profile example prepared for a product being developed to treat osteoarthritis is shown in Table 5.1.

Table 5.1
Target product profile for a fictitious product to treat osteoarthritis.

Key Attributes	Target Product Profile
Disease to be treated	Osteoarthritis
Patient type (e.g., geriatric, paediatric)	Adults over 40 years, including geriatrics
Route of administration	Oral
Efficacy	Analgesic and anti-inflammatory activity better than "gold standard"
Safety/tolerability	No GI side-effects
	No interactions with other agents
Pharmaco-economics	Reduced healthcare costs by preventing disease progression
Dosage/presentation (type/size)	Immediate release tablet
	No more than two strengths
Dose and dose frequency	Once daily
Pack design/type	Blister calendar pack with moisture barrier
	Must be able to be opened by patient
	Tamper evident
Process	Use standard processing equipment for tablets
Aesthetic aspects (colour, flavours, taste, etc.)	Colour to differentiate tablet strengths
	Taste masked to reduce bitterness
Territories to be marketed	U.S., Europe, Japan
Cost of goods	No more than 10% of commercial price
Commercial price	Equivalent or less than "gold standard"

The level of information on the dosage form and pack should provide sufficient clarity of detail to enable the Pharmaceutical Development group to plan their development. These pharmaceutical attributes may be documented separately in a "pharmaceutical product profile". A typical example of a pharmaceutical product profile is shown in Table 5.2 for an intravenous injection product, illustrating the level of detail expected in a Product Design Report.

It is clearly beneficial to conduct some early preformulation studies to characterise the candidate drug and to determine the physicochemical properties considered important in the development of the intended dosage form to support product design. Preformulation data from solubility, stressed stability, excipient compatibility and other preformulation studies may influence the selection of the formulation dosage form and excipients. The results may also influence the choice of manufacturing process, as shown in the example in Table 5.2, where terminal sterilisation by autoclaving has been shown not to be feasible. The preformulation data should also help to establish the critical quality parameters for the product. In Chapter 6 of this book, Gerry Steele discusses in much greater detail the preformulation studies that may be undertaken to support product design.

The formulation developed for early clinical trials (Phase I) is often a simple one and different from the intended commercial dosage form. A parallel development approach can significantly reduce development time by delinking early clinical supply with commercial formulation development. However, the product profile in the Product Design Report is for the intended commercial product. This information is required at the start of development so that the final commercial product and simple clinical formulation can both be developed in parallel to avoid affecting the medical needs or timings. For example, the commercial formulation could be a film-coated tablet, but the early clinical formulation may be a simple oral solution or suspension or a hand-filled capsule. Regulatory authorities will be interested in the linkage between formulations used in early clinical studies and those used in the pivotal

Table 5.2

Example of a pharmaceutical product profile for an intravenous solution.

Key Attributes	Target Product Profile
Dosage form presentation	Single-dose, non-preserved
Primary pack	Type I clear glass vial (10 mL)
	Rubber stopper
	Aluminium overseal
Secondary pack	Carton with patient instruction leaflet
Product strength range	10 to 50 mg in 5 mL
Excipient to be evaluated:	
Tonicity adjustment	Dextrose or saline
Buffer	Phosphate or citrate
Antioxidant	Sodium metabisulphite or acetylcysteine
Manufacturing process	Aseptic manufacture/sterile filtration (terminal sterilisation by autoclaving not possible)

(Phase III) studies and the final commercial product. The objective of many companies is to optimise and finalise the commercial product (formulation and process) for the start of the pivotal clinical studies, to minimise any regulatory concerns.

Meeting Customer Needs

There are various methods and tools available for gathering information about customer needs to establish the product profile. It is not the intention of this book to cover this in great detail, and only an overview is given here.

A primary source of information is usually held within the pharmaceutical company, particularly if the company is already established with marketed products in a particular therapeutic area. Most companies will have a variety of information representing the voice of their customers. Much of this may be negative in the form of complaints and letters from users. These can be valuable sources of information to consider in the development of better products. It is important that all of the company"s internal departments involved in product development are consulted. These internal departments include Pharmaceutical Development, Design Engineering, Manufacturing Operations, Quality Assurance, Safety/Toxicology, Medical and Marketing. They should be involved in the product design and product profile discussions, as they are also key internal customers. However, it is important to recognise that these internal customers' perceptions and requirements may be far removed from those of external customers.

If a company is venturing into a new therapeutic area, or is endeavouring to learn more about the changing needs of the market, external customers and end users in the supply chain need to be consulted for their views about current treatments and shortfalls. There are various ways of achieving feedback. For example, surveys can be conducted by sending out questionnaires or by telephoning key customers and end users to gather perception data. Alternatively, clinics and focus groups can be set up to gain insight into customers' wants and perceptions. Clinicians, doctors, patients or other customers may be asked to attend small focus groups, facilitated by medical, marketing or pharmaceutical personnel, to discuss their likes and dislikes. This type of forum can be useful for demonstrating samples and prototypes of devices and drug delivery systems. Other ways of obtaining feedback include setting up individual interviews with opinion leaders in the field and generally listening to customers' comments at conferences, exhibitions and trade shows. Consultancy organisations are often hired to gather this type of information on behalf of the pharmaceutical company developing a new product.

The Pharmaceutical Development group can play a leading role in determining the pharmaceutical requirements for a new product from key customers. Customers may want more specific packs or delivery systems, and different markets still have their own preferences for different dosage forms.

Quality function deployment (QFD), also referred to as "customer driven engineering" and "matrix product planning", is a useful quality and planning tool which uses a structured approach in defining all the customer needs or requirements and translates these into design requirements for product development.

QFD originated in Japan in the late 1960s and was initially applied to shipbuilding, where large capital investments are made and design and planning need to be thorough. Through the 1970s and 1980s, there was a rapid increase in the application of QFD to all industries in Japan, and in the 1980s and 1990s, it was accepted in the United States and Europe as a means of quality improvement (Akao 1990; Day 1993; Mizuno and Akao 1994)

The QFD basic approach is to start with customer requirements, which are usually vague qualitative items such as easy to use, feels good, lasts a long time. These vague customer requirements are converted into internal company design requirements that are measurable and can be used objectively to evaluate the product. If the company requirements are properly introduced, the product should satisfy all the customer requirements. The company requirements must then be translated into specific parts of the product, and the characteristics of these specific parts should cause the essential functions to be performed.

Customer Requirements ➡ Company Requirements (measures)
➡ Design Characteristics (specific parts)

QFD is accomplished through a series of charts, sometimes referred to as "the House of Quality" because the shape of the charts have a rooflike structure at the top (see Figure 5.1). Ideally, the chart should be developed by a cross-functional team made up from members of the core functions in product development. The first step in building the House of Quality is to list the customer requirements, "the WHATs", down the left-hand side of the matrix (area 1 in Figure 5.1). Each of the WHATs is translated into one or more global customer characteristics or design requirements, "the HOWs", and listed across the top of the matrix (area 2). The design requirements will usually be measurable characteristics which can be evaluated on the completed product. The next step is to complete the relationship matrix in the centre (area 3). The strength of the relationship between each customer requirement and technical requirement is depicted by using different symbols and weightings. For example, "strong" = 9, "medium" = 3 and "weak" = 1. A blank column in the relationships matrix could indicate a design requirement that is not really needed.

Next, the team completes area 4, comprising measurements for the design requirements (HOW MUCH). These objective target values should represent how good the product has to be to satisfy the customer and need not necessarily represent current performance levels. These values are required to provide an objective means of assuring that requirements have been met and to provide targets for further detailed development.

In area 5, the roof of the house, the correlation matrix establishes any potential synergies or conflicts between each design requirement (HOW). The purpose is to identify areas where trade-off decisions may be required. Symbols are often used to describe the strength of the relationship, for example, positive, strong positive, negative and strong negative. From the matrix, it should be possible to identify which of the design requirements support one another and which are in conflict. Positive correlations are important because some resource efficiencies may be gained by not duplicating efforts to attain the same result. Negative correlations are also important because they indicate conditions where trade-offs are suggested. There may be ways of eliminating trade-offs by introducing some degree of innovation, which may lead to competitive advantage and patent opportunities. Trade-off resolution is achieved by adjusting the values of the targets for customer requirements (HOW MUCH).

The competitive assessment is a pair of graphs (areas 6 and 7) which depict item for item how competitive products compare with current company products. This is completed for both the customer requirements (WHATs) and the design requirements (HOWs). The customer competitive assessment is important to understand the customer's perception of the product relative to the competition, whereas the technical competitive assessment is undertaken by the company's product development experts to gain an internal view.

The final step in constructing the QFD chart is to establish the importance ratings. The customer importance rating (area 8) is based on customer assessment and is expressed as a relative scale (typically 1 to 5), with the higher numbers indicating greater importance to the

Figure 5.1 The QFD diagram: "the House of Quality".

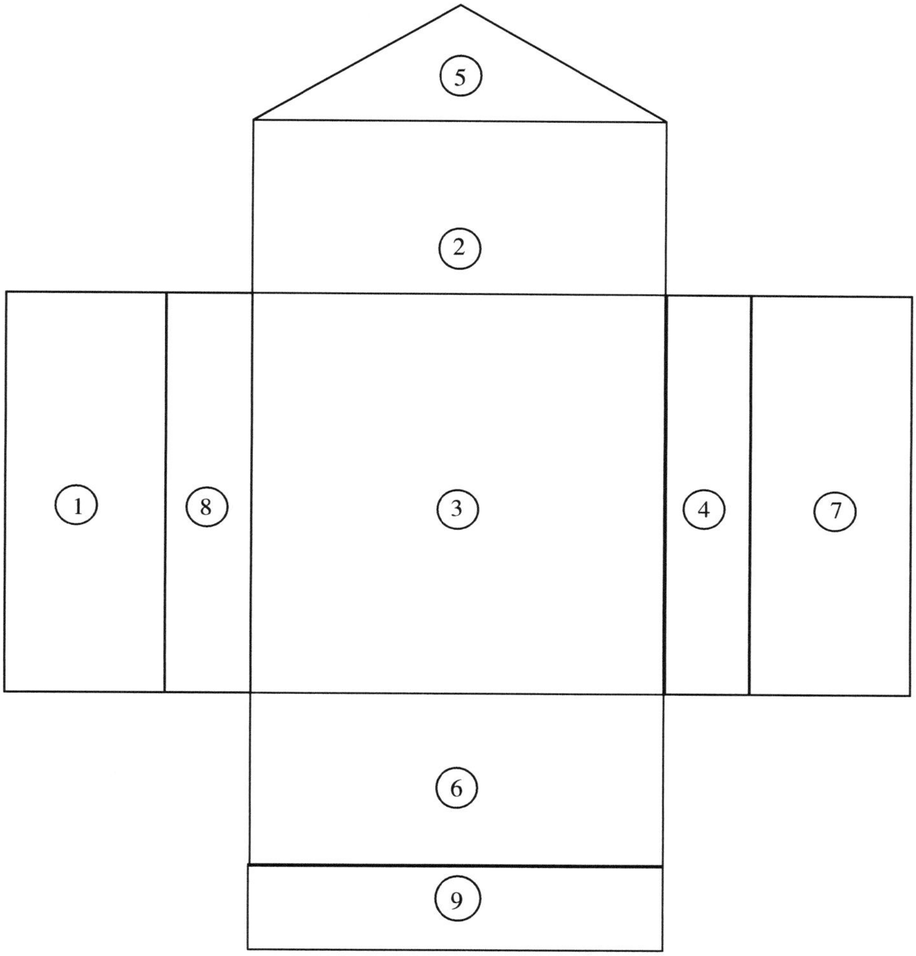

Key:

1. Customer requirements (WHATs)
2. Design requirements (HOWs)
3. Relationship matrix
4. Objective targets for customer's requirements (HOW MUCH)
5. Correlation matrix
6. Customer competitive assessment
7. Technical competitive assessment
8. Customer importance rating
9. Technical importance rating

customer. It is vital that these values represent the true customer needs and not just internal company perceptions. Importance ratings for the design requirements (HOWs) are calculated by multiplying the value of the symbols in the relationship matrix for each cell (9, 3 or 1) by the corresponding customer importance rating and summing the products down the columns (area 9). The importance ratings are useful for prioritising efforts and making trade-off decisions. The values have no direct meaning but rank in relative importance the customer and technical requirements that have to be satisfied.

Figure 5.2 provides a typical example of a completed top level QFD chart for a fictitious metered dose inhaler (MDI) product to be used for the treatment of asthma.

The QFD concept can be further utilised by cascading the voice of the customer through a series of matrices or phases. In the product development process, this involves taking the customer requirements and defining design requirements. Some of the design requirements are translated to the next chart to establish the optimum design characteristics. This is continued to define the optimum manufacturing process requirements and production requirements. In practice, this is achieved by creating new charts in which the HOWs of the previous chart become the WHATs of the new chart, as illustrated in Figure 5.3.

While the QFD charts are a good planning and documentation tool, the real value is in the process of communicating and decision making within a company because the process encourages input from multiple functional disciplines involved in product development. The active participation of the various disciplines should lead to a more balanced consideration of the customer and design requirements and, ultimately, increased customer/end-user satisfaction. Having said that, the perceived complexity of the QFD charts, and getting buy-in from across the company, can be barriers to success. However, QFD should help to maintain a focus on the true requirements and requires more time to be spent at the start of development, thereby ensuring that the company determines, understands and agrees with what needs to be done before rushing into development activities. When appropriately applied, QFD has demonstrated that design changes are less likely later in development and has shown a corresponding reduction in development time to market (Akao 1990).

Design Specifications and Critical Quality Parameters

In addition to the preformulation information, there will be other considerations in the selection of the excipients and packaging components for the product. Taking the intravenous injection example in Table 5.2, it may be important to stipulate that any excipient used must be of parenteral grade, will comply with pharmacopoeial requirements and be restricted to those known to be safe and acceptable to the regulatory authorities. This will reduce the risk, compared to using a novel excipient, which might be questionable to some regulatory authorities. It will also reassure the Safety/Toxicology Department that no extra toxicological studies will be required to approve a new excipient.

Similarly, a list of requirements can be produced for the primary pack, such as the following:

- The pack will be acceptable to regulatory authorities (other approved marketed products already use this type of pack).

- Only packs which can be multiple sourced from more than one supplier/country will be used.

- The pack must have consistency of dimensions and performance.

- The pack will meet function/user tests and specifications.

These dimensions, performance limits and function/user test limits should be specified in the Product Design Report.

Figure 5.2 A fictitious QFD chart for metered dose inhaler.

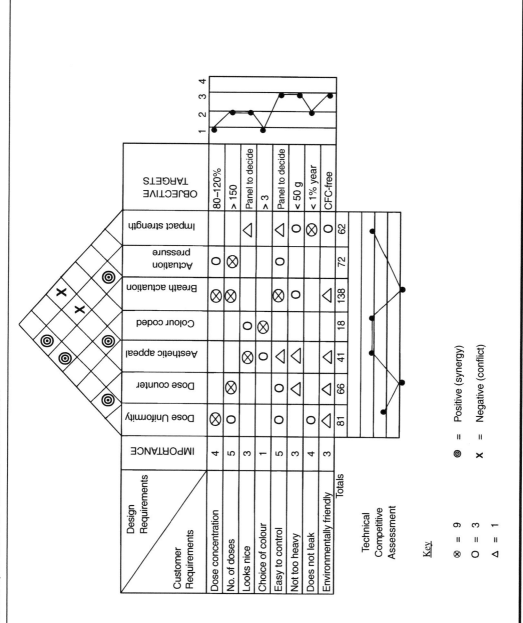

Figure 5.3 QFD: cascading the voice of the customer.

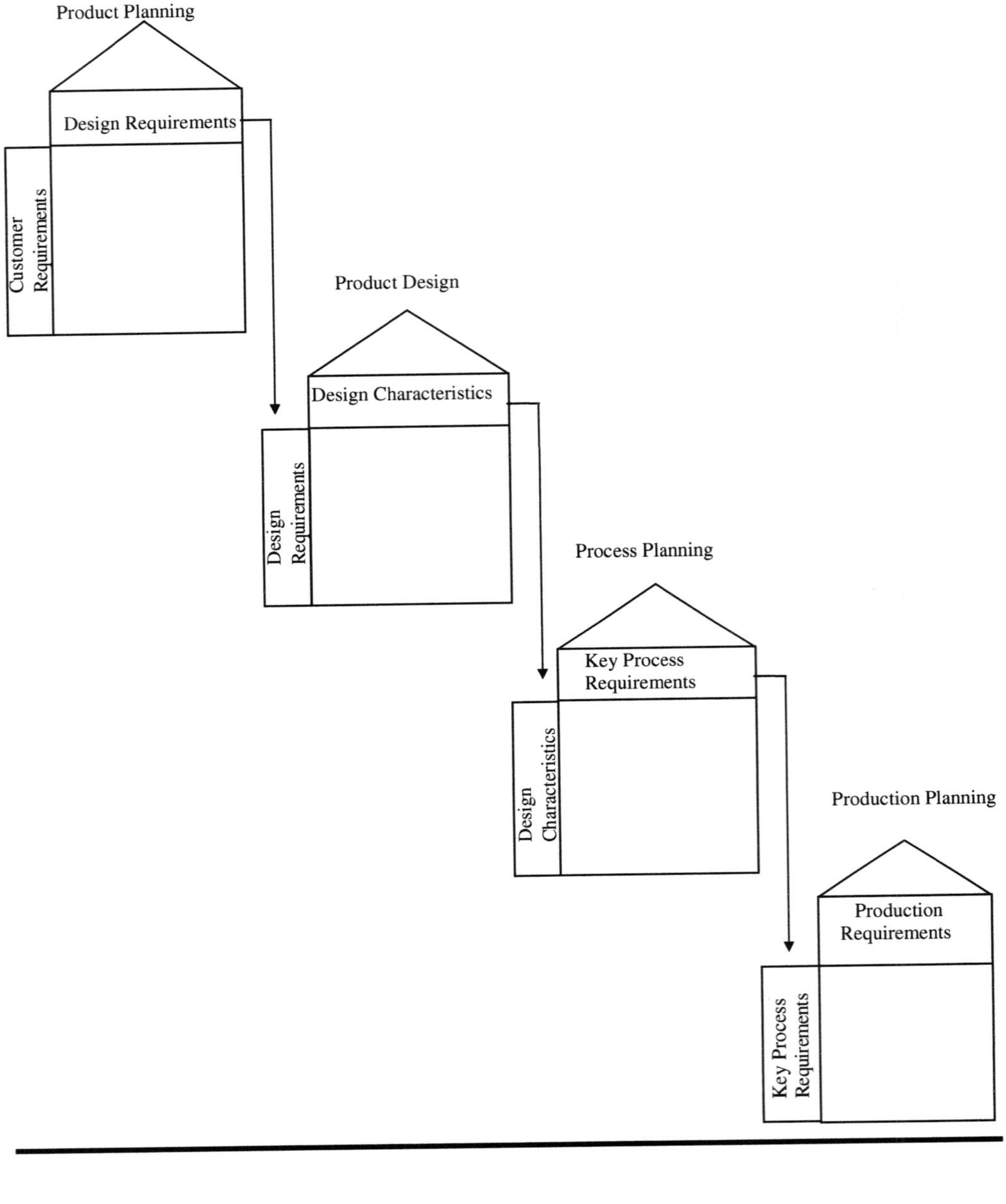

Even though the product has not yet been developed, a high-quality product specification can be proposed with tests and limits that the product should meet at the time of manufacture and at the end of shelf life. For the intravenous product example, tests might include appearance (clear, particle free), pH, osmolality, particulate levels, sterility and endotoxin levels. Appropriate standards or limits can also be proposed based on the knowledge of similar types of products that have already been developed and from standard pharmacopoeial monographs.

Finally, in this section, it is useful to agree on what the minimum acceptable shelf life for the product should be. The product will need to be stable enough to allow time for quality control (QC) testing and quality assurance (QA) release after manufacture; distribution to wholesalers, pharmacists and doctors; and with acceptable time for storage until prescribed and used by patients. Normally, a minimum three-year shelf life at room temperature is targeted. However, if the treatment is very novel, it may be possible to justify a shorter shelf life and/or storage at lower temperatures, if stability is likely to be a problem.

Commercial and Marketing Considerations

Any pharmaceutical company's economic objective must be to maximise its ROI after launch. Therefore, the commercial viability of a new product to be developed needs to be commercially assessed at the product design stage to satisfy the company that it will achieve a satisfactory ROI. Some of the factors that should be considered in the evaluation are as follows:

- Development costs

- Timing to market

- Market size (disease prevalence, diagnosis and treatment rates, market value)

- Competition (current, developing and impact on future market)

- Unmet medical need (effectiveness of current treatment, improvements required)

- Pricing and reimbursement (current and future)

- Cost of goods (target)

The development costs are an estimate of the total costs of development of the product through the various stages of research and development (R&D), including preclinical, clinical, pharmaceutical (drug substance and product) and marketing costs. As a rule, the development costs will increase exponentially with development time (see Figure 1.2, Chapter 1), and the cost of conducting the Phase III clinical studies are usually the most expensive element of the development programme. Estimates of the total cost of all material, labour and overhead costs should be included.

A major consideration for the development costs is whether to contract out some or all of the work (Spurlin et al. 1996). Contract research organisations (CROs) can offer a broad range of services covering all parts of the drug development process. In terms of product development, preformulation studies, including drug substance characterisation, formulation development, stability testing, clinical trial manufacturing and scale-up/technology transfer, are typically outsourced. In fact, most pharmaceutical companies have to contract out some aspect of R&D because of the diverse requirements and multidisciplinary nature of the work. Taken to the extreme, it is possible to create a "virtual" pharmaceutical company run by a committee of project managers responsible for coordinating the outsourcing of every part of the development programme (Stevenson 1997). However, it is unlikely that major pharmaceutical companies would want to take this approach and not have any internal capability.

There are pros and cons to outsourcing, some of which are summarised in Table 5.3. Clearly, contracting out is not simply a commercial decision. The issues identified if outsourcing is done have to be carefully considered. One significant risk of outsourcing is if the relationship with the CRO goes sour or the CRO goes out of business. It may be difficult to find an alternative without having the detailed technical knowledge.

Table 5.3
Advantages and disadvantages of outsourcing.

Advantages	Disadvantages

• More cost effective:
 	
  −Reduced overhead costs
 	
  −Avoid capital expenditure
 	
  −Reduced cost of goods
 	
  −Reduced training costs
 	
• Access to the best expertise, technology and resources not available within company
 	
• Access to patented technology
 	
• Allows optimal use of internal resource (focus on company strengths)
 	
• Free up resource for other purposes
 	
• Management of peaks and troughs
 	
• Shorter time to achieve results—fast track to market
 	
• Shared risk-joint venture
 	
• Increased probability of success?
 	
• Convenient and efficient
	• A big commitment and initial costs
	
	• Questionable quality and regulatory concerns; detailed audits required
	
	• Secrecy/loss of patent opportunities
	
	• Loss of technical expertise and product knowledge
	
	• Stagnation of in-house competence
	
	• Decreased flexibility moving resources between projects
	
	• Short-term gain—no future development of company
	
	• Dependability on partner

The outsourcing company should be aware of the potential additional costs to simply paying for a package of work. Someone from the parent company has to manage the process, and this can involve several stages:

- Selecting the CRO

- Auditing to ensure technical, commercial and quality standards are acceptable

- Establishing a contract and agreement of the work programme

- Attending reviews to discuss progress or technical issues

- Accepting the end result.

These activities are likely to involve significant parent company investment in time, people and costs, if the outsourcing is to be successful. Some of these issues associated with using and controlling contractors are discussed further by Burton (1997).

An estimate of the timing to market is important to know in order to assess the positioning of the new product in relation to competitor products in development and those already marketed. The use of CROs should be able to speed up development by allowing activities to be conducted in parallel. It is also important to predict what the market size is likely to be at the time of launch, based on market trends. Being first to market with a new treatment can be very advantageous in determining a high commercial price. However, if other competitor products are already established, the market price may be restricted unless some significant benefit can be shown over existing treatments. For example, a novel delivery system or device that improves patient compliance might achieve a higher price than a conventional delivery system.

The potential market size can be estimated from current research data, showing the number of patients in the countries of interest and the total value of treatment. Trends in disease prevalence should be noted, whether the number of patients is increasing or decreasing. However, it should also be noted that market research can sometimes be misleading and could result in missed opportunities. A good example to illustrate this point is the introduction of a new therapeutic class of drugs where there was no existing market. Prior to the introduction of the H2-receptor antagonist cimetidine, there was little evidence that many people suffered from gastric ulcers. It was only after an effective treatment was available that people came forward, and an enormous market was established.

One way of assessing the commercial viability for a new product is to subtract the total development costs from the potential market share value. The potential market share value is estimated by multiplying the percentage of the potential number of patients by the potential commercial price for the new product. An alternative approach is to do the calculations based on the cost of the product or one course of treatment:

Estimated commercial return = (commercial price – cost of goods) × predicted sales volume

The commercial price that the company thinks it can obtain for the product, or for a course of treatment, will depend on some of the other factors mentioned above, such as the predicted time of market launch, the competitive positioning and the relative cost of competitor products in the countries to be marketed. The "cost of goods" (CoG) is an estimate of the sum of the cost of the drug substance, excipients, packaging materials, manufacture, labour and overheads, among other things, that contribute to making the product.

It has been estimated that 85 percent of the future cost of a new product can be determined at the product design phase (Matthews 1997). The industry average for the CoG has gradually increased over the last decade from about 10 to 20 percent of the commercial price. A CoG target of 5 to 10 percent is about the industry average, with a maximum of no more than 40 percent. Higher than this would be difficult to justify developing, as the margins would be too small. The choice of the commercial dosage form and manufacturing process can have a significant impact on the CoG. For example, if a product is freeze-dried, the processing costs will be extremely high because of the limited batch sizes and lengthy process involved. A less obvious example is the choice between tablets versus capsules. Cole (1998) compared the relative costs in the development and production of film-coated tablets with a dry-filled hard gelatin capsule for a New Chemical Entity (NCE). The relative costs in terms of development time, raw materials used, production equipment, facilities and validation for the manufacture were considered. There is a general belief that tablets are easier and cheaper to produce than dry-fill capsules, but surprisingly, Cole found that a capsule-manufacturing facility is cheaper to build, validate and operate than a tablet-manufacturing facility. Only when the costs of excipients are considered in isolation does the tablet process have an advantage, mainly because gelatin capsules are relatively expensive.

Technical Issues and Risk Assessment

There may be a variety of issues which should be documented in the Product Design Report to highlight the perceived risks involved in developing the product. Some of these risks will be related to pharmaceutical development and others to clinical, safety/toxicology or other areas.

For pharmaceutical development, risk may be associated with the technical challenges anticipated in developing a novel or complex drug delivery system or manufacturing process. Information from early preformulation and biopharmaceutics studies should indicate the potential problems for drug delivery, formulation development and manufacture.

There may be a lack of in-house expertise resulting in the need to contract out the work or the need to develop an in-house capability. Alternatively, there may be a lack of in-house facilities or equipment to handle the candidate drug. These issues need to be resolved quickly or else time penalties could be incurred. Other areas of risk include the sources of excipients and packaging components. Some excipients or packaging components may only be available from one supplier, with the risk that the supplier could go out of business.

The importance of identifying these issues in a Product Design Report is to make the company aware of the risks it is taking and to make effective plans to overcome problems and manage the risks.

Safety Assessment Considerations

In the interests of rapid product development, it is beneficial to select well-established excipients that already have regulatory approval in registered products. However, there may be situations where there are good reasons to use new excipients. There may be incompatibility problems with the candidate drug and existing excipients or there may be a need to use new excipients in a new drug delivery system. The replacement of chlorofluorocarbons (CFCs) with new hydrofluorocarbon (HFA) propellants in pressurised MDIs has been driven by environmental factors. The cost of safety testing HFA-134a and HFA-227 has been shared by a consortium of pharmaceutical companies who all had a vested interest. However, the search for novel surfactants required to suspend the drug in the new propellants has been left to individual companies, after it was discovered that none of the traditional surfactants were compatible with HFA propellants. This has resulted in many new surfactants being patented, but few have been successfully safety tested and used in marketed products.

The safety-toxicological testing of a new excipient for Europe or the United States is as extensive as that for an NCE and can take four to five years to complete. There are differences in the safety evaluation requirements for different types of formulations: oral, parenteral and topical/transdermal. The International Pharmaceutical Excipients Council (IPEC Europe and IPEC-Americas) have been working on a protocol for the rational safety testing of excipients to aid the introduction of new chemical excipients (see Table 5.4). IPEC is a federation of three independent regional industry associations based in Europe, the United States and Japan who are focused on the applicable law, regulations and business practices of each region with respect to pharmaceutical excipients.

Investment in a new excipient includes the cost of safety testing, investment in manufacturing facilities and other development costs, including stability testing.

Safety testing of a new excipient alone can be expensive. It is estimated that about $40 million is required to allow for the cost of those materials which do not make it to the market. There is a big financial risk that the investment costs will not be recovered during the patent life of a new product. However, it may be possible to reduce these costs and timings. For example, if the new excipient is essential for the development of the new candidate drug, it may be possible to "piggyback" the safety evaluation of the new excipient onto the safety evaluation of the candidate drug itself. This approach could be particularly appropriate for

Table 5.4

Summary of excipient safety testing for different routes of exposure for humans (draft proposal being developed by IPEC–Europe and IPEC–America).

Tests	Oral	Mucosal	Transdermal	Dermal/ Topical	Parenteral	Inhalation/ Intranasal	Ocular
Appendix 1–Base Set							
Acute Oral Toxicity	R	R	R	R	R	R	R
Acute Dermal Toxicity	R	R	R	R	R	R	R
Acute Inhalation Toxicity	C	C	C	C	C	R	C
Eye Irritation	R	R	R	R	R	R	R
Skin Irritation	R	R	R	R	R	R	R
Skin Sensitisation	R	R	R	R	R	R	R
Acute Parenteral Toxicity	–	–	–	–	R	–	–
Application Site Evaluation	–	–	R	R	R	–	–
Pulmonary Sensitisation	–	–	–	–	–	R	–
Phototoxicity/Photoallergy	–	–	R	R	–	–	–
Ames Test	R	R	R	R	R	R	R
Micronucleus test	R	R	R	R	R	R	R
ADME–Intended Route	R	R	R	R	R	R	R
28-Day Toxicity (2 species)–Intended Route	R	R	R	R	R	R	R
Appendix 2							
90-Day Toxicity (Most Appropriate Species)	R	R	R	R	R	R	R
Teratology (Rat & Rabbit)	R	R	R	R	R	R	R
Additional Assays	C	C	C	C	C	C	C
Genotoxicity Assays	R	R	R	R	R	R	R
Appendix 3							
Chronic Toxicity (Rodent, Non-rodent)	C	C	C	C	C	C	C
1 Generation Reproduction	R	R	R	R	R	R	R
Photocarcinogenicity	–	–	C	C	–	–	–

R: Required; C: Conditional

parenteral products. Finally, there may be lesser considerations for excipient safety testing in novel treatments, where there is an overwhelming need to treat patients quickly and effectively, for example, for life-threatening diseases such as cancer.

Environmental, Health and Safety Considerations

There are increasing pressures on the pharmaceutical industry to use environmentally friendly materials in products, which are biodegradable or recyclable and do no harm to the environment. Examples are the replacement of CFCs in pressurised metered dose aerosols and the replacement of polyvinyl chloride (PVC) for alternative packaging materials in some countries. Any special restrictions on the use of materials in the product need to be identified at the product design stage. The choice of appropriate materials to suit product, customer and environment may also have cost implications.

Another aspect is the nature of the candidate drug to be developed. Special handling requirements may be required for a very potent and potentially hazardous compound. There may be implications for the design and purchase of new facilities or equipment or the training of employees in new techniques.

Intellectual Property Considerations

Few pharmaceutical companies would venture into a long and expensive development programme without a strategy for effective patent protection in place to ensure market exclusivity. Patents are legal property which prevent others using the invention (for 20 years in most countries) in exchange for a full public disclosure of information.

The pharmaceutical industry is one of the major users of the patent system, which requires that three criteria are met in order to grant a patent. These criteria are novelty, presence of an inventive step and industrial applicability. Although an invention might be novel, it might not be patentable if it could have been predicted from "prior art", that is, knowledge in the public domain. Hence, there is a need for an inventive step.

At the product design stage of development, the only patent filed is likely to be for the new candidate drug. There may be a patent for a candidate drug and further patents for a new indication or a new pharmaceutical use. For example, Minoxidil, originally developed as an antihypertensive, had been discovered subsequently to be useful for the treatment of male pattern baldness. Patent protection is stronger if multiple patents can be obtained, for example, a single product could have patents covering a range of features from the candidate drug itself to the method of treatment and the delivery system. These new discoveries may only become known during development. Polymorphs (e.g., Cimetidine) and hydrates (e.g., Amoxycillin trihydrate) have been patented, as they have shown to have therapeutic advantages. A new formulation of the drug, delivery device or new pharmaceutical process might allow further patent cover to be granted, to extend the exclusivity beyond that of the primary patent.

The current patent status and potential for future patents to be obtained should be highlighted in the Product Design Report to assess the overall strength of patent protection to cover future development, and, as long as possible, market exclusivity.

CONCLUDING REMARKS

The potential benefits of conducting an initial product design stage prior to commencing product development have been emphasised in this chapter. Experience shows that the most frequent reason for terminating a project in late phase development is not because of lack of efficacy or poor safety but because the product developed does not meet the market (customer) needs. This might have been avoided if more consideration had been given to product design.

The Product Design Report can be a very useful document to focus the company on developing the right product at the right time to the market. Of course, to be of value it is essential that the correct input has been obtained from internal and external customers. For this to happen, a pharmaceutical company's senior management has to support this approach and ensure that time and resources are allowed for the design phase activities. The most successful pharmaceutical companies are effectively using this approach.

It is important that the Product Design Report is reviewed by the project team at milestones in the project life and updated if necessary. It is imperative that some information will change with time, for example, competitor activity. The introduction of a new competitor product to the market with unexpected product attributes may result in a re-evaluation of the desired product profile for the new product being developed. This, in turn, can result in subsequent modifications to the preformulation and formulation development programme. It is hoped that this will not be a complete change in direction, but if it is, the product design review will have alerted the company sooner rather than later to address this, and not to develop a product that is not wanted or needed.

REFERENCES

Akao, Y., ed. 1990. *Quality function deployment*. Cambridge, Mass., USA: Productivity Press.

Berliner, C., and J. Brimson, eds. 1988. *Cost management for today's advanced manufacturing: The CAM-I conceptual design*. Boston: Harvard Business School Press.

Burton, W. 1997. Using and controlling subcontractors. *Medical Device Technol.* (December):14–16.

Cole, G. 1998. Evaluating development and production costs: Tablets versus capsules. *Pharmaceut. Technol. Eur.* (May):17–26.

Day, R. G. 1993. *Quality function deployment: Linking a company with its customers*. Milwaukee: ASQC Quality Press.

Matthews, E. 1997. Economic considerations for device design and development. *Medical Device Technol.* (November):18–26.

Mizuno, S., and Y. Akao, eds. 1994. *QFD: The Customer-driven approach to quality planning and development*, Asian Productivity Organisation, Tokyo. New York: Quality Resources.

Spurlin, S., M. Green, L. Kelner, W. Ideus, K. Cairns, R. Press, and S. Duff. 1996. An insider's guide to outsourcing drug development—10 key steps to getting your money's worth. *Pharmaceut. Technol.* (February):64–76.

Stevenson, R. 1997. Outsourcing and the virtual company. *Chemistry in Britain* (October):29–31.

6

Preformulation as an Aid to Product Design in Early Drug Development

Gerry Steele

AstraZeneca R&D Charnwood
Loughborough, United Kingdom

Preformulation is usually defined as the science of the physicochemical characterization of candidate drugs. However, any studies carried out to define the conditions under which the candidate drug should be formulated can also be termed preformulation. This is a broader definition than was used in Chapter 3, and, as such, it can include studies on preliminary formulations under a variety of conditions. These studies may influence the Product Design and should be conducted at the earliest opportunity at the start of development. In the interest of faster drug development and reduced drug usage, preformulation studies should not be undertaken on a "check-list" basis. Rather, they should be conducted on a need-to-know basis.

Whilst there are many traditional approaches to dosage form design, newer approaches based on expert systems are now becoming available. Expert systems are discussed further in Chapter 8 on Product Optimisation.

SOLID DOSAGE FORMS

Since tablets and capsules account for approximately 70 percent of pharmaceutical preparations, it is important to undertake an investigation into the solid-state properties of candidate drugs during preformulation (Wells 1988). However, other studies are also important, since, for example, the same chemical compound can have different crystal structures (poly-morphs), external shapes (habits) and hence different flow and compression properties.

Cartensen et al. (1993) have usefully, although briefly, reviewed the physicochemical properties of particulate matter, dealing with the topics of cohesion, powder flow, mi-cromeretics, crystallization, yield strengths and effects of moisture and hygroscopicity. Buck-ton (1995) has reviewed the surface characterization of pharmaceuticals with regard to understanding sources of variability. A general overview of the methods available for the phys-ical characterization of pharmaceutical solids has been presented by Brittain et al. (1991). York (1994) has also dealt with these issues and produced a hierarchy of testing techniques for pow-dered raw materials. Finally, there is a book dealing with the physical characterization of pharmaceutical solids, edited by Brittain (1995).

A number of other studies can be performed on a candidate drug to determine other im-portant solid-state properties, for example, particle size, powder flow and compression and polymorphism. Therefore, when a sample undergoes initial preformulation testing the fol-lowing parameters should be noted: particle size, true, bulk and tapped density, surface area, compression properties and, powder flow properties. Some of these factors will be discussed in this chapter; others, however, are dealt with in more detail in Chapter 11 on Solid Oral Dosage Forms.

Particle Size Reduction

The particle size of pharmaceuticals is important since it can affect the formulation charac-teristics and bioavailability of a compound (Chaumeil 1998). For example, sedimentation and flocculation rates in suspensions are, in part, governed by particle size, and inhalation therapy of pulmonary diseases demands that a small particle size (2–5 μm) is delivered to the lung for the best therapeutic effect. Particle size is also important in the tableting field, since it can be very important for good homogeneity in the final tablet. In this respect, Zhang and Johnson (1997) showed that a blended jet-milled compound exhibited a smaller range of potencies when compared to those blends where the compound had a larger particle size. It is therefore important that the particle size be consistent throughout the development studies of a prod-uct to satisfy formulation and regulatory demands (Turner 1987).

Thus, to reduce the risk of dissolution rate-limited bioavailability, and if there is sufficient compound, grinding in a mortar and pestle should be done to reduce the particle size of the compound. If larger quantities are available, then ball milling or micronization can be used to reduce the particle size. The main methods of particle size reduction have been reviewed by Spencer and Dalder (1997), who devised the mill selection matrix shown in Table 6.1.

Ball Milling

In a review of milling, it was stated that ball milling was "the most commonly used type of tum-bling mill in pharmacy" (Parrot 1974). Indeed, it is probably used most often at the preformu-lation stage to reduce the particle size of small amounts of a compound, especially for the preparation formulations to be administered to animals. At the lead optimization (LO) stage, however, only small quantities (e.g., 50 mg) will be available to administer to a test animal. For a review of high purity applications of ball milling, such as pharmaceuticals, see Vernon (1994).

Ball mills reduce the size of particles through a combined process of impact and attrition. Usually they consist of a hollow cylinder that contain balls of various sizes, which is rotated to initiate the grinding process. There are a number of factors that affect the efficiency of the

Table 6.1
Mill selection matrix.

Criteria	Slurry	Fluid Energy	Universal	Cone	Hammer
Particle size	Less than average	Very favourable	Very favourable	Less than average	Average
Particle distribution	Average	Very favourable	Very favourable	Favourable	Favourable
Cleaning	Less than average	Average	Average	Favourable	Less than average
Operating cost	Favourable	Unfavourable	Unfavourable	Very favourable	Favourable
Dust containment	Very favourable	Less than average	Less than average	Very favourable	Favourable
Temperature	Very favourable	Favourable	Less than average	Very favourable	Favourable
Flexibility	Average	Average	Very favourable	Favourable	Favourable

Spencer, R. and Dalder B., Sizing up grinding mills, *Chemical Engineering*, Vol. 104, No. 4, pp. 84–87 (1997). With permission.

milling process and these include rotation speed, mill size, wet or dry milling and amount of material to be milled.

Although ball milling can effectively reduce the particle size of compounds, prolonged milling may be detrimental in terms of compound crystallinity and stability. This has been illustrated in a study that examined the effect of ball mill grinding on cefixime trihydrate (Kitamura et al. 1989). Using a variety of techniques, it was shown that the crystalline solid was converted to an amorphous solid after 4 h in a ball mill. The stability of the amorphous solid was found to be less than that of the crystalline solid, and the samples were discoloured due to grinding.

It is important to check this aspect of the milling process, since amorphous compounds can show increased bioavailability and possible pharmacological activity compared to the corresponding crystalline form. Ball milling may also change the polymorphic form of a compound, as shown by the work of Leung et al. (1999) with aspartame.

Figure 6.1, for example, shows the X-ray powder diffraction (XRPD) patterns of a sample of a compound "as received" and after ball milling. After ball milling for 1 h, the sample was rendered amorphous, and hence a shorter milling period was used.

Micronization

If instrumentation and sufficient compound are available, then micronization can be undertaken. This technique is routinely used to reduce the particle size of active ingredients so that the maximum surface area is exposed to enhance the solubility and dissolution properties of poorly soluble compounds. Because of the enhanced surface area, the bioavailability of

Figure 6.1 XRPD patterns showing the effect of ball milling on a compound.

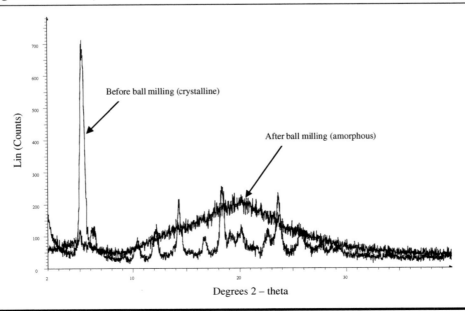

compounds is often improved, e.g., micronization enhanced the bioavailability of felodipine when administered as an extended release tablet (Johansson and Abrahamsson 1997).

The process involves feeding the drug substance into a confined circular chamber where the powder is suspended in a high velocity stream of air. Interparticulate collisions result in a size reduction. Smaller particles are removed from the chamber by the escaping air stream towards the centre of the mill where they are discharged and collected. Larger particles recirculate until their particle size is reduced. Micronized particles are typically less than 10 μm in diameter (Midoux et al. 1999).

Effect of Milling and Micronization

Although micronization of the drug offers the advantage of a small particle size and a larger surface area, it can result in processing problems due to high dust, low density and poor flow properties. Indeed, micronization may be counterproductive, since the micronized particles may aggregate, which may decrease the surface area. In addition, changes in crystallinity of the drug can also occur, which can be detected by techniques such as microcalorimetry (Briggner et al. 1994), dynamic vapour sorption (Ward and Schultz 1995) and inverse gas chromatography (Feeley et al. 1998).

Ward and Schultz (1995) reported subtle differences in the crystallinity of salbutamol sulphate after micronization by air jet milling. They found that amorphous to crystalline conversions occurred that were dependent on temperature and relative humidity (RH). It was suggested that particle size reduction of the powder produced defects on the surface that, if enough energy was imparted, led to amorphous regions on the surface. In turn, these regions were found to have a greater propensity to sorb water. On exposure to moisture, these regions crystallized and expelled excess moisture. This is illustrated in Figure 6.2, which shows the

Figure 6.2 DVS isotherm showing crystallization effects due to moisture.

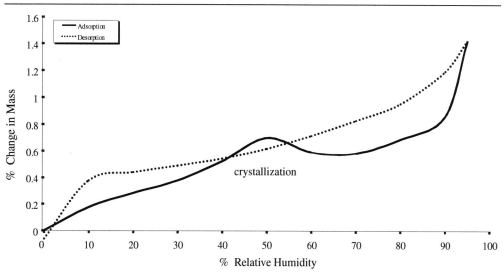

uptake of moisture, as measured by dynamic vapour sorption (DVS), of a micronized development compound. Note how the percent mass change increases and then decreases as the RH is increased between 40 and 60 percent during the sorption phase. This corresponds to crystallization of the compound and subsequent ejection of excess moisture. The compound also exhibits some hysteresis.

This effect can be important in some formulations, such as dry powder inhaler devices, since it can cause agglomeration of the powders and variable flow properties. In many cases, this low level of amorphous character cannot be detected by techniques such as XRPD. Since microcalorimetry can detect < 10 percent amorphous content (the limit of detection is 1 percent or less), it has the advantage over other techniques such as XRPD or DSC. Using the ampoule technique with an internal hygrostat, as described by Briggner et al. 1994, and shown in Figure 6.3, the amorphous content of a micronized drug can be determined by measuring the heat output caused by the water vapour inducing crystallization of the amorphous regions.

Figure 6.4 shows the calibration curve of heat output versus amorphous content of a development compound. In this case, the technique is used to crystallize, or condition, these amorphous regions by exposure to elevated RHs. Thus, if authentic 100 percent amorphous and crystalline phases exist, it is possible to construct a calibration graph of heat output versus percentage crystallinity, so that the amount of amorphous character introduced by the milling process can be quantified.

Figure 6.3 Internal hygrostat and heat output due to crystallization of an amorphous phase measured by isothermal microcalorimetry.

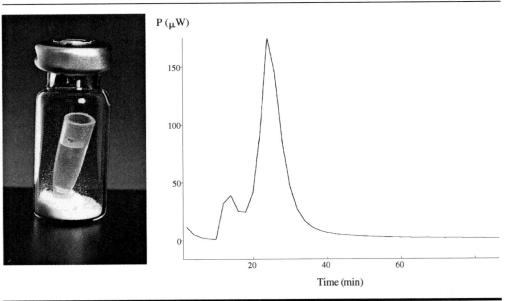

Figure 6.4 Crystallization peak energy versus amorphous content using microcalorimetry.

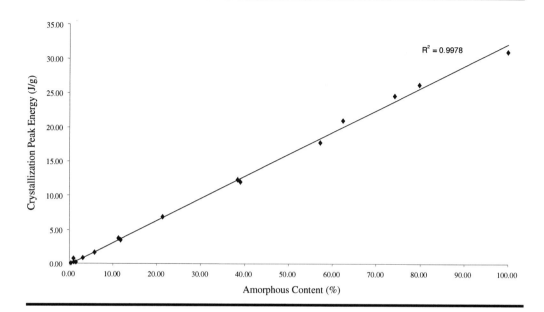

Inverse Gas Chromatography

In addition to the DVS and microcalorimetric techniques for characterizing the surface properties of powders, a recently introduced technique known as inverse gas chromatography (IGC) can also be used. This technique differs from traditional gas chromatography insofar as the stationary phase is the powder under investigation. In this type of study, a range of non-polar and polar adsorbates (probes) are used, e.g., alkanes, from hexane to decane, acetone, diethyl ether or ethyl acetate. The retention volume, i.e., the net volume of carrier gas (nitrogen) required to elute the probe, is then measured. The surface partition coefficient (K_s) of the probes between carrier gas and surfaces of test powder particles can then be calculated. From this, a free energy can be calculated which can show that one batch may favourably adsorb the probes when compared to another, implying a difference in the surface energetics.

The experimental parameter measured in IGC experiments is the net retention volume, V_n. This parameter is related to the surface partition coefficient, K_s, which is the ratio between the concentration of the probe molecule in the stationary and mobile phases shown by

$$K_s = \frac{V_n}{m} \times A_{sp} \tag{1}$$

where m is the weight of the sample in the column, and A_{sp} is the specific surface of the sample in the column.

From K_s the free energy of adsorption $(-\Delta G_A)$ is defined by

$$-\Delta G_A = RT\ln\left(K_s \times \frac{P_{sg}}{P}\right)a\left(\gamma_L{}^D\right)^{1/2} \tag{2}$$

where P_{sg} is the standard vapour state $(101\ \text{KN/m}^2)$ and P is the standard surface pressure, which has a value of $0.338\ \text{mN/m}$.

IGC and molecular modelling have been used to assess the effect of micronization on dl-propranolol (York et al. 1998). The samples were jet milled (micronized) to various particle sizes and $\gamma_s{}^D$ was measured and plotted against their median particle size. This showed that as the particle size decreased due to the micronization process, the surface of the particles became more energetic. Interestingly, it was pointed out that the plateau region corresponded to the brittle-ductile region of this compound. This observation implied a change in the mechanism of milling from a fragmentation to an attrition process. The data for $-\Delta G_A{}^{SP}$ for the tetrahydrofuran (THF) and dichloromethane probes showed that the electron donation of the surface increased as the particle size decreased. Combining these data with molecular modelling, which was used to predict which surfaces would predominate, they showed that the electron-rich naphthyl group dominated the surface of the unmilled material. This led to the conclusion that as the particle size was reduced, this surface became more exposed, leading to a greater interaction with the THF and dichloromethane probes. However, as previously noted, as milling proceeded, the mechanism of size reduction changed, which might lead to exposure of the chloride and hydroxyl moieties.

Therefore, using moisture sorption, microcalorimetric, IGC, molecular modelling and other techniques, the consequences of the particle size reduction process can be assessed. Moreover, surface energetics can be measured directly and predictions made about the nature of the surface, which ultimately could affect properties such as the flow of powders or adhesion of particles (Podczeck et al. 1996b).

Particle Size Distribution Measurement

Washington (1992) has discussed the concepts and techniques of particle size analysis and its role in pharmaceutical sciences and other industries. There are many different methods available for particle size analysis. The techniques most readily available include sieving, optical microscopy in conjunction with image analysis, electron microscopy, the Coulter Counter and laser diffractometers. Size characterization is simple for spherical particles, but not for irregular particles where the assigned size will depend on the method of characterization used. Table 6.2 lists particle size measurement methods commonly used and the corresponding approximate useful size range (Mullin 1993).

Figure 6.5 shows the particle size distribution of a micronized powder determined by scanning electron microscopy (SEM) and laser light scattering. The Malvern Mastersizer is an example of an instrument that measures particle size by laser diffraction. The use of this technique is based on light scattered through various angles, which is directly related to the diameter of the particle. Thus, by measuring the angles and intensity of scattered light from the particles, a particle size distribution can be deduced. It should be noted that the particle diameters reported are the same as those that spherical particles would produce under similar conditions. Table 6.3 shows the data obtained from the laser diffraction analysis shown in Figure 6.5.

Two theories dominate the theory of light scattering; the Fraunhofer and Mie. In the former, each particle is treated as spherical and essentially opaque to the impinging laser light. The

Table 6.2
Particle size techniques and size range.

Method	Size Range (μm)
Sieving (woven wire)	20–125,000
Sieving (electroformed)	5–120
Sieving (perforated plate)	1,000–125,000
Microscopy (optical)	0.5–150
Microscopy (electron)	0.001–5
Sedimentation (gravity)	1–50
Sedimentation (centrifugal)	0.01–5
Electrical zone sensing (e.g., Coulter)	1–200
Laser light scattering (Fraunhofer)	1–1,000
Laser light scattering (quasi-elastic)	0.001–1

From Mullin, J. W., *Anal. Proc.* 30:455–456 (1993). Reproduced by permission of The Royal Society of Chemistry.

Mie theory, on the other hand, takes into account the differences in refractive indices between the particles and the suspending medium. If the diameter of the particles is above 10 μm, then the size produced by utilizing each theory is essentially the same. However, discrepancies may occur when the diameter of the particles approaches that of the wavelength of the laser source. The following are the values reported from diffraction experiments.

- $D(v, 0.1)$ is the size of particles for which 10 percent of the sample is below this size

- $D(v, 0.5)$ is the volume (v) median diameter of which 50 percent of the sample is below and above this size

- $D(v, 0.9)$ gives a size of particle for which 90 percent of the sample is below this size

- $D[4,3]$ is the equivalent volume mean diameter calculated using:

$$D[4,3] = \frac{\Sigma d^4}{\Sigma d^3} \qquad (3)$$

- $D[3,2]$ is the surface area mean diameter; also known as the Sauter mean, where $d =$ diameter of each unit

- Log difference represents the difference between the observed light energy data and the calculated light energy data for the derived distribution

- *Span* is the measurement of the width of the distribution and is calculated using

$$Span = \frac{D(v, 0.9) - D(v, 0.1)}{D(v, 0.5)} \qquad (4)$$

The dispersion of the powder is important in achieving reproducible results. Ideally, the dispersion medium should have the following characteristics:

- Have a suitable absorbancy
- Not swell the particles
- Disperse a wide range of particles
- Slow sedimentation of particles
- Allow homogeneous dispersion of the particles
- Be safe and easy to use

Figure 6.5 SEM of a micronized powder and particle size measured by laser diffraction.

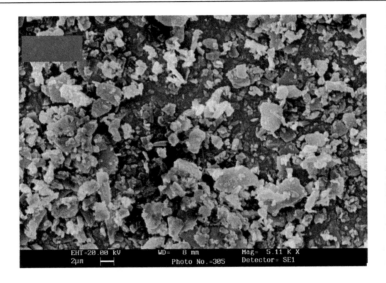

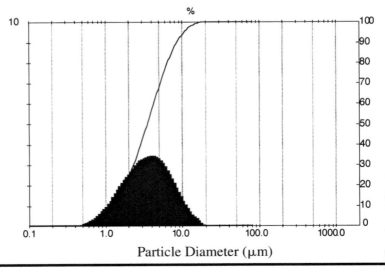

Table 6.3
Particle size distribution of a micronized powder measured using laser diffraction.

Range: 45 mm	Beam: 2.40 mm	Sampler: MS1	Obs*: 15.8%
Presentation: 2$SD	Analysis: Polydisperse		Residual: 0.117%
Modifications: None			

Conc. = 0.0062% Vol	Density = 1.427 g/cm³	S.S.A. = 1.6133 m²/g
Distribution: Volume	D [4, 3] = 4.34 μm	D [3, 2] = 2.61 μm
D (v, 0.1) = 1.29 μm	D (v, 0.5) = 3.50 μm	D (v, 0.9) = 8.54 μm
Span = 2.071E+00	Uniformity = 6.515E-01	

Size (μm)	Volume under%	Size (μm)	Volume under%	Size (μm)	Volume under%	Size (μm)	Volume under%
0.05	0.00	0.65	1.09	4.30	60.67	28.15	100.00
0.12	0.00	0.81	2.58	5.29	71.18	34.69	100.00
0.15	0.00	1.00	5.08	6.52	80.61	42.75	100.00
0.19	0.00	1.23	8.90	8.04	88.21	52.68	100.00
0.23	0.00	1.51	14.24	9.91	93.69	64.92	100.00
0.28	0.00	1.86	21.22	12.21	97.18	80.00	100.00
0.35	0.00	2.30	29.72	15.04	99.08		
0.43	0.03	2.83	39.38	18.54	99.87		
0.53	0.34	3.49	49.86	22.84	100.00		

In terms of sample preparation, it is necessary to deaggregate the samples so that the primary particles are measured. To achieve this, the sample may be sonicated, although there is a potential problem of the sample being disrupted by the ultrasonic vibration. To check for this, it is recommended that the particle dispersion be examined by optical microscopy.

Although laser light diffraction is a rapid and highly repeatable method in determining the particle size distributions of pharmaceutical powders, the results obtained can be affected by particle shape. In this respect, Kanerva et al. (1993) examined narrow sieve fractions of spherical pellets, cubic sodium chloride and acicular anhydrous theophylline. Size distributions were made using laser light diffraction and compared to results using image analysis. The results showed that all determinations using the laser light scattering resulted in a broadened size distribution compared to image analysis. In addition, it has been pointed out that the refractive index of the particles can introduce an error of 10 percent under most circumstances if it is not taken into account (Zhang and Xu 1992).

Another laser-based instrument, relying on light scattering, is the Aerosizer. This instrument is for a particle sizing and is based on a time-of-flight principle as described by Niven (1993). The Aerosizer with aero-disperser is specifically designed to carry deaggregated particles in an air stream for particle sizing. This instrumentation has been evaluated using a salbutamol base, terbutaline sulphate and lactose (Hindle and Byron 1995).

For submicron materials, particularly colloidal particles, quasi-elastic light scattering is the preferred technique. This has been usefully reviewed by Phillies (1990). The particle size distribution of ofloxacin/prednisolone acetate for ophthalmic use has been investigated by image analysis photon correlation spectroscopy (PCS) and single particle optical sizing (SPOS) (Hacche et al. 1992). Using these techniques, it was shown that ball milling yielded a particle size of $\sim 1 \ \mu m$ and that increasing the ball-milling time increased the reproducibility of diameter of particles. PCS was then used to show that extended ball milling reduced the particle size to a constant value.

Surface Area Measurements

The surface areas of drug particles are important because dissolution is a function of this parameter (as predicted by the Noyes-Whitney equation). Surface area can also be quoted if the particle size is difficult to measure (Curzons et al. 1993).

Surface areas are usually determined by gas adsorption (nitrogen or krypton) and although there are a number of theories describing this phenomenon, the most widely used method is the Brunauer, Emmet and Teller, or BET, method. Adsorption methods for surface area determination have been reviewed in detail by Sing (1992). Two methods are used: the multipoint and single-point.

Without going into too much theoretical detail, the BET isotherm for Type II adsorption processes (typical for pharmaceutical powders) is given by:

$$\frac{P}{V(P_0 - P)} = \frac{1}{cV_{mon}} + \left\{ \frac{c-1}{cV_{mon}} \right\} \left\{ \frac{P}{P_0} \right\} \qquad (5)$$

where P is the partial pressure of the adsorbate, V is the volume of gas adsorbed at pressure p, V_{mon} is the volume of gas at monolayer coverage, P_0 is the saturation pressure and c is related to the intercept. Thus by plotting $P/V(P_0 - P)$ versus P/P_0 a straight line of slope $c - 1/cV_{mon}$ and intercept $1/cV_{mon}$ will be obtained. The total surface area is thus:

$$S_t = \frac{V_{mon}NA_{CS}}{M} \qquad (6)$$

where N is the Arogadro's number, A_{cs} is the cross-sectional area of the adsorbate and M is the moleular weight of the adsorbate. It follows that the specific surface area is given by S_t/m, where m is the mass of the sample. According to the U. S. Pharmacopeia (USP), the data are considered to be acceptable if, on linear regression, the correlation coefficient is not less than 0.9975, i.e., r^2 is not less than 0.995.

Figure 6.6 shows the full adsorption-desorption isotherm of two batches of the micronized powder shown earlier in Figure 6.4.

Figure 6.6 Full Type IIb adsorption isotherm for two batches of a micronized powder.

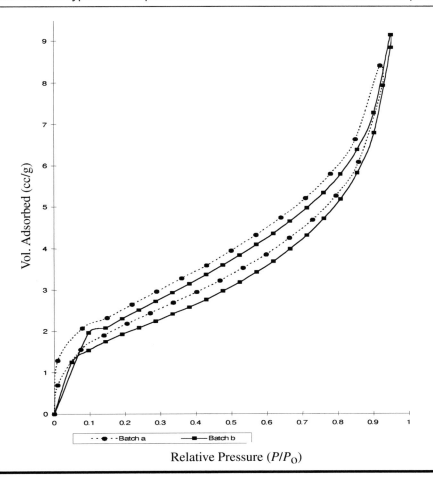

It should be noted that, experimentally, it is necessary to remove gases and vapours that may be present on the surface of the powder. This is usually achieved by drawing a vacuum or purging the sample in a flowing stream of nitrogen. Raising the temperature may not always be advantageous. For example, Phadke and Collier (1994) examined the effect of degassing temperature on the surface area of magnesium stearate obtained from two manufacturers. In this study, helium at a range of temperatures between 23 and 60°C was used in single and multipoint determinations. It was found that the specific surface area of the samples decreased with an increase in temperature. From other measurements using DSC and thermogravimetric analysis (TGA), it was found that raising the temperature changed the nature of the samples. Hence, it was recommended that magnesium stearate should not be degassed at elevated temperatures. Figure 6.7 shows the effect of sample weight and temperature of degassing on a sample of a micronized powder using a Micromeritics Gemini BET analyser. From this plot, it can be seen that the weight of the sample can have a marked effect on the measured surface area of the compound under investigation. Therefore, to avoid reporting erroneous surface areas, the sample weight should not be too low, and in this case, should be greater than 300 mg.

True Density

Density can be defined as ratio of the mass of an object to its volume; therefore, the density of a solid is a reflection of the arrangement of molecules in a solid. In pharmaceutical development terms, knowledge of the true density of powders has been used for the determination of

Figure 6.7 Effect of sample weight and degassing temperature on the surface area of micronized powder.

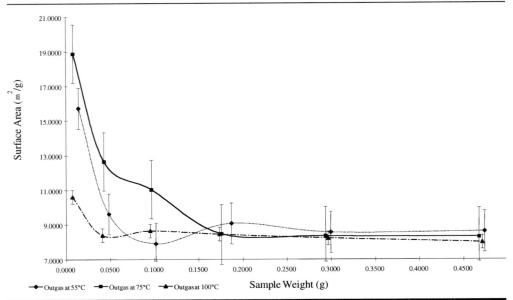

the consolidation behaviour. For example, the well-known Heckel equation (7) requires knowledge of the true density of the compound:

$$\ln\left[\frac{1}{1-D}\right] = KP + A \qquad (7)$$

where D is the relative density, which is the ratio of the apparent density to the true density, K is determined from the linear portion of the Heckel plot and P is the pressure. The densities of molecular crystals can be increased by compression, for example, whilst investigating the compression properties of acetylsalicylic acid using a compaction simulator, increases in the true density were found (Pedersen and Kristensen 1994).

Information about the true density of a powder can be used to predict whether a compound will cream or sediment in a metered dose inhaler (MDI) formulation. The densities of the hydrofluoroalkane (HFA) propellants, 227 and 134a, which are replacing chlorofluorocarbons (CFCs) in MDI formulations, are 1.415 and 1.217 g/cm^{-3}, respectively. Therefore, suspensions of compounds that have a true density less than these figures will cream (rise to the surface), and those that are denser will sediment. Those that match the density of the propellant will stay in suspension for a longer period (Williams III et al. 1998). It should be noted, however, that the physical stability of a suspension is not merely a function of the true density of the material.

The true density is thus a property of the material and is independent of the method of determination. In this respect, the determination of the true density can be determined using three methods: displacement of a liquid, displacement of a gas (pycnometry) or floatation in a liquid. These methods of measuring true density have been evaluated by Duncan-Hewitt and Grant (1986). They concluded that, whereas liquid displacement was tedious and tended to underestimate the true density, displacement of a gas was accurate but needed relatively expensive instrumentation. As an alternative, the floatation method was found to be simple to use and inexpensive. Although more time consuming than gas pycnometry, it was accurate using relatively simple instrumentation.

Gas pycnometry is probably the most commonly used method in the pharmaceutical industry for measuring true density. All gas pycnometers rely on the measurement of pressure changes, as a reference volume of gas, typically helium, is added to, or deleted from, the test cell.

Experimentally, measurements should be carried out in accordance with the manufacturers' instructions. However, it is worth noting that artefacts may occur. For example, Figure 6.8 shows the measured true density of a number of tableting excipients as a function of sample weight. As can be seen, at low sample weights, the measured true density increased, making the measurements less accurate.

Flow and Compaction of Powders

Although at the preformulation stage only limited quantities of candidate drug are available, any data generated on flow and compaction properties can be of great use to the formulation scientist. The data provided can give guidance on the selection of the excipients to use, the formulation type and the manufacturing process to use, for example, direct compression or granulation. It is important that once the habit and size distribution of the test compound have been determined, the flow and compaction properties are evaluated, if the intended dosage form is a solid dosage form. York (1992) has reviewed the crystal engineering and particle

Figure 6.8 True density as a function of sample mass for some excipients.

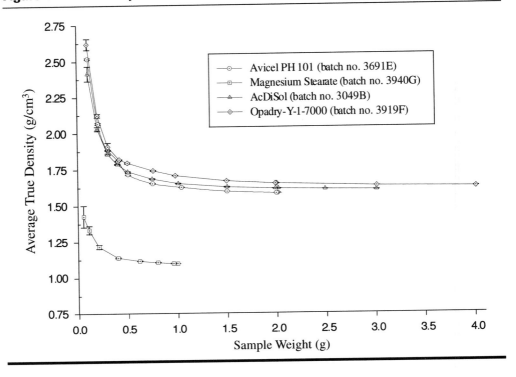

design for the powder compaction process, and Amidon (1999) has reviewed the powder flow methods.

The compression of flow powders is dealt with in more detail in Chapter 11, Oral Solid Dosage Forms. With respect to the preformulation screening of candidate drugs for solid dosage forms, a protocol to examine their compression properties devised by Aulton and Wells (1988) is recommended. Their scheme is shown in Table 6.4. Essentially, the compound is compressed using an infrared (IR) press and die under 10 tons of pressure, and the resulting tablets are tested with regard to their crushing strength.

The interpretation of crushing strengths was as follows. If the crushing strengths are of the order B > A > C, the material probably has plastic tendencies. Materials that are brittle are usually independent of the scheme, whilst elastic material can behave in a variety of ways. For example: (a) A will cap or laminate; (b) B will probably maintain integrity, but will be very weak; and (c) C will cap or laminate (Aulton and Wells 1988).

Figure 6.9 shows a scanning electron micrograph of a compound that had poor compression properties. Notice how the top of the compact has partially detached (capping) and how the compact has separated into layers (lamination).

As shown by Otsuka and Matsuda (1993), it is always worth checking the effect of compression on a powder if the compound is known to be polymorphic. Using the XRPD patterns of chlorpropamide forms A and C, they examined the effect of temperature and

Table 6.4
Compression protocol (Aulton and Wells 1988).

	500 mg drug + 1% magnesium stearate		
	A	**B**	**C**
Blend in a tumbler mixer for	5 min	5 min	30 min
Compress 13 mm diameter compacts in a hydraulic press at	75 MPa	75 MPa	75 MPa
Dwell time of	2 sec	30 sec	2 sec
Store tablets in sealed container at room temperature to allow equilibration	24 h	24 h	24 h
Perform crushing strength on tablets and record load	AN	BN	CN

Aulton, M. A., and Wells, J. E. (1998), *Pharmaceutics: The Science of Dosage Form Design,* edited by M. E. Aulton. Reprinted with permission from Churchill Livingstone.

Figure 6.9. SEM of a compound that undergoes capping and lamination.

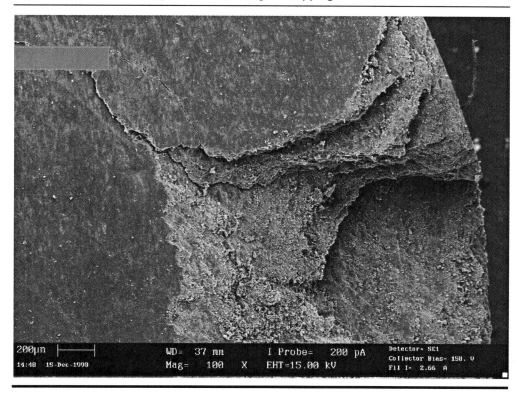

compression force on the deagglomerated powders and found that both forms were mutually transformed.

Computational methods of predicting the mechanical properties of a powder from the crystal structure are now being explored. There appears to be a relationship between indentation hardness and the molecular structure of organic materials. However, a prerequisite for predicting indentation hardness is knowledge of the crystal structure (Roberts et al. 1994). Payne et al. (1996) have used molecular modelling to predict the mechanical properties of aspirin and forms A and B of primodone. The predicted results of Young's modulus were found to be in good agreement with those determined experimentally, and thus compaction measurements might not always be necessary if they are difficult to perform.

Colour

Colour can be useful when describing different batches of drug substance, since it can sometimes be used as an indicator of solvent presence or, more importantly, of degradation. In addition, subtle differences in colour may be due to variations in the particle size distribution. Usually colour is subjective and is based on individual perception; however, more quantitative measurements can be obtained by using, e.g., tristimulus colorimetry (Nyqvist et al. 1980; Vemuri et al. 1985; Nyqvist and Wadsten 1986; Stock 1993).

Stark et al. (1996) have observed colour changes during accelerated stability testing of captopril tablets, flucloxacillin sodium capsules, cefoxitin sodium powder for injection and theophylline CR tablets. Under ambient conditions, only the flucloxacillin sodium and cefoxitin were observed to show any significant colouring. However, under stress conditions of accelerated stability testing, a linear relationship between colour formation and the drug content of the formulations was found, except for the theophylline tablets, where discoloration occurred in the absence of any significant degradation. Interestingly, the rate of colouring was found to obey the Arrhenius equation. The authors proposed that the shelf life of the formulations could be specified using the Commission Internationale de'Ecalarage (CIE) system for colour.

Electrostaticity

Powders can acquire an electrostatic charge during processing, the extent of which is related to the aggressiveness of the process. Table 6.5, from BS5958, gives the range of values that arise due to various processes. According to Kulvanich and Stewart (1987), static electrification of two dissimilar materials occurs by the making and breaking of surface contacts (triboelectrification). Thus, the extent of the electrostatic charge accumulation will increase as the surfaces collide and contact, e.g., by increasing the agitation time and intensity of a powder in a mixer. The net results will therefore increase the spot charge over the particle surfaces and adhesive characteristics. This technique has been used to prepare drug-carrier systems known as an interactive mixture. Kulvanich and Stewart (1987) have reported the effect of particle size and concentration on the adhesive characteristics of a model drug carrier (glass beads coated with hydroxypropyl methylcellulose [HPMC] plus a range of antibiotic sulpha drugs). From their results, they concluded that an increase in size and particle concentration decreased the adhesive tendencies of the drug.

The net charge on a powder may be either electropositive or electronegative. Although the process is not fully understood, it is generally accepted that charging occurs as a result of electron transfer between materials of different electrical properties.

Table 6.5
Mass charge density arising from various operations (BS5958).

Operation	Mass Charge Density (μC/kg)
Sieving	10^{-5} to 10^{-3}
Pouring	10^{-3} to 10^{-1}
Scroll feed transfer	10^{-2} to 1
Grinding	10^{-1} to 1
Micronising	10^{-1} to 10^{2}

Reproduced from BS5958 with permission of BSI under licence number 2001 SK/0091. Complete standards can be obtained from BSI Customer Services, 389 Chiswick High Road, London W4 4AL.

The electrostatic charges on the surface of a powder can affect the flow properties of powders. An electric detector can determine the electric field generated by the electrostatic charges on the surface of the powder. This acts as a voltmeter and allows the direct determination of both polarity and absolute value of the electrostatic field. As an example, the electrostaticity of the experimental compound ITF 296, when sieved at 200 μm, showed an electrostatic field of –60 V due to the charge on the powder surface (Dobetti et al. 1995). As a consequence, the powder formed stacked aggregates, which led to the unsieved powder being less wettable and difficult to handle. Führer (1996) has reviewed interparticulate attraction mechanisms.

Carter et al. (1992) designed and used an apparatus to investigate the triboelectrification process between α-lactose monohydrate and beclomethasone dipropionate and salbutamol sulphate. The results showed that particle size and the type and nature of contact surface resulted in differences in charging tendencies. Further work on this topic by this group (Carter et al. 1998) investigated the charging and its decay on compacts of lactose and salbutamol and polyvinyl chloride (PVC), which are commonly used dry powder inhaler devices. Results showed that PVC gained to the highest charge from a carona electrode. Whilst the PVC and the lactose lost their charge relatively quickly (within 30 min), salbutamol still had a measurable charge after 120 min.

Caking

Caking can occur after storage and involves the formation of lumps or the complete agglomeration of the powder. A number of factors have been identified that predispose a powder to exhibit caking tendencies. These include static electricity, hygroscopicity, particle size, impurities of the powder and, in terms of the storage conditions, stress temperature, RH and storage time can also be important. The caking of 11-amino undeceonoic acid has been investigated, and it was concluded that the most important cause of the observed caking with this compound was its particle size (Provent et al. 1993). The mechanisms involved in caking are based on the formation of five types of **interparticle bonds:**

1. Bonding resulting from mechanical tangling

2. Bonding resulting from steric effects

3. Bonds via static electricity

4. Bonds due to free liquid

5. Bonds due to solid bridges

The caking tendency of a development compound was investigated when it was discovered to be lumpy after storage. An experiment was performed on the compound whereby it was stored at different RHs (from saturated salt solutions) for 4 weeks in a desiccator. Results revealed that caking was evident at 75 percent RH with the compound forming loosely massed porous cakes (Table 6.6). TGA of the samples showed that caked samples lost only a small amount of weight on heating (0.62 percent w/w), which indicated that only low levels of moisture were required to produce caking for this compound.

It is known that micronization of compounds can lead to the formation of regions with a degree of disorder which, because of their amorphous character, are more reactive compared to the pure crystalline substance. This is particularly true on exposure to moisture and can lead to problems with caking, which is detrimental to the performance of the product. It has been argued that these amorphous regions transform during moisture sorption, due to surface sintering and recrystallization at RHs well below the critical RH.

Polymorphism Issues

Because polymorphism can have an effect on so many aspects of drug development, it is important to fix the polymorph (usually the stable form) as early as possible in the development cycle.

A U.S. Food and Drug Administration (FDA) reviewer's perspective of regulatory considerations in crystallization processes for bulk pharmaceutical chemicals has been presented by DeCamp (1996). In this paper, he stated that

Table 6.6
Effect of moisture on the caking of a development compound.

%RH	Moisture Content	Appearance and Flow Properties
0	0.31	Free-flowing powder; passed easily through sieve
11.3	0.24	Ditto
22.5	0.27	Less free-flowing powder
38.2	0.32	Base of powder bed adhered to petri dish; however, material above this flowed
57.6	0.34	Less free flowing
75.3	0.62	Material caked
Ambient	0.25	Base of powder adhered to petri dish

process validation should include at least one, if not more, checks to verify that the process yields the desired polymorph. At the time of a New Drug Application (NDA) submission, it would be expected that occurrences of polymorphism would be established and whether these affect the dissolution rate or the bioavailibility.

He continued that

It is not necessary to create additional solid state forms by techniques or conditions unrelated to the synthetic process for the purpose of clinical trials. However, submission of a thorough study of the effects of solvent, temperature and possibly pressure on the stability of the solid state forms should be considered. A conclusion that polymorphism does not occur with a compound must be substantiated by crystallization experiments from a range of solvents. This should also include solvents that may be involved in the manufacture of the drug product, e.g., during granulation.

Whilst it is hoped that the issue of polymorphism is resolved during prenomination and early development, it can remain a concern when the synthesis of the drug is scaled-up into a larger reactor or transferred to another production site. In extreme cases, and despite intensive research, work may have only produced a metastable form, and the first production batch produces the stable form. Dunitz and Bernstein (1995) have reviewed the appearance of, and subsequent disappearance of, polymorphs. Essentially, this describes the scenario whereby, after nucleation of a more stable form, the previously prepared metastable form could no longer be made.

The role of related substances in the case of the disappearing polymorphs of sulphathiazole has been explored (Blagden et al. 1998). These studies showed that a reaction by-product from the final hydrolysis stage could stabilize different polymorphic forms of the compound, depending on the concentration of the by-product. Using molecular modelling techniques, they were able to show that ethamidosulphthiazole, the by-product, influenced the hydrogen bond network, and hence form and crystal morphology.

In the development of a reliable commercial recrystallization process for dirithromycin, Wirth and Stephenson (1997) proposed that the following scheme should be followed in the production of candidate drugs:

1.   Selection of solvent system

2.   Characterization of the polymorphic forms

3.   Optimisation of process times, temperature, solvent compositions, etc.

4.   Examination of the chemical stability of the drug during processing

5.   Manipulation of the polymorphic form, if necessary

Whilst examples of disappearing polymorphs exist, perhaps more common is the crystallization of mixtures of polymorphs. Many analytical techniques have been used to quantitate mixtures of polymorphs, e.g., XRPD has been used to quantitate the amount of cefepime · 2HCl dihydrate in cefepime · 2HCl monohydrate (Bugay et al. 1996). As noted by these workers, a crucial factor in developing an assay based on a solid-state technique is the production of pure calibration and validation samples. Moreover, whilst the production of the forms may be straightforward, production of homogeneously mixed samples for calibration purposes may not. To overcome this problem, a slurry technique was employed, which satisfied the NDA requirements, to determine the amount of one form in the other. The criteria employed were as follows:

- A polymorphic transformation did not occur during preparation or analysis

- A limit of detection of 5 percent (w/w) of the dihydrate in monohydrate

- Ease of sample preparation, data acquisition and analysis

- Ease of transfer to a quality control (QC) environment

Calibration samples were limited to a working range of 1–15 percent w/w, and to prepare the mixes, samples of each form were slurried in acetone to produce a homogeneous mixture of the two.

With respect to solid dosage forms, there have been a few reports on how processing affects the polymorphic behaviour of compounds. For example, the effect of polymorphic transformations that occurred during the extrusion-granulation process of carbamazepine granules has been studied by Otsuka et al. (1997). Results showed that granulation using 50 percent ethanol transformed Form I into the dihydrate during the process. Wet granulation (using ethanol-water) of chlorpromazine hydrochloride was found to produce a phase change (Wong and Mitchell 1992). This was found to have some advantage, since Form II (the initial metastable form) was found to show severe capping and lamination compared to Form I, the (stable) form produced on granulation. As another example, Yamaoka et al. (1982) reported the cracking of tablets by one form of carbochromen.

Polymorphism is not an issue only with the compound under investigation; excipients also show variability in this respect. For example, it is well known that the tablet lubricant magnesium stearate can vary depending on the supplier. In one study, Wada and Matsubara (1992) examined the polymorphism with respect to 23 batches of magnesium stearate obtained from a variety of manufacturers. Using DSC, they classified the batches into six groups—interestingly, the polymorphism was not apparent by XRPD, IR or SEM observations. In another report, Barra and Somma (1996) examined 13 samples of magnesium stearate from 3 manufacturers. They found that there was variation not only between the manufacturers but also in the lots supplied by the same manufacturer.

SOLUTION FORMULATIONS

Development of a solution formulation requires a number of key pieces of preformulation information. Of these, solubility (and any pH dependence) and stability are probably the most important. Since parenteral products probably represent the most common solution formulation type, these are discussed in more detail. The principles and practices governing the formulation development of parenteral products have been reviewed by Sweetana and Akers (1996) and are discussed in detail in Chapter 9 on Parenteral Dosage Forms. Rowe et al. (1995) have described an expert system for the development of parenteral products.

Solubility Considerations

One of the main problems associated with developing a parenteral or any other solution formulation of a compound is its aqueous solubility. For poorly soluble drug candidates, there are several strategies for enhancing their solubility. These include pH manipulation, co-solvents, surfactants, emulsion formation and complexing agents. More sophisticated delivery systems, e.g., liposomes, can also be used in this way.

pH Manipulation

Since many compounds are weak acids or bases, their solubility will then be a function of pH. Figure 6.10 shows the pH-solubilty curve for a hydrochloride salt with pK_as at 6.58 and 8.16. When the acid-base titration method (Serrajudden and Mufson 1985) was used, the solubility curve showed a minimum between pH 6 and 8. Below this pH region, the solubility

Figure 6.10 pH-solubility curve of a development compound (amine hydrochloride).

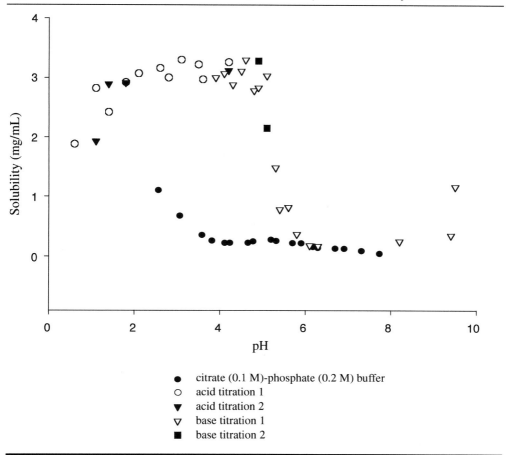

- ● citrate (0.1 M)-phosphate (0.2 M) buffer
- ○ acid titration 1
- ▼ acid titration 2
- ▽ base titration 1
- ■ base titration 2

increased as the pK_a was passed, to reach a maximum between pH 2 and 4 and then decreased due to the common ion effect. As the second pK_a was passed in the alkaline region, the solubility again increased.

When the solubility experiments were performed in 0.2 M citrate-phosphate buffer, the compound solubility decreased, and this illustrates the effect that ionic strength may have on drug solubility. Clearly, the region between pH 2 and 5 represents the area to achieve the best solubility. However, caution should be exercised if the solution needs to be buffered, since this can decrease the solubilty. Myrdal et al. (1995) found that a buffered formulation of a compound did not precipitate on dilution and did not cause phlebitis. In contrast, the unbuffered drug formulation showed the opposite effects. These results reinforce the importance of buffering parenteral formulations instead of simply adjusting the pH.

Co-solvents

The use of co-solvents has been utilized quite effectively for some poorly soluble drug substances. It is probable that the mechanism of enhanced solubility is the result of the polarity of the co-solvent mixture being closer to the drug than it is in water. This was illustrated in a series of papers by Rubino and Yalkowsky (1984, 1985a, b, 1987a, b) who found that the solubilities of phenytoin, benzocaine and diazepam in co-solvent and water mixtures were approximated by the log-linear equation

$$\log S_m = f \log S_c + (1 - f) \log S_w \tag{8}$$

where S_m = the solubility of the compound in the solvent mix, S_w = solubility in water, S_c is the solubility of the compound in pure cosolvent, f = the volume fraction of co-solvent and σ = the slope of the plot of log (S_m/S_w) versus f. Furthermore, they related s to indexes of cosolvent polarity such as the dielectric constant, solubility parameter, surface tension, interfacial tension and octanol-water partition coefficient.

It was found that the aprotic co-solvents gave a much higher degree of solubility than the amphiprotic co-solvents. This means that if a co-solvent can donate a hydrogen bond, it may be an important factor in determining whether it is a good co-solvent. Deviations from log-linear solubility were dealt with in a subsequent paper (Rubino and Yalkowsky 1987). Figure 6.11 shows how the solubility of a development drug increases in a number of water-solvent systems. Care must be taken when attempting to increase the solubility of a compound; a polar drug might actually show a decrease in solubility with increasing co-solvent composition (Gould et al. 1984).

It is often necessary to administer a drug parenterally at a concentration that exceeds its aqueous solubility. Co-solvents offer one way of increasing drug solubility, but the amount of co-solvent that can be used in a parenteral IV formulation is often constrained by toxicity considerations. The formulation may cause haemolysis (Fu et al. 1987), or the drug may precipitate when diluted or injected, causing phlebitis (e.g., Ward and Yalkowsky 1993). Yalkowsky and co-workers (1983) have developed a useful *in vitro* technique, based on ultraviolet (UV) spectrophotometry, for predicting the precipitation of parenteral formulations *in vivo* following injection. Figure 6.12 shows the effect of injection rate on the transmittance at 600 nm of a PEG 400 formulation of a compound being introduced into flowing saline. As shown, the faster the injection rate, the more precipitation was detected by the spectrophotometer. This simple technique can be used to assess whether preciptation of a compound might occur on dilution or injection.

Figure 6.11 Solubility as a function of co-solvent volume for a development compound.

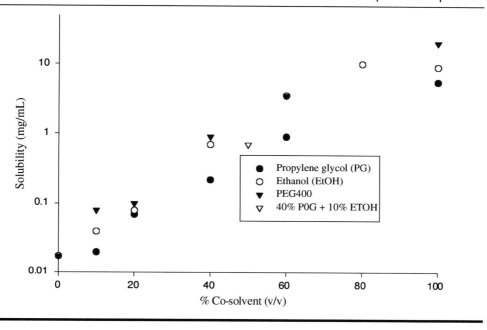

Figure 6.12 Effect of flow rate on the precipitation of a PEG400 solution of a drug compound.

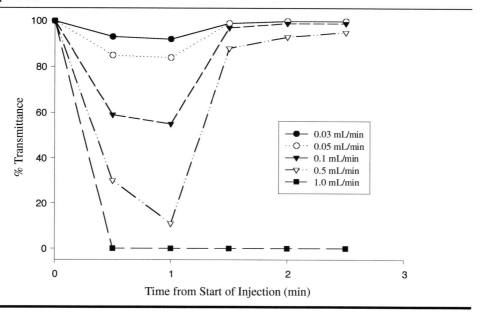

Whilst co-solvents can increase the solubility of compounds, on occasion they can have a detrimental effect on their stability. For example, a parenteral formulation of the novel anti-tumour agent carzelsin (U80,244), using a polyethylene glygol 400 (PEG 400)/absolute ethanol/polysorbate 80 (PET) formulation (ratio 6:3:1, v/v/v), has been reported (Jonkman-De Vries et al. 1995). Whilst this formulation effectively increased the solubility of the compound, this work showed that interbatch variation of PEG 400 could affect the stability of the drug through pH effects.

One point that is often overlooked when considering co-solvents is their influence on buffers or salts. Since these are conjugate acid-base systems, it is not surprising that by introducing solvents into the solution, a shift in the pK_a of the buffer or salt can result. These effects are important in formulation terms, since many injectable formulations that contain co-solvents also contain a buffer to control the pH (Rubino 1987).

Emulsion Formulations

Oil-in-water (o/w) emulsions have been successfully employed to deliver drugs with poor water solubility, e.g, diazepam (Collins-Gold et al. 1990). In preformulation terms, the solubility of the compound in the oil phase (often soybean oil) is the main consideration in using this approach. However, the particle size of the emulsion and its stability (physical and chemical) also need to be assessed. Ideally, the particle size of the emulsion droplets should be in the colloidal range to avoid problems with phlebitis. To achieve this size, a microfluidizer should be used, since other techniques may produce droplets of a larger size, as shown in Table 6.7 (Lidgate 1990). Emulsions are prepared by homogenizing the oil in water in the presence of emulsifiers, e.g., phospholipids, which stabilize the emulsion via a surface charge and a mechanical barrier.

The particle size of emulsions can be measured using PCS (e.g., Whateley et al. 1984), whilst the surface charge or zeta potential can be measured using electrophoretic mobility measurements (Levy and Benita 1989). Physical instability of emulsions can take a number of forms, e.g., creaming, flocculation, coalescence or breaking, whilst chemical instability can be due to hydrolysis of the stabilizing moieties. In order to assess the stability of the emulsion, heating and freezing cycles can be employed, as well as centrifugation (Yalabik-Kas 1985). Chansiri et al. (1999) have investigated the effect of steam sterilization (121°C for 15 min) on

Table 6.7
Size of emulsion droplets produced by various methods.

Method of Manufacture	Particle Size (μm)
Vortex	0.03–24
Blade mixer	0.01–8
Homogenizer	0.02–2
Microfluidizer	0.07–0.2

From Lidgate, D. M. et al., Using a microfluidizer to manufacture parenteral emulsions, *Pharm. Tech. Int.* (1990), pp. 30–33. Reprinted with permission.

the stability of o/w emulsions. They found that emulsions with a high negative zeta potential did not show any change in their particle size distribution after autoclaving. Emulsions with a lower negative value, on the other hand, were found to separate into two phases during auto- claving. Because the stability of phospholipid-stabilized emulsions is dependent on the surface charge, these emulsions are normally autoclaved at pH 8–9.

Stability Considerations

The second major consideration with respect to solution formulations is stability. Notari (1996) has presented some arguments regarding the merits of a complete kinetic stability study. He calculated that with reliable data and no buffer catalysis, 16 experiments were re- quired to provide a complete kinetic stability study. If buffer ions contribute to the hydrolysis, then each species contributes to the pH-rate expression. Thus, for a single buffer, e.g., phos- phate, a minimum of 6 experiments was required. A stock solution of the compound should be prepared in an appropriate solvent and a small aliquot (e.g., 50 μL) added to, e.g., a buffer solution at a set pH. This solution should be maintained at a constant temperature, and the ionic strength may be controlled by the addition of KCl (e.g., $I = 0.5$). After thorough mixing, the solution is then sampled at various time points and assayed for the compound of interest. If the reaction is very fast, it is recommended that the samples are diluted into a medium that will stop or substantially slow the reaction; for example, a compound that is unstable in acid may be stable in an alkaline medium. Cooling the solution may also be useful. Slow reactions, on the other hand, may require longer-term storage at elevated temperature. In this situation, solutions should be sealed in an ampoule to prevent loss of moisture. If sufficient compound is available, the effect of, e.g., buffer concentration, should be investigated.

The first-order decomposition plot of an acid labile compound with respect to pH is shown in Figure 6.13. Clearly, this compound is very acid labile, and even at pH 7, some de- composition is observed. A stable solution formulation would, therefore, be difficult to achieve in this pH range.

A detailed paper on the mechanistic interpretation of pH-rate profiles is that by Loudon (1991). More recently, van der Houwen et al. (1997) have reviewed the systematic interpreta- tion of pH-degradation profiles. The rate profiles obtained when pH is varied can take a num- ber of forms. However, Loudon (1991) makes the point that they "usually consist of linear regions of integral slope connected by short curved segments". Indeed, the linear regions gen- erally have slopes of –1, 0, or +1 and "any pH-rate profile can be regarded as a composite of fundamental curves".

It is also possible that compounds may be formulated in co-solvent systems for geriatric or paediatric use, where administration of a tablet would be difficult (Chang and Whitworth 1984). In addition, co-solvents are routinely employed in parenteral formulations to enhance the solubility of poorly soluble drugs; for example, Tu et al. (1989) have investigated the sta- bility of a non-aqueous formulation for injection based on 52 percent N,N-dimethylac- etamide and 48 percent propylene glycol. By stressing the preparation with regard to temperature, they found that, using Arrhenius kinetics, the time for 10 percent degradation at 25°C would be 885 days. The solution also discoloured when stressed. Furthermore, it is also sometimes useful to assess the effect of ethanol/acid on the stability of compounds that can be taken concurrently, e.g., temazepam (Yang 1994).

Figure 6.13 First-order hydrolysis decomposition of a compound (25°C).

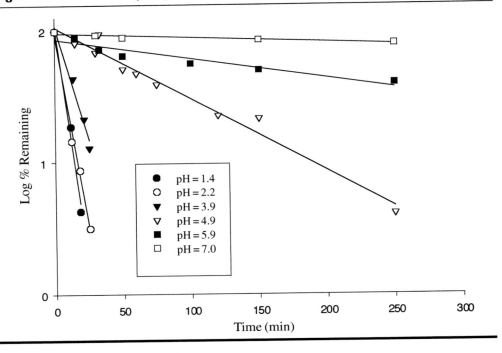

Stability to Autoclaving

For parenteral IV formulations, a sterile solution of the compound is required. A terminal sterilization method is preferred, rather than aseptic filtration, because there is a greater assurance of achieving sterility. As noted by Moldenhauer (1998), the FDA requires a written justification to explain why a product is not terminally sterilized. Therefore, it is mandatory to assess whether the candidate drug is stable to autoclaving as part of any preformulation selection process. Autoclaving (usually 15 min at 121°C) at various pHs is undertaken, after which the solutions should be evaluated for impurities, colour, pH and degradation products. Clearly, if one compound shows superior stability after autoclaving, then this will be the one to choose.

The effect of the autoclave cycle, i.e., fill, heat-up, peak dwell and cool down, on the theoretical chemical stability of compounds intended for IV injection has been investigated by Parasrampuria et al. (1993). Assuming first-order degradation kinetics, i.e., hydrolysis, the amount of degradation was calculated for any point during the above process. Although the results were calculated for first-order kinetics, the authors estimated that the calculations were applicable to other reaction orders, i.e., zero and second. Acceptable reasons for not proceeding with a terminally sterilized product are as follows:

- pH changes

- Colour changes

- Carbonate buffering loss

- Container closure problems

- Drug or excipient degradation

Effect of Metal Ions and Oxygen on Stability

In formulation terms, the removal of oxygen and trace metal ions, and the exclusion of light, may be necessary to improve the stability of oxygen sensitive compounds. Formulation aids to this end include antioxidants and chelating agents and, of course, the exclusion of light where necessary. Antioxidants are substances that should preferentially react with oxygen and hence protect the compound of interest towards oxidation. A list of water and oil soluble antioxidants is given in Table 6.8 (Akers 1982).

Preformulation screening of the antioxidant efficiency in parenteral solutions containing epinephrine has been reported by Akers (1979), who concluded that screening was difficult on the basis of the redox potential, and was complicated by a complex formulation of many components. Indeed, the most recent study on the preformulation screening of antioxidants found that the ability of an antioxidant to consume the oxygen in the formulation was a superior indicator of suitability when compared to redox methods (Ugwu and Apte 1999).

To illustrate the effect of oxygen on a compound that was sensitive to its presence, and its effect on the antioxidant (sodium metabisulphite), we performed the following experi-

Table 6.8
List of water and oil soluble antioxidants.

Water Soluble	Oil Soluble
Sodium bisulphite	Propyl gallate
Sodium sulphite	Butylated hydroxyanisole
Sodium metabisulphite	Butylated hydroxytoluene
Sodium thiosulphate	Ascorbyl palmitate
Sodium formaldehyde sulphoxylate	Nordihydroguaiaretic acid
l and d Ascorbic acid	α-Tocopherol
Acetylcysteine	
Cysteine	
Thioglycerol	
Thioglycollic acid	
Thiolactic acid	
Thiourea	
Dithithreitol	
Glutathione	

Reprinted with permission. *J. Parenteral Sci. Tech.* 36:222–228 (1982).

ments. The formulation (which had been degassed by flushing with nitrogen) was dispensed into ampoules (using a modified Autopak machine) and the headspace was flushed with nitrogen or nitrogen-oxygen mixtures, which are normally used to calibrate gas-liquid chromatographs. The gases used to fill the headspace were oxygen free nitrogen, 1, 3.1 and 5.2 percent v/v oxygen in nitrogen; however, when analyzed by gas-liquid chromatography (GLC), the initial values were higher, giving 1, 1.7, 3.4 and 6.4 percent v/v oxygen in nitrogen, respectively. The amount of oxygen in the headspace was determined using GLC; decomposition of the compound was monitored by UV spectroscopy at 340 nm, because it gave a coloured decomposition product; and metabisulphite was assessed using Ellmans reagent 5,5 dethiobis-(2-nitrobenzoic acid). Figure 6.14 shows the increase in absorbance with time; Figure 6.15a shows the level of oxygen in the headspace; and Figure 6.15b shows the decrease in metabisulphite with time.

It is clear from these data that the metabisulphite consumed oxygen, reducing it in all cases to a constant low value. Nonetheless, only the two lowest oxygen headspace levels were deemed acceptable, illustrating the need to keep the presence of oxygen to an absolute minimum. It should be noted that, if the concentration of metabisulphite is greater than 0.01 M, it hydrolyses to give two molecules of bisulphite.

The reaction of bisulphite with dissolved oxygen is given by

$$2HSO_3^- + O_2 \rightarrow 2SO_4^- + 2H^+$$

Figure 6.14 Plot of absorbance versus time for a development undergoing degradation via oxidation.

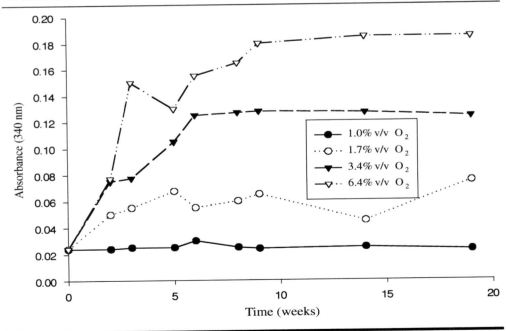

Figure 6.15 (a) Decrease in headspace oxygen with time; (b) decrease in metabisulphite concentration with time for various headspace oxygen levels.

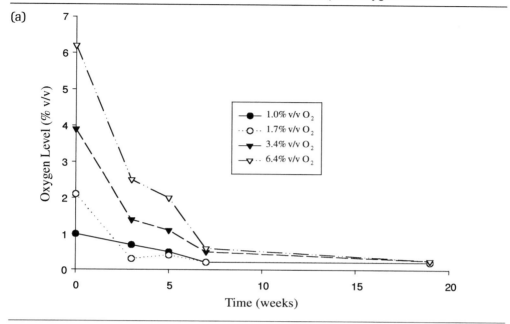

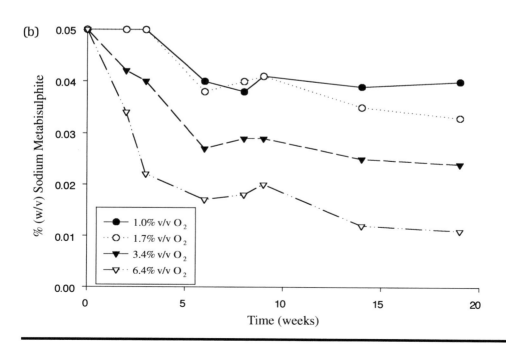

compounds (Asahara et al. 1990). Thus, oxygen-sensitive substances should be screened for their compatibility with a range of antioxidants. It should also be noted that bisulphite has also been known to catalyse hydrolysis reactions (e.g., Munson et al. 1977).

Trace metal ions can affect stability and can arise from the bulk drug, formulation excipients or glass containers. The effect of metal ions on the solution stability of fosinopril sodium has been reported (Thakur et al. 1993). In this case, the metal ions were able to provide, through complexation, a favourable reaction pathway.

Metal ions can also act as degradation catalysts by being involved in the production of highly reactive free radicals, especially in the presence of oxygen. The formation of these radicals can be initiated by the action of light or heat, and propagate the reaction until they are destroyed by inhibitors or by side reactions that break the chain (Scott 1988). Free radical oxygen species can be generated by transition metals in solution such that reactions can be initiated, illustrated by the potentiation of the auto-oxidation of dopamine by metal ions (Poirier et al. 1985).

Ethylenediaminetetraacetic Acid (EDTA) and Chelating Agents

Because of the involvement of metal ions in degradation reactions, the inclusion of a chelating agent is often advocated. The most commonly used chelating agent are the various salts of EDTA. In addition, β-hydroxyethylenediaminetriacetic acid (HEDTA), diethylenetriaminepentaacetic acid (DTPA) and nitrilotriacetate (NTA) have been assessed for their efficiency in stabilizing, e.g., isoniazid solutions (Ammar et al. 1982).

EDTA has pK_a values of $pK_1 = 2.0$, $pK_2 = 2.7$, $pK_3 = 6.2$ and $pK_4 = 10.4$ at 20°C. Generally, the reaction of EDTA with metal ions can be described by

$$M^{n+} + Y^{4-} \rightarrow MY^{(4-n)+} \tag{9}$$

In practice, however, the disodium salt is used because of its greater solubility, hence

$$M^{n+} + H_2Y \rightarrow MY^{(n-4)+} + 2H^+ \tag{10}$$

From equation 13, it is apparent that the dissociation (or equilibrium) will be sensitive to the pH of the solution, therefore, this will have implications for the formulation.

The stability of the complex formed by EDTA-metal ions is characterized by the stability or formation constant, K. This is derived from the reaction equation and is given by

$$K = \frac{\left[(MY)^{(n-4)^+} \right]}{\left[M^{n^+} \right]\left[Y^{4-} \right]} \tag{11}$$

Stability constants (expressed as log K) of some metal ion-EDTA complexes are shown in Table 6.9, and an example of a metal ion-EDTA complex is shown in Figure 6.16.

Equation 14 assumes that the fully ionized form of $EDTA^{4-}$ is present in solution, however, at low pH, other species will be present, i.e., $HEDTA^{3-}$, H_2EDTA^{2-} and H_3EDTA^- as well as the undissociated H_4EDTA. Thus the stability constants become conditional upon pH.

The ratio can be calculated for the total uncombined EDTA (in all forms) to the form $EDTA^{4-}$. Thus the *apparent* stability constant becomes K/α_L, such that

Table 6.9
Metal ion–EDTA stability constants.

Ion	log K	Log K_H	Ion	log K	Log K_H	Ion	log K	Log K_H
Ag^+	7.3	-4.2	Co^{2+}	16.3	4.3	Fe^{3+}	25.1	13.1
Li^+	2.8	-9.2	Ni^{2+}	18.6	6.6	Y^{3+}	18.2	6.2
Na^+	1.7	-10.3	Cu^{2+}	18.8	6.8	Cr^{3+}	24.0	12.0
Mg^{2+}	8.7	-3.3	Zn^{2+}	16.7	4.7	Ce^{3+}	15.9	3.9
Ca^{2+}	10.6	-1.4	Cd^{2+}	16.6	4.6	La^{3+}	15.7	3.7
Sr^{2+}	8.6	-3.4	Hg^{2+}	21.9	9.9	Sc^{3+}	23.1	11.1
Ba^{2+}	7.8	-4.2	Pb^{2+}	18.0	6.0	Ga^{3+}	20.5	8.5
Mn^{2+}	13.8	1.8	Al^{3+}	16.3	4.3	In^{3+}	24.9	12.9
Fe^{2+}	14.3	2.3	Bi^{3+}	27.0	15.0	Th^{4+}	23.2	11.2

Note: Log K_H values calculated for pH 2.5.

$$\alpha_L = \frac{[EDTA]_{allforms}}{[EDTA^{4-}]} \tag{12}$$

Thus

$$K_H = \frac{K}{\alpha_L} \text{ or } K_H = \log K - \alpha_L \tag{13}$$

Figure 6.16 Structure of metal-EDTA complex.

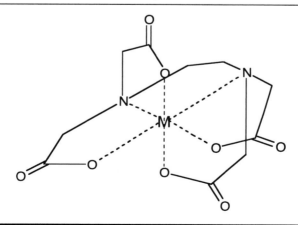

where $\log K_H$ is known as the conditional stability constant. Fortunately, α_L can be calculated from the known dissociation constants of EDTA, and its value can be calculated from

$$\alpha_L = \left\{1 + \frac{[H^+]}{K_4} + \frac{[H^+]}{K_4 K_3} + ...\right\} = 1 + 10^{(pK_4 - pH)} + 10^{(pK_4 + pK_3 pH)} + ... \qquad (14)$$

Thus at pH = 4, the conditional stability constants of some metal-EDTA complexes are calculated as follows:

$\log K_H$ EDTABa^{2+} = 0.6

$\log K_H$ EDTAMg^{2+} = 1.5

$\log K_H$ EDTACa^{2+} = 3.4

$\log K_H$ EDTAZn^{2+} = 9.5

$\log K_H$ EDTAFe^{3+} = 17.9

Thus at pH 4, the zinc and ferric complexes will exist; however, calcium, magnesium and barium will be only weakly complexed, if at all.

The inclusion of EDTA is occasionally not advantageous, since there are a number of reports of EDTA catalyzing the decomposition of drugs (Mendenhall 1984; Nayak et al. 1986). Citric acid, tartaric acid, glycerin and sorbitol can also be considered as complexing agents; however, these are often ineffective. Interestingly, some Japanese formulators often resort to amino acids or tryptophan because of a ban on EDTA in a particular country (Wang and Kowal 1980).

Surface Activity

Many drugs show surface active behaviour because they have the correct mix of chemical groups that are typical of surfactants. The surface activity of drugs can be important if they show a tendency to, e.g, adhere to surfaces, or if solutions foam. The surface activity of compounds can be determined using a variety of techniques, such as surface tension measurements using a Du Nouy tensiometer, Whilhelmy plate and conductance measurements. Figure 6.17 shows the surface tension as a function of concentration (using a Du Nouy tensiometer) of a primary amine hydrochloride solution in water. The surface tension of water decreased due to the presence of the compound, however, there was no break, which would have been indicative of micelle formation. Even when the pH of the solution was adjusted to 7, where a solubility "spike" had been observed, the surface tension was not significantly different to that observed for water alone. Thus, although the compound was surface active, it did not appear to form micelles, probably due to steric effects.

The surface active properties of MDL-201,346, a hydrochloride salt, has been investigated by a number of techniques including conductivity measurements (Streng et al. 1996). It was found that it underwent significant aggregation in water at temperatures greater than 10°C. Moreover, a break in the molar conductivity versus square root of concentation was noted, which corresponded to the critical micelle concentration (CMC) of the compound and aggregation of 10–11 molecules. In addition to surface active behaviour, some drugs are known to form liquid crystalline phases with water, e.g., diclofenac diethylamine (Kriwet and Müller-

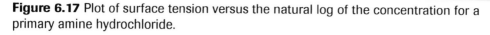

Figure 6.17 Plot of surface tension versus the natural log of the concentration for a primary amine hydrochloride.

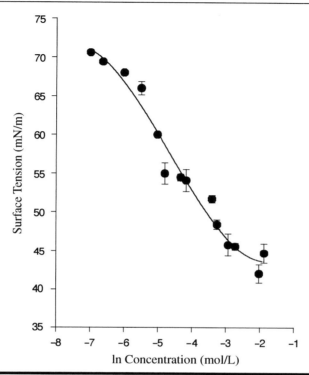

Goymann 1993). Self-association in water (vertical stacking) of the novel anticancer agent brequiner sodium (King et al. 1989) has been reported.

Osmolality

Body fluids, such as blood, normally have an osmotic pressure which is often described as corresponding to that of a 0.9 percent w/v solution of sodium chloride and, indeed, a 0.9 percent w/v NaCl solution is said to be iso-osmotic with blood. Those solutions with an osmotic pressure lower than 0.9 percent w/v NaCl are known as hypotonic, and those greater than this value are said to be hypertonic. The unit commonly used unit to express osmolality is the osmol, and this is defined as the weight in grams per solute, existing in a solution as molecules, ions, macromolecules, etc., that is osmotically equivalent to the gram molecular weight of an ideally behaving non-electrolyte.

Pharmaceutically, osmotic effects are important in the parenterals and ophthalmic fields, and work is usually directed at formulating to avoid the side-effects or finding methods of administration to minimize them. The ophthalmic respose to various concentrations of sodium chloride is shown in Table 6.10 (Flynn 1979).

Table 6.10
Ophthalmic response to various concentrations of sodium chloride.

% NaCl	Ophthalmic Response
0.0	Very disagreeable
0.6	Perceptibly disagreeable after 1 min
0.8	Completely indifferent after long exposure
1.2	"
1.3	Perceptibly disagreeable after 1 min
1.5	Somewhat disagreeable after 1 min
2.0	Disagreeable after 1/2 min

Reprinted with permission. *J. Parenteral Sci. Tech.* 33:292–315 (1979).

Osmolality determinations are usually carried out using a cryoscopic osmometer, which is calibrated with deionized water and solutions of sodium chloride of known concentration. Using this technique, the sodium chloride equivalents and freezing point depressions for more than 500 substances have been determined and reported in a series of papers by Hammerlund and co-workers (e.g., see Hammerlund 1981). Figure 6.18 shows the osmolality of mannitol-water solutions.

FREEZE-DRIED FORMULATIONS

If a drug in solution proves to be unstable to autoclaving, then an alternative formulation approach will be required. Freeze-drying such solutions is often attempted to produce the requisite stability. Preformulation studies can be performed to evaluate this approach and to aid the development of the freeze-drying cycle. Briefly, freeze-drying consists of three main stages: (a) freezing of the solution, (b) primary drying and (c) secondary drying (Williams and Polli 1984). In many cases, the inclusion of excipients is necessary to act as bulking agents or stabilizing agents. Thus, production conditions should be evaluated to ensure that the process is efficient and that it produces a stable product. The first stage, therefore, is to characterize the freezing and heating behaviour of solutions containing the candidate drug. In this respect DSC can be used, as described by Hatley et al. (1996).

To understand the processes taking place during freezing a solution containing a solute, it is worth referring to the phase diagram described by Her and Nail (1994). If, on cooling a solution of a compound, crystallization does not take place, the solution becomes supercooled and thus becomes more concentrated and viscous. Eventually, the viscosity is increased to such an extent that a glass is formed. This point is known as the glass transition temperature (T_g).

Measurement of the glass transition of frozen solution formulation of the candidate drug is an important preformulation determination, since freeze-drying an amorphous system above this temperature can lead to a decrease in viscous flow of the solute (due to a decrease

Figure 6.18 Plot of tonicity versus concentration for mannitol in water.

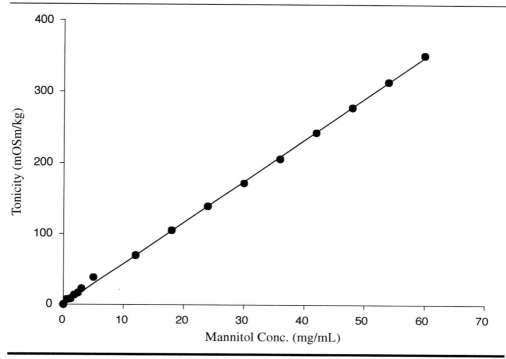

in viscosity) after the removal of the ice. This leads to what is commonly known as "collapse", and for successful freeze-drying, it should be performed below the T_g. Consequences of collapse include high residual water content in the product and prolonged reconstitution times. In addition, the increase in the mobility of molecules above the T_g may lead to in-process degradation (Pikal and Shah 1990).

Figure 6.19 shows the glass transition, as determined by DSC, of a trial formulation of a candidate drug. The glass transition was measured by freezing a solution of the compound in a DSC pan and then heating the frozen solution. It should be noted that T_g is usually a subtle event compared to the ice-melt endotherm, and so the thermogram should be examined very carefully. In some cases, an endotherm due to stress relaxation may be superimposed on the glass transition. It is possible to resolve these events using the related technique, modulated DSC (MDSC) or dynamic DSC (DDSC).

If during freezing the solutes crystallize, the first thermal event detected using DSC will be the endotherm that corresponds to melting of the eutectic formed between ice and the solute. This is usually followed by an endothermic event corresponding to the melting of ice. Figure 6.20 shows this behaviour for a 9% w/v saline solution. Normally, freeze-drying of these systems is carried out below the eutectic melting temperature (see e.g., Williams and Schwinke 1994). Another way of detecting whether a solute or formulation crystallizes on freezing is to conduct subambient X-ray diffractometry (Cavatur and Suryanarayanan 1998).

Figure 6.19 DSC thermogram showing a glass transition of heated frozen drug solution.

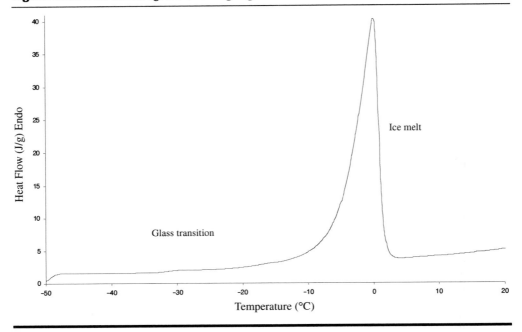

If a lyophilized drug is amorphous, then knowledge of the glass transition temperature is important for stability reasons. Chemically, amorphous compounds are usually less stable than their crystalline counterparts. This is illustrated in Table 6.11, which shows some stability data for an amorphous compound (produced by lyophilization) and the crystalline hydrate form of the compound.

Although the moisture content of the amorphous form was increased, it did not crystallize. Other work showed that at RHs greater than 70 percent, the sample crystallized. It is important to note that moisture has the effect of lowering the glass temperature, which in turn increases the propensity for instability. This appears to be due to water acting as a plasticizer such that molecular mobility is increased, thus facilitating reactivity (Shalaev and Zografi 1996).

Duddu and Weller (1996) have studied the importance of the glass transition temperature of an amorphous lyophilized aspirin-cyclodextrin complex. Using DSC, the glass transition was found to be 36°C, and was followed by an exothermic peak, believed to be due to aspirin crystallization. The glass transition at this temperature was also observed using dielectric relaxation spectroscopy. When the aspirin/hydroxypropyl-β-cyclodextrin (HPCD) lyophile was exposed to higher humidities, the T_g was reduced to a temperature below room temperature, and the product became a viscous gel. Craig et al. (1999) have reviewed the physicochemical properties of the amorphous state with respect to drugs and freeze-dried formulations.

Figure 6.20 DSC thermogram of a frozen 9% w/v saline solution.

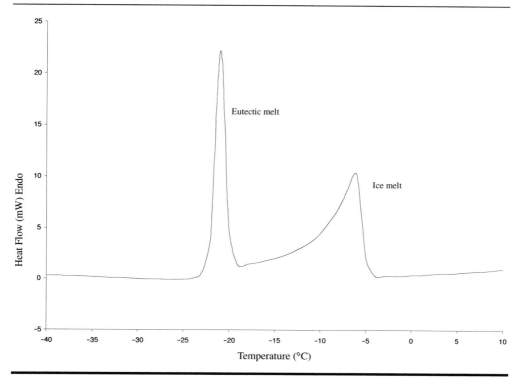

Table 6.11
Stability data for an amorphous (lyophilized)
and crystalline hydrate form of a compound.

	Storage Conditions (°C/%RH)	Time (month)	Moisture Content (%w/w)	Total Impurities (%w/w)
Crystalline		Initial	15.98	0.53
	25/16	1	15.78	0.54
	25/60	1	15.50	0.56
	40/75	1	15.76	0.59
Amorphous		Initial	4.83	0.47
	25/16	1	8.31	0.57
	25/60	1	12.55	0.69
	40/75	1	12.72	1.44

SUSPENSIONS

Data considered to be important for suspensions at the preformulation stage include solubility, particle size and propensity for crystal growth and chemical stability. Furthermore, during development, it will be important to have knowledge of the viscosity of the vehicle to obtain information with respect to settling of the suspended particles, syringibility and physical stability (Akers et al. 1987). In a report on the preformulation information required for suspensions, Morefield et al. (1987) investigated the relationship between the critical volume fraction as a function of pH. They noted that "it is usually desirable to maximize the volume fraction of solids in order to minimize the volume of the dose".

It should be obvious that for a successful suspension, insolubility of the candidate drug is required. Whilst for large hydrophobic drugs like steroids this may not a problem, weak acids or bases, however, may show appreciable solubility. In this instance, reducing the solubility by salt formation is a relatively common way to achieve this end. For example, a calcium salt of a weak acid may be sufficiently insoluble for a suspension formulation. However, difficulties may arise due to hydrate formation with concomitant crystal growth; e.g., Hoelgaard and Møller (1983) found that metronidazole formed a monohydrate on suspension in water. Another way crystals can grow in suspension, that is not due to a phase change, is by Ostwald ripening. This is the result of the difference in solubility between small and large crystals as predicted by

$$\frac{RT}{M}\ln\left(\frac{S_2}{S_1}\right) = \frac{2\sigma}{\rho}\left(\frac{1}{r_1} - \frac{1}{r_2}\right) \tag{15}$$

where R is the gas constant, T is the absolute temperature, S_1 and S_2 are the solubilities of crystals of radii r_1 and r_2 respectively, σ is the specific surface energy, ρ is the density and M is the molecular weight of the solute molecules. Ostwald ripening is promoted by temperature changes during storage, particularly if there is a strong temperature-solubility relationship. Therefore, as the temperature is increased, the small particles of the drug will dissolve, which is followed by crystal growth as the temperature is decreased. Ziller and Rupprecht (1988a) have reported the design of a control unit to monitor crystal growth; however, simple microscopic observation may be all that is necessary to monitor the growth of crystals. If a phase change occurs, then the usual techniques may be used to assess the solid-state form of the compound produced on storage such as DSC, hot stage microscopy (HSM) or XRPD. Polymeric additives may be employed to inhibit drug crystallization; Ziller and Rupprecht (1988b) found that polyvinylpyrrolidone and bovine serum albumin inhibit crystal growth using a variety of compounds.

It is a pharmacopoeial requirement that suspensions should be redispersible if they settle on storage. However, the pharmacopoeias do not offer a suitable test that can be used to characterize this aspect of the formulation. In an attempt to remedy this situation, Deicke and Süverkrüp (1999) have devised a mechanical redispersibility tester, which closely simulates the action of human shaking. The crystal habit may also affect the physical stability of the formulation; Tiwary and Panpalia (1999) showed that trimethoprim crystals with the largest aspect ratio showed the best sedimentation volume and redispersibility.

If the suspension is for parenteral administration, it will need to be sterilized. Terminal heat sterilization can affect both its chemical and physical stability, the latter usually observed as crystal growth or aggregation of the particles (Na et al. 1999). Another measure of suspension stability is the zeta potential, which is a measure of the surface charge. However, various studies have shown that it only useful in some cases. For example, Biro and Racz (1998) found that the zeta potential of albendazole suspensions was a good indicator of stability, whereas Duro et al. (1998) showed that the electrical charge of pyrantel pamoate suspensions was not important for its stabilization.

As noted above, the particle size of suspensions is another important parameter in suspension formulations. The particle size distribution can be measured using a variety of techniques, including laser diffraction. A point to note in laser diffraction is the careful selection of the suspending agent. This was illustrated by Atkinson and White (1992) who used a Malvern Mastersizer to determine the particle size of a 1 percent methylcellulose in the presence of seven surface active agents (Tween 80, Tween 20, Span 20, Pluronic L62, Pluronic F88, Cetomacrogol 1000 and sodium lauryl sulphate). The particle size of the suspensions was measured as a function of time and, surprisingly, Tween 80, which is widely used in this respect, was found to be unsuitable for the hydrophobic drug under investigation. Other surfactants also gave poor particle size data, e.g., Tween 20, Cetomacrogol 1000, Pluronic F88 and sodium lauryl sulphate. This arose from aggregation of the particles, and additionally, these suspensions showed slower drug dissolution in water. Span 20 and Pluronic L62 showed the best results, and therefore the authors cautioned the use of a standard surface active agent in preclinical studies.

Usually, suspensions are flocculated so that the particles form large aggregates that are easy to disperse—normally this is achieved using potassium or sodium chloride (Akers et al. 1987). However, for controlled flocculation suspensions, sonication may be required to determine the size of the primary particles (Bommireddi et al. 1998).

Although high performance liquid chromatography (HPLC) is the preferred technique for assessing the stability of formulations, spectrophotometry can also be used. Girona et al. (1988) used this technique for assessing the stability of an ampicillin-dicloxacillin suspension.

TOPICAL/TRANSDERMAL FORMULATIONS

Samir (1997) has reviewed preformulation aspects of transdermal drug delivery. This route of delivery offers several potential advantages compared to the oral route, such as avoidance of fluctuating blood levels, no first-pass metabolism and no degradation due to stomach acid. However, the transdermal route is limited because of the very effective barrier function of the skin. Large, polar molecules do not penetrate the stratum corneum well. The physicochemical properties of candidate drugs that are important in transdermal drug delivery include molecular weight and volume, aqueous solubility, melting point and log P. Clearly, these are intrinsic properties of the molecule and, as such, will determine whether or not the compounds will penetrate the skin. Furthermore, since many compounds are weak acids or bases, pH will have an influence on their permeation.

One way in which the transport of zwitterionic drugs through skin has been enhanced is by salt formation. This was demonstrated by Mazzenga et al. (1992) who showed that the rank order of epidermal flux of the salts of phenylalanine across the epidermis was hydrobromide > hydrochloride > hydrofluoride > phenylalanine. Thus, like most other delivery routes, it is worth considering salt selection issues at the preformulation stage to optimize the delivery of the compound via the skin.

The formulation in which the candidate drug is applied to the skin is another important factor that can affect its bioavailability. In transdermal drug delivery, a number of vehicles may be used, such as creams, ointments, lotions, gels and so on. The solubility of the compound in the vehicle needs to be determined. Problems can arise from crystal growth if the system is supersaturated; for example, phenylbutazone creams were observed to have a gritty appearance due to crystal growth (Sallam et al. 1986). Indeed, in matrix patches, crystals of estradiol hemihydrate or gestodene up to 800 μm grew during 3 months of storage at room temperature (Lipp and Müller-Fahrnow 1999). As another example, needle-like crystals of the hydrate of betamethasone-17-valerate were found by Folger and Müller-Goymann (1994) when creams were placed on storage.

Chemical and physical stability also need to be considered. For example, Thoma and Holzmann (1998) showed that dithranol showed a distinct instability in the paraffin base due to light, but was stable when protected from light. In terms of kinetics, Kenley et al. (1987) found that the degradation in a topical cream and in ethanol-water solutions were very similar in the pH range 2–6. This suggested that the degradation of this compound occurred in an aqueous phase or compartment that was undisturbed by the oily cream excipients. If the compound decomposes due to oxidation, then an antioxidant may have to be incorporated. Table 6.8 lists the water soluble and oil soluble antioxidants that can be considered for incorporation into a topical formulation.

In an attempt to reduce the photodegradation of a development compound, Merrifield et al. (1996) compared the free acid of compound to a number of its salts, each of which they incorporated into a white soft paraffin base. Their results (Table 6.12) showed that after a 1 h exposure in a SOL2 light simulation cabinet, the disodium salt showed significant degradation.

Martens-Lobenhoffer et al. (1999) have studied the stability of 8-methoxypsoralen (8-MOP) in various ointments. They found that after 12 weeks storage, the drug was stable in Unguentum Cordes and Cold Cream Naturel; however, the Unguentum Cordes emulsion began to crack after 8 weeks. When formulated in a Carbopol gel, 8-MOP was unstable.

The physical structure of creams has been investigated by a variety of techniques, e.g., DSC, TGA, microscopy, reflectance measurement, rheology, Raman spectroscopy and dielectric analysis (see references in Peramal et al. 1997). Focussing on TGA and rheology, Peramal et al. (1997) found that when aqueous British Pharmacopoeia (BP) creams were analyzed by

Table 6.12
Light stability of the salts of a candidate drug in a white soft parrafin base.

Salt/Form	% initial compound after 1 h exposure in SOL2		
	0.1% conc.	0.5% conc.	2.0% conc.
Free acid (micronized)	51.0	80.0	85.9
Free acid (unmicronized)	69.4	nd	nd
Disodium (unmicronized)	9.9	3.6	nd
Ethylenediamine (unmicronized)	51.9	65.1	nd
Piperazine (unmicronized)	79.9	88.2	nd

From Merrifield, D. R. et al., Addressing the problem of light instability during formulation development. In *Photostab. Drugs: Drug Formulations* [Int. Meet. Photostab. Drugs 1995], edited by H. H. Tønneson (1996). Reprinted with permission from Taylor and Francis.

TGA, there were two peaks in the derivative curve. It was concluded that these were due to the loss of free and lamellar water from the cream, and therefore TGA could be used as a QC tool. The lamellar structure of creams can also be confirmed using small angle X-ray measurements (Niemi and Laine 1991). For example, the lamellar spacings of sodium lauryl sulphate and cetostearyl alcohol liquid paraffin creams were found to increase in size (from 8.5 to 17.6 nm) as the water content of the cream increased until, at > 60 percent water, the lamellar structure broke down. This was correlated with earlier work that showed that at this point, the release of hydrocortisone was increased (Niemi et al. 1989).

Atkinson et al. (1992) have reported the use of a laser diffraction method to measure the particle size of drugs dispersed in ointments. In this study, they stressed the fact that a very small particle size was required to ensure efficacy of the drug. In addition, the size of the particles was especially important if the ointment was for ophthalmic use where particles must be less than 25 μm. Whilst the particle size of the suspended particles can be assessed microscopically, laser diffraction offers a more rapid analysis.

INHALATION DOSAGE FORMS

Metered Dose Inhalers

In pressurised metered dose inhaler (pMDI) technology, CFC propellants are being replaced with the ozone-friendly hydrofluoroalkanes (HFA)-134a and -227. In pMDI drug delivery systems, the drugs are formulated as a suspension or as a solution, depending on the solubility of

$$F_3C—CF_2H$$

134a

$$F_3C—\overset{H}{\underset{F}{|}}—CF_3$$

227

the drug in the propellant. Although suspensions offer the advantage of superior chemical stability (Tiwari et al. 1998b), they may have problematic physical stability in terms of crystal growth or poor dispersion properties. In this respect, Tzou et al. (1997) examined whether the free base or the sulphate salt of albuterol (salbutamol) had the best chemical and physical stability for a pMDI formulation. In addition to the older CFC propellants, they examined the stability of the base and sulphate in HFA-134a. Results showed that all of the sulphate formulations were chemically stable for up to 12 months, however, the base was less stable. In terms of physical stability, the base formulations showed crystal growth and agglomeration, illustrating the need for undertaking a salt selection process.

One significant challenge in the transition from the CFCs to HFAs is that the surfactants and polymers used as suspension stabilizers in CFC formulations are not soluble enough in the HFAs to be effective. For example, sorbitan/trioleate (Span 85), commonly used in CFC formulations, is not soluble in HFA-134a or -227; however, other surfactants and polymers have been screened for their effectiveness in stabilizing propellant suspensions with some success. Some solubility of the surfactant in the propellant is a prerequisite and, whilst some suitable agents have been identified, they have not been progressed because of their potential toxicity in the lung. Some apparent solubilities of surfactants in HFA-134a and -227 are shown in Table 6.13 (Vervaet and Byron 1999).

It would of value to know if and how much surfactant or polymer was adsorbed by the particles. In an attempt to understand this process, Blackett and Buckton (1995) used

Table 6.13
Apparent solubilities of some surfactants in HFA-134a and HFA-227.

Surfactant	HLB	Apparent Solubility (%w/w)	
		HFA-134a	**HFA-227**
Oleic acid	1.0	< 0.02	< 0.02
Sorbitan trioleate	1.8	< 0.02	<0.01
Propoxylated PEG	4.0	≈ 3.6	1.5–15.3
			32.0–60.3
Sorbitan monooleate	4.3	< 0.01	< 0.01
Lecithin	7.0	< 0.01	< 0.01
Brij 30	9.7	≈ 1.8	0.8–1.2
Tween 80	15.0	< 0.03	0–10.0
			25.0–89.8
Tween 20	16.7	≈ 0.1	1.4–3.5
PEG 300	20	≈ 4.0	1.5–4.3
			16.1–100
PVP, PVA		> 0.1	
Oligolactic acids		≈ 2.7	

isothermal microcalorimetry. The system investigated was the model CFC Arcton 113, salbutamol sulphate (crystalline and partially crystalline) and oleic acid or Span 85 as stabilizers. Using a perfusion-titration set-up, they titrated suspensions of the drug with solutions of the surfactant and followed heat output as a function of time. It was shown that the heat output and adsorption was different, depending on the crystallinity of the sample, i.e., there was less heat output for the more energetic, partially crystalline sample. From these data, it was hypothesized that the orientation of the surfactant molecule during adsorption was different, depending on the surface energy of the particles in suspension.

Drugs for inhalation therapy via a pMDI (and dry powder inhalers, DPIs) are reduced in size by micronization to particles of approximately 1 to 6 μm, which are capable of penetrating the deep airways and impact at the site of action. As noted earlier, micronization can cause problems due to the reduction in crystallinity and poor flow properties as a result of the milling process (see, e.g., Buckton 1997). The effect of micronization on samples can be assessed by a variety of techniques, e.g., DVS, microcalorimetry and IGC. IGC, for example, has been used to determine the surface properties of two batches of salbutamol sulphate (Ticehurst et al. 1994). This group also investigated the surface properties of α-lactose monohydrate (an excipient used in DPIs, see next section) using this technique to detect batch variation (Ticehurst et al. 1996). It was hypothesized that these differences in surface energetics between the nominally equivalent batches were due to small variations in surface crystallinity or purity. One common way removing the high energy portions from the surface is

Table 6.14
Heat of solution of triamcinolone acetonide recovered from pMDIs after storage.

	Heat of Solution (J/g)		
	Raw Material	**Recovered TAA (3 months, 25°C)**	**Recovered TAA (3 months, 40°C)**
Unmicronized	44.1	39.0	47.7
Ball milled	38.6	29.6	36.4
Micronized	43.7	36.0	35.2

Reprinted from Influence of micronization method on the performance of a suspension triamcinolone acetonide pressurized metered-dose inhaler formulation, by R. O. Williams et al., in *Pharm. Dev. Tech.*, Vol. 4, pp. 167–179. Courtesy of Marcel Dekker, Inc.

to condition the powder with moist air, which crystallizes the amorphous regions (Ahmed et al. 1996).

Williams III et al. (1999a) have reported the influence of ball milling and micronization on the formulation of triamcinolone acetonide (TAA) for MDIs. Both methods reduced the particle size of the powder; however, as shown by solution calorimetry measurements ball milling produced material with a greater amorphous content (Table 6.14). Although the ball-milled material was less crystalline, it was found have the smallest particles and the highest respirable fraction.

It is possible that a number of physical changes can occur due to suspension in the propellant. The first is due to Ostwald ripening, a phenomenon described earlier in this chapter. This arises when the compound shows some solubility in the propellant, resulting in particle growth and caking. In this process, the smallest micronized particles dissolve and then recrystallize on the larger particles. As shown by Phillips et al. (1993), optical microscopy can be used to assess the crystal growth of micronized salicylic acid in CFC pMDIs. In this study, the increase in the axial ratio (length/breadth) of the crystals was measured as a function of time. Although the crystals continued to grow after an initial increase in the axial ratio, after some time it did not change. It was therefore concluded that axial ratios of crystals should always by determined by microscopy to detect any physical instability in the early stages of MDI formulation development. In another paper by this group, Phillips and Byron (1994) have investigated the surfactant promoted crystal growth of micronized methylprednisolone in trichloromonofluoromethane (CFC-11). The effect of drug concentration, surfactant type and composition on the solubility of methylprednisolone was determined and related to the observed crystal growth in suspension. In particular, high concentrations of Span 85 (sorbitan trioleate) were found to increase the solubility of the compound with the consequence of crystal growth. Oleic acid and lower concentrations of Span 85, on the other hand, showed little particle size change. In addition to an increase in particle size, the crystals may also solvate the propellants, and this may also lead to crystal growth. Apart from the obvious increase in particle size of the suspension, there are a number of techniques that can be used to confirm the existence of the solvate. These include DSC, TGA, HSM, XRPD and IR spectroscopy.

An example of this phenomenon is a development compound that was found to have changed from a micronized powder to much larger particles after storage in propellant. When the recovered crystals were analyzed using TGA, a mass loss of 25.5 percent was detected in the range between 40 and 100°C. This thermal event was also evident in the DSC, which showed an endotherm corresponding to solvent loss followed by an exotherm probably due to crystallization. HSM showed that, when heated in silicone oil, a gas was evolved as the temperature was raised. This is illustrated is Figure 6.21. Notice how the crystals broke apart as the gas was released as the temperature was raised.

To confirm that the crystals had solvated the propellant, IR spectroscopy provided a useful test. The main difference between the IR spectra before and after storage was the appearance of a medium-strong peak at 1289 cm^{-1}. By reference to standard tables of IR stretching frequencies, this new peak was assigned as a C-F stretch that, with the other information, led to the conclusion that the compound had solvated the propellant gas (134a).

Figure 6.21 HSM photographs of an inhalation drug before and after suspension in HFA-134a.

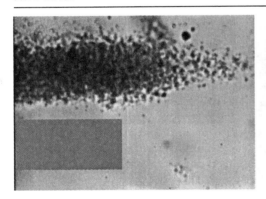

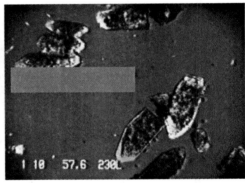

Before suspension   After 6 months' suspension.
                                                        57.6°C

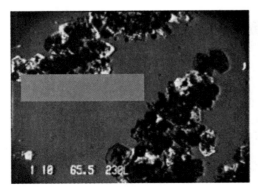

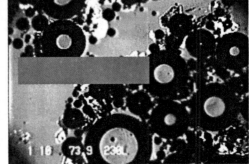

65.5°C   73.9°C

A method for determining the solubility of drugs in aerosol propellants has been described by Dalby et al. (1991). At room temperatures, the propellants are gases. Special procedures are therefore required in separating the excess solid from the solution in the aerosol can; in this case, it is a simple filtration from one can to another. The propellent from the can containing the filtrate is then allowed to evaporate, and the residue is assayed for the drug using, e.g., HPLC. Appreciable drug solubility may lead to particle growth; this may be overcome, however, by the appropriate choice of salt if the compound is a weak acid or base. Table 6.15 shows the data obtained by Williams et al. (1999b) of some steroids in HFA-134a (+ 7.9 percent w/w ethanol) at 5 and 25°C.

For pMDIs, the compatibility of the propellants with the valve elastomers also needs to be evaluated. For example, Tiawari et al. (1998a) investigated the effect of 134a on a number of valve elastomers and found that it adversely affected the performance of the valve. Inhalation dosage forms are discussed in more detail in Chapter 10.

Dry Powder Inhalers

Timsina et al. (1994) have reviewed the use of DPIs for drug delivery to the lungs. Although pMDIs remain the most popular device for the delivery of drugs to the lungs, DPIs have certain advantages over them. For example, DPIs do not rely on the CFC or HFA propellant gases and hence are more "environmentally friendly" than MDIs.

There are number of devices which can deliver drugs to the lungs as dry powders, e.g., Turbuhaler™ or Diskhaler™. DPIs rely on a larger carrier particle, such as α-lactose monohydrate, to which the drug is attached. (The lactose is usually fractionated such that it lies in the size range 63–90 μm.) On delivery, the drug detaches from the lactose and, because the drug is micronized, it is delivered to the lung, whereas the lactose is eventually swallowed. Staniforth (1996) has reviewed the preformulation aspects of DPIs. In that article, he states that measurements of the micromeretic, RH and electrostatic properties of the powder should be the basis of the characterization carried out. It was also shown that the polymorphic form of the lactose used could affect the aerosolization properties of the formulation. The results showed that, as function of flow rate, the β-forms were easily entrained, but held onto the

Table 6.15
Solubility of some steroids in HFA-propellant/ethanol mixtures. at 5 and 25°C.

Compound	Solubility in HFA-134a/Ethanol (μg drug per g solvent)		Solubility in HFA-227/Ethanol (μg drug per g solvent)	
	5°C	25°C	5°C	25°C
Hydrocortisone	134.4	190.1	147.2	175.2
Dexamethasone	99.8	133.5	77.5	145.7
Betamethasone-17-valerate	2549.7	2635.6	2730.7	2733.4
Danazol	640.0	1077.9	633.2	816.4

Reprinted from Study of solubility of steroids in hydrofluoroalkane propellants, by R. O. Williams et al., in *Drug Dev. Ind. Pharm.*, Vol. 25, pp. 1227–1234. Courtesy of Marcel Dekker, Inc.

drug particles most strongly. The anhydrous α-form showed the opposite behaviour, and the α-form (the monohydrate) showed intermediate behaviour.

Micronized particles form strong agglomerates, and the size of these agglomerates, among other things, depends on the surface free energy of the powder. Since micronization can change the surface free energy of a material, the adherence properties of the compound will also be changed. For example, Podczeck et al. (1994, 1995a,b) have performed adhesion and auto-adhesion measurements of salmeterol xinafoate particles of various sizes to compacted lactose monohydrate surfaces using a centrifuge technique. This work was followed by work investigating the adhesion force of micronized salmeterol xinafoate particles to pharmaceutically relevant surface materials (Podeczeck et al. 1996a). Results showed that long contact times with PVC, polyethylene or aluminium should be avoided because the adhesion force between the drug and these surfaces was much higher than between it and the lactose carrier. Thus, detachment and loss of drug in the formulation could occur. In another study, Podczeck et al. (1996b) investigated the adhesion strength of some salts of salmeterol to lactose and other substrates with varying surface roughness, surface free energy and Young's modulus. It was concluded that many of these factors play a part, as do chemical forces, and that only experimental assessment could indicate whether the material was suitable. Boerefijn et al. (1998) have reported the disintegration of weak lactose agglomerates using an agglomerate impact test with high-speed digital video recording. The experiments showed that dry agglomerates were broken apart as a function of the square of the impact velocity.

As noted by Jashnani and Byron (1996), in formulation terms, it is always worth optimising the salt form. In this study, the performance comparisons of dry powder aerosol generation in different environments were determined for the sulphate, adipate (diethanolate) and stearate salts of albuterol. Overall, the stearate emptied and aerosolized best from the inhaler and showed the least sensitivity to environmental factors such as temperature and humidity. Another use of low solubility salts is to mask the taste of those compounds with unpleasant taste when delivered by DPI (or pMDI for that matter). By lowering the solubility, and hence dissolution rate, the taste can often be effectively eliminated.

Because lactose is the most commonly used carrier excipient in DPIs, its compatibility with the candidate drug should be assessed—particularly if it is a primary amine (see section on compatibility, below). The physicochemical characteristics of some alternative carrier particles have been described by Byron et al. (1996). The effect of the surface morphology of lactose carriers on the inhalation properties of pranlukast hydrate has been reported (Kawashima et al. 1998). The lactose carriers investigated were pharmatose 325M, pharmatose 200M (sieved to ~ 60 μm) and fluidized bed granulated lactose. Results showed that with increasing specific surface area and roughness, the effective index of inhalation decreased due the drug being held more tightly in the inhaled airstream. Therefore, characterization of the carrier particles by, e.g., surface area measurements, SEM and other solid-state techniques are recommended preformulation activities for DPIs.

Nebulizer Solutions

Nebulizer formulations are normally solutions, however, suspensions are also used, e.g., the insoluble steroid budesonide has been successfully formulated for delivery by nebulization (Dahlback 1994). Some important preformulation considerations for nebulizers are stability, solubility, viscosity and surface tension (McCallion et al. 1996; Nikander 1997). In terms of solubility, the common ion effect may be important where, e.g., a hydrochloride salt is to be dissolved in saline. In addition, the temperature dependence of the solubility of the drug may be important. Taylor et al. (1992), for example, found that the temperature of a solution of a pentamidine isethionate decreased by up to 13°C, causing the drug to crystallize from solution. The osmolality of solutions has been found to increase during nebulization, although the pH does not appear to do so (Schoeni and Kraemer 1989).

Table 6.16 shows solubility data for an inhalation candidate drug (secondary amine hydrochloride), which was to be delivered by a pMDI and as a nebulizer solution.

These data show the increase in solubility of the compound with respect to temperature and how the presence of the chloride ion depressed its solubility.

If the drug is insoluble, it is important that for a suspension formulation the drug be micronized to a size of less than 2 μm (Dahlback 1994). The particle size distribution of nebulized droplets can be measured using, e.g, laser diffraction (Clark 1995). Validation experiments showed that laser diffraction was robust and reliable and that the diffraction data were a good measure of the particle size of the aerosolized droplets.

Nebulized inhalation drugs are often admixed with others; however, their physical and chemical compatibility should be assessed before proceeding. For a discussion of this aspect of nebulizer therapy, see the review by Jutta (1997).

COMPATIBILITY

Although there has been some debate in the literature about the nature of compatibility testing and the value of results (e.g., see Monkhouse and Maderich 1989, and Monkhouse 1993), it is felt that it still has some relevance to pharmaceutical preformulation. Essentially, there are four major stages in drug-excipient compatibility studies, but before considering such studies, it is worth checking whether there are any known incompatibilities, as is shown in Table 6.17 (Monkhouse 1993).

Whilst the Maillard reaction between lactose and primary amines is well known, the same reaction between the secondary amine fluoxetine hydrochloride (Prozac®) and lactose has recently been reported (Wirth et al. 1998). In the solid-state water content, lubricant concentration and temperature were also found to influence the degradation. In addition to the chemical reactions noted above, the drug may also interact to form a molecular compound. For example, solid-state interactions between trimethoprim and antimicrobial paraben esters to form a 1:1 molecular compound has been reported (Pedersen et al. 1994).

When conducting compatibility studies, there are four steps to consider:

Table 6.16
Solubility of an inhalation candidate drug in water and isotonic saline as a function of temperature.

	Solubility (μg/mL)		
Solvent	**4°C**	**25°C**	**40°C**
Water	1789	2397	6837
Saline	< 30	61	157

Table 6.17
Known reactivities of some functional groups.

Functional Group	Incompatibilities	Type of Reaction
Primary amine	Mono and disaccharides	Amine-aldehyde and amine-acetal
Ester, cyclic, lactone	Basic components	Ring opening ester-base hydrolysis
Carbonyl, hydroxyl	Silanol	Hydrogen bonding
Aldehyde	Amine carbohydrates	Aldehyde-amine Schiff base or glycosylamine
Carboxyl	Bases	Salt formation
Alcohol	Oxygen	Oxidation to aldehydes and ketones
Sulphfhydryl	Oxygen	Dimerization
Phenol	Metals	Complexation
Gelatin capsule shell	Cationic surfactant	Denaturation

From Monkhouse, D. C., Excipient compatibility possibilities and limitations in stability prediction. In *Stability testing in the EC, Japan and the USA. Scientific and regulatory requirements,* edited by W. Crim and K. Krummen (1993). Reprinted with permission from Wissenschaftlidie Verlassgellschaft mbH.

1. Sample preparation

2. Statistical design

3. Storage conditions

4. Method of analysis

Traditionally, a binary mixture of drug with the excipient being investigated is intimately mixed, and the ratio of drug to excipient is often 1:1; however, other mixtures may also be investigated. Powder samples, one set of which is moistened, are then sealed into ampoules to prevent moisture loss. These are then stored at a suitable temperature and analyzed at various time points using HPLC, DSC and TGA, as appropriate. Alternatively, the drug in suspension with excipients may be investigated (Waltersson 1986). Table 6.18 shows data for 250 mg of a primary amine hydrochloride mixed with 250 mg of spray-dried lactose and dispensed into clear, neutral glass ampoules. Half of the ampoules were sealed without further treatment, and to the others, 25 μL of distilled water was added prior to sealing. The ampoules were then stored at 25°C for 1, 4 and 12 weeks.

As expected, there is clear evidence of incompatibility between the amine hydrochloride and the spray-dried lactose. However, the results also showed that moisture was the catalyst for decomposition, as no degradation was observed in the dry state even after 12 weeks storage at 90°C. At the time of this writing, Serrajuddin et al. (1999) have devised a protocol for compatibility testing (Table 6.19).

Ahlneck and Lundgren (1985) and Ahlneck and Waltersson (1986) have described methods for the evaluation of solid-state stability and compatibility between drugs and excipients. Three methods were studied and compared isothermally and non-isothermally: suspension, storage of powders and compacts at specified humidities and elevated temperatures.

Table 6.18
Compatibility study between a primary
amine hydrochloride and spray-dried lactose.

Water Added (μL)	Storage Temp. (°C)	Storage Time (weeks)	Colour	Moisture by TGA	% Drug Recovered
0	25	1	White	2.6	101.2
		4	White	2.6	99.4
		12	White	2.6	102.8
	70	1	White	2.6	105.0
		4	White	2.6	101.8
		12	Off-white	2.5	100.3
	90	1	White	2.6	102.5
		4	White	2.6	98.5
		12	Off-white	2.2	100.2
25	25	1	White	2.6	93.6
		4	White	6.8	102.6
		12	White	5.0	88.4
	70	1	Brown	3.2	91.4
		4	Brown/Black	N/I*	99.7
		12	Brown/Black	N/I	74.4
	90	1	Brown	4.0	98.5
		4	Brown/Black	N/I	90.0
		12	Black	N/I	51.4

*N/I: Thermogram not interpretable due to extensive sample degradation.

It was concluded that the suspension technique was good for fast screening of chemical instability. The other solid state procedures were found to be better predictors of the solid dosage form.

Depending on the number of excipients to be investigated, compatibility tests can be speeded up by using factorial or reduced factorial design experiments. Preformulation compatibility experiments utilizing such designs have been reported by, e.g., Dürig and Fassihi (1993). However, it should be remembered that drug instability or incompatibility can be the result of multiple excipient interactions, which is more difficult to address in a practical manner. Furthermore, the processing method used to formulate the drug can affect results, again complicating the matter.

The storage conditions used to examine compatibility can vary widely in terms of temperature and humidity, but a temperature of 50°C for storage of compatibility samples is considered appropriate. Some compounds may require higher temperatures to make reactions proceed at a rate that can be measured over a convenient time period. Methods of analysis also

Table 6.19
Compatibility protocol.

	Experiment																
	1	2	3	4	5	6	7	8	9	10	11	12	13	14	15	16	17
Drug substance	200	25	25	25	25	25	25	25	25	25	25	25	25	25	25	25	25
Lactose		175				170				170			170				
Mannitol			175				170				170			170			
Microcrystalline cellulose				175				170				170			170		
Dibasic calcium phosphate dihydrate					175				170				170			170	
Magnesium stearate						5	5	5	5								
Sodium stearyl fumarate										5	5	5	5				
Stearic acid														5	5	5	5

From Selection of a solid dosage form composition through drug-excipient compatibility testing. Serrajuddin, A. T. M., A. B. Thakur, R. Ghoshal, M. G. Fakes, S. A. Ranadive, K. R. Morris, and S. A. Varia. *J. Pharm. Sci.* 88:696–704. Copyright 1999 John Wiley and Sons, Inc. Reprinted by permission of Wiley-Liss, Inc., Jossey-Bass, Inc., a subsidiary of John Wiley & Sons, Inc.

vary widely, ranging from thermal techniques (DSC) to chromatographic techniques (TLC, HPLC) to microcalorimetry.

DSC has been used extensively for compatibility studies (for example, see Holgado et al. 1995). Although only milligram quantities of drug are needed for a DSC experiment, the interpretation of the thermograms may be difficult, and conclusions may be misleading on the basis of DSC experiments alone (van Dooren 1983, Charznowski et al. 1986). Nonetheless, the technique remains popular, and the protocol that has been adopted is that proposed by van Dooren (1983), who suggested the following scheme:

1. Run the New Chemical Entity (NCE) and excipients individually.

2. Run mixtures of the NCE and excipients immediately after mixing.

3. Run the NCE and excipients individually after 3 weeks at 55°C.

4. Run the NCE-excipient mix after 3 weeks at 55°C.

5. Run the single components and mixtures after 3 weeks at 55°C only if the curves of the mixtures before and after storage at this temperature differ from each other.

An excipient that is particularly desired may be investigated further by examining different weight ratios with the drug. This method of compatibility testing has been criticized by Chrzanowski et al. (1986) who found that the DSC compatibility method was an unreliable compatibility predictor for fenretinide and three mefenidil salts with various direct compression excipients. They concluded that an isothermal stress (IS) method (which requires a specific, quantitative assay method, e.g., HPLC, for either test substance or its degradation products) was preferred for its accuracy over DSC in compatibility testing. In addition, the IS method gave quantitative information. Disadvantages of the IS system compared to DSC are that the tests tend to consume more compound than the DSC test and are conducted over longer storage times, 1–2 months at 60 to 80°C. However, the whole point of DSC is speed of prediction. So DSC may be of use if the amount of drug available is small and an idea of compatibility is required (Venkataram et al. 1995). On the other hand, although DSC may be used to predict that interactions may occur, it provides little insight into the nature of the interaction (Hartauer and Guillory 1991).

Microcalorimetry has also been used in excipient compatibility studies (Phipps et al. 1998). In their study, 1:1 mixtures were prepared using a ball mill and examined for incompatibility by sealing samples in glass crimped vials using a microcalorimeter at 50°C at a set RH. After an equilibration period of between 1 and 4 days, thermal data were collected over 15 h. Generally, the data from the thermal activity monitor (TAM) was comparable to the corresponding HPLC analysis. However, it was less successful in prediction when mixtures contained a hygroscopic component. Other work by Selzer et al. (1998) has shown that microcalorimetry can be used to detect incompatibility. Microcalorimetry only detects heat flow, however, and they made the point that physical events such as crystallinity changes would be superimposed on the heat output signal. They also found that experimental temperatures close to ambient could not be employed because the enthalpy change was not large enough.

In solid dose form technology, Monkhouse (1993) has argued that it may be a better idea to make tablets with proven excipient blends in a compaction simulator using representative compression forces. This, it was claimed, would use a small amount of the candidate drug and also take into account factors such as mixing, granulation and compression. Then, only if the tablet were proven to be unstable, should retrospective examination of the incompatibility be undertaken to identify the excipients that are incompatible. Indeed, according to this author, any formulations that do not contain lactose and magnesium stearate should be successful! Other investigators may have different experiences and may not have access to a compaction simulator.

REFERENCES

Ahlneck, C., and P. Lundgren. 1985. Methods for the evaluation of solid state stability and compatibility between drug and excipient. *Acta Pharm. Suec.* 22:305–314.

Ahmed, H., G. Buckton, and D. A. Rawlins. 1996. Use of isothermal microcalorimetry in the study of small degrees of amorphous content of a hydrophobic powder. *Int. J. Pharm.* 130:195–201.

Akers, M. J. 1979. Preformulation screening of antioxidant efficiency in parenteral solutions. *J. Parenteral Drug Assoc.* 33:346–356.

Akers, M. J. 1982. Antioxidants in pharmaceutical products. *J. Parenteral Sci. Tech.* 36:222–228.

Akers, M. J., A. L. Fites, and R. L. Robinson. 1987. Formulation design and development of parenteral suspensions. *J. Parenteral Sci. Tech.* 41:88–96.

Amidon, G. E. 1999. Physical test methods for powder flow characterization of pharmaceutical materials. A review of methods. *Pharm. Forum* 25:8298–8305.

Ammar, H. O., S. A. Ibrahim, and A. El-Mohsen. 1982. Effect of chelating agents on the stability of injectable isoniazid solutions. *Pharmazie* 37:270–271.

Asahara, K., H. Yamada, S. Yoshida, and S. Hirose. 1990. Stability prediction of nafamostat mesylate in an intravenous admixture containing sodium bisulfite. *Chem. Pharm. Bull.* 38:492–497.

Atkinson, T. W., and S. White. 1992. Hydrophobic drug substances: The use of laser diffraction particle size analysis and dissolution to characterize surfactant stabilized suspensions. *Spec. Publ. R. Soc. Chem.* 102:133–142.

Atkinson, T. W., M. J. Greenway, S. J. Holland, D. R. Merrifield, and H. P. Scott. 1992. The use of laser diffraction particle size analysis to predict the dispersibility of a medicament in a paraffin based ointment. *Spec. Publ. R. Soc. Chem.* 102:139–152.

Aulton, M., and J. A. Wells. 1988. In *Pharmaceutics. The Science of Dosage Form Design.* edited by M. E. Aulton. Edinburgh: Churchill Livingstone.

Barra, J., and R. Somma. 1996. Influence of the physicochemical variability of magnesium stearate on its lubricant properties: Possible solutions. *Drug Dev. Ind. Pharm.* 22:1105–1120.

Biro, E. J., and I. Racz. 1998. The role of zeta potential in the stability of albendazole suspensions. *S.T.P. Pharma Sci.* 8:311–315.

Blackett, P. M., and G. Buckton. 1995. A microcalorimetric investigation of the interaction of surfactants with crystalline and partially crystalline salbutamol sulphate in a model inhalation aerosol system. *Pharm. Res.* 12:1689–1693.

Blagden, N., R. J. Davey, R. Rowe, and R. Roberts. 1998. Disappearing polymorphs and the role of reaction byproducts: The case of sulphathiazole. *Int. J. Pharm.* 172:169–177.

Boerefijn, R., Z. Ning, and M. Ghadiri. 1998. Disintegration of weak lactose agglomerates for inhalation applications. *Int. J. Pharm.* 172:199–209.

Bommireddi, A., L. Li, D. Stephens, D. Robinson, and E. Ginsberg. 1998. Particle size determination of a flocculated suspension using a light scattering particle analyzer. *Drug Dev. Ind. Pharm.* 24:1089–1093.

Briggner, L.-E., G. Buckton, K. Bystrom, and P. Darcy. 1994. Use of isothermal microcalorimetry in the study of changes in crystallinity induced during the processing of powders. *Int. J. Pharm.* 105:125–135.

Brittain, H. G., S. J. Bogdanowich, D. E. Bugey, J. DeVincetis, G. Lwen, and A. W. Newman. 1991. Physical characterization of pharmaceutical solids. *Pharm. Res.* 8:963–973.

Brittain, H. G., ed. 1995. *Physical characterization of pharmaceutical solids.* New York: Marcel Dekker.

Buckton, G. 1995. Surface characterisation: Understanding sources of variability in the production and and use of pharmaceuticals. *J. Pharm. Pharmacol.* 47:265–275.

Buckton, G. 1997. Characterisation of small changes in the physical properties of powders of significance for dry powder inhaler formulations. *Adv. Drug Del. Rev.* 26:17–27.

Bugay, D. E., A. W. Newman, and W. P. Findlay. 1996. Quantitation of cefepime-2HCl dihydrate in cefepime-2HCl monohydrate by diffuse reflectance IR and powder X-ray diffraction techniques. *J. Pharm. Biomed. Anal.* 15:49–61.

Byron, P. R., V. Naini, and E. M. Phillips. 1996. Drug carrier selection—Important physicochemical characteristics. *Respir. Drug Delivery V.* 103–113.

Cartensen, J. T., C. Ertell, and J.-E. Geoffroy. 1993. Physico-chemical properties of particulate matter. *Drug Dev. Ind. Pharm.* 19:195–219.

Carter, P. A., G. Rowley, E. J. Fletcher, and E. A. Hill. 1992. An experimental investigation of triboelectrification in cohesive and non-cohesive pharmaceutical powders. *Drug Dev. Ind. Pharm.* 18:1505–1526.

Carter, P. A., G. Rowley, E. J. Fletcher, and V. Stylianopoulos. 1998. Measurement of electrostatic charge decay in pharmaceutical powders and polymer materials used in dry powder inhaler devices *Drug Dev. Ind. Pharm.* 24:1083–1088.

Cavatur, R. K., and R. Suryanarayanan. 1998. Characterization of frozen aqueous solutions by low temperature X-ray powder diffractometry. *Pharm. Res.* 15:194–199.

Chang, H.-K., and C. W. Whitworth. 1984. Aspirin degradation in mixed polar solvents. *Drug Dev. Ind. Pharm.* 10:515–526.

Chansiri, G., R. T. Lyons, M. V. Patel, and S. T. Hem. 1999. Effect of surface charge on the stability of oil/water emulsions during steam sterilization. *J. Pharm. Sci.* 88:454–458.

Chaumeil, J. C. 1998. Micronization: A method of improving the bioavailability of poorly soluble drugs. *Meth. Find. Exp. Clin. Pharm.* 20:211–215.

Chrzanowski, F. A., L. A. Ulissi, B. J.Fegely, and A. C. Newman. 1986. Preformulation excipient compatibility testing. application of a differential scanning calorimetry method versus a wet granulation simulating isothermal stress method. *Drug Dev. Ind. Pharm.* 12:783–800.

Clark, A. R. 1995. The use of laser diffraction for the evaluation of the aerosol clouds generated by medical nebulizers. *Int. J. Pharm.* 115:69–78.

Collins-Gold, L. C., R. T. Lyons, and L. C. Bartlow. 1990. Parenteral emulsions for drug delivery. *Adv. Drug Del. Rev.* 5:189–208.

Craig, D. Q. M., P. G. Royall, V. L. Kett, and M. L. Hopton. 1999. The relevance of the amorphous state to pharmaceutical dosage forms: Glassy drugs and freeze dried systems. *Int. J. Pharm.* 179:179–207.

Curzons, A. D., D. R. Merrifield, and J. P. Warr. 1993. The assessment of crystal growth of organic pharmaceutical material by specific surface measurement. *J. Phys. D: Appl. Phys.* 26:B181–B187.

Dahlback, M. 1994. Behaviour of nebulizing solutions and suspensions. *J. Aerosol Med.* 7 (Suppl.) S13–S18.

Dalby, R. N., E. M. Phillips, and P. R. Byron. 1991. Determination of drug solubility in aerosol propellants. *Pharm. Res.* 8:1206–1209.

DeCamp, W. H. 1996. Regulatory considerations in crystallization processes for bulk pharmaceutical chemicals: A reviewers perspective. *Proceedings of the 1995 Conference on Cryst. Growth Org. Mater.*, edited by Mayerson et al., pp. 65–71. Washington DC: American Chemical Society.

Deicke, A., and R. Süverkrüp. 1999. Dose uniformity and redispersibility of pharmaceutical suspensions I: Quantification and mechanical modelling of human shaking behaviour. *Eur. J. Pharm. Biopharm.* 48:225–232.

Dobetti, L., A. Grassano, and R. Forster. 1995. Physicochemical characterization of ITF 296, a novel anti-ischemic drug. *Boll. Chim. Pharm.* 134:384–389.

Duddu, S. P., and K. Weller. 1996. Importance of glass transition temperature in accelerated stability testing of amorphous solids: Case study using a lyophilized aspirin formulation. *J. Pharm. Sci.* 85:345–347.

Duncan-Hewitt, W. C., and D. J. W. Grant. 1986. True density and thermal expansivity of pharmaceutical solids: Comparison of methods and assessment of crystallinity. *Int. J. Pharm.* 28:75–84.

Dunitz, J. D., and J. Bernstein. 1995. Disappearing polymorphs. *Acc. Chem. Res.* 28:193–200.

Dürig, T., and A. R. Fassihi. 1993. Identification of stabilizing and destabilizing effects of excipient-drug interactions in solid dosage form design. *Int. J. Pharm.* 97:161–170.

Duro, R., C. Alverez, R. Martinez-Pachecon, J. L. Gomez-Amoza, A. Concheiro, and C. Souto. 1998. The adsorption of cellulose ethers in aqueous suspensions of pyrantel pamoate: Effects of zeta potential and stability. *Eur. J. Pharm. and Biopharm.* 45:181–188.

Feeley, J. C., P. York, B. S. Sumby, and H. Dicks. 1998. Determination of surface properties and flow characteristics of salbutamol sulphate, before and after micronisation. *Int. J. Pharm.* 172: 89–96.

Flynn, G. L. 1979. Isotonicity-collagative properties and dosage form behaviour. *J. Parenteral Drug Assoc.* 33:292–315.

Folger, M., and C. C. Müller-Goymann. 1994. Investigations on the long-term stability of an O/W cream containing either bufexamac or betamethasone-17-valerate. *Eur. J. Pharm. Biopharm.* 40:58–63.

Fu, R. C.-C., D. M. Lidgate, J. L. Whatley, and T. McCullough. 1987. The biocompatibility of parenteral vehicles—In vitro/in vivo screening comparison and the effect of excipients on hemolysis. *J. Parenteral Sci. Tech.* 41:164–168.

Führer, C. 1996. Interparticulate attraction mechanisms. *Drug Pharm. Sci.* 71:1–15.

Girona, V., C. Pacareu, A. Riera, R. Pouplana, M. Castillo, and J. Bolos. 1988. Spectrophotometric determination of the stability of an ampicillin-dicloxacillin suspension. *J. Pharm. Biomed Anal.* 6:23–28.

Gould, P. L., M. Goodman, and P. A. Hanson. 1984. Investigation of the solubility relationship of polar, semi-polar and non-polar drugs in mixed co-solvent systems. *Int. J. Pharm.* 19:149–159.

Hacche, L., M. A. Dickason, R. M. Oda, B. A. Firestone. 1992. Particle size analysis for ofloxacin, prednisolone acetate, and an ophthalmic suspension containing the ofloxacin/steroid combination. *Part. Sci. Tech.* 10:37–47.

Hammerlund, E. R. 1981. Sodium chloride equivalents, cryoscopic properties, and hemolytic effects of certain medicinals in aqueous solution IV: Supplemental values. *J. Pharm. Sci.* 70:1161–1163.

Hartauer, K. J., and J. K. Guillory. 1991. A comparison of diffuse reflectance FT-IR spectroscopy and DSC in the characterization of a drug excipient interaction. *Drug Dev. Ind. Pharm.* 17:617–630.

Hatley, R. H. M., F. Franks, S. Brown, G. Sandhu, and M. Gray. 1996. Stabilization of a pharmaceutical drug substance by freeze-drying: A case study. *Drug Stabil.* 1:73–85.

Her, L.-H., and S. L. Nail. 1994. Measurement of the glass transition temperatures of freeze concentrated solutes by differential scanning calorimetry. *Pharm. Res.* 11:54–59.

Hindle, M., and P. R. Byron. 1995. Size distribution control of raw materials for dry powder inhalers using the aerosizer with aero-disperser. *Pharm. Tech.* 19:64–78.

Hoelgaard, A., and N. Møller. 1983. Hydrate formation of metronidazole benzoate in aqueous suspensions. *Int. J. Pharm.* 15:213–221.

Holgado, M. A., M. Fernandez-Arevalo, J. M. Gines, I. Caraballo, and A. M. Rabasco. 1995. Compatibility study between carteolol hydrochloride and tablet excipients using differential scanning calorimetry and hot stage microscopy. *Pharmazie* 50:195–198.

Jashnani, R. N., and P. R. Byron. 1996. Dry powder aerosol generation in different environments: Performance comparisons of albuterol, albuterol sulfate, albuterol adipate and albuterol stearate. *Int. J. Pharm.* 130:13–24.

Johansson, D., and B. Abrahamsson. 1997. In vivo evaluation of two different dissolution enhancement principles for a sparingly soluble drug administered as extended-release (ER) tablet. *Proc. 24th Int. Symp. Controlled Release Bioact. Mater.*, pp. 363–364.

Jonkman-De Vries, J. D., H. Rosing, R. E. C. Henrar, A. Bult, and J. H. Beijnen. 1995. The influence of formulation excipients on the stability of the novel antitumor agent carzelesin (U-80,244) *PDA J. Pharm. Sci. Tech.* 49:283–288.

Jutta, J. C. 1997. Compatibility of nebulizer solubility admixtures. *Ann. Pharmacother.* 31:487–489.

Kanerva, H., J. Kiesvaara, E. Muttonen, and J. Yliruusi. 1993. Use of laser light diffraction in determining the size distributions of different shaped particles. *Pharm. Ind.* 55: 849–853.

Kawashima, Y., T. Sergano, T. Hino, H. Yamamoto, and H. Takeughi. 1998. Effect of surface morphology of carrier lactose on dry powder inhalation property of pranlukast. *Int. J. Pharm.* 172:179–188.

Kenley, R. A., M. O. Lee, L. Sakumar, and M. F. Powell. 1987. Temperature and pH dependence of fluocinolone acetonide degradation in a topical cream formulation. *Pharm. Res.* 4:342–347.

King, S., O. Ying, A. M. Basita, and G. Torosian. 1989. Self-association and solubility behavior of a novel anticancer agent, brequinar sodium. *J. Pharm. Sci.* 78:95–100.

Kitamura, S., A. Miyamae, S. Koda, and Y. Morimoto. 1989. Effect of grinding on the solid-state stability of cefixime trihydrate. *Int. J. Pharm.* 56:125–134.

Kriwet, K., and C. C. Muller-Goymann. 1993. Binary diclofenac diethylamine-water systems: Micelles, vesicles, and lyotropic liquid crystals. *Eur. J. Pharm. Biopharm.* 39:234–238.

Krzyzaniak, J. F., and S. H. Yalkowsky. 1998. Lysis of human red blood cells 3: Effect of contact time on surfactant-induced haemolysis. *PDA J. Pharm. Sci. Tech.* 52:66–69.

Kulvanich, P., and P. J. Stewart. 1987. The effect of particle size and concentration on the adhesive characteristics of a model drug-carrier interactive system. *J. Pharm. Pharmacol.* 39:673–678.

Leung, S. S., B. E. Padden, E. J. Munson, and D. J. W. Grant. 1998. Solid state characterization of two polymorphs of aspartame hemihydrate. *J. Pharm. Sci.* 87:501–507.

Levy, M. Y., and S. Benita. 1989. Design and characterization of a submicronized o/w emulsion of diazepam for parenteral use. *Int. J. Pharm.* 54:103–112.

Lidgate, D. M., R. C. Fu, and J. S. Fleitman. 1990. Using a microfluidizer to manufacture parenteral emulsions. *Pharm. Tech. Int.* 30–33.

Lipp, R., and A. Müller-Fahrnow. 1999. Use of X-ray crystallography for the characterization of single crystals grown in steroid containing transdermal drug delivery systems. *Eur. J. Pharm. Biopharm.* 47:133–138.

Loudon, G. C. 1991. Mechanistic interpretation of pH-rate profiles. *J. Chem. Ed.* 68:973–984.

Martens-Lobenhoffer, J., R. M. Jens, D. Losche, and H. Gollnick. 1999. Long term stability of 8-methoxypsoralen in ointments for topical PUVA therapy ("Cream-PUVA"). *Skin Pharmacol. Appl. Skin Physiol.* 12:266–270.

Mazzenga, G. C., B. Berner, and F. Jordan. 1992. The transdermal delivery of zwitterionic drugs II: The flux of zwitterion salt. *J. Controlled Release* 20:163–170.

McCallion, O. N. M., K. M. G. Taylor, P. A. Bridges, M. Thomas, and A. J. Taylor. 1996. Jet nebulisers for pulmonary drug delivery. *Int. J. Pharm.* 130:1–11.

Mendenhall, D. W. 1984. Stability of parenterals. *Drug Dev. Ind. Pharm.* 10:1297–1342.

Merrifield, D. R., P. L. Carter, D. Clapham, and F. D. Sanderson. 1996. Addressing the problem of light instability during formulation development. In *Photostab. Drugs: Drug Formulations* [Int. Meet. Photostab. Drugs 1995], edited by H. H. Toφnneson. London: Taylor and Francis, pp. 141–154.

Midoux, N., P. Hosek, L. Pailleres, and J. R. Authelin. 1999. Micronization of pharmaceutical substances in a spiral jet mill. *Powder Tech.* 104:113–120.

Moldenhauer, J. E. 1998. Determining whether a product is steam sterilizable. *PDA J. Pharm. Sci. Tech.* 52:28–32.

Monkhouse, D. C., and A. Maderich. 1989. Whither compatibility testing. *Drug Dev. Ind. Pharm.* 2115–2130.

Monkhouse, D. C. 1993. Excipient compatibility possibilities and limitations in stability prediction. In *Stability testing in the EC, Japan and the USA. Scientific and regulatory requirements*, edited by W. Crim and K. Krummen. Paperback APV, 32, pp. 67–74. Stuttgart: Wissenschaftlidie Verlassgellschaft mbH.

Morefield, E. M., J. R. Feldkamp, G. E. Peck, J. L. White, and S. L. Hem. 1987. Preformulation information for suspensions. *Int. J. Pharm.* 34:263–265.

Mullin, J. W. 1993. Crystal size and size distribution: The role of test sieving. *Anal. Proc.* 30:455–456.

Munson, J. W., A. Hussain, and R. Bilous. 1977. Precautionary note for use of bisulphite in pharmaceutical formulations. *J. Pharm. Sci.* 66:1775–1776.

Myrdal, P. B., P. Simamora, Y. Surakitbanharn, S. H. Yalkowsky. 1995. Studies in phlebitis. VII: In vitro and in vivo evaluation of pH-solubilized levemopamil. *J. Pharm. Sci.* 84:849–852.

Na, G. C., Jr., H. S. Stevens, B. O. Yuan, and N. Ragagopalan. 1999. Physical stability of ethyl diatrizoate nanocrystalline suspension in steam sterilization. *Pharm. Res.* 16:569–574.

Nayak, A. S., A. J. Cutie, T. Jochsberger, and A. I. Kay. 1986. The effect of various additives on the stability of isoproternol hydrochloride solutions. *Drug Dev. Ind. Pharm.* 12:589–601.

Niemi, L., L. Turakka, and P. Kahela. 1989. Effect of water content and type of emulgator on the release of hydrocortisone from o/w creams. *Acta Pharm. Nord.* 1:23–30.

Niemi, L., and E. Laine. 1991. Effect of water content on the microstructure of an o/w cream. *Int. J. Pharm.* 68:205–214.

Nikander, K. 1997. Some technical, physicochemical and physiological aspects of nebulization of drugs. *Eur. Respir. Rev.* 7:168–172.

Niven, R. W. 1993. Aerodynamic particle-size testing using a time-of-flight aerosol beam spectrometer. *Pharm. Technol.* 17:64–78.

Notari, R. E. 1996. On the merits of a complete kinetic stability study. *Drug Stabil.* 1:1–2.

Nyqvist, H., P. Lundgren, and I. Jansson. 1980. Studies on the physical properties of tablets and tablet excipients. Part 2. Testing of light stability of tablets. *Acta Pharm. Suec.* 17:148–156.

Nyqvist, H., and T. Wadsten. 1986. Preformulation of solid dosage forms: Light stability testing of polymorphs as part of a preformulation program. *Acta Pharm. Technol.* 32:130–132.

Otsuka, M., and Y. Matsuda. 1993. Physicochemical characterization of phenobarbital polymorphs and their pharmaceutical properties. *Drug Dev. Ind. Pharm.* 19:2241–2269.

Otsuka, M., H. Hasegawa, and Y. Matsuda. 1997. Effect of polymorphic transformation during the extrusion-granulation process on the pharmaceutical properties of carbmazepine granules. *Chem. Pharm. Bull.* 45:894–898.

Parasrampuria, J., L. C. Li, A. Dudleston, and H. Zhang. 1993. The impact of an autoclave cycle on the chemical stability of parenteral products. *J. Parenteral Sci. Tech.* 47:177–179.

Parrot, E. L. 1974. Milling of pharmaceutical solids. *J. Pharm. Sci.* 63:813–829.

Payne, R. S., R. J. Roberts, R. C. Rowe, M. McPartlin, and A. Bashal. 1996. The mechanical properties of two forms of primidone predicted from their crystal structures. *Int. J. Pharm.* 145:165–173.

Pedersen, S., and H. G. Kristensen. 1994. Change in crystal density of acetylsalicyclic acid during compaction. *S. T. P. Pharma. Sci.* 4:201–206.

Pedersen, S., H. G. Kristensen, and C. Cornett. 1994. Solid-state interactions between trimethoprim and parabens. *S. T. P Pharma Sci.* 4:292–297.

Peramal, V. L., S. Tamburie, and D. Q. M. Craig. 1997. Characterisation of the variation in the physical properties of commercial creams using thermogravimetric analysis and rheology. *Int. J. Pharm.* 155:91–98.

Phadke, D. S., and J. L. Collier. 1994. Effect of degassing temperature on the specific surface area and other physical properties of magnesium stearate. *Drug Dev. Ind. Pharm.* 20:853–858.

Phillies, G. D. J. 1990. Quasielastic light scattering. *Anal. Chem.* 62:1049A-1057A.

Phillips, E. M., P. R. Byron, and R. N. Dalby. 1993. Axial ratio measurements for early detection of crystal growth in suspension-type metered dose inhalers. *Pharm. Res.* 10:454–456.

Phillips, E. M., and P. R. Byron. 1994. Surfactant promoted crystal growth of micronized methylprednisolone in trichloromonofluoromethane. *Int. J. Pharm.* 110:9–19.

Phipps, M. A., R. A. Winnike, S. T. Long, and F. Viscomi. 1998. Excipient compatibility as assessed by isothermal microcalorimetry. *J. Pharm. Pharmacol.* 50 (Suppl):9.

Pikal, M. J., and S. Shah. 1990. The collapse temperature in freeze-drying: Dependence on measurement methodology and rate of water removal from the glassy phase. *Int. J. Pharm.* 62:165–186.

Podczeck, F., J. M. Newton, and M. B. James. 1994. Assessment of adhesion and autoadhesion forces between particles and surfaces. I. The investigation of autoadhesion phenomena of salmeterol xinafoate and lactose monohydrate particles using compacted powder surfaces. *J. Adhesion Sci. Technol.* 8:1459–1472.

Podczeck, F., J. M. Newton, and M. B. James. 1995a. Assessment of adhesion and autoadhesion forces between particles and surfaces. Part II. The investigation of adhesion phenomena of salmeterol xinafoate and lactose monohydrate particles in particle-on particle and particle-on-surface contact. *J. Adhesion Sci. Technol.* 9:475–486.

Podczeck, F., J. M. Newton, and M. B. James. 1995b. Adhesion and autoadhesion measurements of micronized particles of pharmaceutical powders to compacted powder surfaces. *Chem. Pharm. Bull.* 43:1953–1957.

Podczeck, F., J. M. Newton, and M. B. James. 1996a. The adhesion force of micronized salmeterol xinafoate to pharmaceutically relevant materials. *J. Phys. D: Appl. Phys.* 29:1878–1884.

Podczeck, F., J. M. Newton, and M. B. James. 1996b. The influence of physical properties of the materials in contact on the adhesion strength of particles of salmeterol base and salmeterol salts to various substrate materials. *J. Adhesion Sci. Technol.* 10:257–268.

Poirier, J., J. Donaldson, and A. Barbeam. 1985. The specific vulnerability of the substantia nigra to MPTP is related to the presence of transition metals. *Biochim. Biophys. Res. Commun.* 128:25–33.

Provent, B., D. Chulia, and J. Carey. 1993. Particle size and caking tendency of a powder. *Eur. J. Pharm. Biopharm.* 39:202–207.

Roberts, R. J., R. C. Rowe, and P. York. 1994. The relationship between indentation hardness of organic solids and their molecular structure. *J. Mater. Sci.* 29:2289–2296.

Rowe, R. C., M. J. Wakerly, R. J. Roberts, R. U. Grundy, and N. G. Upjohn. 1995. Expert systems for parenteral development. *PDA J. Pharm. Sci. Tech.* 49:257–261.

Rubino, J. T. 1987. The effects of cosolvents on the action of pharmaceutical buffers. *J. Parenteral Sci. Tech.* 41:45–49.

Rubino, J. T., and S. H. Yalkowsky. 1985. Solubilization by cosolvents. Part 3. Diazepan and benzocaine in binary solvents. *Buu. Parenter. Drug Assoc.* 39:106–111.

Rubino, J. T., and S. H. Yalkowsky. 1987a. Cosolvency and deviations from log-linear solubilization. *Pharm. Res.* 4:231–235.

Rubino, J. T., and S. H. Yalkowsky. 1987b. Cosolvency and cosolvent polarity: *Pharm. Res.* 4:220–230.

Rubino, J. T., J. Blanchard, and S. H. Yalkowsky. 1984. Solubilization by cosolvents. Part 2. Phenytoin in binary and ternary solvents. *Buu. Parenter. Drug Assoc.* 38:215–221.

Sallam, E., H. Saleem, and R. Zaru. 1986. Polymorphism and crystal growth of phenylbutazone in semisolid preparations. Part One: Characterisation of isolated crystals from commercial creams of phenylbutazone. *Drug Dev. Ind. Pharm.* 12:1967–1994.

Samir, R. D. 1997. Preformulation aspects of transdermal drug delivery systems. In *Transdermal topical drug delivery systems*, edited by T. K. Ghosh and W. R. Pfister. Buffalo Grove, Ill., USA: Interpharm Press; pp. 139–166.

Schoeni, M. H., and R. Kraemer. 1989. Osmolality changes in nebulizer solutions. *Agents Actions* 31:225–228.

Scott, G. 1988. Antioxidants. *Bull. Chem. Soc. Jpn.* 61:165–170.

Selzer, T., M. Radau, and J. Kreuter. 1998. Use of isothermal heat conduction microcalorimetry to evaluate stability and excipient compatibility of a solid drug. *Int. J. Pharm.* 171:227–241.

Serrajuddin, A. T. M., and D. Mufson. 1985. pH-solubility profiles of organic bases and their hydrochloride salts. *Pharm. Res.* 2:65–68.

Serrajuddin, A. T. M., A. B. Thakur, R. Ghoshal, M. G. Fakes, S. A. Ranadive, K. R. Morris, and S. A. Varia. 1999. Selection of solid dosage form composition through drug-excipient compatibility testing. *J. Pharm. Sci.* 88:696–704.

Shalaev, E. Y., and G. Zografi. 1996. How does residual water affect the solid-state degradation of drugs in the amorphous state? *J. Pharm. Sci.* 85:1137–1141.

Sing, K. S. W. 1992. Adsorption methods for surface area determination. In *Particle size analysis*, edited by N. G. Stanley-Wood and R. W. Lines. *Proceedings of the 25th Anniversary Conference (1991) the Royal Society of Chemistry*, pp. 13–32.

Smith, A. 1982. Use of thermal analysis in predicting drug-excipient interactions. *Anal. Proc.* 554–556.

Spencer, R., and B. Dalder. 1997. Sizing up grinding mills. *Chem. Eng.* 84–87.

Staniforth, J. N. 1996. Pre-formulation aspects of dry powder aerosols. *Respir. Drug Delivery* V, 65–73.

Stark, G., J. P. Fawcett, I. G. Tucker, and I. L. Weatherall. 1996. Intrumental evaluation of color of solid dosage forms during stability testing. *Int. J. Pharm.* 143:93–100.

Stock, N. 1993. Direct non-destructive colour measurement of pharmaceuticals. *Anal. Proc.* 30:41–43.

Streng, W. H., D. H.-S. Yu, and C. Zhu. 1996. Determination of solution aggregation using solubility, conductivity, calorimetry, and pH measurements. *Int. J. Pharm.* 135:43–52.

Sweetana, S., and M. J. Akers. 1996. Solubility principles and practices for parenteral drug dosage form development. *PDA J. Parenteral Sci. Tech.* 50:330–342.

Taylor, K. M. G., G. Venthoye, and A. Chawla. 1992. Pentamidine isethionate delivery from jet nebulisers. *Int. J. Pharm.* 85:203–208.

Thakur, A. J., K. Morris, J. A. Grosso, K. Himes, J. K. Thottathil, R. L. Jerzewski, D. A. Wadke, and J. T. Cartensen. 1993. Mechanism and kinetics of metal ion mediated degradation of fosinopril sodium. *Pharm Res.* 10:800–809.

Thoma, K., and C. Holzmann. 1998. Photostability of dithranol. *Eur. J. Pharm. Biopharm.* 46:201–208.

Ticehurst, M. D., R. C. Rowe, and P. York. 1994. Determination of the surface properties of two batches of salbutamol sulphate by inverse gas chromatography. *Int. J. Pharm.* 111:241–249.

Ticehurst, M. D., P. York, R. C. Rowe, and S. K. Dwivedi. 1996. Characterisation of the surface properties of α-lactose monohydrate with inverse gas chromatography used to detect batch variation. *Int. J. Pharm.* 141:93–99.

Timsina, M. P., G. P. Martin, C. Marriot, D. Ganderton, and M. Yianneskis. 1994. Drug delivery to the respiratory tract using dry powder inhalers. *Int. J. Pharm.* 101:1–13.

Tiwari, D., D. Goldman, S. Dixit, W. A. Malick, and P. L. Madan. 1998. Compatibility evaluation of metered dose inhaler valve elastomers with tetrafluoroethane (P134a), a non-CFC propellant. *Drug Dev. Ind. Pharm.* 24:345–352.

Tiwari, D., D. Goldman, W. A. Malick, and P. L. Madan. 1998. Formulation and evaluation of albuterol metered dose inhalers containing tetrafluoroethane (P134a), a non-CFC propellant. *Pharm. Dev. Tech.* 3:163–174.

Tiwary, A. K., and G. M. Panpalia. 1999. Influence of crystal habit on trimethoprim suspension formulation. *Pharm. Res.* 16:261–265.

Tu, Y.-H., D. -P. Wang, and L. V. Allen. 1989. Stability of a nonaqueous trimethoprim preparation. *Am. J. Hosp. Pharm.* 46:301–304.

Turner, J. L. 1987. The regulatory perspective to particle size specification. *Anal. Proc.* 24:80–81.

Tzou, T.-S., R. R. Pachta, R. B. Coy, and R. K. Schultz. 1997. Drug form selection in albuterol-containing metered-dose inhaler formulations and its impact on chemical and physical. *J. Pharm. Sci.* 86:1352–1357.

Ugwu, S. O., and S. P. Apte. 1999. Systematic screening of antioxidants for maximum protection against oxidation: An oxygen polarograph study. *PDA J. Pharm. Sci. Tech.* 53:252–259.

Van der Houwen, O. A. G. J., M. R. de Loos, J. H. Beijnen, A. Bult, and W. J. M. Underberg. 1997. Systematic interpretation of pH-degradation profiles. A critical review. *Int. J. Pharm.* 155:137–152.

Vemuri, S., C. Taracatac, and R. Skluzacek. 1985. Color stability of ascorbic acid tablets measured by a tristimulus colorimeter. *Drug Dev. Ind. Pharm.* 11:207–222.

Venkataram, S., M. Khohlokwane, and S. H. Wallis. 1995. Differential scanning calorimetry as a quick scanning technique for solid state stability studies. *Drug Dev. Ind. Pharm.* 21:847–855.

Vernon, B. 1994. Using a ball mill for high-purity milling applications. *Powder Bulk Eng.* 53–62.

Vervaet, C., and P. R. Byron. 1999. Drug-surfactant-propellant interactions in HFA-formulations. *Int. J. Pharm.* 186:13–30.

Villiers, M. M., and L. R. Tiedt. 1996. An analysis of fine grinding and aggregation of poorly soluble drug powders in a vibrating ball mill. *Pharmazie* 51:564–567.

Wada, Y., and T. Matsubara. 1992. Pseudo-polymorphism and crystalline transition of magnesium stearate. *Thermochim. Acta* 196:63–84.

Waltersson, J. O. 1986. Factorial designs in pharmaceutical preformulation studies. Part 1. Evaluation of the application of factorial designs to a stability study of drugs in suspension form. *Acta Pharm. Suec.* 23:129–138.

Wang, Y.-C. J., and R. R. Kowal. 1980. Review of excipients and pH's for parenteral products used in the United States. *J. Parenteral Drug Assoc.* 34:452–462.

Ward, G. H., and R. K. Schultz. 1995. Process-induced crystallinity changes in albuterol sulfate and its effect on powder physical stability. *Pharm. Res.* 12:773–779.

Ward, G. H., and S. H. Yalkowsky. 1993. Studies in phlebitis. VI: Dilution-induced precipitation of amiodarone HCl. *J. Parenteral. Sci. Technol.* 47:161–165.

Washington, C. 1992. *Particle size analysis in the pharmaceutics and other industries.* Chichester, UK: Ellis Horwood.

Wells, J. I. 1988. *Pharmaceutical preformulation. The physicochemical properties of drug substances.* Chichester, UK: Ellis Horwood.

Whateley, T. L., G. Steele, J. Urwin, and G. A. Smail. 1984. Particle size stability of intralipid and mixed total parenteral nutrition mixtures. *J. Clin. Hosp. Pharm.* 9:113–126.

Williams, N. A., and G. P. Polli. 1984. The lyophilization of pharmaceuticals: A literature review. *J. Parenteral Sci. Tech.* 38:48–56.

Williams, N. A., Y. Lee, G. P. Polli, and T. A. Jennings. 1986. The effects of cooling rate on solid phase transitions and associated vial breakage occurring in frozen mannitol solutions. *J. Parenteral Sci. Tech.* 40:135–141.

Williams, N. A., and J. Guglielmo. 1993. Thermal mechanical analysis of frozen solutions of mannitol and some related stereoisomers: Evidence of expansion during warming and correlation with vial breakage during lyophilization. *J. Parenteral. Sci. Tech.* 47:119–123.

Williams, N. A., and D. L. Schwinke. 1994. Low temperature properties of lyophilized solutions and their influence on lyophilization cycle design: Pentamidine isothionate. *J. Pharm. Sci. Technol.* 48:135–139.

Williams, R. O., III, M. Repka, and J. Liu. 1998. Influence of propellant composition on drug delivery from a pressurized metered dose inhaler. *Drug Dev. Ind. Pharm.* 24:763–770.

Williams, R. O., III, J. Brown, and J. Liu. 1999a. Influence of micronization method on the performance of a suspension triamcinolone acetonide pressurized metered-dose inhaler formulation. *Pharm. Dev. Tech.* 4:167–179.

Williams, R. O., III, T. L. Rodgers, and J. Liu. 1999b. Study of solubility of steroids in hydrofluoroalkane propellants. *Drug Dev. Ind. Pharm.* 25:1227–1234.

Wirth, D. D., and G. A. Stephenson. 1997. Purification of dirithromycin. Impurity reduction and polymorph manipulation. *Org. Proc. Res. Dev.* 1:55–60.

Wirth, D. D., S. W. Baertschi, R. A. Johnson, S. R. Maple, M. S. Miller, D. K. Hallenbeck, and S. M. Gregg. 1998. Maillard reaction of lactose and fluoxetine hydrochloride, a secondary amine. *J. Pharm. Sci.* 87:31–39.

Wong, M. W . Y., and A. G. Mitchell. 1992. Physicochemical characterization of a phase change produced during the wet granulation of chlorpromazine hydrochloride and its effects on tableting. *Int. J. Pharm.* 88:261–273.

Yalabik-Kas, H. S. 1985. Stability assessment of emulsion systems. *S. T. P. Pharma.* 1:978–984.

Yalkowsky, S. H., and J. T. Rubino. 1985. Solubilization by cosolvents. Part 2. Organic solvents in propylene glycol–water mixtures. *J. Pharm. Sci.* 74:416–421.

Yalkowsky, S. H., S. C. Valvani, and B. W. Johnson. 1983. *In vitro* method for detecting precipitation of parenteral formulations after injection. *J. Pharm. Sci.* 72:1014–1017.

Yamaoka, T., H. Nakamachi, and K. Miyata. 1982. Studies on the characteristics of carbochromen hydrochloride crystals. II. Polymorphism and cracking in the tablets. *Chem. Pharm. Bull.* 30:3695–3700.

Yang, S. K. 1994. Acid catalyzed ethanolysis of temazepam in anhydrous and aqueous ethanol solution. *J. Pharm. Sci.* 83:898–902.

York, P. 1992. Crystal engineering and particle design for the powder compaction process. *Drug Dev. Ind. Pharm.* 18:677–721.

York, P. 1994. Powdered raw materials: Characterizing batch uniformity. *Respir. Drug Delivery* IV, 83–91.

York, P., M. D. Ticehurst, J. C. Osborn, R. J. Roberts, and R. C. Rowe. 1998. Characterisation of the surface energetics of milled dl-propranolol hydrochloride using inverse gas chromatography and molecular modelling. *Int. J. Pharm.* 174:179–186.

Zhang, Y,. and K. C. Johnson. 1997. Effect of drug particle size on content uniformity of low-dose solid dosage forms. *Int. J. Pharm.* 154:179–183.

Zhang, H.-J., and G.-D. Xu. 1992. The effect of particle refractive index on size measurement. *Powder Tech.* 70:189–192.

Ziller, K. H., and H. Rupprecht. 1988a. Control of crystal growth in drug suspensions. Part 1. Design of a control unit and application to acetaminophen suspensions. *Drug Dev. Ind. Pharm.* 14:2341–2370.

Ziller, K. H., and H. H. Rupprecht. 1988b. Control of crystal growth in drug suspensions. Part 2. Influence of polymers on dissolution and crystallization during temperature cycling. *Pharm. Ind.* 52:1017–1022.

7

Biopharmaceutical Support in Formulation Development

*Bertil Abrahamsson and
Anna-Lena Ungell*

Astra Zeneca
Mölndal, Sweden

The pharmaceutical formulation plays an important role in the delivery of a drug to the body. The clinical benefit of a drug molecule can thereby be optimised by delivering the right amount at the right rate to the right site at the right time. For example, extended-release (ER) formulations have been used for a long time to control the rate of absorption and thereby keep drug levels within the therapeutic interval during an entire dosage interval. More examples of biopharmaceutical properties that can be provided by oral formulations are given in Table 7.1. In the future, the pharmaceutical possibilities for improving clinical utility may be extended to include site-specific drug delivery systems that reach systemic targets, such as cancer cells and the central nervous system (CNS), or gene delivery to cell nuclei. Such areas of drug delivery are, however, outside the scope for the present chapter.

In order to achieve the potential clinical benefits that can be provided by a formulation, as exemplified in Table 7.1, biopharmaceutical input is needed from the start of preformulation, through formulation development, to documentation for regulatory applications. The main objective is to obtain and verify desirable drug delivery properties for a pharmaceutical formulation. The key activities are as follows:

- Characterisation of relevant physicochemical, pharmacokinetic/dynamic prerequisites provided by the drug molecule

- Identification of the relevant biopharmaceutical targets and hurdles in formulation development

239

- Definition of test methods/study designs needed to obtain the biopharmaceutical targets in the formulation development and correct interpretation of the study results obtained

- Choice of suitable drug form, formulation principles and excipients

In addition, understanding of the physiological processes that may interact with the biopharmaceutical function of the dosage form is crucial.

Successful biopharmaceutical input during development can make a significant contribution to clinical efficiency and tolerability of a drug product. In certain cases, such as poorly absorbable drugs or drugs that are degraded in the gut, the biopharmaceutical aspects can make the difference between a new useful product or an aborted development programme of a potentially very useful drug compound. Additionally, appropriate use of biopharmaceutics will also contribute to a time and cost-efficient development process.

The present chapter is limited to presentations and uses of different biopharmaceutical test methods in formulation development, such as

- *in vitro* dissolution testing,

- bioavailability studies,

- *in vitro/in vivo* (IVIVC) correlation of drug dissolution,

- use of animal models in *in vivo* studies of formulations and

- *in vivo* imaging of formulations by gamma scintigraphy.

This chapter is strongly focussed on oral drug delivery. The relevant principles and methods involved in biopharmaceutical characterisation of a drug molecule, mainly applied in the preformulation phase, are described in Chapter 4, "Biopharmaceutical Support in Candidate Drug Selection".

Table 7.1
Examples of biopharmaceutical properties of oral dosage forms.

Biopharmaceutical Target	Formulation Function
Increase amount absorbed/ reduced variability of amount absorbed	Dissolution or permeability enhancement Protection from degradation in GI tract
Control rate of absorption	Extended release
	Pulsed release
Control site of delivery	Gastric retention
	Colon release
	Mucoadhesive

IN VITRO DISSOLUTION

In vitro dissolution testing of solid dosage forms is the most frequently used biopharmaceutical test method in formulation development. It is used from the start of dosage form development and in all subsequent phases. Examples of different purposes of dissolution testing in research and development are as follows:

- Investigation of drug release mechanisms, especially for ER formulations

- To obtain a predefined target release profile and robust formulation properties regarding influences of physiological factors (e.g., pH and food) on the drug release

- Generation of supportive data to bioavailability studies as an aid in interpretation of *in vivo* results

- Validation of manufacturing processes

- Investigation of effects of different storage conditions

- Batch quality control (QC)

- A surrogate for bioequivalence studies

An *in vitro* dissolution method for batch QC is always defined for a new solid dosage form product. However, this method may not be sufficient for all the different aims of dissolution testing that might arise. The choice of dissolution method and test conditions should therefore be adapted to best serve their purpose. For example, simplicity and robustness are crucial properties of a QC method; whereas physiological relevance may overrule these factors when a method is used for *in vivo* predictions.

Standard *in vitro* dissolution testing models two processes; the release of drug substance from the solid dosage form and drug dissolution. Drug release will be determined by formulation factors such as disintegration/dissolution of formulation excipients or drug diffusion through the formulation. Drug dissolution will be affected by the physicochemical substance properties (e.g., solubility, diffusivity), solid-state properties of the substance (e.g., particle surface area, polymorphism) and formulation properties (e.g., wetting, solubilisation). *In vitro* dissolution testing should thus provide predictions of both the drug release and the dissolution processes *in vivo*. Therefore, in most situations, the use of *in vitro* dissolution will be meaningless if the method used does not provide some correlation with *in vivo* data or resemblance with the physiological conditions in the gastro-intestinal (GI) tract. In order to reach this goal, the choice of dissolution apparatus and test medium should be carefully considered. Another important aspect in the development and definition of a new method is that it must be designed and operated in such a way that drug release and dissolution are not sensitive to minor variations in the operating conditions.

This chapter will provide some practical considerations for developing and using *in vitro* dissolution methods. Aspects of study design and evaluation of *in vitro* dissolution data will also be discussed. For additional information on *in vitro* dissolution testing, the "FIP Guidelines for Dissolution Testing of Solid Oral Products" (1997), *Handbook of Dissolution Testing* (Hansson 1991), pharmacopoeias and regulatory guidelines are recommended.

Dissolution Apparatus

The most well-established apparatuses are those described in the pharmacopoeias. Four methods, mainly intended for oral solid dosage forms, are described in the U.S. Pharmacopeia (USP) XXIV: the rotating basket method (USP I), the rotating paddle method (USP II), the reciprocating cylinder (USP III) and the flow-through method (USP IV). All of these methods, except for the reciprocating cylinder, are also described in the European Pharmacopoeia (EP), although the equipment specifications are not identical to those in the USP. These methods are schematically presented in Figures 7.1 a–d.

- **USP I.** The dosage form is placed in a cylindrical basket that is covered by a mesh. The basket is immersed in the dissolution medium and rotated at a speed of between 25 and 150 rpm. The standard beaker has a volume of 1 L, but 4 L vessels are also available. The mesh size in the basket wall can also be varied.

- **USP II.** The dosage form moves freely in the same type of glass beaker as used for USP I. A paddle is rotated at a speed of 25 to 150 rpm. The dosage form may be placed in a steel helix in order to avoid floating.

- **USP III.** The formulation is placed in a cylindrical glass tube with steel screens in the bottom and the top. The mesh size of the tubes may vary. This tube is moved up and down in a larger tube that contains the dissolution fluid. The amplitude of the inner tube movements is 5–40 dips/min, and the volume of the outer tube is 300 mL. Tubes containing 100 mL and 1 L are also available. The inner tube can be moved during the dissolution process between different outer tubes, which may hold different dissolution fluids.

- **USP IV.** The formulation is placed in a thermostated flow-cell. The dissolution fluid is pumped through the cell in a pulsating manner at a constant rate, typically between 4 and 16 mL/min. Before the inlet flow reaches the formulation, it is passed through a bed of glass pellets to create a laminar flow. A filter is placed in the cell at the outlet side of the formulation. The cell is available in different sizes/designs, and tablet holders are available as an option.

USP XXIV and the EP describe four additional apparatuses mainly intended for transdermal or dermal delivery: the paddle over disc (USP V, EP), the extraction cell method (EP), the cylinder method (USP VI, EP) and the reciprocating holder method (USP VII). A large number of other non-compendial methods have been described. Most of them could be categorised as

- modified USP methods,

- rotating flask methods (Koch 1980) and

- dialysis methods (El-Arini et al. 1990).

An example of a commercially available (VanKel, Cary, N.C., USA) alternative to the standard USP II method is one that consists of a glass vessel that has been modified by introducing a peak in the bottom (see Figure 7.2). This modification has been introduced to create appropriate stirring in all parts of the vessel and thereby avoid formation of poorly agitated heaps of undissolved material.

Figure 7.1 Different dissolution apparatuses:

(a) the rotating basket (USP I) dissolution apparatus.

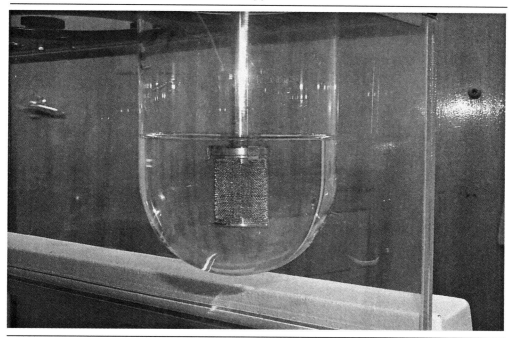

(b) The rotating paddle (USP II).

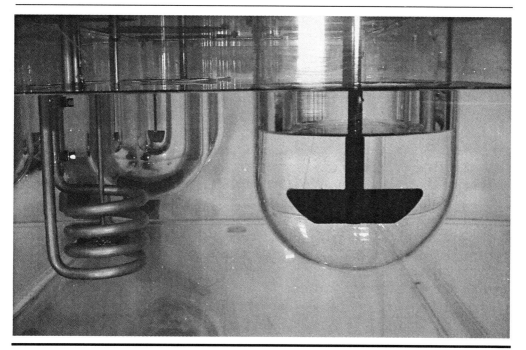

Figure 7.1 continued

(c) The reciprocating cylinder (USP III) dissolution apparatus.

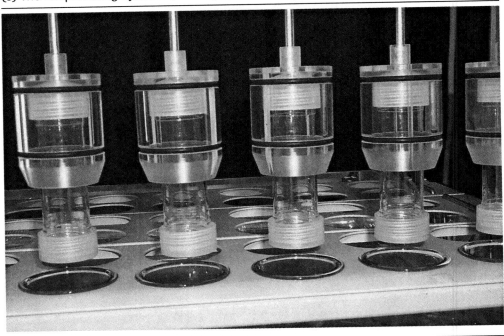

(d) Flow-through cell (USP IV).

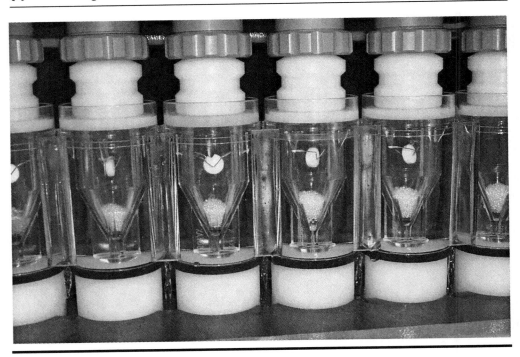

Figure 7.2 Standard and modified (peak vessel) USP II dissolution apparatuses including illustrations of the different flow patterns within the beakers and photographs taken at a paddle stirring rate of 100 rpm showing a heap of pellets beneath the paddle in the standard method compared to the desirable dispersion of pellets in the modified method.

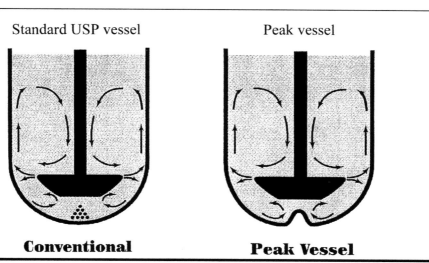

The choice of dissolution apparatus will be specific for each formulation, and the following factors should be considered:

- Correlation to *in vivo* data

- Risk for hydrodynamic artefacts

- Regulatory guidelines

- Drug solubility

- Need to change the dissolution medium during dissolution testing

- Ease of operation, in-house know-how and suitability for automation

As a general guideline in the choice of dissolution test apparatus, the simplest and most well-established method should be chosen, with respect to both in-house know-how and regulatory aspects. In most cases, this is the USP II paddle method or the USP I rotating basket method. However, if satisfactory performance cannot be obtained by these methods, others should be considered. Primarily, the USP III and USP IV methods, and non-compendial methods could also provide relevant advantages.

Correlation of the *in vitro* dissolution to the *in vivo* dissolution is a crucial property of a dissolution test. The major difference in this respect between different apparatus is the hydrodynamic conditions. It has been argued for some of the methods, such as the USP IV flow-through cell or a rotating flask with baffles, that an *in vivo*–like situation is created in the *vitro* test. However, this hypothesis has not been verified by any experimental means for any method, and it is clear that no apparatus mimics the full complexity of the motility patterns in the GI tract. A recommended approach is therefore to evaluate different apparatuses on a case-by-case basis using IVIVC studies (see "Bioavailability Studies", p. 257) to reveal which method provides the most desirable results.

The potential for hydrodynamic artefacts (e.g., floating, clogging of material to screens, adhesion to equipment of the formulation or variable flow conditions in the vicinity of the formulation due to other reasons) is strongly formulation dependent and thus has to be evaluated for each type of formulation. In order to detect artefacts, careful visual inspection of the dissolution test equipment is crucial. Video recordings can be used to aid such investigations.

The present regulatory guidelines in the United States and Europe propose the use of USP I and USP II as the methods of choice. Other methods, both compendial and non-compendial, could be acceptable, but the rationale for not using USP I and II must be clearly stated and supported by experimental data. In generic product development, complete dissolution methods, including the apparatus, are provided for many products in the USP and should thus be a first choice in a regulatory context. It should be noted, however, that this is not applicable in all cases. A dissolution method that is well functioning for a certain formulation type may provide high variability, artefacts or poor IVIVC for other dosage forms. Thus, in particular, for ER formulations or dosage forms containing dissolution enhancing principles, different dissolution tests may be needed for different formulations, although the drug substance is the same.

For sparingly soluble substances, the volume in standard vessel methods may not be sufficient to dissolve the dose. In this case, the USP IV flow-through method is beneficial, since it provides a continuous renewal of the dissolution fluid. However, the maximum flow rate will limit the apparent solubility in this procedure. Sufficient solubility will not be obtained for a rapidly releasing formulation of a drug with very low solubility in relation to the dose.

In certain cases, it is desirable to change the dissolution medium during the dissolution test. For example, a more physiologically relevant medium is desired with changes of the conditions (e.g. pH) corresponding to the differences along the GI tract. Both USP III and USP IV permit such changes without significant interruptions of the dissolution process.

Irrespective of the chosen apparatus, the equipment must be set up and handled in a way that both minimises the variability of the dissolution and avoids artefacts. The most common source to such variability or artefacts is hydrodynamic factors, but unwanted chemical reactions or temperature shifts could also occur. Alterations of hydrodynamics, as well as changes of temperature, can both affect the dissolution of a drug substance and the release of a substance from the dosage form. Chemical reactions in the test medium may cause degradation of the drug substance or some formulation excipient which may affect the dissolution, or may lead to misinterpretation of the results. Examples of different sources to variability for the USP apparatuses are summarised below:

- **USP I**—clogging of basket screen, positioning of basket

- **USP II**—adherence of formulation to the beaker wall, floating, "entrapment" of solid material in the stagnant area beneath the paddle, positioning of the paddle

- **USP III**—floating, adherence to tube wall or bottom screen, clogging of screens, disappearance of undissolved material through the screens

- **USP IV**—clogging of filter, variations in flow rate

Some other factors that potentially could cause problems are not specific for a certain apparatus. These general factors include vibrations, variations in agitation rate, impurities due to poor cleaning or to trace amounts of metals from dissolution equipment, variations in dissolution fluid components and poor quality of dissolution media components. Another factor relevant for lipophilic compounds is migration of the drug substance into fillers and plastic material.

Choice of Agitation Intensity

All compendial dissolution apparatus can be operated at different agitation intensities. The three most outstanding aspects to consider when deciding at which level the tests should be performed are

1. correlation to *in vivo* data,

2. variability of dissolution results and

3. regulatory guidelines and pharmacopoeial recommendations.

The U.S. regulatory agency recommends a stirring rate of 50–100 rpm for USP I and 50–75 rpm for USP II.

The above-proposed agitation intensities should be used if IVIVCs cannot be improved or the variability in dissolution data can be improved by other settings. The major problem associated with a too low agitation is that solid material is not sufficiently well dispersed, which will delay the dissolution. On the other hand, the possibility to discriminate between different formulations/batches with different dissolution properties might be lost at a too intensive agitation.

Sometimes a dissolution test is performed with the aim to investigate the robustness of the release properties towards potential changes of the physiological conditions *in vivo*. In this case, tests at different agitation intensities should be considered to model different intestinal motilities. The use of more than one apparatus may also be considered.

Choice of Dissolution Test Media

The choice of dissolution medium is highly dependent on the purpose of the dissolution study, but the following aspects should always be considered:

*   Correlation to *in vivo* data

*   Resemblance of physiological conditions in the GI tract

*   Regulatory and pharmacopoeial recommendations

*   Drug solubility and stability properties at different pH values

*   Known sensitivity of the formulation function for different medium factors

Attainment of IVIVC is a key aspect in the choice of dissolution test medium. However, it is not recommended to choose a test medium based only on correlation to *in vivo* data. The dissolution test medium should also be relevant for the physiological conditions in the GI tract. Components and physicochemical characteristics of the GI fluids that might be considered in the choice of dissolution medium were discussed in Chapter 4. The *in vivo* conditions are not static, but the fluids are constantly changing along the GI tract due to absorption of water and nutrients, secretions of enzymes, carbonate, salts and bile and digestive processes. It is therefore clear that it is not realistic to reconstitute the full complexity of the *in vivo* conditions in an *in vitro* test. An approach has to be taken where the most relevant factors are included, based on knowledge of the solubility of the drug substance and the release mechanism of the dosage form. Examples of some dissolution test media that have been proposed to be physiologically relevant are given in Table 7.2 (USP 2000; Dressman et al. 1998).

Another important aspect in the selection of a dissolution test medium is the need to consider the saturation solubility of drug in the test medium in relation to the drug dose tested. Drug dissolution will depend on the amount of drug in the solution if the dissolved amount of drug in the test medium approaches the saturation solubility. This can be understood from the Noyes-Whitney equation (see equation 1 in Chapter 4, "Biopharmaceutical Support in Candidate Drug Selection"); the dissolution rate will be affected by the drug concentration in the dissolution medium (Ct) if Ct is not much less than the saturation solubility (Cs). This is not a desirable situation since, if Ct controls the rate of dissolution, the test may not be discriminative for factors related to the formulation performance. Another disadvantage, if Ct is significant in relation to Cs, is that the dissolution rate will be dose dependent, and different results will be obtained for different strengths of the same formulation. Finally, it can be assumed, in most cases, that Ct does not affect the *in vivo* dissolution rate due to the continuous removal of drug from the GI lumen by the drug absorption process that keeps the drug concentrations in the GI tract at a level far below Cs. Consequently, it is desirable to choose a

Table 7.2
Examples of dissolution test media including physiological components.

USP simulated gastric fluid	2 g/L NaCl
	3.2 g/L pepsin
	0.06 M HCl
USP simulated intestinal fluid	0.05 M KH_2PO_4
	0.015 M NaOH
	10.0 g/L pancreatin
	pH adjusted to 6.8 by HCl or NaOH
Simulated gastric fluid–fasted state (Dressman et al. 1998)	0.01–0.05 M HCl
	2.5 g/L Na lauryl sulphate
	2 g/L NaCl
Simulated intestinal fluid–fasted state (Dressman et al. 1998)	0.029 M KH_2PO_4
	5 mM Na taurocholate
	1.5 mM lecithin
	0.22 M KCl
	pH adjusted to 6.8 by NaOH

dissolution test method that provides a high enough saturation solubility to avoid dependence on *Ct*. *Cs* should be at least 3–5 times higher than *Ct* when the total dose has been dissolved. Such conditions have been termed "sink conditions". In the first instance, maximum volume or flow of test medium should be used to obtain sink conditions. Adjustment of the pH to a level that provides optimal solubility should be considered for proteolytic drugs without neglecting the aspects of physiological relevance. For drugs with a very low solubility in relation to the administered dose, the above-described approaches will not provide sufficient drug solubility in the test media. In those cases, a surfactant should be added to the test medium in amounts above its critical micelle concentration (CMC) in order to solubilise the drug. The solubility can thereby be increased several hundred orders of magnitude. This approach is also favoured due to the occurrence *in vivo* of drug solubilising micelles formed in the presence of bile acids. However, the use *in vitro* of bile acids in standard methods is not recommended due to variations in quality and high costs, and it will still be almost impossible to simulate the *in vivo* complexity. Therefore, synthetic surfactants are the first choice, and sodium lauryl sulphate (SLS) has been especially recommended (Shah et al. 1989). Due to the risk of specific interactions between the formulation and SLS (of no *in vivo* relevance) or poor solubilisation capacity for certain drugs, other synthetic surfactants may be considered on a case-by-case basis. An example of the first case is illustrated in Figure 7.3 where the *in vitro* dissolution-time profiles of a poorly soluble compound, felodipine, are shown for three different hydrophilic matrix ER tablets (A–C) when three different surfactants (SLS, CTAB [cetyl-trimethylammonium bromide], Tween) were used to obtain sink conditions (Abrahamsson et al. 1994). SLS interacted with the gel forming excipient, which led to much less of a difference in drug dissolution rate between the three different tablets, compared to the use of the other surfactants. It is also important to realise that attainment of sink conditions does not guarantee that the *in vitro* results correlate to the *in vivo* performance, due to other effects. The discriminating power of a dissolution test may be lost if the solubility of the drug is too favourable in the dissolution medium. For example, an *in vitro* dissolution method including SLS in amounts providing sink conditions was used to test three other felodipine ER tablets. No difference was obtained *in vitro* for the three tablets, which contained different forms of the drug substance, whereas one of the tablets provided almost no bioavailability *in vivo* due to poor dissolution (Johansson and Abrahamsson 1997). Thus, general recommendations of the amount and type of solubiliser to be used in an *in vitro* test medium may be misleading, and the test medium should preferably be based on correlation to relevant *in vivo* data for poorly soluble substances.

Based on the knowledge of the substance solubility, release mechanisms from the dosage forms and known interactions with key excipients, certain components may be of special importance to include or exclude in the dissolution test medium. This has to be considered on a case-by-case basis. Two examples are given below.

Example 1

Hard gelatine capsules have the potential to be cross-linked during storage, which leads to formation of non-water soluble capsules. However, this does not affect the *in vivo* dissolution due to the presence of enzymes that digest the gelatine. Thus, the presence of pepsin and pancreatin in simulated gastric and intestinal fluids, respectively, may be especially important in the dissolution testing of hard-gelatine capsules (Digenis et al. 1994).

Figure 7.3 *In vitro* dissolution-time profiles of a poorly soluble compound, felodipine, for three different hydrophilic matrix extended release tablets (A–C) when three different surfactants (SLS, CTAB, Tween) were used in the dissolution test medium at levels providing "sink conditions".

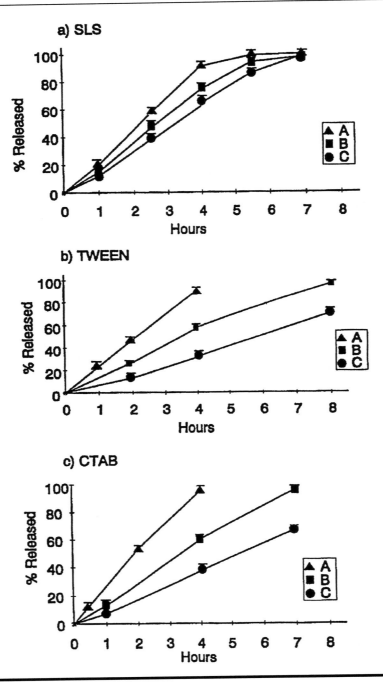

Example 2

The ionic concentration in the test medium can affect both the drug solubility and the release mechanism for modified-release formulations. One example of the latter case is hydrophilic gel matrix tablets, a type of ER tablet that forms a gel layer in contact with the GI fluids. Solutes will affect the hydration of the gel matrix and, thereby, affect the drug release rate.

It has been shown for such tablets that the correlation to *in vivo* data can be completely lost by use of inappropriate ionic compositions in the test medium (Abrahamsson et al. 1998a). For ER formulations with osmotically driven drug release, a decreased drug release rate approaching no release will occur for high ionic concentrations in the test medium, and misleading *in vitro* results may be obtained if a relevant ionic composition is not used (Lindstedt et al. 1989).

The concern for variability in dissolution results is of special significance when setting up a specification test method to be used for batch release but may also be considered for other tests. In order to reduce variability in dissolution results due to the test medium, the quality aspects of the dissolution media components that could affect the drug dissolution and release must be identified, and appropriate qualities of the components should be defined. This is especially important for the use of surfactants to provide micellar solubilisation in the test medium (Crison et al. 1997). Another potential source of variability is impurities in the components that may alter the solubility or catalyse degradation of labile drugs. It is also important to see that the dissolution test medium is stable, i.e., that the components are not degraded or precipitated during the dissolution test period. This is of no concern for plain buffer systems but is more relevant for complex media including physiological components.

Dissolved air in the dissolution medium could, under certain circumstances, be located as air bubbles on the surface of the dosage form or released solid material. This will clearly affect the dissolution process by reducing wetting and the available surface area for dissolution in an uncontrolled way. In order to avoid this problem, the dissolution media has to be deaerated. A method for deaeration based on heating and filtration can be found in USP XXIV. Other methods have also been described (Diebold and Dressman 1998). It is, however, important to realise that the reaeration of deaerated water is a rapid process. The oxygen content increases significantly during filling of the *in vitro* dissolution test vessel as well as during the dissolution experiment (Diebold and Dressman 1998) (see Figure 7.4).

Other Study Design Aspects

The design aspects of dissolution testing include, primarily, the choice of sampling intervals and number of tablets to be tested. Batch control often includes the testing of 6 individual units, whereas testing for regulatory purposes most often requires the testing of 12 individual units. In batch control of immediate-release (IR) formulations, one test point is most commonly used to assure complete dissolution (e.g., 80 or 85 percent of the total dose) at a specified time point (e.g., after 30–60 min), whereas three time points are required for ER formulations. For more slowly dissolving IR formulations, or poorly soluble drugs, a two-point dissolution test, i.e., sampling at two different times, has been proposed (FDA 1997b). For regulatory purposes, when *in vitro* dissolution is used as a surrogate for bioequivalence studies, multiple time point determinations may also be required for IR formulations; if not, complete dissolution is not obtained within 15 min. For ER formulations, a more frequent sampling schedule than three time points is recommended during development, or as surrogate for *in vivo* bioequivalence studies, to reveal the full character of the dissolution profile. For example, the biphasic release pattern or a significant lag phase may not be detected if too few samples are collected.

Figure 7.4 Oxygen concentration in deaerated dissolution test medium at different times in the USP I and II apparatuses at an agitation speed of 100 rpm.

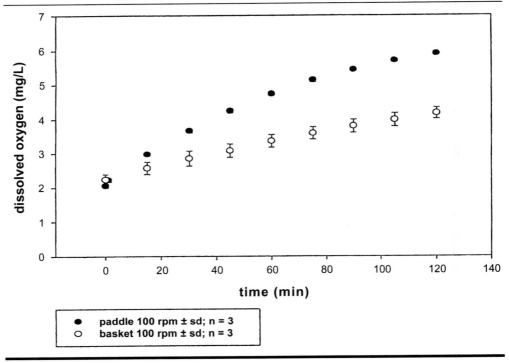

● paddle 100 rpm ± sd; n = 3
○ basket 100 rpm ± sd; n = 3

Another design aspect of dissolution tests occurs when several parameters in the dissolution test method are varied. This could be the situation when looking for the best correlation to *in vivo* data, testing the robustness of the dissolution method or testing the robustness of the dissolution properties of a certain formulation towards different physiological factors. The traditional approach has been to vary one factor at a time, while keeping the others at a constant level. The main disadvantages of this design approach are the numerous experiments needed when many factors have to be investigated, and the risk of suboptimisation when there are interactions between different study variables. Statistical experimental design has been applied to dissolution testing during recent years as a method of reducing these problems. For full information regarding design and evaluation of such experiments, statistical textbooks such as *Statistics for Experimenters* (Box et al. 1978) are recommended, since the aim of the present chapter is only to provide a short introduction to this topic.

The basic principle of experimental design is to vary all factors concomitantly according to a randomised and balanced design, and to evaluate the results by multivariate analysis techniques, such as multiple linear regression or partial least squares. It is essential to check by diagnostic methods that the applied statistical model appropriately describes the experimental data. Unacceptably poor fit indicates experimental errors or that another model should be applied. If a more complicated model is needed, it is often necessary to add further experimental runs to correctly resolve such a model.

An example of a design aimed at validation of a dissolution method is given below (Gottfries et al. 1994). Seven factors were included, and each one was tested at two different levels plus one centre point (i.e., all factors are set at a level in the middle between the high and low levels). In this case, there were $2^7 = 128$ number of unique experiments that could be performed, excluding the centre point, in order to cover all possible combinations of the low and high level settings of the seven different factors. Such a large number of experiments is seldom practically and economically justified. However, in statistical design, it is possible to do fractional designs, i.e., a limited number of all possible experiments is chosen according to balanced design. In the present case, only 16 experiments, excluding the centre point, were performed, and the settings in all experimental runs are presented in Table 7.3. The centre point was replicated four times in order to assess experimental variability. The most common ways to present the results are shown in Figure 7.5 and 7.6. In Figure 7.5, the bars represent the effect on the amount of drug dissolved after 4 h of each variable when varying the setting from the centre to the upper level. The most predominant effects were provided by the stirring rate (St), temperature (T), ionic strength (Ion), the square of T, interaction between St and buffer volume (Buf) and interaction between T and Ion. Figure 7.6 is a surface response plot that displays the dissolution response at different levels of two selected variables while others are held constant at the mid-level. It is also possible to use an obtained model to predict dissolution results for any experimental setting within the tested domain. In this case, dissolution profiles were simulated for all possible combinations of settings within a series of predetermined limits in order to determine acceptable limits for methodological variation.

Examples of applications of statistical designs for optimising correlations with *in vivo* data and for the testing of a formulation under different experimental conditions to elucidate the sensitivity of the drug release towards different physiological factors have also been published (Abrahamsson et al. 1999; Abuzarur-Aloul et al. 1997).

Assessment of Dissolution Profiles

It is often desirable to present the dissolution results by some response variable. The most common descriptor is the amount dissolved at a certain time point. For rapidly dissolving dosage forms, it may be sufficient to provide the amount dissolved, for example, at 15 or 30 min. For dosage forms where it is relevant to study the whole profile, more sophisticated methods are needed, since the use of a single point neglects all other data points.

Any model can be applied to *in vitro* dissolution data and fitted by linear or non-linear regression, as appropriate. Sometimes a first-order model [$A(t) = A - Ae^{-kt}$ where $A(t)$ is the amount dissolved after time t, A is the initial amount and k is the first-order dissolution rate constant] or even a zero-order model ($A(t) = A - Akt$) is sufficiently sophisticated to determine a dissolution rate that is representative for the whole process. However, a more general equation that is commonly applied to dissolution data is the Weibull equation (Langenbucher 1976):

$$A(t) = A_\infty \times \left[1 - e^{-\left(\frac{t - t_{\text{lag}}}{\tau_d}\right)^\beta} \right]$$

$$(1)$$

where $A(t)$ is the amount dissolved at time t, A_∞ is the final plateau level of amount dissolved in the dissolution-time curve and t_{lag} is the duration of an initial period of no dissolution. τ_d

Table 7.3
Worksheet illustrating a statistical experimental design for evaluating the effect on the dissolution of variations of the test conditions in an *in vitro* dissolution method.

Exp. No.	Stirring Sp. (rpm)	pH	Conc. of CTAB (%)	Temp. (°C)	Basket Pos. (cm)	Ionic Strength of Buffer (M)	Buffer Vol. (mL)
1	110.0	6.0	0.50	34.0	2.0	0.05	510.0
2	110.0	6.0	0.30	34.0	2.0	0.15	490.0
3	110.0	7.0	0.50	34.0	0.0	0.15	490.0
4	110.0	7.0	0.30	34.0	0.0	0.05	510.0
5	110.0	7.0	0.50	40.0	2.0	0.15	510.0
6	110.0	6.0	0.50	40.0	0.0	0.05	490.0
7	110.0	7.0	0.30	40.0	2.0	0.05	490.0
8	110.0	6.0	0.30	40.0	0.0	0.15	510.0
9	100.0	6.5	0.40	37.0	1.0	0.10	500.0
10	100.0	6.5	0.40	37.0	1.0	0.10	500.0
11	100.0	6.5	0.40	7.0	1.0	0.10	500.0
12	100.0	6.5	0.40	37.0	1.0	0.10	500.0
13	100.0	6.5	0.40	37.0	1.0	0.10	500.0
14	90.0	7.0	0.50	34.0	2.0	0.05	490.0
15	90.0	6.0	0.50	34.0	0.0	0.15	510.0
16	90.0	6.0	0.30	34.0	0.0	0.05	490.0
17	90.0	7.0	0.30	34.0	2.0	0.15	510.0
18	90.0	6.0	0.30	40.0	2.0	0.05	510.0
19	90.0	7.0	0.30	40.0	0.0	0.15	490.0
20	90.0	7.0	0.50	40.0	0.0	0.05	510.0
21	90.0	6.0	0.50	40.0	2.0	0.15	490.0
A1	110.0	7.0	0.50	40.0	0.0	0.15	490.0
A2	90.0	6.0	0.30	40.0	0.0	0.05	490.0
A3	110.0	7.0	0.50	40.0	0.0	0.05	510.0
A4	90.0	6.0	0.50	34.0	0.0	0.05	510.0
A5	90.0	7.0	0.50	34.0	2.0	0.15	490.0
A6	100.0	6.5	0.40	34.0	1.0	0.10	500.0
A7	100.0	6.5	0.40	40.0	1.0	0.10	500.0
A8	100.0	6.5	0.40	37.0	1.0	0.10	490.0
A9	100.0	6.5	0.40	37.0	1.0	0.10	510.0

Reprinted from *International Journal of Pharmaceutics*, Vol. 106, J. Gottfries et al., Validation of an extended release tablet dissolution testing system using design and multivariate analysis, Pages 141–148, Copyright 1994, with permission from Elsevier Science.

is a rate parameter, more specifically it is a scale factor of the time axis. Two curves differing only in τ_d appear as being stretched or compressed along the time axis. Finally, β is a parameter that characterises the shape of the curve. At β values of 0 and 1, the dissolution-time curve follows zero- and first-order kinetics, respectively.

Figure 7.5 Scaled and centred coefficients for felodipine *in vitro* dissolution after 4 h (Y4). The height of the bars illustrates the change in response estimated for a relative increase of each factor from the mid-point level to the high level in the factorial design. The different factors were stirring speed (St), pH, concentration cetyltrimethylammonium bromide (CT), temperature (T), basket position (BP), ionic strength (Ion), buffer volume (Buf), square of T (T × T), interaction terms between St and Buf (St × Buf) and between T and Ion (T × Ion).

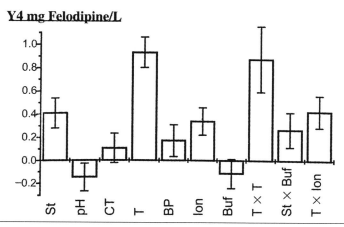

Y4 mg Felodipine/L

Another approach to obtain a parameter that describes the dissolution rate is to use statistical moments to determine the mean dissolution time (MDT) (von Hattingberg 1984). This method has the advantage of being applicable to all types of dissolution profiles, and it does not require fitting to any model. The only prerequisite is that data points are available close to the final plateau level. The MDT can be interpreted as the most likely time for a molecule to be dissolved from a solid dosage form. In the case of zero- and first-order dissolution processes, the MDT corresponds to the time when 50 and 63.2 percent have been released, respectively. The MDT is determined from:

$$\mathrm{MDT} = \frac{{}^{i}\sum t_i \times \Delta M_i}{M_0} \tag{2}$$

where t_i is the midpoint of the *i*th time period during which the fraction ΔM_i has been released and M_0 is the final amount released. The length of each time period is given by the sampling intervals.

A special case occurs when two dissolution profiles are compared. This is often the case when a change has been introduced in the composition, manufacturing process or manufacturing site. The aim is then to maintain the same dissolution properties as for the original version. Such comparisons of dissolution profiles are performed by calculating a similarity factor, f_2, which is calculated as follows from cumulative mean data (Shah et al. 1998):

Figure 7.6 Response surface of felodipine dissolved *in vitro* after 4 h expressed as drug concentration at different ionic strengths and temperatures.

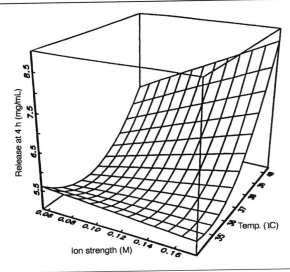

Reprinted from *International Journal of Pharmaceutics*, Vol. 106, J. Gottfries et al., Validation of an extended release tablet dissolution testing system using design and multivariate analysis, Pages 141–148, Copyright 1994, with permission from Elsevier Science.

$$ f_2 = 50 \times \log \left\{ \left[1 + \left(\frac{1}{n} \right) \sum_{t=1}^{n} (R_t - T_t)^2 \right]^{-0.5} \times 100 \right\} \qquad (3) $$

where n is the number of time points in the dissolution-time curve and R_t and T_t are the cumulative amount dissolved at time t for the reference and test formulation, respectively. The number of time points, n, should be at least 3, but only including one value close to the final plateau level ($\geq$85 percent). From a regulatory perspective, f_2-values greater than 50 ensure that the profiles are similar enough (FDA 1997b) and if $f_2 = 100$, the test and reference products have identical dissolution-time curves. An f_2-value of 50 corresponds to an average difference between the test and reference curves of 10 percent. This test is not relevant for very rapidly dissolving formulations (i.e., complete release within 15 min), since differences in the dissolution profiles between formulations that are so rapid is of no *in vivo* relevance.

Validation of *In Vitro* Dissolution Methods

High quality and valuable *in vitro* dissolution tests are obtained by a rational design of test method as described above. However, there are different means to validate the method, i.e., to verify that the method functions as intended. These include

- dissolution tests with USP calibrator tablets,

- robustness testing and

- comparison with *in vivo* results.

Disintegrating as well as non-disintegrating USP calibrator tablets are available with a specified dissolution profile for each apparatus. These tablets are used to control the dissolution apparatus and to allow it to operate as intended, i.e., so that the hydrodynamic conditions are satisfactory. However, it should be noted that certain formulations might be more sensitive to such factors than are the calibrator tablets.

Another important aspect in validation of a new dissolution method is to investigate how sensitive the dissolution results of the product, for which the method has been developed, are for minute variations in operating conditions. Examples of factors to consider in such a test are temperature of test medium, rotational speed, volume, sampling procedure, medium compositions and testing performed by different operators. Based on such robustness tests of the method, limits can be defined for acceptable variations of test conditions. Statistical design may be useful to apply in situations such as those demonstrated earlier in this chapter.

Comparison of *in vitro* dissolution results with corresponding *in vivo* data for different formulations in order to verify that the *in vitro* methods predict the *in vivo* dissolution properties (see the section "*In Vitro/In Vivo Correlations*") is preferably used already in the design of the test method. However, if not so, the *in vivo* validity of the method should be investigated at a later stage, especially for modified release formulations and poorly soluble drugs.

BIOAVAILABILITY STUDIES

In bioavailability studies, the drug plasma concentrations, and potentially the amount of drug/metabolites in urine, are followed over an appropriate time interval after administration in order to derive drug absorption parameters. There are basically two different aspects of the function of the formulation that can be evaluated: (a) rate of drug dissolution and/or release and (b) extent of drug that is made available for absorption.

The drug dissolution or release rate will directly determine the absorption rate in cases where this is the rate-limiting step in the absorption process. The formulation may also affect the extent of absorption, for example

- when dissolution enhancers are used for poorly soluble compounds

- when absorption enhancers are used for poorly permeable drugs

- when the drug release is incomplete from the formulation

- when the formulation provides a means of avoiding degradation in the GI tract.

The importance and need to study these factors increases if the substance has problematic absorption properties, or if the aim is to develop an advanced formulation, such as a modified release product, or if a dosage form affects the biopharmaceutical properties in any other way.

Bioavailability studies are performed during formulation development at different stages and for several reasons:

- to obtain and verify the desirable dissolution and release properties

- to study the influence of physiological factors such as food

- to establish bioquivalence between clinical trial and commercial formulations after changes of a formulation

- to develop and validate IVIVCs for *in vitro* dissolution test methods

Although all of these different types of studies aim to investigate the influence of the dosage form on the rate and extent of absorption, different designs and means to evaluate the data are applied. This chapter describes different ways to assess the formulation function from plasma concentration data obtained in bioavailability studies. Certain study design aspects will also be pointed out. For a more basic understanding of pharmacokinetics, specialised textbooks should be consulted, such as *Clinical Pharmacokinetics—Concepts and Applications* (Rowland and Tozer 1995).

Aspects of Study Design

Single-Dose Studies

Single-dose Studies are most sensitive for evaluation of absorption properties and should generally be used for evaluation of formulations. The main exception is if the regulatory guidelines require repeated dosing studies. The drug should be administered under fasting conditions (overnight) together with 200 mL of water. No food should generally be allowed for 4 h after intake, and the subjects should thereafter follow a standardised meal schedule during the study day.

Cross-Over Designs

In cross-over designs, the same subjects receive test and reference formulations to avoid the influence of any interindividual differences that could affect the plasma concentration-time profile. For drugs with a very long half-life (several weeks), a parallel group design (i.e., each formulation is studied in different groups of subjects) may be applied for practical reasons to shorten the duration of the study. A parallel group design could also be used if the inter-individual (between subjects) variability of the bioavailability variables is of the same magnitude as the intraindividual (within-subject) variability. Additionally, other standard design principles such as randomisation should be used, as described in more detail in statistical textbooks.

Wash-out Period

A wash-out period, i.e., a minimum number of days between administration of each formulation, is needed in order to avoid influence of the previous administration on the plasma concentration profile of the following formulation. As a rule of thumb, the wash-out period should be at least five times the elimination half-life of the drug under investigation.

Reference Formulation

In almost all studies, a reference formulation is needed, either as a comparator for assessment of relative performance compared to the test formulation, or as a simple vehicle, to characterise the drug substance pharmacokinetics. If the aim is to investigate the influence of certain formulations on the rate and extent of absorption, which is the case in early development or IVIVC studies, an oral solution of the drug is the first choice as a reference formulation. Stability of the solution, regarding drug compound degradation and precipitation, is an important factor to verify before study start. Inclusion of a parenteral reference formulation, if feasible, provides additional information, as will be further discussed below.

Number of Subjects

The number of subjects to be included in the study will be determined by the inherent variability in drug substance pharmacokinetics, the magnitude of effects that are of interest, the desired confidence in conclusions, costs, time, ethical aspects and where relevant, regulatory guideline recommendations. Three different situations may be identified that require different algorithms to determine the sample size:

1. The aim is to determine the absorption characteristics for a certain formulation, for example, in an IVIVC study. In this case, the question for the pharmaceutical scientist is how precise the mean estimates of primary variables must be, i.e., how wide confidence intervals around the mean are acceptable.

2. The aim is to investigate the difference between two or more formulations. In this case, the question is how large a difference between the formulations can be of interest to detect at a certain statistical significance level.

3. The aim is to establish bioequivalence between two formulations by obtaining a confidence interval for the difference within specified limits. In this case, the main question is how large a risk the investigator is willing to take to obtain non-conclusive results. Inclusion of more subjects will decrease the width of the confidence interval and thereby reduce the risk of not meeting the acceptance criteria.

Calculations of a suitable number of subjects are most often made by statisticians. However, for an understanding of these calculations, any basic statistical textbook is recommended for the first two cases, and in the case of bioequivalence studies, another reference (Hauschke et al. 1999) is suggested.

Plasma Sampling

The plasma sampling schedule has to be designed so that the desired accuracy of the primary bioavailability variables can be obtained. In cases of evaluation of formulation performance, it is crucial to have frequent sampling during the absorption phase. In addition, at least three samples should be obtained during the major terminal elimination phase in order to obtain a relevant measure of the rate constant for this phase, which is needed for a correct estimate of the extent of absorption. Numerous late plasma samples, when the drug concentration is below the limit of quantification of the bioanalythical assay, should be avoided.

Food

Food may not only affect drug substance pharmacokinetics, such as first-pass metabolism or drug clearance; it may also influence drug dissolution, or by other means, the function of the dosage form. For example, with food, drug residence time in the stomach will be increased, the pH will be changed, motility will be altered and bile and pancreatic secretions will increase. All of these factors could potentially affect drug release and dissolution from a solid formulation. It is therefore relevant to study the influence of food on rate and extent of drug dissolution/release during development. Such a study should include an oral solution, to allow for a distinction between the effects of food on formulation and drug substance. The dosage forms are typically administered immediately after intake of the food. Since almost all medications are administered in the morning, studies are usually performed together with a breakfast. The composition of the meal has to be well defined, since variations can introduce unwanted variability.

Generally, a heavy breakfast (approximately 1000 calories and 50 percent of the energy content from fat) should be used, since this is supposed to stress potential food effects. A proposal for a standardised composition of a heavy breakfast is displayed in Table 7.4 (FDA 1997c).

Assessments

Evaluation of drug plasma concentrations is an indirect way of estimating the rate and amount of drug dissolution and/or absorption. Several assumptions are therefore needed, irrespective of which of the metrics described below are applied:

- In cross-over studies, drug substance pharmacokinetics, including first-pass metabolism, distribution and clearance, should be identical within the same subject, between administrations of different formulations.

- Linear pharmacokinetics within the investigated rate of delivery (dose/time units) of the drug to the body, i.e., the plasma concentration–time profile, should be identical for different doses after correction for dose. The most common reason for nonlinear pharmacokinetics is dose-dependent first-pass metabolism. This phenomenon does not just occur at high doses, but has also been shown for the slow delivery rates obtained by ER formulations.

In cases where the *in vivo* dissolution/release rate is going to be quantified in some way from plasma concentrations, it is important to emphasise that this is only relevant if this is the rate-limiting step in the absorption process. If other factors are affecting the absorption rate,

---

Table 7.4
Example of a standardised breakfast to be used in food interaction studies.

2 eggs fried in butter	4 ounces of hash brown potatoes
2 strips of bacon	8 ounces of whole milk
2 slices of toast with butter	

estimations of the *in vivo* dissolution will be confounded. Examples of such confounding factors in determination of the *in vivo* dissolution rate are

- gastric emptying (assuming negligible absorption over the gastric mucosa);

- low drug permeability over the gastric wall;

- degradation in the GI tract;

- complex-binding of the drug to any component in the GI tract; and

- entero-hepatic circulation, i.e., intact drugs are excreted by the bile into the intestine.

In vivo evaluation of formulations thus requires a high level of knowledge regarding the drug substance absorption properties obtained both by *in vitro* and *in vivo* methods described in this chapter and in Chapter 4, and also by basic pharmacokinetic studies, a review of which is outside the scope of the present chapter.

Standard Bioavailability Variables

The standard bioavailability variables after a single-dose administration are the maximum plasma concentration (C_{max}), the time to reach C_{max} (t_{max}) and the area under the plasma concentration—time curve from time zero to infinity (AUC).

C_{max} and t_{max} are used as characteristics of the absorption rate and may thereby be affected by the drug dissolution and release, as discussed above. However, both variables are affected by several pharmacokinetic properties other than the absorption rate (Ka) as shown in equations 4 and 5, which describe C_{max} and t_{max}, respectively, for a first-order absorption process;

$$C_{max} = \frac{F \times D \left(\dfrac{Ka}{Ke}\right)^{-Ke(Ka-Ke)}}{Vd} \tag{4}$$

$$t_{max} = \frac{2.303 \times \log\left(\dfrac{Ka}{Ke}\right)}{Ka - Ke} \tag{5}$$

where F is the extent of oral drug bioavailability expressed as a fraction, D is the administered dose, Ke is the first-order elimination rate constant, according to one compartment model, and Vd is the volume of distribution.

Thus, C_{max} and t_{max} are not useful as pure measures of the absorption rate but can be used in comparisons between different formulations. Another disadvantage is that they are single-point estimates, which does not take into account all data sampled during the absorption process. In the case of rapid dissolution processes, it is difficult to accurately localise the true maximum, and frequent plasma sampling during the absorption phase is especially crucial in getting reasonably good estimates. The main merit of C_{max}, besides simplicity, is its potential clinical relevance, i.e., when the peak plasma concentration is related to maximal pharmacological effects or adverse effects.

AUC is used to evaluate the extent of absorption which may be affected by the formulation, as discussed above. AUC is a composite variable determined not only by the extent of bioavailability (F) but also by the systemic drug clearance (Cl) and the dose (D) as described by:

$$AUC = \frac{D \times F}{Cl} \tag{6}$$

Thus, AUC is only of interest as a relative variable, where the AUC for a test formulation is related to a reference. If the AUC-ratio is determined for a formulation in relation to an oral solution, the influence of the dosage form on the extent of absorption can be determined, that is, if $AUC_{solid}/AUC_{solution} \neq 1.00$, the deviation from 1 can be attributed to the formulation, provided that the above-stated assumptions hold. AUC is also a primary variable in bioequivalence studies.

The calculation of AUC is commonly determined by the linear trapezoidal rule. In this procedure, the sum of the areas of a series of trapezoids which are formed between the data points for two adjacent times is calculated (see Figure 7.7). This approximate method requires that blood sampling be frequent enough so that the curvature of the plasma concentrations between two data points is negligible. For example, in the ascending part, the plasma concentration curve has a convex profile, and a straight line will provide an overestimation of the AUC. Applying a modified version, the log trapezoidal rule, can reduce this problem. The area under each segment between two data points for the linear trapezoidal (equation 7) and logarithmic trapezoidal (equation 8) methods are determined by:

$$AUC(t_n, t_{n+1}) = \left(\frac{C_n + C_{n+1}}{2} \right) \times (t_{n+1} - t_n) \tag{7}$$

Figure 7.7 Drug plasma concentration–time curve illustrating formation of trapezoids, in calculation of the area under the curve (AUC).

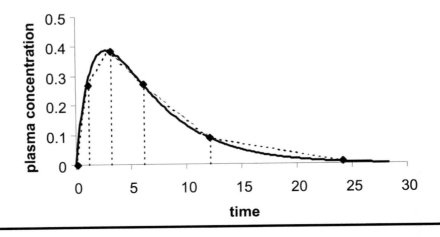

$$\mathrm{AUC}(t_n, t_{n+1}) = \left(\frac{C_n - C_{n+1}}{\ln\dfrac{C_n}{C_{n+1}}} \right) \times \left(t_{n+1} - t_n \right) \qquad (8)$$

where C_n is the drug concentration for the nth plasma sample obtained at time t_n. It is imperative in single-dose studies, which are generally most suitable for evaluation of dosage form performance, to determine the AUC from time zero to infinity. This requires that the remaining area from the last measured data point (Ct_{last}) to infinity be extrapolated, and is made from the following equation:

$$\mathrm{AUCt}_{\mathrm{last}-\infty} = \frac{Ct_{\mathrm{last}}}{Ke} \qquad (9)$$

where Ke is the elimination rate constant which is determined from the slope of the terminal log-linear plasma concentration–time profile (see Figure 7.8) by linear regression. In order to obtain a reliable estimate of AUC, the extrapolated area ($\mathrm{AUCt}_{\mathrm{last}-\infty}$) should not exceed 10 percent of the total AUC.

$C_{\max}$ and AUC are also used as primary variables in bioequivalence studies, i.e., studies aiming to establish that a test and a reference product provide similar enough plasma concentration–time profiles to be exchanged without altering the clinical effects. Such studies are, for example, performed in NDA programmes to compare the clinical trial formulations with the "to-be-marketed" product, at post-approval changes of composition, manufacturing process or site of a product and to document a generic versus the original product. More details regarding performance and evaluation of such studies can be found in appropriate guidelines (FDA 1999; EMEA 1998).

Model Dependent Analysis

An absorption rate, which could reflect dosage form performance, as discussed above, could be determined from plasma concentration data by fitting the data to a pharmacokinetic model. The absorption rate could be a zero-order or first-order rate constant, i.e., the amount absorbed is constant over time, or, the absorption rate decreases exponentially over time, respectively. The choice of model also depends on how many phases in the log-plasma concentration–time profile are identified after the peak concentration, i.e., how many compartments are needed to describe the plasma concentration–time profile. The model may also include a lag time ($t$lag) before absorption starts. A comprehensive description of different models can be found in Gabrielsson and Weiner (1997). Model dependent analysis could also be used to determine the standard bioavailability variables such as $C_{\max}$, $t_{\max}$ and AUC. Fitting the plasma concentration data to the suitable model is done by non-linear regression. Computer programs designed for pharmacokinetic modelling are available, such as NONLIN (Pharsight Corp., Mountain View, Calif., USA). More detail regarding performance and evaluation of non-linear regressions for this purpose can be found elsewhere (Gabrielsson and Weiner 1997).

In the case of one-compartment disposition pharmacokinetics, i.e. when the declining part of the plasma concentration–time curve can be approximated by a one log-linear phase, a first-order rate constant (Ka) can be determined according to:

Figure 7.8 Logarithmic drug plasma concentration–time curve for an oral administration illustrating the elimination rate constant (*Ke*) and first-order absorption rate constant (*Ka*).

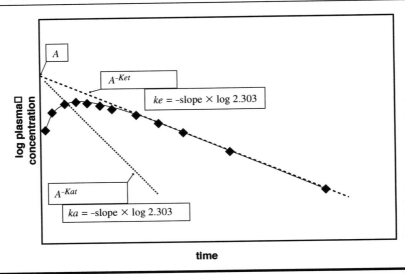

$$Ae^{-Kat} = Ae^{-Ket} - Ct \tag{10}$$

where *A* is determined from the intercept with the y axis of the extrapolated log-linear elimination phase (see Figure 7.8), *Ke* is the first-order rate constant that describes the elimination phase, and *C* is the plasma concentration at time *t*. The difference between the extrapolated elimination phase and the actual plasma concentration ($Ae^{-Ket} - Ct$) is plotted versus time, which thus equals Ae^{-Kat} and describes the absorption phase. The *Ka* can then be determined from the slope of the line in a log-linear plot as shown in Figure 7.8.

Moment Analysis

Moment analysis provides the means to determine a model independent characteristic of the absorption rate or dissolution rate (Riegelman and Collier 1980). A single value characterising the rate of the entire dissolution or absorption process is obtained, which is called the mean absorption or dissolution time (MAT and MDT, respectively). These parameters can be determined without any assumptions regarding absorption or disposition pharmacokinetics, apart from the general prerequisites of linear pharmacokinetics and absence of intraindividual variability described above. MAT/MDT can be interpreted as the most probable time for a molecule to become absorbed/dissolved, based on a normal Gaussian distribution.

If these processes follow zero- or first-order kinetics, MAT/MDT corresponds to 50 and 63 percent absorbed/dissolved, respectively. MDT is especially useful for correlations with *in vitro* data since this *in vivo* variable corresponds to the MDT determined from *in vitro* dissolution data, as described in the section "*In Vitro* Dissolution".

MAT and MDT for a test formulation are determined from drug plasma concentrations–time data obtained in a single dose study according to the following equations;

$$MRT = \frac{AUMC_{0-\infty}}{AUC_{0-\infty}} \tag{11}$$

$$MAT = MRT_{test} - MRT_{IV} \tag{12}$$

$$MDT = MRT_{test} - MRT_{oral\ solution} \tag{13}$$

where MRT is the mean residence time, which includes the complete time from intake to elimination of the drug. $AUMC_{0-\infty}$ is the area under the curve of the product of time t and the plasma concentration versus time from zero to infinity, and $AUC_{0-\infty}$ is the area under the plasma concentration–time curve, as defined above. Thus, administration of an oral or intravenous (IV) reference administration is needed to calculate MAT and MDT, respectively, except when the drug substance follows one-compartment pharmacokinetics. In this case, the MAT can be determined without a reference according to the following formula:

$$MAT_{test} = MRT_{test} - \left(\frac{1}{Ke}\right) \tag{14}$$

i.e., MRT and *Ke* are determined from the plasma concentration–time profile for the test formulation according to the procedures described above.

In Vivo *Dissolution/Absorption-Time Profiles*

A full-time course *in vivo* dissolution- or absorption-time profile is generally the most informative way of evaluating formulation performance from the plasma concentration–time data. The methods described in the present chapter all have the advantage over the modelling of zero- or first-order rate constants, in that no assumptions have to be made regarding the kinetics of the absorption phase. Some of the methods provide an estimate of the absorption-time profile, rather than the *in vivo* dissolution-time profile. However, in the context of evaluating formulation performance, the former measure is fully valid, provided that the drug dissolution/release is the rate-determining step in the absorption process.

The method of choice for determination of *in vivo* dissolution- or absorption-time profiles is *deconvolution*. In deconvolution, three components are defined: input, weighting and response functions, as exemplified in Figure 7.9. The input function corresponds to the entry of drug into the body, i.e., the *in vivo* dissolution- or absorption-time profiles for the oral test formulation. The weighting function corresponds to the time course of the drug within the body, as described by the plasma concentration—time profile after administration of an oral or IV reference solution, and the response function is described by the plasma concentration–time curve for the test formulation. In deconvolution, the input function is determined from data that describe the weighting and response functions, i.e., the *in vivo* dissolution- or absorption-time profile is calculated from the plasma concentration–time data of the test formulation and a reference solution. It is also possible to calculate the response function from available data of the input and weighting functions, i.e., the plasma concentration–time profile for a solid oral dosage form is simulated from *in vitro* dissolution data and plasma concentration–time data for a solution. This latter procedure is called *convolution*. The three

Figure 7.9 Illustrations of the different functions included in deconvolution/ convolution.

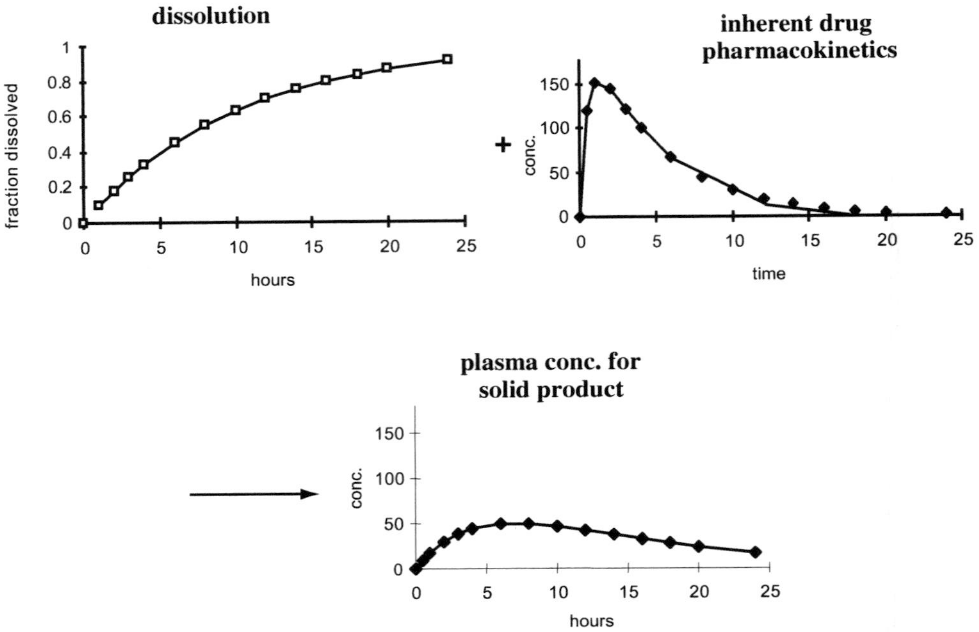

most common definitions of the input, weighting and response functions in deconvolution/ convolution are presented in Table 7.5.

Different deconvolution algorithms have been described (Tucker 1983). However, further descriptions in the present chapter will be limited to numerical deconvolution (Langenbucher 1982). The merits of this equation compared to others are the relative simplicity of the algorithm and the lack of any modelling of the plasma concentration–time data to be used in

Table 7.5
Definitions of the different functions in deconvolution/convolution.

Input (I)	Weighting (W)	Response (R)
	Plasma concentration–time profile for:	Plasma concentration–time profile for:
Dissolution-time profile or solid formulation	Oral solution	Solid formulation
Absorption-time profile or solid formulation	IV solution	Solid formulation
Absorption-time profile for oral solution	IV solution	Oral solution

the assessment of the input profile. The fractional amount dissolved or absorbed (I) is calculated by the following deconvolution algorithm:

$$I_1 = \frac{R_1 T}{W_1} \tag{15}$$

$$I_2 = \frac{\dfrac{R_2}{(T - I_1)W_2}}{W_1}$$

$$I_3 = \frac{\dfrac{R_3}{(T - I_1)(W_3 - I_2)W_2}}{W_1}$$

$$I_n = \frac{\dfrac{R_n}{(T - I_1)(W_n - I_2)(W_{n-1} - \ldots - I_{n-1})W_2}}{W_1}$$

where W_i and R_i are the plasma concentrations for the ith time representing the weighting and response functions, respectively. These plasma concentration–time profiles are divided into finite intervals of equal time T before the plasma concentrations can be entered into the equation described above. Interpolations are generally needed between the measured data points to obtain such data. A common method for performing such interpolations is the point-area method (Vaughan and Dennis 1978).

A drawback of deconvolution algorithms is that they are not stable. Small inconsistencies or noise in the data could, in some cases, lead to input time profiles that oscillate by increasing amplitude, i.e., no meaningful interpretation of such results can be made. Such problems could be overcome by changing the time interval T, by suitable interpolation or by smoothing/modelling of the plasma concentration data used as weighting and response functions.

The plasma concentration for a solid product can be estimated from *in vitro* dissolution data and plasma concentration–time data for a reference formulation by rearranging equation 15 to a convolution algorithm:

$$R_1 = I_1 W_1 T \tag{16}$$

$$R_2 = (I_1 W_2 + I_2 W_1)T$$

$$R_3 = (I_1 W_3 + I_2 W_2 + I_3 W_1)T$$

$$R_n = (I_1 W_n + I_2 W_{n-1} + \cdots + I_n W_1)T$$

The convolution algorithm (equation 16) is stable, in contrast to deconvolution procedures.

Two other methods have been described that require modelling of the disposition pharmacokinetics but not of the absorption phase. For drugs with disposition pharmacokinetics that can be approximated by a one-compartment model, i.e., the declining part of the plasma concentration–time curve can be approximated by a one log-linear phase, the following equation can be applied to determine the fractional amount absorbed (A) at different times t after administration (Wagner and Nelson 1963):

$$A(t) = \frac{Ct + \left(Ke \times AUC_{0-t}\right)}{\left(Ke \times AUC_{0-\infty}\right)} \tag{17}$$

where *Ke* and AUC have been defined previously in this chapter. This equation is known as the *Wagner-Nelson method*. The main advantage of this method is that the absorption-time profile can be determined without administration of any reference formulation, provided that the elimination rate constant can be accurately determined from the post-absorption phase of the plasma concentration–time curve of the test formulation. Another merit of the Wagner-Nelson method is the simple calculation procedure compared to other methods. An important limitation of the Wagner-Nelson method is that the amount absorbed is expressed as the fraction of the total amount absorbed, i.e., the asymptotic plateau level of the absorption-time profile will always be 1.0. Thus, no conclusions can be drawn from such data regarding completeness of drug release or dissolution.

For drugs that are best described by a two-compartment pharmacokinetic model, the absorption-time profile can be determined by the *Loo-Riegelman method* (Loo and Riegelman 1968). However, this method requires administration of an IV bolus dose to determine the disposition pharmacokinetics. Therefore, this method does not provide any clear advantages compared to deconvolution.

Fractional Amount Absorbed

The fractional *amount of drug absorption* (*Fa*) can be defined as the amount of intact drug that permeates the gastric wall. It is related to the absolute bioavailability (*F*), i.e., the fraction of the administered drug that reaches the systemic circulation, according to the following equation:

$$F = Fa \times Fh \times Fg \tag{18}$$

where *Fh* and *Fg* are the fractions of the administered drug that escape first-pass metabolism, before entering the systemic circulation, in the liver and the gut wall, respectively. *Fa* is of special relevance for elucidation of formulation performance, because it is affected by the completeness of dissolution/release, the success in avoiding degradation in GI tract and/or potential effects of the formulation on drug permeability.

Fa can be estimated from plasma concentration–time data and urine data. In the former case, administration of a reference IV solution is needed, in addition to administration of the test formulation. *Fa* can be approximately determined from the following series of algorithms:

$$Fa = \frac{F}{1 - E_h} \tag{19}$$

$$F = \left(\frac{AUC_{oral}}{AUC_{IV}}\right) \times \left(\frac{dose_{IV}}{dose_{oral}}\right) \tag{20}$$

$$E_h = \frac{Cl_{h_{blood}}}{Q_h} \tag{21}$$

$$Cl_{h_{blood}} = Cl_{h_{plasma}} \times blood{:}plasma\ concentration\ rat \tag{22}$$

$$Cl_{h_{plasma}} = Cl_{tot} - CLr \qquad (23)$$

$$Cl_{tot} = \frac{dose_{IV}}{AUC_{IV}} \qquad (24)$$

$$CLr = fe \times Cl_{tot} \qquad (25)$$

$$fe = \frac{Au}{F \times dose} \qquad (26)$$

where E_h is the hepatic elimination ratio, $Cl_{h_{blood}}$ is the hepatic blood clearance and Q_h is the hepatic blood flow, which is assumed to be 1.5 L/min in man. The partition of drug between blood and plasma has to be experimentally determined. Cl_{tot} is the total systemic plasma clearance, CLr is the renal plasma clearance, fe is the fraction of drug excreted unchanged in urine and Au is the total amount of drug excreted unchanged in urine. It should be realised that this is only an approximate method since neither the blood flow nor the blood/plasma drug ratio is measured during the absorption process. In addition, it has to be assumed that all first-pass metabolism is performed by the liver. Systemic clearance is only provided by the liver and kidneys, and hepatic metabolism is linear within the concentration range encompassed by high levels during the first-pass through the liver and lower levels returned from the systemic circulation.

If a radioactively labelled drug is administered intravenously and orally, the fraction absorbed (Fa) can be more simply estimated from the oral/intravenous ratio, corrected for dose, of total radioactivity in the urine. This requires that urine collection continue over a time period long enough to provide almost complete emptying of the radioactivity. Furthermore, in order to get reasonable precision, a significant amount of metabolites and/or unchanged drug has to be excreted by the kidneys. Finally, it has to be assumed that the parent drug molecule is not degraded in the GI tract and is subsequently absorbed as the metabolite.

IN VITRO/IN VIVO CORRELATIONS

The correlation between *in vitro* and *in vivo* dissolution, or other *in vivo* characteristics, is useful during several stages of formulation development. For example, in early formulation development, it may be desirable to establish the *in vivo* relevance of the dissolution method used for screening of different candidate formulations. During later development phases, IVIVCs can be used to validate the batch control dissolution test method, or as a guide when setting the dissolution specification limits. IVIVC may also form a basis for replacing bioequivelence studies with simpler *in vitro* dissolution studies for modified release formulations, both during development and in connection with later post-approval changes (EMEA 1999; FDA 1997a).

It should be possible to establish IVIVCs provided that the following prerequisites are fulfilled:

- Drug release or dissolution is the rate-limiting step in the absorption process.

- The *in vitro* dissolution method provides *in vivo* relevant results.

- Unbiased estimates of the *in vivo* dissolution-time profiles are obtained from plasma concentration–time data (see "Bioavailability Studies" section).

The drug release or dissolution can only be expected to fulfil the first prerequisite given above in cases of modified release formulations and poorly soluble drugs. In other cases, such as rapidly dissolving formulations of highly soluble drugs, or drugs with low permeability over the GI wall, gastric emptying and transport over the gastric mucosa, respectively, will determine the absorption kinetics. Thus, IVIVCs are not possible to obtain in those cases, since permeability and gastric emptying are not at all modelled by an *in vitro* dissolution test method.

It is important to realise that an established IVIVC is not a general characteristic of a drug compound that can freely be applied to all kinds of oral formulations. An IVIVC is, rather, specific for a certain type of formulation. The main limitation of IVIVCs is the problem of defining how large the changes made to a specific formulation can be without affecting the applicability of an established correlation.

Reports have been published in the case of ER tablets, showing that the relationship between *in vitro* and *in vivo* data could be altered by changing the quality of a critical excipient (Abrahamsson et al. 1994). The most conservative approach is to apply IVIVC only to formulation changes that are covered by the formulations included in the establishment of a correlation. However, provided that good knowledge exists regarding drug absorption properties, function of the dosage form and role of critical excipients, as well as the *in vitro* dissolution under various physiologically relevant conditions, somewhat wider applications are possible with reasonable confidence.

Three different types of correlation have been defined, levels A, B and C, as described in Table 7.6. The following part of this chapter will describe how these levels are established and their respective roles, merits and disadvantages.

Valuable additional information on IVIVCs can be found in Brockmeier (1986) and in Young et al. (1997).

Level A

Level A correlation is generally the most desirable form, since the *in vitro* method completely mimics the *in vivo* results, and a direct correspondence exists at each time point. The achievement of an *in vitro* method that models the entire *in vivo* process confers confidence in the method's capability as a surrogate for *in vivo* studies. This allows for predictions from *in vitro* data of complete absorption-time and plasma concentration–time profiles in early formulation development as well as in later phases, when relevant *in vitro* specification limits are settled. In addition, it is only level A correlations that are accepted by regulatory agencies as a basis for replacing *in vivo* bioequivalence studies with *in vitro* dissolution tests.

The development and evaluation of a level A correlation consists of the following steps:

I.   Design and assessment of *in vitro* dissolution studies and human bioavailability studies

   •   choice/development of formulations

   •   study design aspects

   •   assessment of *in vivo* absorption/dissolution-time data

II.   Establishment of an IVIVC

   •   relationship between *in vitro* and *in vivo* data

Table 7.6
Different types of *in vitro/in vivo* correlations of drug dissolution.

Type	Description	Example
Level A	*In vitro* and *in vivo* dissolution-time profiles are superimposable	
Level B	Relationship established between MDT*vitro* and MDT*vivo* determined by statistical moment analysis	
Level C	Relationship established between single-point *in vitro* dissolution rate characteristic and bioavailability variables	

III. Evaluation of predictability

- prediction of drug plasma concentrations from *in vitro* model

- comparisons of predicted and measured bioavailability variables by calculation of the prediction error

Design and Assessment of In Vitro *Dissolution Studies and Human Bioavailability Studies*

It is possible to establish a level A correlation based on data from only one formulation. However, this will not be sufficient for regulatory purposes in most cases, and an established correlation should preferably be validated by additional data. The most common approach is therefore to include several formulations with different *in vitro* release rates. Formulations with different release rates for IVIVC studies may be obtained by (a) choosing batches with different rates due to batch-to-batch variation, (b) altering the manufacturing process in a way that affects dissolution rate, (c) altering the amount or quality of critical excipients or (d) altering the particle size or crystal form of the active drug substance. The ideal formulations for an IVIVC study should provide differences in the release rate of a magnitude that could be detected *in vivo* on top of the inherent pharmacokinetic variation. Furthermore, the mechanism of the variation of release rate should be known, and the modifications performed to obtain the different batches should be relevant for variations that may occur in normal production.

The *in vivo* bioavailability studies should generally be single dose, cross-over studies with administration under fasting conditions, of formulations with different release rates, and a reference solution. The primary response variable in bioavailability studies aimed at establishing IVIVCs is the assessment of an *in vivo* dissolution-time or an absorption-time profile. Further details regarding assessment of such data are given in the section "Bioavailability Studies". The number of subjects to be included should be based on the desired precision in the mean estimate of the dissolution-time profile.

The *in vitro* dissolution programme may comprise tests under several conditions to find the optimal method (see the section "*In Vitro* Dissolution") or may only include testing by use of a tentative production control method. It is crucial that frequent sampling be applied to appropriately characterise the entire dissolution-time curve, since tentative test points in a product specification are generally not sufficient. An adequate number of individual tablets should be tested. For regulatory purposes, 12 individual dosage units from each batch are usually required.

Establishing an IVIVC

When the obtained *in vitro* and *in vivo* dissolution-time curves for all included formulations are superimposable without further mathematical modelling, no additional steps are needed to establish an IVIVC. However, at times, some scaling of the *in vitro* data must be done to obtain superimposable curves. The same scaling factor should be used for all formulations. Linear scaling is recommended, especially in cases where few formulations (<3) are included in the IVIVC, although the use of non-linear scaling functions has also been proposed. The scaling may be performed in two dimensions, either as a time scaling or as a scaling of the amount dissolved, at a certain time point. In the first case, the *in vitro* and *in vivo* time curves are made superimposable by the scaling of the time axis (see Figure 7.10a). The rationale for this approach is that the drug release/dissolution follows the same type of kinetics *in vitro* and *in vivo*, but the differences between the *in vitro* milieu and physiological conditions affect the rates. Another reason for time scaling may be lag times *in vivo* due to gastric emptying which cannot be reflected by an *in vitro* test. An easy way to obtain a scaling function is to plot the time points from the *in vitro* and *in vivo* dissolution-time curves when equal amounts of drug have been dissolved, and subsequently fit a linear function to the data by linear regression. This function should then be used to transform the *in vitro* dissolution-time points to obtain an *in vivo* relevant dissolution-time curve. Another principle for scaling between *in vitro* and *in vivo* dissolution data is to adjust the y axis, i.e., the *in vitro* dissolution data, by the linear scaling factor ($y = kx$) to reach the same level when the dissolution process has been completed (see Figure 7.10b). Thus, the scaling factor k is determined from the ratio of the asymptotic plateau levels obtained in the *in vitro* and *in vivo* dissolution-time curves. The rationale for using this approach is that there may be differences in the extent of bioavailability between test

Figure 7.10 (a) Cumulative *in vitro* and *in vivo* dissolution-time curves illustrating the time-scaling procedure of an *in vitro* dissolution-time curve to obtain an *in vivo* predictive *in vitro* model. (b) Cumulative *in vitro* and *in vivo* dissolution-time curves illustrating a case where an *in vivo* predictive *in vitro* model can be obtained by scaling of the amount dissolved based on the ratio between the asymptotic plateau levels (dashed lines).

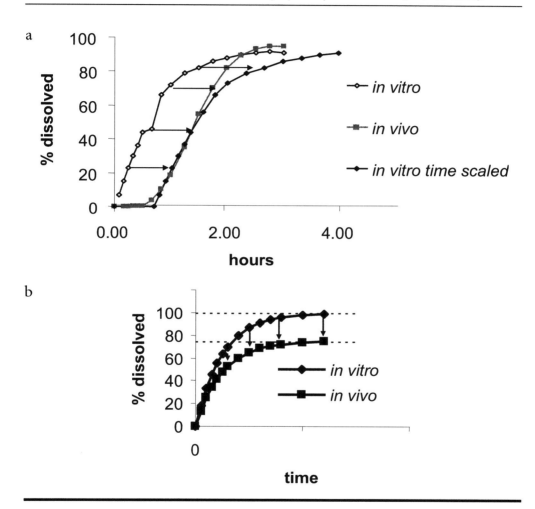

and reference formulations that cannot be attributed directly to the formulation performance, but more to indirect effects (e.g., first-pass metabolism) due to the differences in the rate of administration or site of absorption.

Evaluation of IVIVCs

The *in vivo* predictability of an *in vitro* model with or without a scaling function should be evaluated. A subjective assessment can be made by comparing the modelled *in vitro* dissolution data and the corresponding *in vivo* dissolution-time curves in a graph. However, a more stringent approach, applied in regulatory contexts, is to predict the plasma concentration–time profiles from the *in vitro* model and compare them to measured *in vivo* data. The latter step is performed by comparing the estimated and measured primary bioavailability variables, Cmax and AUC.

The plasma concentration–time data of a test formulation can be predicted from a dissolution-time profile, obtained from the *in vitro* model, and measured plasma concentrations for a reference formulation in the IVIVC bioavailability study (e.g., an oral solution), by use of convolution (see previous section). The difference in Cmax and AUC based on predicted and measured plasma concentrations can be numerically assessed for each formulation by a simple estimation of the relative difference, denoted prediction error (PE), as follows:

$$\%PE = \left(\frac{\text{observed value} - \text{predicted value}}{\text{observed value}} \right) \times 100 \qquad (27)$$

This evaluation may be performed either by use of the same data, as included in the establishment of an IVIVC (internal predictability), or by use of other data sets (external predictability). The criteria for concluding a level A IVIVC in a regulatory context requires, in the case of internal predictability, an average percentage PE of ≤ 10 percent for C_{max} and AUC, respectively, and the percentage PE for each formulation regarding these two bioavailability variables should not exceed 15 percent (FDA 1997a).

Level B

A level B correlation is based on comparisons between MDT *in vitro* and MDT *in vivo*, or MAT. MDT and MAT are average rate characteristics, which take into account all data points. They are determined by statistical moment analysis, as described in the sections "*In Vitro* Dissolution" and "Bioavailability Studies" for *in vitro* and *in vivo* data, respectively.

In order to establish a level B correlation, *in vitro* and *in vivo* data for at least three formulations with different release properties are required. Each formulation provides one pair of *in vitro* and *in vivo* MDT values. A level B correlation can be concluded if a linear relationship is obtained between the *in vitro* and *in vivo* MDT values by use of linear regression.

Level B correlations can be used when level A correlations are not possible, due to different dissolution profiles *in vitro* and *in vivo*. The establishment of a level B correlation implies that the dissolution method can discriminate between formulations that are different *in vivo*. This provides an increased confidence in the suitability of a product control method or a method to be used for optimisation during development. It is also possible to use a level B correlation for the scaling of the *in vitro* dissolution rate to obtain a more *in vivo* relevant estimate of the dissolution process. For example, if MDT*vivo* $\propto$ 2MDT*vitro*, the dissolution process is on average twice as fast *in vivo* compared to *in vitro*. The main disadvantage of level B correlations compared to level A correlations is lack of the possibility to predict the entire *in vivo* dissolution- and plasma concentration–time profiles from *in vitro* data. Therefore, level B correlations have very limited use in regulatory contexts.

Level C

A level C correlation establishes a single-point relationship between a measure of the *in vitro* dissolution rate, e.g., the time when 50 percent of the dose has been dissolved (*t*50 percent), and a bioavailability variable, e.g., C_{max} or AUC. Thus, a corresponding approach is applied as for level B correlations. An advantage of level C correlations, compared to level A and B correlations, is that no reference formulation is needed in the *in vivo* studies. Another advantage of a level C correlation is that the *in vitro* dissolution data are directly related to a bioavailability variable that can be more easily interpreted in a clinical context, compared to dissolution-time profiles and MDT. Level C correlations could also be useful for rapidly releasing formulations to assess at which level a formulation variable, such as tablet disintegration time or drug particle size, becomes a rate-limiting step in the absorption process and starts to affect the bioavailability variables. An example of such usage of a level C correlation is given in Figure 7.11. In this case, an initial phase is found where the *in vivo* variable is independent of the *in vitro* dissolution rate, followed by a linear relationship at slower dissolution rates. This could be useful in establishing the discriminating power of the dissolution test,

Figure 7.11 Mean maximal plasma concentrations (C_{max}) versus time when 50 percent has been dissolved *in vitro* for seven different immediate release formulations. Two linear relationships have been identified, and the cross-section between the two lines indicates the critical dissolution rate at which the dissolution becomes the rate-limiting step in the absorption process.

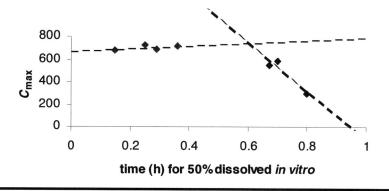

optimising the formulation during development and establishing biopharmaceutically relevant specifications for drug particle size or other critical manufacturing variables.

The disadvantages of single-point level C correlations are; that

- it is not possible to predict entire plasma concentration–time profiles from *in vitro* data

- the single-point estimates, such as *t*50 percent and *C*max, do not take into account the majority of data points obtained in the *in vitro* and *in vivo* studies

- the bioavailability variable is influenced by several other pharmacokinetic drug properties that are not intended to be modelled by the dissolution test.

Single-point level C correlations, therefore, also have a limited use for regulatory purposes.

ANIMAL MODELS

Man is the ultimate model for *in vivo* evaluations, such as bioavailability studies or other investigations of new formulations. However, the use of animal models can provide some important advantages:

- The possibility to perform early *in vivo* studies during preclinical drug development before studies in man are possible

- The use of advanced sampling techniques and other manipulations of experimental conditions not possible in man

- Studies which are cheaper and faster than studies in man

Animal models may thus not only be used as a screening tool before studies are performed in humans, but also for later mechanistic evaluations of findings obtained in human studies.

The main limitation of the usage of animal models is that no single species resembles all physiological properties of man. This introduces a risk that the results obtained in the animal model are not relevant for the situation in man. In the evaluation of oral dosage forms, the main aspects to consider are physiological features of the GI tract, such as dimensions, residence times in different segments, motility patterns, secretions, physical and physicochemical characteristics of GI fluids, the presence of enzymes that could metabolise drugs, and critical excipients, since these factors could directly affect the formulation performance. In cases where the main study variable is the drug plasma concentration, other factors such as the presence of active drug transporters over the GI wall or species differences in first-pass metabolism may also confound the extrapolation of animal data to man. These problems can be handled by choosing the best possible animal model and an appropriate study design and by integrating knowledge of differences between animal and man in the interpretation of obtained results.

Choice of Animal Model

The great majority of studies are performed in dogs. They are, together with other animals such as pigs and monkeys, generally the most suitable species due to many anatomical and physiological similarities with man. Pigs and monkeys, however, have some practical disadvantages compared to dogs, such as being more difficult to train, the need for larger space, ethical concerns and high costs. Rabbits are also used to some extent, despite some fundamental physiological differences to humans. Smaller animals such as rodents, common in other preclinical experiments, are often too small to allow administration of solid formulations.

The initial approach should be to first identify which formulation properties are critical for its *in vivo* function. Thereafter, all potential physiological factors that may influence this function should be identified and the correlation between the animal and man regarding those factors should be considered. For example, in the case of a pH-dependent enteric-coat formulation, the dissolution of the coating layer will clearly be a critical formulation variable. The pH in the stomach and small intestine, as well as gastric emptying, will all be critical variables. If the correlation of such parameters with man is poor for all available animal models, there is no rationale for performing such studies if the deviations cannot be accounted for when interpreting the results.

Physiological and anatomical characteristics for different species are summarised in Table 7.7 (Dressman and Yamada 1991). Some additional information of relevance for the use of animal models in formulation studies can be found in other review articles (Kararli 1995; Ritschel 1987).

The most frequently used animal is the dog, which can in many cases be an acceptable model due to its similarity to man regarding anatomy, motility pattern, GI residence times and many secretory components. However, cases exist where favourable results in dogs have not been verified in subsequent human studies. Examples of differences that could lead to pitfalls in formulation development studies are:

- No basal acid secretion in the stomach during fasted state, and thereby often close to neutral pH in contrast to the acidic human pH. However, an acidic pH may be induced in some individuals without intake of food. This has to be specially considered, for example, when drug solubility is pH dependent and for enteric-coated formulations, for which drug release is dependent on the pH in the GI tract.

- The dog has a higher bile salt concentration than man, which could potentially lead to too favourable conditions for dissolution of very low water soluble drugs.

- Fed state could be introduced by coprophagy, which may lead to the tablets and capsules being retained in the stomach for a long time.

- The residence time in the colon is much shorter than in man, making the dog a poor model for long-acting ER formulations, due to the risk of incomplete drug release before the formulation is expelled from the body.

- The microbiological activity in the distal parts of the intestine is much less than in man, which has implications for drugs or excipients that are metabolised by gut flora enzymes, or drug release principles, based on this process.

Table 7.7
Comparison of anatomical and physiological data for the cecum and colon of humans, dogs, swine, and rhesus monkeys (Dressman and Yamada 1991).

Parameter	Human	Dog	Swine	Monkey
Length (autopsy) (m)	7	4	15–20	5 cm (duod.)
(*in vivo*) (m)	3	1.5		
Duodenal diameter (cm)	3–4	2–2.5	2.5–3.5	1.5–2
Villi: length	0.5–1.5		0.5–1	
shape	Filamentous	Long, slender		Ridges, leaflike
Peyer's patches: location	Ileum	Duodenum, jejunum, ileum	Jejunum, ileum, colon	Ileum
Secretions				
Bile: major acid	Cholic	Cholic	Hyocholic	
conc. by gallbladder	×5	×8–10	×2	
flow rate (L/day)	0.8–1	0.1–0.4		
Pancreatic juice flow rate (mL/min)	1	2–3	1	
Intestinal pH: fasted	6.1 [5.6–6.4][a]	6.5–7.5	7.2 (duodenum)	7–9; 5.5–6.0
fed	5.4 [5.0–5.8][a]	6.5–6.9		
Cecum:				
length (cm)	7	12–15	20–30	5–6
diameter (cm)	6		8–10	
volume (L)	about 1	0.25	1.5–2.2	
Colon:				
length, overall (m)	0.9–1.5	0.6–0.75	4–4.5	0.4–0–5
length, asc. colon (cm)	20		Long, coiled	10
diameter (cm)	6	Similar to SI	8–10	
haustrae	Present	Absent	Present	Present
Microbial metabolism, colon	Volatile fatty acids Vitamins	Very minor	Volatile fatty acids Vitamins	
pH, colon	6 (upper)			
	7.5 (lower)			

[a] Lower duodenum

Reprinted from Animal models for oral drug absorption, by J. B. Dressman and K. Yamada in *Pharmaceutical Bioequivalence*, edited by P. G. Welling, F. L. S. Tse, and S. V. Dighe, pp. 235–266 by courtesy of Marcel Dekker, Inc.

Study Design Aspects in Bioavailability Studies

Most investigations in animals aimed at evaluating new formulations are bioavailability studies, i.e., the rate and extent of dissolution/release is determined from plasma concentration–time data. There may be differences in drug absorption, first-pass metabolism, distribution and elimination between animals and man, which will lead to different plasma concentration–time profiles. However, this is a minor problem in the evaluation of dosage forms, provided that an oral drug solution is included in the study as a reference. Thereby, it is possible to eliminate the influence of pharmacokinetic factors other than those purely related to the formulation function. The same methods and assumptions should be applied as described in the section "Bioavailability Studies".

In most animal studies, the dose is given as the amount of drug in relation to body weight. In an evaluation of dosage form, it is preferable to administer the doses intended for humans in order to avoid development of specific low-dose formulations for animal studies. Two prerequisites of specific significance for the usefulness of this approach are (a) no toxicological effects at the given dose and (b) no saturation of any process involved in the drug absorption.

In the *administration of* solid *dosage forms* to dogs, the formulation is placed into the posterior pharynx followed by closing the dog's mouth. A feeding tube is subsequently inserted into the trachea, and 50 to 75 mL of water is administered. Liquid formulations are administered directly through a feeding tube. For administration to pigs or monkeys, applicators are often used to insert the dosage form. Small solid formulations (<5 mm) may also be administered to rats in this manner.

Many animals, including dogs, rats, rabbits and monkeys eat excrement, which is called *coprophagy*. This could alter the physiological conditions in the GI tract, such as fasting/fed motility, secretions and microflora, and thereby lead to an uncontrolled study situation. Furthermore, drug or metabolites that have been excreted by faeces could be re-absorbed, which will obscure interpretation of bioavailability data. Coprophagy has thus to be prevented by using cages with bottom screens and by placing plastic collars around the animals neck, preventing the animal from reaching its anus.

Additional information on design of bioavailability studies in animals can be found in Ritschel (1987).

IMAGING STUDIES

Non-invasive imaging can be used to study the dosage form after administration in man or animals. The amount of radioactivity administered in such studies is at such a low level that no known hazards exist for study subjects. Several factors of relevance for the function of the formulation can thus be monitored directly *in vivo*. Potential study variables are given below:

- Residence time in different parts of the GI tract

- Location of a formulation within the GI tract at a certain time point

- Transit/emptying times in the GI tract

- Distribution of multiple units or liquid vehicles in the GI tract

- "Pharmacoscintigraphy"—relation of drug plasma concentrations to location of dosage form

- Disintegration/erosion of solid formulations

- Release of a marker substance from the formulation

More detailed overviews of different applications of imaging in *in vivo* studies of formulations can be found in Wilding et al. (1991) and in Digenis et al. (1998a, b).

The imaging data can be used either as the main study variable, for example, in case of regional GI treatments, or to provide complementary information to bioavailability data. In the latter case, the information obtained regarding the location and performance of the formulation provides information that could often be crucial for correct interpretation of the bioavailability data, especially in the case of modified release formulations. Data obtained from imaging studies are generally not required by regulatory agencies, but they may well be used as supportive information in an NDA file.

Gamma scintigraphy has been established as the method of choice for *in vivo* imaging studies of formulations. Other methods such as positron emission tomography (PET), magnetic resonance imaging (MRI), ultrasound and X ray have a much more limited applicability. In gamma scintigraphy, the formulation is visualised by gamma radiation emitted from trace amounts of one or two radionuclides that have to be included in the dosage form. These types of studies in humans or animals are often performed at specialised Contract Research Organisations or at university hospitals. They involve several disciplines, besides traditional biopharmaceutical and pharmaceutical competence, such as radiochemical, nuclear medicinal or other imaging expertise. However, it is crucial that the pharmaceutical/biopharmaceutical scientist, who understands the critical manufacturing variables and the biopharmaceutical function of a dosage form, cooperates with the radiation and imaging expertise in the design and evaluation of such studies. Furthermore, manufacturing and *in vitro* testing of labelled formulations may often be an in-house activity at the company developing the formulation of interest. The present chapter will include an introduction of the basic principles of gamma scintigraphy, different aspects of labelling of formulations and performance of *in vivo* studies.

Basic Principles of Gamma Scintigraphy

The physical principles of gamma scintigraphy are based on the fact that a radionuclide emits electromagnetic gamma rays at decay to stable isotopes. The decay of a radionuclide is logarithmic, and the half-life $(t_{1/2})$ is a key characteristic determined by the following equation:

$$A_t = A_0 e^{-kt} \tag{28}$$

where At and A_0 are the radioactivity at time zero and after t time units after time zero, respectively, k is a first-order decay constant, expressed in the same time unit as t. The decay half-life equals $\ln 2 / k$. The amount of radioactivity is expressed in Bequerel (Bq), which corresponds to decay/second or Curie (Ci), where $1 \text{ Ci} = 3.7 \times 10^{10}$ Bq. The gamma rays travel at the speed of light and permeate effectively through the formulation, body tissue and air, although some energy is lost when the photon hits atoms. Such attenuation of the gamma radiation follows the following equation:

$$I_l = I_0 \times e^{-\mu l} \tag{29}$$

where I_l is the intensity of the radiation after travelling the length l through a material with an attenuation coefficient μ, and I_0 is the intensity of the radiation before it hits the material. Typical lengths (l) in water and lead, which reduce the intensity to half of its initial value $(I_0/2)$ for radionuclides used in formulation studies, are about 0.5 m and 1 mm, respectively.

A schematic picture of a gamma camera is shown in Figure 7.12. The radiation enters the gamma camera through a collimator, which is a lead shield with many small holes. The purpose of the collimator is to limit the field of view and thereby prevent radiation from non-target areas, such as naturally existing background radiation, from reaching the detectors. When the gamma ray has passed the collimator, it hits an NaI(Tl) crystal and a light impulse is created. An array of photomultipliers is used to determine the position of the light. The signal is then digitalised, and a picture can be produced, or other quantifications can be performed with computer programs. Two radionuclides can be monitored simultaneously if they produce different peak photon energies. This makes it possible to concomitantly administer two formulations with different labellings for head-to-head comparisons under identical conditions. Primarily, an image is obtained which consists of a two-dimensional matrix of, for example, 64×64 units called pixels. The radioactivity gathered during the sampling period within each pixel will provide different colours on an image where most often black-blue-red-yellow-white corresponds to different intensities from very low to maximum. Examples of gamma camera images of a labelled multiple unit formulation at different times after intake are given in Figures 7.13a–c. The data behind the construction of the gamma camera image may be further analysed to obtain various quantifications, as described further below. The spatial resolution, i.e., the minimum distance between two labelled objects that can be distinguished by the camera, is dependent on the radionuclide, collimator and distance from the object to the detector. A normal value of the spatial resolution obtained in phantom studies to mimic the *in vivo* situation is about 0.5 cm.

Figure 7.12 Schematic drawing of a gamma camera.

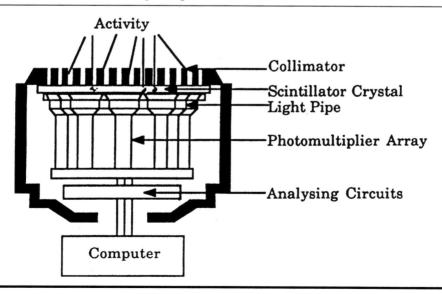

Figure 7.13 Example of a series of gamma camera images of pellet formulation obtained at 0.5 h (a), 10 h (b) and 24 h (c).

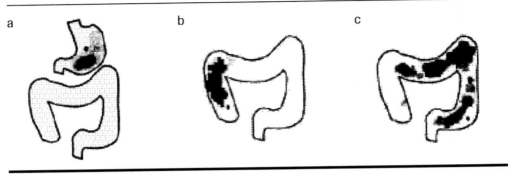

a   b   c

Labelling of Formulations

Labelling Principles

Radionuclides are generally introduced in the formulation by physical mixture rather than chemical bonding. The simplest procedure is to mix a radionuclide solution with other excipients, i.e., in a normal granulation step, thereby getting an even distribution of the marker in the formulation. A formulation, or one of its intermediate states, could also be soaked in a solution of the radionuclide. Other methods are including the radiomarker as discrete particles formed by binding to a resin, precipitation as a poorly soluble salt or oxide, coating with non-dissolving material or polymeric material, or by combinations thereof. Such particulate marker material could be included at well-defined positions within the formulation, or by random distribution of a multitude of particles. A formulation may include two radionuclides with different energies in order to follow more than one process at the same time.

The two main aspects in the radiolabelling of a formulation that will guide the choice of labelling principle are (a) that the labelling should provide an unbiased estimate of the decided imaging study variables and (b) that the function of the dosage form is unaltered. For example, if the purpose is to study the location of a solid dosage form at various times in the GI tract, it is critical that the marker is not released from the formulation. In addition, if the formulation is of a disintegrating type, it should be possible to conclude when this has happened to avoid the location of a free marker being interpreted as the position of the formulation. If the aim is to study drug release from the formulation, the radionuclide should be released from the formulation at a rate that corresponds to the drug of interest. The greatest risk for altered formulation performance by the labelling is if "micro-scale" manufacturing equipment has to be used or if other non-standard manufacturing conditions exist in order to minimise radioactive exposure to laboratory personnel.

In Vitro Evaluation

Before performing an *in vivo* study, *in vitro* testing must be used to see if the intended function of the radiolabelling has been met and that the properties of the formulation are unaffected by the labelling. In these tests, the amount of radionuclide released from the formulation should be determined at physiologically relevant conditions. The amount of released radionuclide could be determined by liquid scintigraphy for assessment of radionuclide in solution and/or by assessing the remaining radioactivity in the solid dosage form by an ionic chamber detector.

Choice of Type and Amount of Radionuclide

Several radionuclides are suitable for use in imaging studies of formulations as outlined in Table 7.8. In the choice of radionuclide, the following aspects should be considered:

- Half-life of radionuclide

    - duration of gamma measurements

    - time needed for manufacturing and QC in advance of study start

- Energy of radionuclide

    - sensitivity of gamma camera crystal to detect radiation

    - combination of two radionuclides with different energies for simultaneous measurements

- Suitability of physicochemical properties of available chemical forms of the radionuclide

    - provide unbiased estimates of desired imaging variables

    - no systemic absorption

Most radionuclides are available as complexes (e. g., ^{99m}Tc-diethylenetriaminepentaacetic acid [DTPA]), or as oxides. The chemical and physicochemical state of the radionuclide should not be altered by either the formulation excipients and/or the physiological conditions in the

Table 7.8
Radionuclides suitable for labelling of formulations, including
decay half-life ($t_{1/2}$) and peak photon energy.

Radionuclide		$t_{1/2}$	Energy (keV)	Comments
Technetium	^{99m}Tc	6.0 h	140	
Indium	^{111}In	2.8 days	173–247	
Iodine	^{131}I	8 days	364	
Chromium	^{51}Cr	28 days	320	
Samarium	^{153}Sm	46.7 h	69–103	Obtained by neutron activation
Erbium	^{170}Er	7.5 h	112–308	"
Ytterbium	^{175}Yb	4.2 days	114–396	"
Barium	^{138}Ba	84 min	166	"

GI tract. Such effects could lead to the radionuclide disappearing from the formulation in an unintended manner, thereby obscuring data evaluation. The amount of radioactivity included in a formulation is determined by the precision and variability that is required in the gamma scintigraphic measurements and by the acceptable level of radiation exposure to study subjects.

Safety Aspects in Manufacturing and Analysis of Radiolabelled Formulations

Radiation exposure is one of the most well-studied hazards to human health, but it has not been possible to link any increased incidence of impaired health at the levels of exposure that are allowed for laboratory personnel. However, higher radiation exposure is harmful, which has several important implications. First, key prerequisites are that personnel involved in the handling of radioactive material are properly educated in how to avoid unnecessary exposure to people and the environment, that appropriate protective and dosimetry devices are used and that a plan is implemented for the handling and disposal of material. Second, it is usually not possible to use normal laboratory or pilot plant-scale equipment, since such batch sizes will require the handling of excessive amounts of radioactivity. Therefore, "micro-scale" equipment may be developed for certain processes.

Neutron Activation

Neutron activation is an elegant way to avoid restrictions and hurdles introduced by the handling of radioactive material in the manufacturing of formulations. Especially favourable is the possibility to use standard equipment and operation conditions. In this procedure, small amounts of a stable isotope, typically a few milligrams, are included in the formulation. The labelled formulation is subsequently exposed to a neutron flux, and the stable isotope is thereby transformed to a radioactive isotope upon capture of a neutron. The most commonly used isotopes for this purpose are listed in Table 7.8. Several of the listed radionuclides are available in both enriched and natural forms; the use of the former, however, requires a less stable isotope to be included and/or less neutron radiation, at the disadvantage of higher costs. The main potential problem connected with neutron activation of dosage forms is the risk of affecting tablet function or causing degradation of the active compound as well as of excipients. Therefore, this has to be checked on a case-by-case basis before the start of in an *in vivo* study. Another potential problem is the creation of radionuclides, other than the intended one, which will obscure data interpretation and increase radiation exposure. If the undesirable isotopes have a significantly shorter half-life than the labelling isotope, this problem can be handled by waiting for a suitable time period such that the activity of the unintended isotope has declined, whereas significant activity remains for the desired radionuclide. One example of a common stable isotope that unintentionally can form radionuclides by neutron flux is sodium (^{24}Na, $t_{1/2} = 15$ h).

Reviews of different applications of neutron activation in studies of dosage forms can be found in Digenis and Sandefer (1991).

Conduct of In Vivo Studies

Practical Procedures

The subject is positioned in front of a gamma camera, or between two cameras, one in front of the subject and one behind (see Figure 7.14). The latter principle is needed when making quantifications of radioactivity at different positions in the GI tract in order to avoid influence

Figure 7.14 A gamma camera investigation with two opposite cameras.

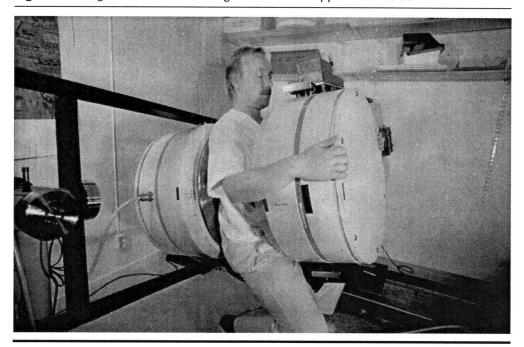

of the position-dependent attenuation of gamma radiation, whereas a one camera system is generally sufficient for locating single units. Systems with cameras that circulate around the subject for creation of three-dimensional images are also available, but their use in formulation studies in man are restricted by the higher amounts of radioactivity needed in the formulation to obtain reliable data. The field of vision usually covers the entire GI tract in most subjects, but sometimes the position of the camera has to be adjusted to cover the lower parts of the abdomen.

The data collection can be dynamic, i.e., the subject is constantly located in front of the gamma camera system, and signals are constantly gathered into images within very short time frames (often <1 min). This procedure may be advantageous to follow very rapid processes. In most cases, radiation is gathered over a finite time period to generate pictures. The time period for collecting radiation to one picture, typically 30 sec to 1 min, is mainly determined by quality requirements on picture/variability in quantitative data and the risk of moving artefacts.

Data Evaluation

It is almost always of interest to determine the localisation, emptying times from one segment to another or transit times through a segment of the formulation in the GI tract. An example of the gastric emptying and colon transit time of a non-disintegrating tablet and small pellets after administration with a breakfast are given in Figures 7.15 a,b. Normally, it is possible to identify the stomach, terminal ileum, caecum, ascending/transversal/descending/sigmoidal

Figure 7.15 Gastric emptying time after administration with breakfast (a) and colon residence time (b) for a non-disintegrating tablet and pellet formulation in eight individual subjects (Abrahamsson et al. 1996).

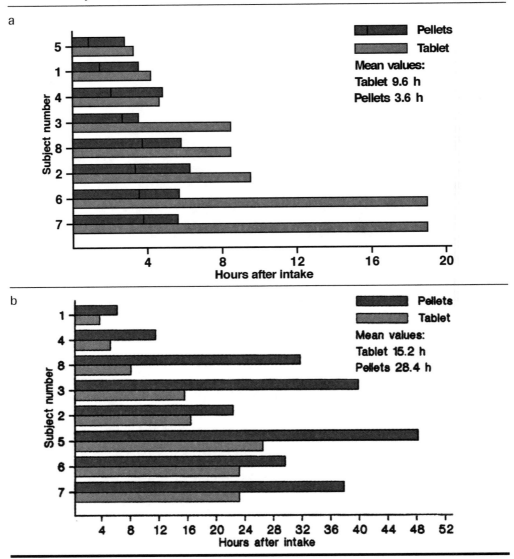

colon or rectum. In contrast to other parts of the GI tract, it is more difficult to obtain a precise position in the small intestine due to the anatomy.

The location of a single unit in the GI tract is determined from the position of the gamma camera image. Since no image of the GI anatomy is obtainable, an external radioactive marker may be positioned at a well-defined anatomical position as a reference point in the determination of the radiolabelled formulation. Another approach for facilitating determination of position is to administer a radiolabelled reference solution, which will provide images of certain intestinal parts, such as the stomach. In the case of solid multiple particles, or liquid formulations, the emptying, transit or arrival time is a continuous process over a certain time interval. This is exemplified in Figure 7.16, which shows the amount of food and a floating antacid remaining in the stomach at different times. The emptying or arrival processes from, or to, a certain region are determined by defining a region encompassing the area of interest. The number of counts obtained within this region is determined at several time points after correction for background radiation. The number of counts is often expressed as a percentage, defining the value obtained in the stomach immediately after administration as 100 percent. A rate constant, for example, the gastric emptying time, can then be determined from the emptying-time profile by applying moment analysis (see the section "*In Vitro* Dissolution"), a model containing a rate constant or by just determining the time point when 50 percent has been emptied, based on the type of data presented in Figure 7.16. The gastric emptying of solids and liquids is often approximated by zero- and first-order kinetics, respectively, although individual data, especially for particles, often shows more discontinuous profiles. The transit times through a segment are determined as the difference between the arrival time to the subsequent compartment and the emptying from the preceding region. For example, the small intestinal transit time is determined from the difference between the colon arrival and the gastric emptying times.

In quantification of the amount of radionuclide remaining in a formulation, for the monitoring of a release process, a region of interest is defined around the formulation, and a quantification of the number of counts within this region is determined at different times after correction for background radiation. Since the formulation may be positioned at different depths in the body at different times, which will affect the number of counts, obtaining simultaneous measurements by a posterior and anterior camera is necessary to avoid artefacts. The geometric mean of the number of counts obtained by the two cameras is used as the characteristic of the release process. The data may be expressed in a percentage, where the number of counts obtained within the formulation immediately after intake is defined as 100 percent. It is important to have frequent data sampling, since a certain number of images have to be discarded due to formulation movements during data collection or other anomalies and arte-

Figure 7.16 The gastric emptying of a meal and a floating antacid formulation after concomitant administration.

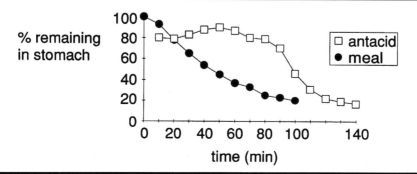

Figure 7.17 Tablet erosion (circles) and cumulative drug absorption (diamonds) for a hydrophilic matrix ER tablet after administration under fasting (a) and non-fasting (b) conditions in one subject. The two dashed vertical lines represent gastric emptying and colon arrival, respectively. The figures illustrate the correspondence between tablet erosion and drug absorption. In addition, the figures also show that the more rapid absorption after intake with food is caused by an increased erosion rate (Abrahamsson 1998b).

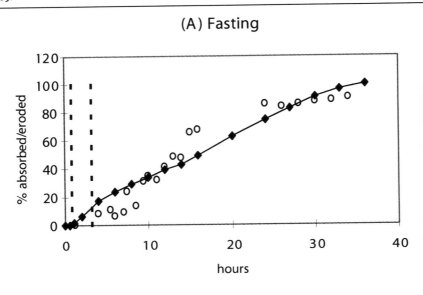

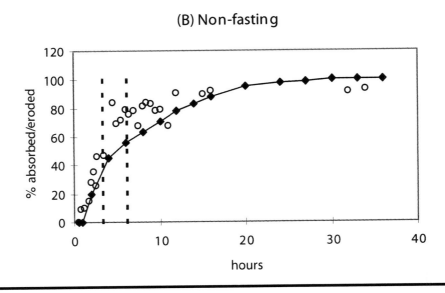

facts. A special problem in data evaluation could occur if release of radiolabelled material gather together with the remaining formulation, which, for example, may happen in the terminal ileum due to normal physiological function.

An example of determination of tablet erosion of a hydrophilic ER matrix tablet is given in Figures 7.17 a, b, where determinations were made after administration under fasting and non-fasting conditions. The scintigraphic erosion data revealed the underlying reason for an increase of the drug absorption rate obtained after non-fasting compared to fasting administration.

REFERENCES

Abrahamsson, B., D. Johanson, A. Torstensson, and K. Wingstrand. 1994. Evaluation of solubilizers in the drug release testing of hydrophilic matrix extended-release tablets of felodipine. *Pharm Res.* 11:1093–1097.

Abrahamsson, B., M. Alpsten, U. E. Jonsson, P. J. Lundberg, M. Sandberg, M. Sundgren, A., Svenheden, and J. Tölli, 1996. Gastro-intestinal transit of a multiple-unit formulation (metoprolol CR/ZOK) and a non-disintegrating tablet with the emphasis on colon. *Int. J. Pharm.* 140:229–235.

Abrahamsson, B., M. Alpsten, B. Bake, A. Larsson, and J. Sjögren, J. 1998a. *In vitro* and *in vivo* erosion of two different hydrophilic gel matrix tablets. *Eur. J. Pharm. Biopharm.* 46:69–75.

Abrahamsson, B., M. Alpsten, B. Bake, U. E. Jonsson, M. Lepkowska-Eriksson, and A. Larsson. (1998b). Drug absorption from nifedipine hydrophilic matrix extended-release (ER) tablet—Comparison with an osmotic pump tablet and effect of food. *J. Controlled Release* 52:301–310.

Abuzarur-Aloul, K., K. Gjellan, M. Sjölund, M. Löfqvist, and C. Graffner. 1997. Critical dissolution test of oral system based on statistically designed experiments. I. Screening of critical fluids and *in vitro/in vivo* modelling of extended release coated spheres. *Drug Dev. Indust. Pharm.* 23:749–760.

Box, G. E. P., W. G. Hunter, and J. S. Hunter. 1978. *Statistics for experimenters.* New York: Wiley, pp. 291–432.

Brockmeier, D. 1986. *In vitro/in vivo* correlation of dissolution using moments of dissolution and transit times. *Acta Pharm. Technol.* 32:164–174.

Crison, J. R., N. D. Weiner, and G. L. Amidon. 1997. Dissolution media for *in vitro* testing of water-insoluble drugs: Effect of surfactant purity and electrolyte on *in vitro* dissolution of carbamazepine in aqueous solutions of sodium lauryl sulfate, *J. Pharm. Sci.* 86:384–388.

Diebold, S. M., and J. B. Dressman. 1998. Dissolved oxygen as a measure for de- and re-aeration of aqueous media for dissolution testing. *Dissolution Technol.* 5:13–16.

Digenis, G. A., and E. Sandefer. 1991. Gamma scintigraphy and neutron activation techniques in the *in vivo* assessment of orally administered dosage forms. *Crit. Rev. Therapeu. Drug Carrier Systems* 7:309–345.

Digenis, G. A., T. B. Gold, and V. P. Shah. 1994. Cross-linking of gelatin capsules and its relevance to their *in vitro-in vivo* performance. *J. Pharm. Sci.* 83:915–921.

Digenis, G. A., E. P. Sandefer, R. C. Page, and W. J. Doll. 1998a. Gamma scintigraphy: An evolving technology in pharmaceutical formulations development—Part 1. *Pharm. Sci. Technol. Today* 1:100–107.

Digenis, G. A., E. P. Sandefer, R. C. Page, and W. J. Doll. 1998b. Gamma scintigraphy: An evolving technology in pharmaceutical formulations development—Part 2. *Pharm. Sci. Technol. Today* 1:160–165.

Dressman, J. B., and K. Yamada. 1991. Animal models for oral drug absorption. In *Pharmaceutical Bioequivalence*, edited by P. G. Welling, F. L. S. Tse, and S. V. Dighe. New York: Marcel Dekker, pp. 235–266.

Dressman, J. B., G. L. Amidon, C. Reppas, and V. P. Shah. 1998. Dissoluting testing as a prognostic tool for oral drug absorption: Immediate release dosage forms. *Pharm. Res.* 15:11–22.

El-Arini, S. K., G. K. Shiu, and J. P. Skelly. 1990. Theophylline-controlled release preparations and fatty food: An *in vitro* study using the rotating dialysis cell method. *Pharm. Res.* 7:1134–1140.

EMEA. 1998. *Note for guidance on the investigation of bioavailability and bioequivalence.* London: European Agency for the Evaluation of Medicinal Products.

EMEA. 1999. *Note for guidance on quality of modified release products A: Oral dosage forms. B: Transdermal dosage forms Section 1 (Quality).* London: European Agency for the Evaluation of Medicinal Products.

FDA. 1997a. *Guidance for industry—Extended release oral dosage forms: Development, evaluation, and application of In vitro/in vivo correlations.* Rockville, Md., USA: Food and Drug Administration.

FDA. 1997b. *Guidance for industry—Dissolution testing of immediate solid oral release dosage forms.* Rockville, Md., USA: Food and Drug Administration.

FDA. 1997c. *Guidance for industry—Food-effect bioavailability and bioequivalence studies.* Rockville, Md., USA: Food and Drug Administration.

FDA. 2000. *Guidance for industry—BA and BE studies of orally administered drug products—General considerations.* Rockville, Md., USA: Food and Drug Administration.

FIP. 1997. Guidelines for dissolution testing of solid oral products. *Dissolution Technol.* 4:5–14.

Gabrielsson, J., and D. Weiner. 1997. *Pharmacokinetic/pharmacodynamic data analysis: Concepts and applications.* Stockholm, Sweden: Swedish Pharmaceutical Press.

Gottfries, J., J. Ahlbom, V. Harang, E. Johansson, M. Josefson, T. Morsing, A. Pettersson, and A. Torstenson. 1994. Validation of an extended release tablet dissolution testing system using design and multivariate analysis. *Int. J. Pharm.* 106:141–148.

Hansson, A. 1991. *Handbook of dissolution testing.* Springfield, Ore. USA: Aster Publishing Corp.

Hauschke, D., M. Kieser, E. Diletti, and M. Burke. 1999. Sample size determination for proving equivalence based on the ratio of two means for normally distributed data. *Statistics Med.* 18:93–105.

Johansson, D., and B. Abrahamsson. 1997. *In vivo* evaluation of two different dissolution enhancement principles for a sparingly soluble drug administered as extended release (ER) tablet. *Proceedings of the International Symposium on Controlled Release of Bioactive Materials*, Controlled Release Society, 24:363–364.

Kararli, T. T. 1995. Comparison of the gastrointestinal anatomy, physiology, and biochemistry of humans and commonly used laboratory animals. *Biopharm. and Drug Disposition* 16:351–380.

Koch, H. P. 1980. The Resotest apparatus. A universally applicable biopharmaceutical experimental tool. *Meth Find Exp. and Clin. Pharmacol.* 2:97–102.

Langenbucher, F. 1976. Parametric representation of dissolution-rate curves by the RRSBW distribution. *Pharm. Ind.* 38:472–477.

Langenbucher, F. 1982. Numerical convolution/deconvolution as a tool for correlating *in vitro* with *in vivo* drug availability. *Pharm Ind.* 44:1166–1172

Lindstedt, B., G. Ragnarsson, and J. Hjärtstam. 1989. Osmotic pumping as a release mechanism for membrane-coated drug formulations. *Int. J. Pharm.* 56:261–268.

Loo, J. C., and S. Riegelman. 1968. New method for calculating the intrinsic absorption rate of drugs. *J. Pharm. Sci.* 57:918–928.

Riegelman, S., and P. Collier. 1980. The application of statistical moment theory to the evaluation of *in vivo* dissolution time and absorption time. *J. Pharmacokinet. Biopharm.*8:509–530.

Ritschel, W. A. 1987. *In vivo* animal models for bioavailability assessment. *S.T.P. Pharma.* 3:125–141.

Rowland, M., and T. N. Tozer. 1995. *Clinical pharmacokinetics—Concepts and applications.* Philadelphia: Williams & Wilkins.

Shah, V. P., J. J. Konecny, R. L. Everett, B. McCullough, A. C. Noorizaden, and J. P. Skelly. 1989. *In vitro* dissolution profile of water insoluble drug dosage forms in the presence of solubilizers. *Pharm. Res.* 6:162–168.

Shah, V. P., Y. Tsong, P. Sathe, and J. P. Liu. 1998. *In vitro* dissolution profile comparison—Statistics and analysis of the similarity factor, f_2. *Pharm. Res.* 15:889–896.

Tucker, G. T. 1983. The determination of *in vivo* drug absorption rate. *Acta Pharmaceu. Technol.* 29:159–164.

USP. 2000. *U.S. Pharmacopeia XXIV.* Rockville, Md., USA: United States Pharmacopeial Convention, Inc.

Vaughan, P., and M. Dennis. 1978. Mathematical basis of point-area deconvolution method for determining *in vivo* input function. *J. Pharm. Sci.* 67:663–665.

von Hattingberg, H. M. 1984. Moment analysis *in vitro* and *in vivo*. *Meth. Find. Exp. Clin. Pharmacol.* 6:589–595.

Wagner, J. G., and E. Nelson. 1963. Per cent absorbed time plots derived from blood level and/or urinary excretion data. *J. Pharm. Sci.* 52:610–611.

Wilding, I. R., A. J. Coupe, and S. S. Davis. 1991. The role of gamma-scintigraphy in oral drug delivery. *Adv. Drug Delivery Rev.* 7:87–117.

Young, D, J. G. Devane, and J. Butler. 1997. *In vitro–in vivo correlations.* New York, London: Plenum Press.

Part III

FROM PRODUCT DESIGN TO COMMERCIAL DOSAGE FORM

8

PRODUCT OPTIMISATION

Mark Gibson

AstraZeneca R&D Charnwood
Loughborough, United Kingdom

PRODUCT OPTIMISATION PURPOSE AND SCOPE

The major objective of the product optimisation stage is to ensure that the product selected for further development (the intended commercial product) is fully optimised and complies with the design specification and critical quality parameters described in the Product Design Report (refer to Chapter 5). The key outputs from this stage of development will be

- a quantitative formula defining the grades and quantities of each excipient and the quantity of candidate drug;

- defined pack;

- defined drug, excipient and component specifications; and

- defined product specifications.

The approach to product optimisation will depend on the nature of the product to be developed. It will always involve testing a range of options, for example: a variety of excipients from different sources, with different grades and concentrations, and in different combinations, or a range of pack sizes or different packaging materials. Additionally, it could involve testing a range of particle size distributions of the candidate drug or of the excipients. Particle size may be critical for drug delivery or formulation processing. For example, material with a mean particle size distribution of 2–5 μm will be required for effective pulmonary delivery of aerosol suspensions and dry powders, whereas an even smaller particle size range (nanoparticles) may be required for the dissolution of poorly water soluble drugs in parenteral formulations.

At the early stages of optimisation, preformulation studies are usually conducted to screen excipients or packaging materials and to select those compatible with the candidate drug, using accelerated stress testing procedures. More details about the preformulation techniques, which can be employed for compatibility studies, are discussed in Chapter 3. The importance of doing compatibility studies is for reducing the number of excipients and formulation options to test in further product optimisation studies.

The final stage of optimisation will normally involve generating sufficient stability data on one or more variants to select the best variant. The optimal product will usually be selected based on technical merit. However, there may be a need to consider other factors, such as the use of novel excipients and the associated safety/toxicological implications, supplier and sourcing issues or the ability to patent the formulation or not. Some of these issues are discussed further below.

The manufacturing process used during product optimisation should be designed with large-scale manufacture in mind. Ideally, the process should be as representative as possible to the eventual commercial-scale manufacture. This is because the manufacturing process may affect product performance characteristics, and could influence the results of clinical studies. Although product and process design and optimisation have been depicted as separate stages in the development framework, in practice, they are often combined or closely linked. For example, it is important in pack optimisation to select a pack which is suitable for use in production and will satisfy the demands of a high-speed automated filling line. Alternatively, the pack may have to be able to withstand stresses during processing which could involve extremes of temperature or pressure, during autoclaving or freeze-drying, for example. Process design and process optimisation considerations are discussed later in this chapter.

At the completion of product optimisation, when the best product variant has been selected, it is a good idea to summarise the work conducted in a Product Optimisation Report. The report should reference the primary data from preformulation, product optimisation and stability studies, cross-referencing other investigational reports where necessary. It should clearly justify the recommendations for the quantitative formula and the excipient, component and product specifications. Such a document can be very useful to aid smooth technology transfer into production and for writing regulatory submissions.

EXCIPIENT AND PACK OPTIMISATION CONSIDERATIONS

Excipient Selection

Historically, pharmaceutical excipients have been regarded as inert additives, but this is no longer the case. Each additive must have a clear justification for inclusion in the formulation and must perform a defined function in the presence of the active and any other excipients included in the formulation. Excipients are included for all sorts of reasons. They may function, for example, as an antimicrobial preservative, a solubility enhancer, a stability enhancer or a taste masker, to name a few.

The International Pharmaceutical Excipients Council (IPEC) have defined a pharmaceutical excipient as

> any substance other than the active drug or prodrug which has been appropriately evaluated for safety and is included in a drug delivery system to either:

1. aid processing of the system during manufacture, or

2. protect, support or enhance stability, bioavailability or patient acceptability, or

3. assist in product identification, or

4. enhance any other attribute of the overall safety and effectiveness of the drug product during storage or use.

In the 1960s, excipients were commodity items and tended to be of natural origin, but today many are synthetic or have been physically modified. Performance testing was done by the user, not the supplier. This has now changed with the introduction of recognised quality and performance standards for raw materials, which are defined in various pharmacopoeias (Moreton 1999). The rationale for these changes is linked to the requirement to ensure that the patient is provided with the correct dose as safely and consistently as possible. This can only be achieved if the raw materials are of a consistent standard, together with the active and consistent processing.

Unfortunately, the standards for the same raw material can vary in different pharmacopoeias, and so the choice of pharmacopoeia will depend on the intended market for the product (see later comments about harmonisation of standards). Suppliers should provide materials that comply with the specified pharmacopoeial standards. Monographs for excipients provide minimum tests and specifications, which can save time and resource negotiating new specifications with the regulatory authorities. Even so, the user may have to do additional tests to show that the excipient is suitable for use in a particular product or drug delivery system.

The basic selection and acceptance criteria for excipients to be used in a product being developed should have been defined in the Product Design Report section on "Design Specifications and Critical Quality Parameters". In practice, each excipient must be shown to be compatible with the formulation and pack and effectively perform its desired function in the product. At the same time, the product design acceptance criteria should be complied with, such as the following: the excipient should be well established, and its intended route of administration should be safe and acceptable to the regulatory authorities; the excipient should comply with pharmacopoeial requirements, be globally acceptable and meet the proposed design specification.

The case for using well-established excipients (and packs) that have already been administered to humans by the intended route, and in similar dosage forms, has been emphasised previously in the section on "Safety Assessment Considerations" in Chapter 5. New chemical excipients (i.e., that have not been used in registered pharmaceutical products before) usually require a full development programme, including comprehensive toxicological testing, to gain "approval" by the regulatory authorities.

There are clearly cost and time savings of using well-established excipients that have already been approved for use in other registered products and that have an established safety profile. The regulatory status of excipients can easily be checked by consulting the FDA's (U.S. Food and Drug Administration) Inactive Ingredient Guide, the Japanese Pharmaceutical Excipients Directory or other similar sources of information (see Table 8.1). These sources should provide information about registered products already approved, which contain a particular excipient with quantities used, or a list of all products by dosage form that have contained a particular excipient.

Excipients are normally considered to be acceptable if they are listed in the major pharmacopoeias from the United States, Europe and Japan. There has been much progress in harmonising the monographs for key excipients in these pharmacopoeias. For products being

Table 8.1
Sources of information for excipients and packaging materials.

Source	Information	Comments
Various pharmacopoeias, e.g., United States/National Formulary; British, European, Japanese, Pharmacopoeias; Martindale, The Extra Pharmacopoeia; The Merck Index; The British Pharmaceutical Codex	Include standards and monographs for drugs, excipients, containers/closures and medical devices	Updated regularly; many available in book format or CD-ROM; can be obtained through various publishers including Interpharm
FDA Inactive Ingredient Guide	Lists excipients used in FDA-approved drug products marketed for human use by route of administration and dosage form	Published by FDA, Division of Drug Resources (DDIR); available through FDA Web site; updated regularly
Handbook of Pharmaceutical Excipients	Excipient monographs containing data on uses, properties, safety, excipient interactions, standards; also a supplier's directory	A joint publication of the American Pharmaceutical Society and the Royal Pharmaceutical Society of Great Britain
Handbook of Pharmaceutical Additives	Excipients used in prescription and OTC products approved by the FDA or recommended by USP/NF, BP and Ph.Eur.; details manufacturers, composition, properties, function and applications, toxicology and regulatory status of additives	Compiled by M. and I. Ash; Published by Gower, Aldershot, UK, and Vermont, USA
Japanese Pharmaceutical Excipients Directory	Monographs on excipients used in pharmaceutical and cosmetic products	Edited by the Japan Pharmaceutical Excipients Council; available through Interpharm
Le Dictionnaire VIDAL	A codex of French approved medicines includes quantitative composition of many products	
ABPI Compendium of Data Sheets and Summaries of Product Characteristics	Data sheets prepared by pharmaceutical companies on prescription and OTC products, including quantitative details of formulation ingredients and packaging used	Published annually by Datapharm Publications Ltd., London
Physicians' Desk Reference	Compendium of FDA approved pharmaceutical products; details formulation, pack, administration and use; identification guide	Published by Medical Economics Co., N.J., USA, in participation with individual manufacturers; also PDRs for ophthalmology and non-prescription drugs; CD-ROM or hard copy

developed for Japan, excipients must comply with the Japanese pharmacopoeia. If other pharmacopoeial grades are used, a detailed explanation of how these are equivalent or better quality is usually required. However, even if the excipient is listed in all the major pharmacopoeias, additional toxicological studies may still be required to qualify an excipient under certain circumstances, such as (1) excipients used previously in humans but not by the intended route or (2) increased concentration of an excipient above that previously used by the intended route. In either case, more extensive testing will be required so that the tests and specifications applied are shown to be capable of controlling the identity, strength, quality and purity of the excipient commensurate with its intended use. In Japan, excipients which have not been used previously in Japan will be treated as new excipients, even if they have been used in other countries.

Some assurance can be gained about the quality and safety of an excipient if a Drug Master File (DMF) is available and the DMF holder provides permission to reference it. This is a document submitted to the FDA by a vendor which provides detailed information, including toxicological data and specification tests, about a specific excipient (or packaging material, drug substance or manufacturing site). A DMF is never approved, but it will be reviewed by the FDA if it is associated with a product licence application. For more information about DMFs, refer to the FDA Guideline for Drug Master Files (September 1989).

Some food and colour additives may have (generally recognised as safe) (GRAS) status, which also gives some assurance that they could be used in pharmaceutical products with minimal additional safety testing. This is especially the case if the excipient is not likely to be absorbed systemically from the formulation.

However, there will always be situations where the introduction of a new excipient is inevitable. The candidate drug, for instance, may be incompatible with the current range of excipients. Another reason might be the phasing out of existing excipients for safety or environmental concerns, such as chlorofluorocarbons (CFCs) in metered dose aerosols. There may be a need to introduce a new excipient for a novel drug delivery system or to overcome disadvantages with the currently available materials.

A common factor which often influences the selection of excipients and excipient suppliers is a company's historical preference for certain excipients based on proven technical, commercial and quality criteria. Many pharmaceutical companies have a list of preferred suppliers that have already been audited and approved. There are significant advantages of selecting excipients that the company already uses, in terms of time and costs. Limiting the range of standard excipients on a company's inventory should minimise overhead because of the reduced auditing, analytical testing and development required. Also, a greater knowledge can be developed about the characteristics of excipients that have been extensively used. Technology transfer from research and development (R&D) to the final manufacturing site should be easier and faster if the excipients are already in the inventory, and the release specifications and analytical methods are already known to the quality control (QC) department. However, a downside to having a limited company inventory is the reduced options of excipient choice placed on the formulator when faced with a new formulation or drug delivery challenge.

For products intended for global marketing, selection of excipients that meet the regulatory requirements can often be more challenging than the technical issues. Obtaining marketing approval for a new product requires the regulatory acceptance of the new candidate drug and the excipients used in the formulation. The specifications for excipients must comply with the pharmacopoeial standard for the particular country. Unfortunately, there is a diversity of specification tests and limits for the same excipients in the different pharmacopoeias. This issue has long been recognised, and there is an ongoing programme to harmonise or unify the different requirements for some excipients in the three major pharmacopoeias, Europe, Japan and the United States. This programme is referred to as ICH, or International Conference on Harmonisation of drugs. However, the process of establishing agreed international excipient specifications has proved to be extremely slow. Inevitably, some excipients for which pharmacopoeial standards are in conflict may be discounted from consideration, even though they perform well in terms of functionality.

Another issue for global marketing is the differences of opinion about the safety of some excipients in different countries. For example, ethylenediaminetetraacetic acid (EDTA) is permitted in most countries for use in intravenous (IV) injections as a metal ion sequestering agent, but not in Japan. Colours, artificial sweeteners and bovine-derived products are other examples where safety concerns vary significantly from country to country (Tovey 1995). All dyes available for food and drug use are banned in at least one country. However, it may be essential to add a colouring agent to a product to distinguish one product from another or to differentiate between a number of product strengths.

Colouring agents may also be required for developing placebos to match coloured products for blinding in clinical trials. Nedocromil sodium nasal, ophthalmic and respiratory products are examples which all required colour matching because of the inherent yellow colour of the drug substance. This can be especially challenging when a range of drug concentrations is required, with each concentration having a different colour intensity. For the above reasons, it is not always possible to develop a single formulation for the world-wide market.

The sourcing of excipients can be another important selection and optimisation criterion. It is generally desirable to have excipient sources available in the country where product manufacture is taking place, to avoid stockpiling material to compensate for possible transport and import delays. Even better is if there are multiple sources of the same type of excipient so that if one supplier fails to deliver or discontinues delivery, an alternative can be used. This might rule out the use of some suppliers or excipients. In order to cater to different manufacturing sites in different countries which might use slightly different equipment, it is important that the product and process developed are robust enough to cater to small differences in excipient characteristics and performance from different sources.

In conclusion, during product optimisation, excipients will be selected based on a variety of acceptance criteria. The quantities included in the formulation will be finalised, based on the performance characteristics of the excipient in the final product. At this stage it is important to fix the specifications of the excipients to ensure that the materials used, and hence the product, will be consistent throughout development. Setting specifications is discussed in a following section.

Pack Selection and Optimisation Considerations

A logical approach to packaging optimisation is, first of all, to define the packaging function, followed by selection of the materials, then testing the performance of the packaging to ensure that it will meet all the product design and functional requirements that were identified in the Product Design Report.

Product optimisation of the pack should initially focus on defining the primary packaging (sometimes referred to as "primary container" or "immediate container"). This is most relevant to regulatory authorities because it is the primary packaging that is in direct contact with the drug product, including the closure, liner, and any other surface contacting the product.

The secondary packaging is that outside the primary pack, and by definition is not in direct contact with the drug product. Secondary packaging is often a carton or a blister, which may also function to protect the product from light or moisture. For example, it may be preferable to use a carton and a clear ampoule or vial, rather than an amber container for a photosensitive parenteral product, to allow users to inspect the contents of the package for contamination or signs of instability. There may be a requirement to have sterile secondary packaging, for example, for a sterile product likely to be used in an operating theatre by a surgeon. The pharmaceutical company developing such a product should identify this requirement in the product design stage to ensure that the pack and sterilisation process are considered during development. In the majority of cases, the purpose of the secondary packaging is simply to be elegant in its appearance, provide clear labelling instructions and project a good marketing image.

Important selection and optimisation criteria for the primary packaging may include the following:

- Satisfies environmental and legislative requirements for world-wide markets

- Availability of a DMF

- Ability to source from more than one supplier/country

- Acceptable cost of goods (particularly if a sophisticated device)

- Consistency of dimensions

- Consistency of pack performance

- Ability to meet function/user tests, customer requirements and specifications

For some excipients, the global acceptability of some packaging materials varies from country to country. This can often stem from environmental concerns and the negative impact from the need to dispose of packaging waste. For example, polyvinyl chloride (PVC) is used widely to manufacture bottles and blisters for pharmaceutical products, but there is a growing concern about its safe use and disposal in some countries (Hansen 1999). Incineration is the preferred method of disposal for PVC, with the downside that it emits toxic gases. Materials that are readily biodegradable, or that can be recycled, are preferred. This is not always possible with some types of synthetic materials.

Multiple sourcing of some synthetic polymeric materials may not always be possible, or desirable, because each supplier may have its own range of additives for the basic packaging material. It is therefore important that, once the packaging material has been established for a product, there is an understanding between the pharmaceutical company and the supplier not to alter the polymer formula or processing conditions without consultation. Any changes should become apparent if the supplier has filed a DMF with the regulatory authorities. Some sophisticated drug delivery systems, such as valves for metering pumps used for nasal and pulmonary delivery, can contain a multitude of components made of different materials and grades. It is important that the pharmaceutical company is made aware of any changes during development so that the implications for product performance and stability can be considered.

The role of the pack will include the following:

- Containment and protection of the product: to ensure stability over shelf-life, protection to withstand the influences of climate, distribution, warehousing and storage during use, protection for child safety.

- Presentation to the user (e.g., doctors, patients, parents): provides relevant information, identification, visually attractive appearance and assurance against tampering.

- Administration of the product: provides convenient and consistent dose delivery.

Protection of the Product

The formulation must be protected from the environmental elements of heat, light, moisture, gaseous and sometimes chemical or microbial attack, as well as physical protection during transport and handling. A product licence will not be granted unless the product quality, safety and stability of the formulation in the commercial pack of choice over the declared shelf-life has been demonstrated to the regulatory authorities. They will be looking for acceptable stability data when the product is stored under anticipated normal conditions, in addition to acceptable data from "accelerated" or stressed conditions. This might include, for example, storage of the product in different orientations or in adverse conditions of extremes of temperature and humidity. Appropriate stressed stability studies should demonstrate the integrity of the container and closure and any possible interaction between product and container. However, there is a possibility that components may be leached from packaging under accelerated/stressed conditions, which may not occur under normal conditions of use. Accelerated studies can be very useful for compatibility testing and screening materials, but they should be accompanied by long-term stability studies under normal conditions of use to confirm the suitability.

Other stress tests worth considering to establish the robustness of the product and pack include vibration and impact testing. Successful testing should instil confidence that the product can be transported and, to some extent, be physically abused (dropped) in the hands of users.

Two specific instances where the regulatory authorities will usually request extensive information are sorption of active(s) or excipient(s) from liquid and semi-solid formulations and leaching of pack components into liquid or finely divided solid preparations, over the proposed shelf-life of the product.

Plastics and rubber materials used in containers and closure systems can contain certain additives, for example, plasticisers, stabilisers, lubricants and mould-release agents. It is worth asking the material suppliers what polymer additives are involved so that these can be analysed when conducting compatibility studies. The regulatory authorities require that these additives should not be capable of extraction into the formulation or leach from the container/closure to contaminate the product. Mercaptobenzothiazole (MCBT) is a common additive to rubber compositions used in closures for multidose parenteral containers, which is extremely toxic. For synthetic polymeric materials, the leaching of additives can result in morphological changes to the packaging materials. These changes may in turn affect physical properties such as hardness, stiffness, tensile strength or viscoelasticity, which can be vital for pack performance. Leaking can be a problem because of the viscoelastic nature of some injection closure compositions. Other less obvious properties may also be affected, such as gas permeability and absorption. Permeation of gases or water vapour through the container material can affect formulation stability if the candidate drug is susceptible to hydrolysis or oxidation.

Drug and excipient interactions with the container may involve leaching, permeation, sorption, chemical reaction or modification of the physical characteristics of the polymer or the product. During product optimisation, formulation factors, such as the pH, concentration of ingredients, composition of the vehicle (solvents and surface active agents), area of contact and contact time, will need to be evaluated. Also, processing variables such as temperature might be important. There are cases where the drug may absorb into components of the pack. This can be a particular problem with protein/polypeptide drugs onto glass and plastic packaging components. The best known example of excipient adsorption or absorption is the loss of antimicrobial preservative from solutions to container/closure systems, most notably the rubber bungs of multidose injection containers, or the rubber gaskets used in metered dose nasal pumps. The effective concentration in solution can be reduced to such an extent that the product is no longer protected from microbial growth.

There is also the possibility of constituents from label adhesives migrating through polyethylene or polypropylene containers. This is something to be aware of when carrying out stressed compatibility testing and long-term stability testing.

Packaging for sterile products must be effectively contained and sealed to prevent microbial contamination, and must be robust enough to withstand any sterilisation process required. The sterilisation process can affect the leaching of components from the container into the product or affect the physical properties of the container. For example, autoclaving can soften plastic containers, and gamma irradiation can cause certain polymers to cross link.

Other protective elements have also become important in recent years, namely those of child resistance and tamper evidence. Child-resistant packaging originated in the United States in the 1970s and was then introduced into Europe, adopted mainly in the United Kingdom and Germany. There has been an ongoing debate between pharmaceutical manufacturers, container suppliers and regulatory authorities on how to ensure that there is a practical balance between child safety and the pack being sufficiently user-friendly so that the elderly and arthritic can obtain their medication. Tamper-evident containers are closed containers fitted with a device that shows irreversibly whether the container has been opened. Tamper evidence is particularly important for sterile products, and has become increasingly desirable for other products, to demonstrate that the product has not been interfered with.

The FDA has published comprehensive information on container closure systems in a guidance for industry document, "Submitting Documentation for Packaging for Human Drugs and Biologics" (February 1987), shortly to be superseded by a new draft guidance for industry, "Submission of Documentation in Drug Applications for Container and Closure Systems used for the Packaging of Human Drugs and Biologics" (July 1999).

Presentation to the User/Administration of the Product

For traditional dosage forms, such as tablets and capsules, the role of the pack is mainly for protection of the product during storage and presentation to the user. The design is not so critical for administration of the dose or performance of the product in the hands of the administrator (doctor or patient). For other dosage forms, such as inhalers for respiratory drugs and self-injection devices for parenteral products (e.g., insulin), the pack is an integral part of the drug product. These are often referred to as "drug delivery systems" because the packaging system or device in the hands of the administrator provides a means of ensuring that the correct amount of active drug product is delivered to the site of action as easily, reliably and conveniently as possible.

With metered dose inhalers (MDIs) for example, the FDA consider the drug product to be the canister, the valve, the actuator, the formulation, any associated accessories (e.g., spacers) and any protective secondary packaging. This is because the clinical efficacy of MDIs may be directly dependent on the design, reproducibility and performance characteristics of the packaging and closure system. For these types of products, and other more sophisticated drug delivery systems, it is important that these product performance aspects are addressed during the product optimisation stage. During development and before initiating critical clinical studies, the performance characteristics of the MDI (e.g., dosing and particle size distribution of the spray), in addition to the compatibility with the formulation, need to be thoroughly investigated.

When developing a product for Europe which uses both device and medicinal product components (such as metered-dose or powder-filled inhalers or prefilled syringes), the pharmaceutical company must establish whether the product will have to conform to the Essential Requirements of European legislation applied to medical devices (Medical Device Directive 93/42/EEC). If the medicinal product has a separate device element that could be refilled/reused, or the device and medicinal substance are presented separately, the device component will be subject to medical device controls, in addition to an application being made to the medicines authority (Tarabah and Taxacher 1999). To obtain a CE mark for a medical device registered in Europe, there will be implications for the pharmaceutical company (and its suppliers) to have suitable quality systems in place (e.g., EN46001). Obviously, this should be established early on in product design to enable the appropriate routes for authorisation to be obtained. Similar regulations apply for medicinal devices which will be marketed in the United States (cGMP, 21 CFR Part 820).

The packaging must also be convenient to use in order to promote good patient compliance, that is, to encourage patients to take their medication at the correct times. User acceptance of the pack and/or delivery device can lead to that product being preferred in the market place. Product optimisation studies may involve testing a range of pack options using a volunteer panel to establish the most user-friendly or patient-compliant packs that can be easily opened and closed. If a novel pack has been designed in-house by the pharmaceutical company, there is the possibility of filing a patent to gain market exclusivity for a number of years. Some examples of new innovations in pharmaceutical packaging development to improve drug delivery systems are described by Williams (1997).

SOURCES OF INFORMATION

Knowing where to find information about excipients and packaging materials, as well as development and regulatory guidelines, is critical to the preformulation and formulation scientist during the product design and optimisation stages of development. Typical information that is often required for excipients and packaging materials include the chemical composition, function, chemical and physical properties, regulatory and safety status, manufacturers and suppliers, qualitative and quantitative composition of marketed products, stability data, known incompatibilities and so on. Having this information can save much valuable time in the laboratory generating the data from scratch.

There are also a lot of guidelines and regulations from various regulatory authorities and standard organisations to be aware of that affect product development. Some of the regulatory documents are legal requirements (regulations) such as the Code of Federal Regulations (FDA), and some are regulatory requirements which are stipulated within licence applications, such as pharmacopoeial monographs. Others are guidelines which must be followed or, if not, a very strong scientific argument must be provided for justification. For example, many of the documents published by the FDA as guidance are being held up by the assessors as a regulatory requirement. Companies have ignored these to their peril.

There is a host of reference sources available from literature, reference books, Web sites and publications from various regulatory authorities and standard organisations. This section is not meant to be exhaustive, but should provide some general guidance to those developing new formulations.

If the excipient or packaging material has been used previously in marketed products by your own pharmaceutical company, and the supplier has been audited, most of the information about these materials should already be available within the company. More often than not, excipients not listed in the company inventory will have to be considered. Some useful reference sources which may provide details of specific excipients and packaging materials are given in Table 8.1. These sources can be used to gain information about the choice and status of materials available. It should be possible to easily check whether the material of interest is well established, safe and meets regulatory authorities' requirements, or not. Some of the reference sources reveal quantitative compositions of products, giving an indication of acceptable levels that have been used previously in approved products.

Other leads can be found by browsing pharmaceutical and packaging technology journals or visiting trade shows and exhibitions.

Once a lead has been found on an excipient or packaging material of interest, the next useful step is often to contact the supplier for further information. It is usually in their interest to persuade pharmaceutical companies to use their materials because of the potential commercial return if the product is successful. Often, suppliers will assist customers with any enquiries and provide any missing information. They may provide small amounts of samples to try, in attempts to satisfy you that their materials should be used. However, if a new supplier or material is seriously anticipated, it is wise to arrange for an audit of the supplier to ensure that it meets your company's appropriate quality standards, before becoming too committed. Also, it is advisable that more than one batch be evaluated to ensure the material is consistent. Be aware that sample materials are not always representative of purchased materials. They may have a different impurity profile, for example, or might have slightly different physicochemical properties which might give misleading performance results.

The rapid development in information technology (IT) in recent years has revolutionised the availability and speed of retrieval of information. Many reference sources are now available on CD-ROM, which are generally much easier to store, access and search than books and journals. The introduction of the World Wide Web (WWW), with a user-friendly graphical interface based on hypertext links, provides easy access via the Internet to a wealth of information and databases which are kept continually updated (D'Emanuele 1996). Some of the useful Web sites for sources of information about pharmaceutical development and regulatory guidelines are listed in Table 8.2. The Web site addresses are correct at the time of this writing.

EXPERT SYSTEMS

The development of a new medicinal product from a new chemical entity is a very time consuming and costly process. The formulator will usually start with a design specification. This could be very general, or it could be quite specific, perhaps expressed in terms of performance levels to be met in a number of predefined tests. In order to develop the formulation that will meet the product specification, the formulator will have to take into account several different technical issues such as the physicochemical properties of the candidate drug, the compatibility of the drug with pharmaceutical excipients and packaging and the manufacturing process to be used. The formulator might have to go through several formulation optimisation steps before the ideal product is achieved.

Pharmaceutical formulation development is thus a highly specialised and complex task that requires specific knowledge and often years of experience. This type of knowledge is very difficult to document and is therefore often passed on by word of mouth from experienced senior formulators to new personnel. The loss of senior formulators from a company through retirement or transfers to other companies can lead to the loss of irreplaceable knowledge. Formulation "expert systems" have been developed to provide a mechanism of capturing and utilising this knowledge and expertise.

Table 8.2
Information technology (IT) sources of information and development guidelines.

Source	Information	Comments
Food and Drug Administration (FDA)	Guidance for industry notes on various aspects of pharmaceutical product development, registration in the USA and inspections	Web site: http://www.fda.gov/
Committee for Proprietary Medicinal Products (CPMP) and European Medicines Evaluation Agency (EMEA)	Guidance for industry notes on various aspects of product development and registration in Europe, e.g., "Excipients in the dossier for application for marketing authorisation of a medicinal product (III/3196/91)"	Web sites: http://www.eudra.org/ emea/cpmp and http://www.eudra.org/w3/emea.html
National Institute of Health Sciences, Japan	Guidance notes on registration of pharmaceutical products in Japan	Web site: http://www.nihs.go.jp/
International Conference on Harmonisation (ICH)	Guidelines and information on harmonised requirements for product development and registration	Web sites: http://www.ifpma.org and http://www.chugai.co.uk
Web site for other regulatory authorities	Local regulatory guidance	http://www.pharmweb.net/
UK Medical Devices Agency (MDA)	Medical device regulations and guidance notes for industry on European Directives for medical devices	Web site: http://www.medical-devices.gov.uk/
International Medical Device Registration	A compilation of all the regulations affecting medical device registration world-wide	Book edited by M. E. Donawa. Published by Interpharm
Parenteral Drug Association (PDA) and British Parenteral Society (BPS)	Technical reports and guidelines prepared by industry on various parenteral topics, e.g., Sterile Pharmaceutical Packaging, compatibility and stability (PDA)	PDA Archive containing research papers, technical reports and conference proceedings available on CD-ROM; updated annually
International Federation of Pharmaceutical Manufacturers (IFPMA)	Information on pharmaceutical manufacturers	Web site: http://www.mcc.ac.uk/pharmweb/ifpma.html

Several different definitions for an expert system have been used (Partridge and Hussain 1994; Turban 1995). They all state that an

> expert system is an advanced computer program that mimics the knowledge and reasoning capabilities of an expert in a particular discipline.

In essence, the programmer will build a system based on the expertise of one or more experts so that it can be used by the layperson to solve difficult or ambiguous problems. The intent of an expert system is not to replace the human expert but to aid or assist that person.

An expert system consists of three main components:

1. *The user interface*, which is necessary for the expert system to interact with the user and vice versa

2. *The inference engine*, the procedure which generates the consequences, conclusions, or decisions from the existing knowledge extracted from the knowledge base

3. *The knowledge base*, the set of production rules that is supplied by the human expert and encoded into rules so that the system can understand the information

Expert systems can be developed using a variety of techniques including conventional computer languages (PASCAL and C), artificial intelligence languages (PROLOG, LISP and SMALLTALK), and specialised tools known as shells or toolkits.

Expert systems shells are computer programs written in both conventional and specialised languages which are capable of forming an expert system when loaded with the relevant knowledge. The development time of an expert system using a shell is much faster than using conventional languages and has therefore proved to be the method of choice. Shells used in product formulation vary from the relatively small and simple systems, such as Insight 2+ and Knowledge Pro, to the large and flexible Product Formulation Expert System (PFES) from Logica (UK). PFES was developed from research work conducted by a consortium of Shell Research, Logica (UK) and Schering Agrochemicals under the UK Alvey programme, 1985–1987 (Turner 1991).

To build a pharmaceutical formulation expert system, the formulation process has to be broken down into a number of discrete elements in order to provide distinct problem-solving tasks, each of which can be reasoned about and manipulated. However, as the formulation process is so complex, none of these tasks can be treated independently. A means of representing interactions and communicating information between tasks is therefore required. For example, one task may result in certain preferences that must be taken into account by subsequent tasks. To achieve this level of communication between tasks, the information in an expert system has to be highly structured and is therefore often represented as a series of production rules. An example of a production rule is as follows:

IF (condition)

THEN (action)

UNLESS (exception)

BECAUSE (reason)

Using a pharmaceutical example, this production rule would read:

IF the drug is insoluble

THEN use a soluble filler

UNLESS the drug is incompatible with the filler

BECAUSE instability will occur

The knowledge used in the production rules can come from many sources, including human experts, textbooks, past formulations, company Standard Operating Procedures (SOPs) and development reports. The knowledge contained within these can be broken down into different types: facts which are the objects and concepts about which an expert reasons, and rules and heuristics, which are often referred to as the expert's rules of thumb. The differences between rules and heuristics is that rules are always true and valid, whereas heuristics are the expert's best judgement in a particular situation and therefore may not always be true (Rowe 1997). The knowledge will be input into the expert system shell by a knowledge engineer. The knowledge engineer is an information technology expert who, through a series of interviews with the formulation experts, will capture all the steps involved in the formulation process. The knowledge engineer will then encode these tasks into a series of production rules which he will build into the expert system. This process of knowledge acquisition can be very time consuming and therefore very expensive.

Reference to the use of expert systems in pharmaceutical product formulation first appeared on 27 April 1989 in the London *Financial Times* (Bradshaw 1989). This article was closely followed by one in the same year by Walko (1989). Both these authors were describing the work being undertaken by ICI (now Zeneca) Pharmaceuticals and Logica UK Ltd. to develop an expert system for formulating pharmaceuticals using PFES. Since these first publications, many companies and academic institutions have published on work being conducted in this area, as shown in Table 8.3.

Table 8.3
Published work on pharmaceutical formulation expert systems.

Formulation	Company	System	Reference
Tablets	ICI (now Zeneca)	PFES	Rowe (1993a,b)
	Cadila Laboratories	PROLOG	Ramani et al. (1992)
	University of Heidelberg (GSH)	C/SMALLTALK	
Capsules	Sanofi Research Division	PFES	Bateman et al. (1996)
	Capsugel/University of London	C	Lai et al. (1995, 1996)
	University of Heidelberg (GSH)	C/SMALLTALK	
Parenterals	ICI (now Zeneca)	PFES	Rowe et al. (1995)
	University of Heidelberg (GSH)	C/SMALLTALK	
Aerosols	University of Heidelberg (GSH)	C/SMALLTALK	

A flow diagram of the Zeneca tablet formulation expert system is shown in Figure 8.1. The formulator enters the physicochemical information known about the drug, the specification for the formulation and the formulation strategy (e.g., whether to use one or two fillers in the product). The system then goes through a series of steps from which the filler, the binder, the lubricant, the disintegrant, the glidant and the surfactant and their relative proportions will be chosen. A formulation will then be recommended to the formulator. A series of defined tests can be carried out on the formulation in order to ensure that it meets the original specification. If it fails to satisfy the necessary requirements, the formulation can be optimised by feeding back the results into the system. The system has been designed to give a report on the decision processes used, that is, the production rules that fired during the development of the formulation.

The following benefits have been seen from the development and use of formulation expert systems (Rowe and Upjohn 1993):

- Protection of commercial knowledge. The expert system acts as a knowledge archive for formulation information, thereby overcoming the problems of staff turnover.

- Harmonisation of formulation processes and excipient usage, giving a guarantee of a consistent approach to formulation within the same company.

- Training aid for novice formulators. Inexperienced formulators can quickly learn about a product or formulation area using an expert system. A spin-off from this is to release the time of more experienced formulators currently involved in the training process.

- Cost reduction. Based on the reduced time required for formulating and speed of development, Boots claim that they have saved 30 formulator days per year since the introduction of their sunscreen formulation expert system (Wood 1991).

- Improved communication. The formulator and decision-making process is transparent to everyone in the company.

In spite of the many perceived benefits, the development of expert systems per se over recent years has been surprisingly slower than one would expect. One possible explanation for this is that when the systems were first introduced, their capabilities were overestimated and they were seen as the panacea to all formulation problems. This was obviously not the case, but as a result, the systems are viewed with some degree of scepticism. Several reviews on the issues and limitations with the development of an expert system have been published (Dewar 1989; Tinsley 1992; Rees 1996).

Further information on expert systems and the use of artificial intelligence software in pharmaceutical formulation can be found in the literature (Rowe and Roberts 1998).

EXPERIMENTAL DESIGN

The concept of experimental design originated in the agricultural industry and was developed by Sir Ronald Fisher. His first article appeared in the *Journal of the Ministry of Agriculture* in 1926, followed by a book *The Design of Experiments* in 1935. The concept of experimental design gradually spread to other industries, with the first publication of pharmaceutical relevance appearing in 1952 (Hwang 1998). The popularity of experimental design techniques

Figure 8.1 Flow diagram of the Zeneca tablet formulation.

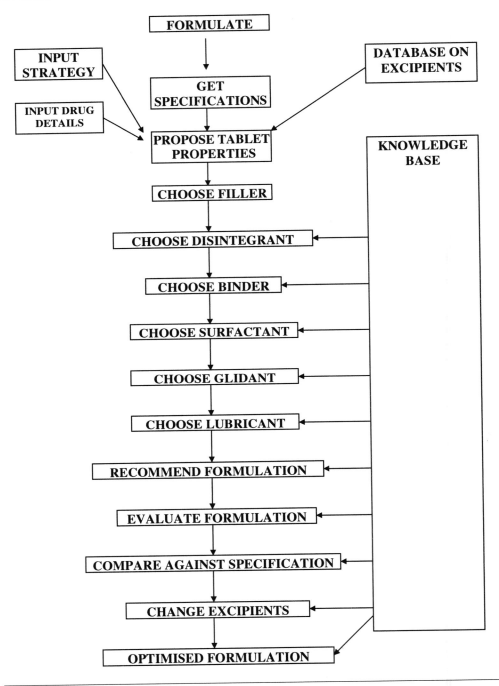

within the pharmaceutical sciences can perhaps be gauged by the number of relevant publications appearing in the pharmaceutical press; a search of International Pharmaceutical Abstracts elicited 41 publications since 1990 in which design of experiments (DOE) techniques were used for either formulation or process optimisation.

Pharmaceutical scientists are now almost universally aware of the disadvantages of traditional "one factor at a time" experimentation and recognise the advantages of a structured statistical approach to product development, as described below. Despite this, the routine use of experimental design in pharmaceutical development has only recently become widespread. The slow uptake of DOE techniques may have been a consequence of the lack of suitable user-friendly software packages. Until recently, scientists were forced to rely on SAS-literate statisticians, with the mechanics of data analysis being something of a "black box". This situation is changing with a number of easy to use software packages, such as Modde and Design Expert, being available. The impact of this development cannot be overstated; with relatively little statistical training, scientists are able to build their own experimental designs and analyse their data. Good statistical support remains of paramount importance, however, for all but the simplest of experimental designs, so that potential pitfalls are not overlooked. The key message from experience of using experimental design in pharmaceutical development is the importance of the pharmaceutical scientist and the statistician working side by side.

Benefits of Experimental Design

The potential benefits of using a structured statistically valid experimental design rather than using traditional "one factor at a time" experimentation are summarised below and are illustrated by the examples given later in this section.

- *Savings in time, money and drug substance.* This is particularly important in early formulation development when both time and drug substance are usually at a premium. The use of a suitable screening design, such as a fractional factorial, can allow the main effects of a number of variables to be evaluated in a minimal number of experiments.

- *Identification of interaction effects.* One of the most important benefits of experimental design is that interaction effects between variables can be identified and quantified, as well as the main effects of the individual variables. This is vitally important in instances where the effect of one variable is dependent on the level of another.

- *Characterisation of response surface.* By defining how a response variable responds to changes in process variables, a process can be selected that is in a plateau region, thus avoiding carrying out a process close to an optimisation precipice. In addition, a knowledge of how a process responds to changes in one or more operating variables is invaluable in instances where process deviations occur.

The Practical Use of DOE Techniques

A detailed discussion of the statistical principles underlying DOE techniques is beyond the scope of this book. Rather, some literature examples are presented which serve to illustrate the potential utility of DOE in all stages of pharmaceutical development.

Screening Studies

Partial factorial designs are widely used in early preformulation and formulation development, since they allow a large number of variables to be evaluated using a relatively small number of experiments. Variables may be either quantitative or qualitative; for example, the presence or absence of a particular component at a fixed level could be an experimental variable. In full factorial experimental designs, every combination of variables is evaluated. This can lead to a large number of experiments, for example, a design which included four variables each at two levels would require 16 experiments. In a half factorial design this number would be reduced to eight. Clearly, there is a price to pay for this resource saving; some information on interaction effects will be lost by the process of confounding interaction effect terms with main effect terms. Nevertheless, the experiment can be structured such that those two-way interaction effects which are suspected to be most significant can be included in the model. Furthermore, fractional factorial experiments can be easily expanded by addition of the missing experimental runs. Hwang et al. (1998) described a tablet formulation optimisation study in which a fractional factorial design was used to identify the formulation factors which were critical to achieving a high-quality product. Nine experimental factors were evaluated with only 16 experiments. Only main effects could be detected using such a small number of experimental runs, but statistical analysis of the data showed that only one factor required further optimisation. This factor was then studied in detail in a subsequent optimisation study. Plackett-Burnham designs, which are based on the two-level factorial approach, are widely used for screening studies where the main effects of a larger number of variables require evaluation in a limited number of experiments.

Optimisation Studies

The use of a full factorial experimental design can provide a detailed understanding of the experimental response surface. This type of design can be used when the number of variables to be investigated is small. Fransson and Hagman (1996) describe the use of a three-factor, two-level full factorial experimental design to evaluate the effects of light intensity, oxygen level and phosphate content on methionine oxidation of human insulin-like growth factor. Although the basic design required eight experiments, a further four experiments were carried out to provide an estimate of the inherent experimental variability. An interaction term was identified between the phosphate concentration and light intensity, with the effect of light being much greater when the phosphate concentration was high. The same technique was used by Bodea and Leucuta (1997) in the optimisation of a sustained-release pellet formulation. Again, significant interaction effects were detected.

One of the limitations of two-level factorial designs is the assumption of linearity of the effects. In reality, it is rather unlikely that the factor/response relationship will be linear. This relationship can be characterised more fully by the use of three-level factorial experiments, but this adds considerably to the number of experimental runs required. Various other experimental designs can be used if a detailed knowledge of the response surface is required. For example, Vojnovic et al. (1996) describe the use of a Doehlert experimental design in the optimisation of a high shear granulation process. In this case, the authors were using experimental design to identify an experimental region in which the quality of the product was relatively insensitive to small changes in processing variables, thus verifying the robustness of the process.

An alternative method of optimisation is the simplex search method. This is a model independent procedure in which the results of earlier experiments are used to define subsequent experiments. This type of optimisation is based on a systematic "trial and error" search for the optimum rather than statistical principles but can nevertheless be a useful method for defining the experimental region of interest.

Mixture Designs

Mixture designs are used in situations where the levels of individual components in a formulation require optimisation, but where the system is constrained by a maximum value for the overall formulation. This is most easily illustrated by considering the optimisation of a solution formulation containing a number of components each at a given percentage w/w. Clearly, the sum of all the components of the formulation, including water, must equal 100 percent. The experimental runs to be carried out depend on the model to be fitted. Marti-Mestres et al. (1997) describe the use of a simplex centroid design to optimise the relative proportions of three surfactants in a shampoo formulation. In this case, the total surfactant concentration was fixed at 18 percent, with the remainder being water and a number of minor components whose concentrations were also fixed and therefore not considered as experimental variables. Seven experimental runs were used to generate a quadratic model; a further three runs were carried out using other combinations of variables within the experimental region, in order to check the fit of the model. Three response factors were used to evaluate the quality of the formulations, and contour plots were developed illustrating acceptable formulations in terms of the individual responses. These contour plots were superimposed to yield a relatively small area of the experimental region in which all three response factors were satisfactory. Vojnovic and Chicco (1997) used a similar approach but used an axial design to evaluate the solubility of theophylline in a four-component solvent system.

It is evident that the use of suitably designed experiments can be an invaluable aid to the optimum use of resource at all stages of product development. In early development, screening studies enable the rapid assessment of the effect of several variables on the key characteristics of the product. More elaborate experimental designs can be used at the formulation, pack and process optimisation stages to ensure that the effect of all components and process variables are fully understood. Finally, prior to process validation, the use of experimental design techniques is invaluable in ensuring that the process is robust and that the operating region is not close to an "optimisation precipice". The software tools are now available to enable the pharmaceutical scientist to exploit the potential benefits of DOE, and the use of this approach should be considered in all experimental investigations.

STABILITY TESTING

The purpose of stability testing is to provide evidence of how the quality of a drug substance or formulated product varies with time under the influence of a variety of environmental factors such as temperature, light and humidity. The ultimate goal of stability testing is the application of appropriate testing to allow the establishment of recommended storage conditions, retest periods and shelf lives.

It is necessary to establish the "fitness for purpose" of the product throughout a proposed shelf-life, that is, to establish that all those attributes affecting product performance in use are not unacceptably changed during the period of storage up to the proposed expiry date. Testing must include factors affecting drug potency, formation of degradation products and the microbiological and physical integrity of the product. It may also be required to measure other quality parameters considered to be important, such as the organoleptic and aesthetic properties of the product.

Stability studies are carried out during all stages of development of new drug substances, formulated products, and where appropriate, novel formulation excipients. However, the stability design and type of testing will depend on the stage of the development process and the nature of the drug and product under test. The types of stability studies carried out during development will typically include the following:

- Accelerated stress stability testing

- Stability to support safety and clinical studies

- Stability to support product licence applications

Accelerated Stress Stability Testing

These are studies in which samples are stored under conditions designed to stress the drug substance or product. Techniques that can be used, and test conditions, are further discussed in Chapter 6, "Preformulation Studies as an aid to Product Design in Early Drug Development". Generally, samples are exposed to extremes of temperature or humidity. Also, exposure to intense light, metal ions and oxygen may be investigated. The aim of these studies is to provide information about the possible routes of degradation of the drug substance and what chemical and physical factors will affect degradation. For the drug product, the compatibility of the candidate drug with potential formulation excipients and packaging, routes of degradation in potential formulations and the identity of the major degradation products can be established. This information will provide important guidance to the formulator on the formulation factors that will affect product stability. Stability data from accelerated studies can also be used to predict shelf-lives at ambient conditions as discussed below.

Stability to Support Safety and Clinical Studies

Although real-time data provide the ultimate test of the defined shelf-life, the prediction of stability by the use of accelerated stress stability studies is vital in reducing the time to establish shelf-lives for products used in safety and clinical studies. By applying the principles of chemical kinetics to data from accelerated storage tests, predictions can be made of the rate of decomposition at ambient temperatures. The Arrhenius relationship is often assumed for this modelling. However, this approach can sometimes fail to give good predictions when applied, because more complex decomposition is occurring, involving both chemical and physical factors. In these cases, more complex predictive models can be applied, but it may be that only real-time data can be used.

The regulatory authorities recognise that modifications are likely to be made to the method of preparation of the new drug substance and formulation, and changes to the formulation itself, during the early stages of development (Phases I and II). The emphasis should generally be placed on providing information to develop a stable formulation, and to support a shelf-life suitable for the duration of the initial clinical studies.

During Phases I and II, stability testing is required to evaluate the stability of formulations used in these clinical studies. The duration of the stability study will depend on the length of the clinical studies, usually 1–2 years. Data generated should be of the appropriate quality for submission to regulatory authorities, to support a Clinical Trials Application (CTA) or Investigational New Drug (IND) submission, for example. The information may also be used to provide supporting data for a Product Licence Application. These stability studies will monitor changes in product performance characteristics and identify formulation degradants produced under actual conditions of storage. Stability data should be sufficient to obtain the additional information needed to develop the final formulation, and to select the most appropriate primary container and closure.

Stability to Support Product Licence Applications

In stability testing to support a product licence application (usually conducted during Phase III), the emphasis should be on testing the proposed commercial formulation stored in the proposed market packaging, and using the final manufacturing process at the proposed commercial production site. Alternatively, the process must be representative of the final manufacturing process at a scale which should be at least 10 percent of that proposed for full commercial scale manufacture. Ideally, drug substance used should be synthesised using the final process. Stability data will be required on at least three batches of drug substance, and for product batches made from three different batches of drug substance and different batches of excipients and packaging materials. If packaging components in contact with the product are obtained from more than one supplier, and they are not considered to be equivalent, then product packed in components from both suppliers should be tested.

Detailed regulatory guidelines are available to provide assistance to companies making regulatory submissions, including recommendations regarding the design, conduct and use of stability studies. These guidelines include, for example, the FDA guidance "Submitting Documentation for the Human Drugs and Biologics" (February 1987), shortly to be superseded by the FDA draft guidance for industry "Stability Testing of Drug Substances and Drug Products" (June 1998) and the Committee for Proprietary Medicinal Products (CPMP) notes for guidance on "Stability Testing: Testing of New Drug Substances and Products" (CPMP/ICH/ 380/95). Information is readily available from the Internet Web sites of various national and international regulatory authorities and manufacturers' associations:

- FDA (http://www.fda.gov/cder/guidance/index.html)
- CPMP (http://www.fda.gov/cder/guidance/index.html)
- ICH (http://www.ifpma.org)

Much progress has been achieved by ICH in harmonising the requirements for stability testing in the three areas of Europe, Japan and the United States. Thus, information generated in any one of these three areas should be mutually acceptable in both of the other two areas, thereby avoiding unnecessary duplication of effort. The FDA has incorporated many of the ICH recommendations into its own guidance for industry document "Stability Testing of Drug Substances and Drug Products". Examples are included where bracketing or matrixing could be acceptable—for different strengths of the same product, different pack sizes and different batch sizes, for example. A bracketing design can be usefully adopted to reduce the number of product strengths to be tested, but still cover the range of commercial product strengths. Similarly, a carefully designed matrix of testing can be used to reduce the number of product variants and time points tested, saving a lot of time and resource.

DEVELOPING SPECIFICATIONS

A specification is defined by ICH as

> a list of tests, references to analytical procedures, and appropriate acceptance criteria which are numerical limits, ranges, or other criteria for the tests described. It establishes the set of criteria to which a drug substance or drug product should conform to be considered acceptable for its intended use.

Specifications will be required for the pharmaceutical active ingredient, any excipients used in the formulation, packaging components, and for the finished product (at time of manufacture and over the shelf-life). In all cases, the specifications tests and limits will evolve during development, as illustrated in Table 8.4. It is clearly beneficial to have full specifications in place for the start of the Phase III pivotal clinical studies, when the product and process should have been optimised, to ensure that there is equivalence between the product used in Phase III and the commercial product.

Raw Material Specifications

The requirements for developing, testing and setting of specifications for raw materials, whether they are New Chemical Entities (NCEs), pharmacopoeial active materials, excipients or packaging materials, are essentially the same. Most emphasis is placed on establishing excipient and packaging specifications here because this usually involves an external supplier and the pharmaceutical company working together.

Table 8.4
Development of specifications.

	Phase I	Phase II	Phase III	Commercial Product
Active	Batch analysis; certificate of analysis; test methods developing	Draft specification; test methods developed and validated	Full specification; test methods developed and validated	Full specification; test methods developed and validated
Excipient	Certificate of analysis and methods developing on functional properties	Draft specification; test methods developed and being validated	Full specification; test methods developed and validated	Full specification; test methods developed and validated
Packaging	Certificate of analysis and limited testing depending on functional properties	Draft specification; test methods developing and being validated	Full specification; test methods developed and validated	Full specification; test methods developed and validated
Finished Product	Batch analysis; draft specification; test methods being developed	Refined draft specification; test methods developed (provisional) and partially validated	Full specification; test methods developed and validated	Full specification; test methods developed and validated

The initial concept and basic requirements for both excipient and packaging specifications should have been identified at the product design stage. For example, the design requirements for an antioxidant to be used in an IV injection may be of parenteral grade, GRAS status or previously approved for use by regulatory authorities but must be compatible with the active pharmaceutical ingredient under development. Similarly, the primary pack should meet the basic product design requirements and be acceptable to regulatory authorities, available from multiple sources and reputable suppliers, a suitable volume for use and sealed to maintain sterility; the container-closure system should be compatible with the formulation.

If compatibility testing of the pharmaceutically active ingredient, excipients and primary packaging components are satisfactory, development specifications are prepared for excipients and packaging materials to be used. These will contain essential information about the materials to be used, including the grade, proposed use, specific physical properties and any testing required for investigational purposes. The quality of the raw materials used is vital to the effectiveness and quality of the finished product.

At the early stages of development, for example, to support Phase I studies, pharmaceutical companies often accept excipient and packaging raw materials based on a certificate of analysis (CofA) or Certificate of Conformance provided by the supplier. This is especially the case if it is a reputable supplier of an established material used by the industry. This reduces the pressure on the pharmaceutical company's Analytical Department to develop methods to test the materials at this early stage. The supplier may also provide useful information such as details of the critical dimensions and drawings for packaging materials.

With a new supply source or a new material, a pharmaceutical company will usually want to audit the supplier, prior to accepting the material on a CofA. They may even want to repeat some of the tests on the CofA until there is confidence on compliance with the specification. The pharmaceutical company will want to seek assurance from the supplier that they are quality conscious at every stage of their process, and have the facilities and internal systems and procedures in place to be able to support this.

As product development progresses, the critical qualities of the raw materials will be identified which affect final product quality, and results of investigational studies will be obtained, to enable the specifications to be developed and refined.

Typical tests performed on raw materials, including the active pharmaceutical ingredient, excipients and packaging components, are as follows:

- Appearance, e.g., visual inspection, free from visible contamination
- Identity tests, e.g., comparison with a standard or by direct analysis, conformance with supplier's drawing
- Chemical tests where appropriate, e.g., for active, related substances, impurities
- Microbiological tests where appropriate, e.g., bioburden, absence of specific microorganisms
- Relevant physical properties, e.g., leak test, tensile strength, moisture vapour transmission, closure removal torque
- Dimensional analysis, e.g., for filling tolerances
- Investigational tests, e.g., reproducibility of dosing devices, particle size distribution of excipients

Official compendia may provide tests and standards for listed excipients and for glass and plastic containers.

Packaging and excipient specification functional tests are developed based on the functional requirements of these in the product. For example, the pack may have to prevent liquid loss, prevent moisture ingress, maintain sterility or deliver a defined dose. An excipient such as an antimicrobial preservative must be able to preserve the formulation in the presence of the active and other formulation ingredients and in the intended pack. Excipient and packaging optimisation must satisfy performance criteria, ensuring that packaging dimensional specifications and performance specifications can be consistently met at the extremes of the limits, and during processing, handling and transport. The evaluation of the sterilisation process is particularly important for sterile products. Robustness to the sterilisation process should be assessed, because it is possible that the thermal, electromagnetic or chemical energy could adversely affect the properties of the materials in question. For example, there may be an irreversible loss in product viscosity, the embrittlement of polypropylene or the loss in thermoplastic quality of polyethylene.

Once several batches of raw materials have been reviewed and tested to demonstrate that they will conform with the functional and quality requirements, the full excipient and packaging specifications can be finalised. Excipient and pack performance should be evaluated from a stability evaluation of the product and feedback from experience in clinical trials. Ideally, the specifications should be finalised for the start of Phase III clinical trials. If for some reason, the excipient or packaging material has to be changed for Phase III supplies, then some or all of the steps involved in the selection of materials, compatibility and stability studies may have to be repeated.

Product Specifications

Product specifications will also evolve during development (see Table 8.4). In the early stages, testing is typically performed on only a small number of samples due to the small scale of manufacture available. There may only be one or two product batches made to support Phase I and early Phase II studies. The specification limits also tend to be wide, due to the limited data available. The specification limits are tightened as more information is gained from testing more batches, and the scale of manufacture is increased.

The product release specification contains tests and limits that apply after manufacture to release the product for use, whereas the product specification contains tests and limits with which the product must comply throughout its shelf-life. The limits may differ from the product release limits to allow for changes during storage, for example, to allow for some drug degradation. Both product release and shelf-life specifications are required for European regulatory submissions, but in Japan and the United States, they are currently only interested in shelf-life specifications. Some companies have internal or in-house specifications which are different (usually tighter) than regulatory specifications. However, this can lead to confusion about which specification the product must comply with. Since the FDA only accepts the existence of the regulatory specifications, it is better to have "action limits" corresponding to the internal specification, rather than two sets of specifications.

When developing product specifications, test methods and limits, the critical parameters must be identified and controlled which affect the quality, safety, performance and stability of the drug product. Several issues have to be considered, such as appropriate regulatory requirements and guidelines, e.g., ICH, relevant compendial monographs and standards and the capability of the manufacturing process and analytical methods used. Appropriate limits will also be influenced by safety/toxicology considerations. For example, impurities, degradation products, extractables and leachables and preservatives should be qualified in safety studies.

Regulatory authorities such as the FDA publish specification guidelines with the expectation that pharmaceutical companies will comply with them. If there are difficulties in achieving the guideline requirements, or in the interpretation of them, it is advisable to discuss those points with the FDA. The internal regulatory group is usually the point of contact with external regulatory bodies. There are helpful ICH guidelines available on specifications, test procedures and acceptance criteria which describe the attributes that should usually be included for a variety of dosage forms. Other ICH guidelines are available, describing impurities and residual solvents.

There are various general compendial monographs available on dosage forms, such as tablets and inhalation dosage forms, as well as compendial test methods and limits listed in the various pharmacopoeias. In spite of the progress made with harmonisation, there are still some significant differences in the test procedures and limits recommended in the major pharmacopoeias. Often, the testing applied is aimed to cover the most stringent requirements.

During process optimisation, the capability and robustness of the manufacturing process is assessed (as described later in this chapter on process robustness), to confirm that the specifications can be met at the extremes of the limits. The capability of the test method, accuracy, precision and reproducibility will also affect the limits that can be achieved.

With all test methods and limits there must be a sound technical justification to support them based on data generated for product and process optimisation, clinical batches and stability studies. A specification set too wide is likely to be challenged by regulatory authorities. However, a tight specification may result in some batches failing, and, once registered, it is very difficult to gain approval to widen again. It is considered best practice to freeze the specifications as late as possible so that as much confirmatory data are available from all batches made to justify the limits. It is also very important to document the justifications for the specifications, and any changes during development, so that the complete specification development can be accounted for. This information will be required for the development report to support FDA Pre-approval Inspection (PAI) and regulatory submissions.

PROCESS DESIGN, PROCESS OPTIMISATION AND SCALE–UP

The primary objective of the process design and optimisation stages of product development is to ensure that manufacturing operations supporting Phase III studies, and ultimately commercial manufacture, are carried out under optimal conditions. The product should consistently comply with specifications.

Process design is the initial stage of process development where an outline of the clinical trial and commercial manufacturing processes are identified on paper, including the intended scale(s) of manufacture. This should be documented in a Process Design Report.

The Process Design Report should include all the factors that need to be considered for the design of the process, including the facilities and environment, equipment, manufacturing variables and any material handling requirements. A list of factors to consider is given in Table 8.5.

It is important to involve Production during the product design stage in the selection of equipment and the process. The eventual technology transfer is likely to be smoother if the same type of equipment employed by R&D is also available in Production on a larger scale. If a completely novel approach to manufacture is being considered, it is important that Production is made aware of this and can plan ahead to deal with the new process. This might involve the purchase of new equipment which will have to be validated.

Table 8.5
Process design considerations.

Factor	Requirement	Purpose
Facility	• Organisation and layout	GMP
	• Space	Health and safety
	• Environmental control	Product sensitivity to:
	• Temperature	• Temperature
	• Humidity	• Moisture
	• Air quality	• Particulates/micro-organisms
	• Electrical zoned (flame proof)	Allow solvents for cleaning
	• Barrier protection	Operator protection
Equipment	• Type and design, e.g., bottom- or top-mounted mixing elements, baffles, heating/cooling jacket, etc.	Suitability for process Mixing efficiency
	• Materials of construction	Compatibility, extractives
	• Range of sizes	Ease of scale-up
	• Access to internal parts	Ability to clean/maintenance
Material Transfer	• Product protection	Clean/sterile product
Transfer	•Operator protection	Hazardous materials
Manufacturing variables	• Order of addition of active and excipients	Mixing effectiveness
	• Temperature	Stability/dissolution
	• Speed	Mixing effectiveness
	• Time	Mixing effectiveness
	• Differences in excipient batches	Robustness of process

Other process design factors to consider are the need for any in-process controls during manufacture, with details of the tests and proposed limits. For example, the thickness, hardness, friability and weight of tablets might be measured during the filling of a tablet product. The tests and limits applied will be based on experience gained from product development, optimisation and stability studies. Depending on the product being developed and type of process, it may be necessary to conduct preliminary feasibility studies before the Process Design Report can be written.

Process Optimisation

Process optimisation will define and investigate critical process parameters, varying these within practical constraints to establish limits for the process parameters, within which acceptable product can be manufactured. Depending on the product being developed and type of process, it may be necessary to conduct preliminary feasibility studies before proceeding to process optimisation.

A useful approach to process optimisation is to identify all the critical process parameters that could potentially affect product quality or performance and prepare a Process Optimisation Protocol. Typically, data used to identify critical process parameters will be derived from laboratory or pilot-scale batches, and do not need to be confirmed on full-scale batches unless the control of the particular parameter can only be evaluated on a production scale. There is good incentive to use the production facilities at the earliest opportunity, drug availability permitting, to iron out any transfer difficulties. Manufacture of the stability batches to support Phase III studies, and also the Phase III clinical batches, at the final commercial site should minimise any questions from the FDA during PAI about possible differences between R&D and Production process used.

The Process Optimisation Protocol should outline the programme of work required to evaluate the effect of changes in the critical variables on product quality. This is in order to establish the working limits within which the process consistently produces product which meets specification. Critical parameters may include

- defining the order of addition of the active and excipients;

- defining the optimum equipment settings, e.g., mixing speed;

- optimising time-dependent process parameters;

- defining the optimum temperature range;

- evaluating the effects of different excipient/active batches (within specification);

- setting in-process targets and controls; and

- development of cleaning procedures for the process.

On completion of the work programme, a Process Optimisation Report should be written. This will summarise the results of the activities specified in the protocol and provide a rationale to define the operating limits for the process and the critical parameters affecting product quality or performance. The report should also conclude that the specifications for the raw active, excipients, components, in-process and product can be met.

Process Capability and Robustness

Several pitfalls that are sometimes encountered with process development can hinder successful technology transfer to production, i.e., if the process has not been designed or optimised with production in mind or a representative scale of production has not been used for the optimisation studies. For example, the sterilisation of a viscous ophthalmic gel by autoclaving at R&D on a 2 kg scale did not require any mixing of the bulk product for efficient heating and cooling. However, when transferred to production at a 100 kg scale, the heating and cooling times were found to be extensive and the bulk contained hot spots because no stirring mechanism had been specified in the vessel.

Another pitfall is to design a process where the operating limits for one or more critical parameters are too narrow and cannot be consistently achieved. It is not acceptable if the process can be performed only by "experts" in R&D. Many pharmaceutical companies apply some measurement of process and equipment capability to demonstrate the reproducibility and consistency of the process in meeting specification limits. The Process Capability Index (CpK) is often used to measure the reproducibility as a function of the specification limits. It is normally, calculated from either of the two equations below, whichever gives the lowest number:

$$CpK = \frac{\text{upper limit of specification} - \text{mean}}{3 \times \text{standard deviation}}$$

or

$$CpK = \frac{\text{mean} - \text{lower limit of specification}}{3 \times \text{standard deviation}}$$

Some generally accepted rules, determined from experimental data, relate the CpK value with robustness. For example, a CpK of less than 0.8 is an indication that the process is not capable, as the acceptance criteria cannot be met routinely. Further work will need to be done to develop a more robust process. CpK values between 0.9 to 1.0 indicate a marginal process, between 1.0 and 1.25 are satisfactory, between 1.25 to 1.5 are good, and values greater than 1.5 are excellent. Using these measurements, it is possible to evaluate process variables and identify which variable has the least or most effect. However, a possible pitfall is to obtain excellent CpK values, but not to have an acceptable process because the mean value is not on target. The process developed needs to be reliable and consistently meet product specifications, to demonstrate it is manufacturable. Another pitfall is to aim for a CpK value much higher than 1.5, which is probably a waste of effort. The process does not have to be "bombproof".

Scale-Up

In reality, product and process development and scale-up will be progressing concurrently in order to meet the demands of Phase I and II clinical and long-term safety supplies. The process used for initial clinical supply manufacture will probably be relatively small scale (laboratory scale). As more drug substance becomes available, and the clinical requirements increase, the product batch size will increase to pilot scale, and the process may have to be modified during scale-up. If drug substance is available and very large Phase III studies are anticipated, it may be essential to scale-up to production scale and transfer the process to the commercial production site.

The objective of scale up is to ensure that the process is scaled up to provide product which will comply with specification. Scale-up may encompass changes in process equipment and operation, with an associated increase in output, for example, in the following situations:

- An increase in batch size of 10-fold or greater on identical equipment

- Use of larger or high-speed versions of identical types of equipment

- Increase in output rate by more than 50 percent for identical equipment

- Changes in equipment type for a given process step

Whenever scale-up is to be undertaken, it is strongly recommended that an experimental batch is manufactured to demonstrate that the process is still acceptable and the product is manufacturable on the increased scale. It must meet all the appropriate in-process and product specification acceptance criteria.

Technology Transfer

The actual transfer of the manufacturing process from R&D to Production, along with the necessary knowledge and skills to be able to make the product, is referred to as "technology transfer". The ultimate objective for successful technology transfer is to have documented proof that the process is robust and effective in producing product complying with the registered specifications and Good Manufacturing Practice (GMP) requirements.

The approach taken by different pharmaceutical companies to technology transfer varies widely from a "hand over the wall" to a more structured team approach. Clearly, the latter approach is more likely to result in successful technology transfer. In some companies, a third party is involved in the process, a specialised Technology Transfer group, who liaise between R&D and Production to ensure a smooth transfer. Companies vary in the way they divide responsibilities for Technology Transfer and the point of handover of responsibility, but there do not appear to be any clear advantages, provided the guidelines below are followed:

- Responsibilities are clear and well defined.

- Representation from Production and the Technology Transfer group are involved early, e.g., during product and process design/optimisation.

- Good communications are maintained with good R&D/Production interface. Time is spent face to face in factory and laboratory.

- There is good scientific basis for product/process design.

- Equipment used at laboratory/pilot scale is similar to production equipment.

- There is good documentation of product/process development and technology transfer.

VALIDATION AND LAUNCH

Clinical Trials Process Validation

At early clinical stages (Phases I and II), where only limited GMP batches of product will have been produced, and where product and process changes make batch replication difficult, only limited process validation may be possible. In such cases, the regulatory authorities will expect to see data from extensive in-process and end-product testing to demonstrate that the batch is adequately qualified, yielding a finished product which meets specification and quality characteristics.

For critical processes such as sterilisation or aseptic manufacture, even for the earliest human studies, the regulatory authorities will expect the process to be qualified, to attain a high degree of assurance that the end-product will be sterile. If drug availability is an issue, the aseptic processing of sterile products may be validated using media fills to simulate the process.

At later development stages, when process optimisation has been completed and clinical batches are being manufactured under replicated conditions, the regulatory authorities will expect more process validation. The actual process used and results obtained must be documented so that it can be duplicated. Normally, the product must meet predetermined product specifications and acceptance criteria on three occasions. The benefit of validating the process successfully is to reduce the amount of product testing.

Validation of Commercial Process

Process validation is a requirement of the FDA Current Good Manufacturing Practices Regulations for Finished Pharmaceuticals, 21 CFR Parts 210 and 211, and of the Good Manufacturing Practice Regulations for Medical Devices, 21 CFR Part 820, and therefore, is applicable to the manufacture of pharmaceuticals and medical devices intended for the United States.

In response to several enquiries from pharmaceutical companies, the FDA has published a useful document entitled "Guideline on General Principles of Process Validation". The guideline has recently been updated (Draft, January 1999). The document includes the principles and practices that are acceptable to the FDA and has a section that describes the types of activities that should be considered when conducting process validation. It is strongly recommended that the procedures in this guideline are reviewed and followed. Otherwise, alternative procedures should be discussed with the FDA in advance to avoid disappointment (and a waste of time and expenditure) if they are later found not to be acceptable. Likewise, in Europe in 1999, the European Agency for the Evaluation of Medicinal Products (EMEA) and the Committee for Proprietary Medicinal Products (CPMP) issued a draft guidance on process validation with the aim of drawing together and presenting more clearly the requirements for effectively validating pharmaceutical manufacturing processes.

The FDA definition of process validation is

> to establish documented evidence which provides a high degree of assurance that a specific process will consistently produce a product meeting its pre-determined specifications and quality characteristics.

Documented evidence is achieved by preparing written validation protocols prior to doing the work, and writing final reports at the completion of the work. Information must be in writing, otherwise it does not exist, according to the FDA. The process equipment used should undergo installation qualification (IQ) and operational qualification (OQ) to establish confidence that the equipment was installed to specification and purpose and is capable of operating within established limits required by the process. Performance characteristics which may be measured could be uniformity of speed for a mixer or the temperature and pressure of an autoclave, for example.

Performance qualification (PQ) is to provide rigorous testing to demonstrate the effectiveness and reproducibility of the process. PQ should not be initiated until the IQ/OQ has been completed and the process specifications have been essentially proven through laboratory, pilot and scale-up batch manufacture. The PQ protocol should specify the approved procedures and tests to be conducted and the data to be collected. Acceptance criteria should be defined prior to starting the work. To gain a high degree of assurance that the process is reproducible, at least three successive replicated process runs are required to ensure statistical significance. It is expected that the conditions for the different runs will encompass upper and lower processing limits, widely known as "worst-case" conditions, to pose the greatest chance of product failure. This will demonstrate whether the process limits are adequate to assure that the product specifications are met. PQ should ideally be undertaken at the scale at which commercial production will take place, although it may be acceptable to use different batch sizes for the three replicated batches if scale has been shown not to be an issue.

Approval of the process for use in routine manufacturing should be based upon a review of all the validation documentation outlined in a Validation Master Plan, including data from IQ/OQ/PQ and product/package testing.

Pre-approval Inspection

Once the clinical and safety evaluation studies for a new medicinal product have shown it to be safe, effective and of acceptable quality, the pharmaceutical company will usually want to submit a Marketing Authorisation Application (MAA) or New Drug Application (NDA) to the regulatory authorities. The chemistry, manufacturing and controls (CMC) section will form a major part of the application. For an MAA in Europe, a development pharmaceutics section is required to describe how the product was developed, and to explain the rationale for the selection of the formulation, pack, manufacturing process and specifications. Also required for Europe are expert reports for each of the pharmaceutical, safety and clinical parts of the application. These have to be written by experienced scientists nominated by the pharmaceutical company who have to critically appraise the development programme for the product. The pharmaceutical expert must acknowledge the acceptability of the CMC part of the application.

A current prerequisite to NDA approval in the United States is to have successfully passed a FDA PAI. In the future, the Mutual Recognition Agreement (MRA), if agreed on, may eliminate the need for FDA inspections in Europe and Japan.

The PAI will essentially be targeted at the commercial manufacturing facility to gain assurance that the facilities, equipment, procedures and controls to manufacture the product are in place and conform with the NDA submission. The FDA will also want to check for compliance with current Good Manufacturing Practice (cGMP).

The FDA may also want to audit R&D to gain assurance that the product development has been done satisfactorily. In particular, the FDA may wish to see data that support the manufacturing process and controls from preformulation, product/process optimisation, clinical trials process validation and stability studies.

It will check for equivalence, for both the drug substance and pharmaceutical product, between that used in the pivotal clinical studies, the pivotal stability studies and commercial production. This is usually achieved by inspecting product and control data such as clinical trial batch records, in-process and end-product test results and raw material, component and product specifications. During an R&D PAI the FDA will also check for general compliance with cGMP, will inspect the facilities and equipment used and check the appropriateness of control systems and procedures.

It is in the interest of pharmaceutical companies to be in a state of readiness for a PAI. Staff should be aware of all procedures, policies and regulations and have current training records. A good documentation storage and retrieval system is essential to be able to locate and retrieve records and reports efficiently. It is now considered essential to have prepared a Development Report for the FDA to aid the PAI. The purpose of the report is to summarise all the product development and to demonstrate the equivalence of the manufacturing process and controls used for the pivotal clinical and stability batches and the commercial product. The typical contents of the Development Report requested by the FDA are as follows:

- Active and key excipients: physicochemical characteristics, particle size, purity, batch analysis

- History of formulation and pack development: design rationale with critical characteristics affecting manufacture

- History of process development: design rationale with critical process parameters

- Specifications: rationale and supporting data for in-process and product

- Product stability summary: equivalence of controls with commercial

- Technology transfer batch history: list all batches made for development, safety, clinical and transfer

- Evaluate cause of failures and remedies

The Development Report should be concise and structured. Clearly, it cannot be finalised until development is complete, but the preparation is much easier if summary reports have been compiled during development, such as the product and process optimisation reports. The Development Report needs to be available to the FDA prior to the inspection, ideally, to give the FDA inspection team confidence that the product has been developed satisfactorily, perhaps resulting in a shorter inspection.

A successful PAI and regulatory approval of the NDA is usually followed by product launch. Launch activities need to be planned carefully and well in advance to ensure that no time is wasted after approval to sell the product on the market. Some companies plan to sell the PQ lots, especially if the product is very expensive. The product insert and label claim will also have to be approved by the regulatory authorities. It may be better to wait for confirmation of approval before printing the labels and pack inserts; everything else can be prepared in advance. The launch stock is then packaged and labelled, QC released and then distributed for sale. Leading pharmaceutical companies can achieve this in 1–2 weeks post-approval, with good preparation and planning.

Post-approval Changes

It is inevitable that pharmaceutical companies will want to acknowledge changes after regulatory submissions have been submitted. Requests for post-approval changes could be for reasons outside the company's control, for example, because the source of raw materials changed, compendial specifications were revised or because suppliers of processing equipment made modifications. Alternatively, the change could be because the company wants to transfer a product to another manufacturing site. Sometimes changes are forced because the manufacturing process has not been properly evaluated and it is found not to be robust enough until a few production runs have been made. Such a situation may be a consequence of the company striving for the earliest submission date, with an attitude of "we'll fix it later"!

However, all of these changes require regulatory approval and this can take significant time and result in lost sales, it is therefore important that the company understands the consequences of post-approval changes prior to making a submission. The regulatory authorities, notably the FDA, have issued guidelines on the process for making changes in an initiative known as SUPAC or "Scale-Up and Post-approval Changes". SUPAC is designed to enable changes to be made to manufacturing processes with reduced regulatory input by providing guidance on what additional testing is required for specific changes.

There are a number of SUPACs, some approved (e.g., Immediate-Release Dosage Forms, Modified-Release Dosage Forms and Semi-Solid Dosage Forms) and some still being developed (e.g., Sterile Products). SUPAC establishes the regulatory requirements for making changes to the composition or components of the dosage form, the batch size, the manufacturing process or equipment or the site of manufacture. Different levels of change are defined and require different actions, for example:

- Level I—unlikely to have a detectable impact on product quality, e.g., a change in the mixing time within the validated range; action: notify FDA in the annual report

- Level II—could have a significant impact, e.g., a change of mixing time outside the validated limits; action: submit updated batch records, generate and submit long-term stability in annual report, generate dissolution profile data and notify the FDA of changes for approval

- Level III—likely to have a significant impact, e.g., a change from direct compression to wet granulation; action: (1) submit updated batch records, 3 months accelerated stability data, dissolution data, *in-vivo* bioequivalence study (unless *in-vitro/in-vivo* correlation verified), long-term stability data; and (2) notify the FDA of all changes for approval

In Europe, there are different arrangements from country to country when changes to MAAs are to be made. It is a legal requirement in the European Community (EC) that all marketed products comply with the details of the MAA. Changes may or may not require prior approval, depending on the type of change. For example, a Type I variation or minor change, such as a change in batch size, may not require prior approval. Details are submitted to all member states where the product is sold and are deemed approved if there are no objections within 30 days. Type II variations, or quite major changes, have to be submitted to all member states where the product is marketed, and the change must be approved or rejected within 90 days. A significant change such as a change of strength or indication would probably require a new application. Companies can make an early submission and avoiding regulatory delays by knowing in advance what changes are allowed without pre-approval.

ACKNOWLEDGEMENTS

I am very grateful to Joanne Broadhead for her contribution on experimental design and to Dawn Adkin for her contribution on expert systems.

REFERENCES

Bateman, S. D., J. Verlin, M. Russo, M. Guillot, and S. M. Laughlin. 1996. The development and validation of a capsule formulation knowledge-based system. *Pharm. Technol.* 20 (3):174–184.

Bodea, A., and S. E. Leucuta. 1997. Optimisation of propranolol hydrochloride sustained release pellets using a factorial design. *Int. J. Pharm.* 154:49–57.

Bradshaw, D. 1989. The computer learns from the experts. *Financial Times*, 27th April, London.

D'Emanuele, A. 1996. The communications revolution. *Int. Pharm. J.* 10 (4):129–134.

Dewar, J. 1989. Expert systems trends revealed. *Systems Int.* 17 (7):12–14.

FDA. 1987. *Guidance for industry on sterile products produced by asephic processing.* Rockville, Md., USA: Food and Drug Administration.

FDA. 1989. *Chemistry guidance document on drug master files (1).* Rockville, Md., USA: Center for Drug Evaluation and Research Food and Drug Administration.

FDA. 1999. *Guideline on general principles of process validation.* Rockville, Md., USA: Food and Drug Administration.

Fisher, Sir R. A. 1926. The arrangements of field experiments. *Y. J. Min.*

Fisher, Sir R. A. 1960. *The design of experiments,* 7th ed. Edinburgh: Oliver and Boyd.

Fransson, J., and A. Hagman, 1996. Oxidation of human insulin-like growth factor I in formulation studies II. Effects of oxygen, visible light and phosphate on methionine oxidation in aqueous solution and evaluation of possible mechanisms. *Pharm. Res.* 13 (10):1476–1481.

Hansen, O. G. 1999. PVC in Scandinavia. *Med. Device Technol.* (January):31–33.

Hwang, R. 1998. Formulation/process optimisation using design of experiments. Paper presented at WorldPHARM 98, Philadelphia, Pa., 22–24 September.

Hwang, R., M. K. Gemoules, D. S. Ramlose, and C. E. Thomasson, 1998. A systematic formulation optimisation process for a generic pharmaceutical tablet. *Pharm. Tech.* (May):48–64.

Lai, S., F., Podczeck, J. M. Newton, and R. Daumesnil, 1995. An expert system for the development of powder filled hard gelatin capsule formulations. *Pharm. Res.* 12 (9):S150.

Lai, S., F. Podczeck, J. M. Newton, and R. Daumesnil, 1996. An expert system to aid the development of capsule formulations. *Pharm. Tech. Eur.* 8 (9):60–68.

Marti-Mestres, G., F., R. Nielloud, R. Marti, and H. Maillols, 1997. Optimisation with experimental design of nonionic, anionic and amphoteric surfactants in a mixed system. *Drug Dev. Ind. Pharm.* 23 (10):993–998.

Moreton, C. R., 1999. Aspects relating to excipient quality and specifications. *Pharmaceut. Technol. Eur.* (Dec.):26–31.

Partridge, D., and K. M. Hussain, 1994. *Knowledge based information systems.* London: McGraw-Hill.

Ramani, K. V., M. R. Patel, and S. K. Patel, 1992. An expert system for drug preformulation in a pharmaceutical company. *Interfaces* 22 (2):101–108.

Rees, C. 1996. *Neural computing—Learning solutions* (user survey). London: UK Department of Trade and Industry.

Rowe, R. C. 1993a. An expert system for the formulation of pharmaceutical tablets. *Manufact. Intelligence* 14:13–15.

Rowe, R. C. 1993b. Expert systems in solid dosage development. *Pharm. Ind.* 55:1040–1045.

Rowe, R. C. 1997. Intelligent software systems for pharmaceutical product formulation. *Pharm. Tech.* 21:178–188.

Rowe, R. C., and R. J. Roberts, 1998. Intelligent software for product formulation. London: Talyor and Francis Ltd.

Rowe, R. C., and N. G. Upjohn, 1993. Formulating pharmaceuticals using expert systems. *Pharm. Tech. Int.* 5:46–52.

Rowe, R. C., M. G. Wakerly, R. J. Roberts, R. U. Grundy, and N. G. Upjohn, 1995. Expert system for parenteral development. *PDA J. Pharm. Sci. Technol.* 49:257–261.

Tarabah, F., and G. Taxacher, 1999. Drug-device products *Med. Device Technol.* (May):44–48.

Tinsley, H. 1992. Expert systems in manufacturing, an overview. *Manufact. Intelligence* 9:7–9.

Tovey, G. D. 1995. Excipient selection for world-wide marketed dosage forms. *In Excipients and delivery systems for pharmaceutical formulations*, edited by D. R. Karsa, and R. A. Stephenson. London: The Royal Society of Chemistry.

Turban, E. 1995. *Decision support systems and expert systems*. Englewood Cliffs, N.J., USA: Prentice-Hall.

Turner, J. 1991. Product formulation expert system. *DTI Manufact. Intelligence Newslett.* 8:12–14.

Vojnovic, D., D. Chicco, and H. El. Zenary, 1996. Doehlert experimental design applied to optimisation and quality control of granulation process in a high shear mixer. *Int. J. Pharm.* 145:203–213.

Vojnovic, D., and D. Chicco, 1997. Mixture experimental design applied to solubility predictions. *Drug Dev. Ind. Pharm.* 23 (7):639–645.

Walko, J. Z. 1989. *Turning Dalton's theory into practice, Innovation*. London, ICI Europa Ltd., pp. 18–24.

Williams, D. E. 1997. Pharmaceutical packaging—Its expanding role as a drug delivery system. *Pharmaceut. Technol. Eur.* 9 (4):44–46.

Wood, M. 1991. Expert systems save formulation time. *Lab. Equip. Digest* (November):17–19.

9

Parenteral Dosage Forms

Joanne Broadhead

AstraZeneca R&D Charnwood
Loughborough, United Kingdom

The dictionary definition of parenteral is non-enteral or non-oral and, therefore, strictly speaking, the term *parenteral* includes all products administered other than by the oral route. The pharmaceutical convention, however, is to use the term parenteral to describe medicines administered by means of an injection. The most common routes of parenteral administration are intravenous (IV), subcutaneous and intramuscular, but there are a variety of lesser used routes, such as intra-arterial. In addition, products such as subcutaneous implants are usually classed as parenterals.

There are, arguably, a greater variety of formulations administered by the parenteral route than by any other. These include emulsions, suspensions, liposomes, particulate systems and solid implants as well as the ubiquitous simple solution. What sets parenteral products apart from most other dosage forms, (with the exception of ocular products), is the absolute requirement for sterility, regardless of the formulation type. This requirement must be uppermost in the pharmaceutical scientist's mind from the first stages of formulation conception, so that the formulation and manufacturing process can be developed in tandem to produce an optimised sterile product.

This chapter aims to provide a practical guide to the development of parenteral products, initially reviewing the basic principles of formulating a straightforward parenteral solution. Subsequent sections will examine the formulation options available when a more sophisticated formulation is warranted, for example when the candidate drug exhibits poor aqueous solubility, is a macromolecule or requires a more sophisticated delivery system. *In vitro* and *in vivo* testing methods for parenteral products will be touched on and the chapter concludes with a discussion of the manufacturing and regulatory issues unique to parenteral products. While, of necessity, the individual topics will be covered only briefly, the objective is to provide the reader with the basic information necessary to evaluate the formulation options available and to provide appropriate references to sources of further and more detailed information.

GUIDING PRINCIPLES FOR SIMPLE PARENTERAL SOLUTIONS

This section summarises the principles which should be followed when developing simple solution formulations; these, after all, comprise the majority of marketed parenteral products. The information presented has been gleaned from standard textbooks and references, but where appropriate an attempt has been made to summarise the industry "norms". For further detailed information on the concepts discussed in this section, the reader is referred to Avis et al. (1992).

Selection of Injection Volume

Pharmacopoeias classify injectables into small-volume parenterals (SVPs) and large-volume parenterals (LVPs). The U.S. Pharmacopeia (USP) defines SVPs as containing less than 100 mL and LVPs as containing more than 100 mL. Many regulatory standards, for example, those for subvisible particulates, have first been developed for LVPs prior to their later application to all parenterals. SVPs can be given rapidly in a small volume; this type of injection is known as a bolus. They may also be added to LVPs, such as 5 percent dextrose and 0.9 percent sodium chloride infusion/injection, for administration by IV infusion. Some antibiotics are sold as LVPs, which eliminates the need for the extemporaneous addition of the drug to the infusion fluid prior to administration. The selection of bolus or infusion will depend on the pharmacokinetics of the drug and the distinction can be somewhat blurred. Infusions can be as brief as 15 minutes or may continue for several days. Generally speaking, if a medicament is to be administered by infusion, the simplest approach is to formulate it as a concentrate which will subsequently be diluted by the practitioner or pharmacist prior to administration.

Intramuscular or subcutaneous injections are almost always administered a bolus. Typically, the injection volume is less than 1–1.5 mL by the subcutaneous route and usually no more than 2 mL by the intramuscular route, although higher volumes (up to 4 mL) can be administered if essential (Ford 1988). Jorgensen et al. (1996) have shown a correlation between pain and the volume of a subcutaneous injection with volumes of 1–1.5 mL causing significantly more pain than volumes of 0.5 mL or less. Clearly, it is preferable to minimize injection volume wherever possible, particularly if chronic administration is anticipated. When the total volume to be administered cannot be reduced to an acceptable level, two or more injections at multiple sites may be required.

One of the first steps in the formulation of a solution product is, therefore, to select the administration volume and concentration. This may be dictated primarily by physiological considerations, such as maximum injection volume as discussed above, or by pharmaceutical considerations. For example, if solubility is low, a larger volume/lower concentration formulation may be required, whereas if stability is improved at higher concentrations, then the converse would be true.

pH and Tonicity Requirements

pH Considerations

Clearly, a parenteral product should be formulated with a pH close to physiological, unless stability or solubility considerations preclude this. Often, the pH selected for the product is a compromise between the pH of maximum stability, solubility and physiological acceptability.

The first step in selecting a suitable formulation pH will be the generation of pH/stability and pH/solubility profiles. This type of information is often available in the preformulation data package. The target pH for maximum physiological acceptability is approximately pH 7.4. In practice, however, a reasonably wide pH range can be tolerated, particularly when dosing is via the IV route, and dilution with blood is rapid. In these circumstances pHs ranging from 2 to 12 can be tolerated (although formulations at the extremes of this range are not recommended). The dilution rate is slower when administration is via the intramuscular route and decreases further when the subcutaneous route is used. For this reason, pH ranges of 3 to 11 and 3 to 6, respectively, are recommended for these routes (Strickley 1999). Many products are formulated at a slightly acidic pH because of solubility or stability considerations, and the vast majority of licensed products have a pH between 3 and 9. A pH outside this range should be avoided if possible, since a pH of greater than 9 can cause tissue necrosis, whereas a pH of less than 3 may cause pain and phlebitis (DeLuc and Boylan 1992). Nevertheless, products with extreme pH values are encountered; Dilantin Injection (phenytoin sodium) is formulated at pH 12, whereas Robinul Injectable (glycopyrrolate) is formulated at pH 2–3. Both products are for intramuscular administration. When a pH at the extreme of the acceptable ranges is necessary, and administration is via the subcutaneous or intramuscular route, it is advisable to conduct *in vivo* studies to assess the level of pain on injection (see the section "Pain"). An important consideration in terms of the tolerability of a formulation is its buffering capacity of; this may be more important than the pH *per se*. The pH of commercially available 0.9 percent w/v Sodium Chloride Infusion, for example, can be as low as 4, but the lack of any buffering capacity means that it will have negligible effect on the pH of the blood into which it is infused, even when administration is rapid.

The use of buffers often can (and should) be avoided if the active ingredient is itself a salt which can be titrated with acid or base to a suitable pH for parenteral administration. Buffers may legitimately be required when the pH must be controlled at that of maximum stability or solubility. In the former case, the buffer concentration should be kept to a minimum so that after injection, the buffering capacity of physiological fluids will outweigh the buffering capacity of the formulation. Where buffers are used to improve solubility, the buffer concentration may need to be a little higher to prevent precipitation after injection. *In vitro* models have been developed which can be used to screen formulations for the potential to precipitate after injection. These are discussed further in the section "*In Vitro* and *In Vivo* Testing Methods".

The buffers most commonly encountered in parenteral products are phosphate, citrate or acetate. Phosphate is useful for buffering around physiological pH, whereas acetate and citrate are used when the required pH is lower. Table 9.1 summarises the buffers which are encountered in approved parenteral products. Typically, buffer concentrations are in the 10–100 millimolar range. In most cases, the sodium salts of acidic buffers are used, although potassium salts are occasionally encountered. Hydrochloride salts of basic buffers are usually used. It is preferable to avoid the combination of anionic drugs with cationic buffers (or vice versa) due to the risk of forming an insoluble precipitate.

Table 9.1
Buffers used in approved parenteral products.

Buffer	pH Range
Acetate	3.8–5.8
Ammonium	8.25–10.25
Ascorbate	3.0–5.0
Benzoate	6.0–7.0
Bicarbonate	4.0–11.0
Citrate	2.1–6.2
Diethanolamine	8.0–10.0
Glycine	8.8–10.8
Lactate	2.1–4.1
Phosphate	3.0–8.0
Succinate	3.2–6.6
Tartrate	2.0–5.3
Tromethamine (TRIS, THAM)	7.1–9.1

Data abstracted from Powell et al. (1998), Flynn (1980) and Strickley (1999).

Tonicity Considerations

Wherever possible, parenteral products should be isotonic; typically, osmolarities between 280 and 290 mOsm/L are targeted during formulation. Isotonicity is essential for LVPs, but again, a wider range of osmolarities can be tolerated in SVPs, since either rapid dilution with blood will occur after injection, or the product itself will be diluted with an LVP prior to administration. Hypertonic solutions are preferable to hypotonic solutions because of the risk of haemolysis associated with the latter. Fortunately, hypotonic formulations can be easily avoided by the use of excipients, often sodium chloride, to raise osmolarity. Mannitol, dextrose or other inert excipients can also be used for this purpose and may be preferable if the addition of sodium chloride is likely to have an adverse effect on the formulation. Gupta et al. (1994a), for example, found that the presence of 0.9 percent w/w sodium chloride reduced the solubility of their candidate drug (Abbott-72517.HCl) by a factor of 3. Tonicity adjusters frequently have dual functionality; for example, mannitol often functions both to increase the osmolarity and to act as a bulking agent in lyophilized formulations.

CHOICE OF EXCIPIENTS

As with all pharmaceutical products, the most important "rule" to bear in mind when formulating parenterals is the "keep it simple" principle. Wherever possible, formulations should be developed using excipients which have an established use in parenteral products administered by the same route as the product under development. Both the excipient concentration, rate of administration and total daily dose should fall within the boundaries established by precedent in existing marketed products. The (U.S. Food and Drug Administration) FDA Inactive Ingredient Guide is a good place to start a search for information about a potential excipient, as it consists of an alphabetical list of all excipients in approved or conditionally approved drug products, and includes the route of administration of the products containing them. The *Physicians' Desk Reference* (PDR) provides an essential source of detailed information on products available on the U.S. market and includes the quantitative formulation of each product. This enables both the rate of administration and total daily dose of excipients in existing products to be calculated. The PDR can be obtained in a CD-ROM format which has a word search facility, thus providing a convenient means of searching for products containing a specific excipient. The PDR is also available in a web-based format, but unfortunately, this version does not have the word search capability. In addition to these reference sources, two excellent recent publications have specifically examined excipient usage in parenteral products on the U.S. market. Powell et al. (1998) have developed a compendium which provides a comprehensive list of excipients present in commercial formulations, together with their concentrations and the routes of administration of products containing them. Nema et al. (1997) carried out a similar review; their article presents the data as summary tables, enabling the frequency of use and concentration range of a particular excipient to be obtained at a glance. As this book goes to press, the first part of a review article entitled "Parenteral Formulations of Small Molecule Therapeutics Marketed in the United States (1999)" has been published in the *PDA Journal of Pharmaceutical Science and Technology* (Strickley 1999). This article provides information similar to the publications of Powell et al. and Nema et al., but collates the information in terms of formulation type and includes the structure of the active ingredients. It also lists the concentration of excipients administered following dilution as well as the concentration in the supplied preparation, thus saving formulators the trouble of performing these calculations themselves! Subsequent parts of this article are awaited with interest.

The information sources described above thus provide an invaluable resource to the parenteral formulator. The publications of Nema et al., (1997), Powell et al. (1998) and Strickley (1999) provide an instant, comprehensive and up-to-date reference source on U.S. licensed formulations, which can save the formulator many hours of trawling through the *Physicians' Desk Reference*! It is unfortunate that the same level of detail is not available for products outside the United States where manufacturers are not obliged to disclose the quantitative details of their formulations.

When considering the use of unusual excipients, or exceptionally high concentrations of "standard" excipients, it is important to bear in mind the indication for which the product is intended. An excipient which may be acceptable as a last resort in a treatment for a life-threatening condition should not be considered for a product to be administered chronically or for a less serious condition. A good example of this is the use of the solvent Cremophor EL in parenteral formulations of cyclosporin. This surfactant is associated with a range of toxic effects, and its use would not be envisaged unless all other more acceptable formulation strategies had been exhausted and the potential benefit of the treatment is such that the risk associated with the excipient is outweighed.

Another important consideration for excipients to be used in parenteral products is their quality, particularly in microbiological terms. Commonly used parenteral excipients can often be obtained in an injectable grade which will meet strict bioburden and endotoxin limits. Pharmacopoeial grades of other excipients may be acceptable, but it is prudent to apply in-house microbiological specification limits, where none are present in the pharmacopoeias. For non-pharmacopoeial excipients, the best approach is always to purchase the highest grade available and apply internal microbiological specification limits.

STERILITY CONSIDERATIONS

The requirement for sterility in parenteral products is absolute and must be borne in mind at all stages of formulation and process development. The regulatory environment now requires that parenteral products be terminally sterilized unless this is precluded, usually by reason of instability (see the section "Manufacturing of Parenteral Products").

For a solution product, one of the earliest investigations carried out during formulation development will be a study of the stability to moist heat sterilization. The results of this study may impact the formulation selection; for example, the stability to autoclaving may be affected by solution pH. Where stability is marginal, attempts should be made through the formulation process to stabilize the product such that it can withstand the stresses of moist heat sterilization. The regulatory authorities will expect to see good justification for new products that are *not* terminally sterilized. In many cases, however, the product will simply not withstand the stresses associated with autoclaving, and in this case, the usual alternative is filtration through sterilizing grade filters followed by aseptic processing. For the formulation scientist, it is important to select a suitable filter early on in development and ensure that the product is compatible with it.

Whilst the vast majority of parenteral products are rendered sterile either by moist heat sterilization or by filtration through sterilizing grade filters, other methods of sterilization should be considered, particularly in the development of non-aqueous formulations or novel drug delivery systems. For implants, for example, gamma irradiation is an option that should be explored early on in development.

Preservatives should not usually be included in parenteral formulations except where a multidose product is being developed. The Committee for Proprietary Medicinal Products (CPMP) "Notes for Guidance on Inclusion of Antioxidants and Antimicrobial Preservatives in Medicinal Products" states that the physical and chemical compatibility of the preservative (or antioxidant) with the other constituents of the formulation, the container and closure must be demonstrated during the development process. The minimum concentration of preservative should be used, which gives the required level of efficacy, as tested using pharmacopoeial methods. Certain preservatives should be avoided under certain circumstances, and preservatives should be avoided entirely for some specialised routes. The guidelines also require that both the concentration and efficacy of the preservative are monitored over the shelf life of the product. In multidose injectable products, the efficacy of the preservative must be established under simulated in-use conditions. Table 9.2 shows some of the most commonly encountered preservatives in licensed products and their typical concentrations.

STRATEGIES FOR FORMULATING POORLY SOLUBLE DRUGS

Increasingly, formulation scientists are being asked to develop parenteral formulations of compounds with solubilities in the order of nanograms or micrograms per millilitre. This presents enormous challenges, particularly given the limited range of excipients which have been used historically in injectable products. This section briefly describes some of the strategies which can be considered and highlights some of the issues associated with each. For a more detailed review of this area, the reader is referred to the recent review by Sweetana and Akers (1996).

Table 9.2
Preservatives used in approved parenteral products.

Preservative	Typical Concentration (%)
Benzyl alcohol	1–2
Chlorbutanol	0.5
Methylparaben	0.1–0.18
Propylparaben	0.01–0.02
Phenol	0.2–0.5
Thiomersal	≤0.01

Data abstracted from Nema et al. (1999) and Powell et al. (1999).

pH Manipulation

As discussed in the section "Guiding Principles for Simple Parenteral Solutions", the acceptable pH range for parenteral products is reasonably wide. Where the poorly soluble compound is a salt, pH manipulation may be all that is necessary to achieve adequate solubility. The potential for precipitation after administration should be considered when using this approach, however. When administration is via the intramuscular and subcutaneous routes, consideration must be given to the possibility of pain on injection, particularly when the product is intended for chronic use. This may preclude the use of pH extremes and favour alternative formulation strategies.

Co-solvents

Co-solvents are reportedly used in 10 percent of FDA approved parenteral products although the range is limited to glycerin, ethanol, propylene glycol, polyethylene glycol and N,N-dimethylacetamide (Sweetana and Akers 1996). Some marketed formulations containing co-solvents are shown in Table 9.1. The use of co-solvents is often one of the earliest options considered by the formulator when solubility is an issue. Quite often, mixtures of co-solvents are used so that the dose or concentration of individual solvents can be minimized, and any synergistic effects can be maximised. The concentration of co-solvent(s) which is acceptable will vary depending on the route, rate of administration and whether the product is to be given chronically. Again, the formulator will do well to be guided by the established precedent in marketed products and is once again referred to the publications of Powell et al. (1998) and Strickley (1999).

Non-aqueous Vehicles

Poorly soluble drugs for intramuscular administration can be formulated in a non-aqueous vehicle; this can have the additional benefit of providing a slow release of the active moiety. Oily vehicles have been used historically; the most commonly encountered is sesame oil, and six products containing it are listed in the PDR (Nema et al. 1997). Federal regulations, however, now require the specific oil to be included in the product labelling, because of the risk of allergic reactions to certain vegetable oils. This and the irritancy of oily vehicles has led to their decreased use. Formulations consisting entirely, or almost entirely, of organic solvents have also been developed, and examples are included in Table 9.3.

Surfactants

Surfactants, generally the polyscrbates, are frequently encountered in parenteral products but generally at very low levels (<0.05 percent) and most commonly to prevent aggregation in formulations of macromolecules (see the section "Strategies for the Formulation of Macromolecules"). Few IV products contain significant levels of surfactant; two notable exceptions are Cordarone IV and Etoposide IV which contain 10 and 8 percent respectively, of polysorbate (Tween) 80. Both products require dilution before administration, such that the maximum concentration of polysorbate 80 in the infusion solution is 1.2 and 0.16 percent, respectively. It

Table 9.3
The formulations of some co-solvent containing marketed products.

Active Ingredient	Route	Vehicle Composition	Special Instructions
Diazepam	IM/IV	40% Propylene glycol 10% Ethyl alcohol 5% Benzoate buffer 1.5% Benzyl alcohol	Inject slowly (at least 1 min/mL) if giving IV. Do not use small veins.
Co-trimoxazole	IV	40% Propylene glycol 10% Ethyl alcohol 0.3% Diethanolamine 1% Benzyl alcohol 0.1% Sodium metabisulphite	Must be diluted with 5% dextrose infusion. Discard if cloudy or if there is evidence of crystallization.
Etoposide	IV	65% w/v PEG 300 30.5% w/v Alcohol 8% w/v Polysorbate 80 3% w/v Benzyl alcohol 0.2% w/v Citric acid	Must be diluted. At concentrations >0.4 mg/mL, precipitation may occur.
Loxapine	IM	70% Propylene glycol 5% Polysorbate 80	
Lorazepam	IV/IM	80% Propylene glycol 18% Ethanol 2% Benzyl alcohol	Dilute twofold for IV injection.

is worth noting, however, that the polysorbate component of Cordarone IV has been implicated in a few cases of acute hepatitis which have developed within hours of the start of administration. Somewhat higher levels of surfactants can be tolerated in products intended for the subcutaneous or intramuscular route. Aquasol A (vitamin A palmitate as retinol) for intramuscular administration, for example, contains polysorbate 80 at a level of 12 percent.

Complexing Agents

Complexing agents, in this context, are molecules that have the ability to form soluble complexes with insoluble drugs. The most well-known examples are the cyclodextrins which have been widely studied as agents for solubilization and stabilization. They are able to increase the aqueous solubility of some poorly soluble drug molecules by orders of magnitude, as a result of their ability to form inclusion complexes. Cyclodextrins are oligosaccharides obtained from the enzymatic conversion of starch. Depending on the number of glucopyranose units, they are named as α (six units), β (seven units) or γ (eight units). These parent molecules can then be further substituted at the hydroxyl groups to alter the properties of the molecule. The nature of the substituents and the degree of substitution will influence the aqueous solubility, complexing capacity and safety of the molecules. An excellent review of the characteristics of cyclodextrins has recently been published (Thompson 1997). In addition, Stella and Rajewski (1997) have reviewed the use of cyclodextrins in drug formulation and delivery, and this provides an excellent summary of the "status quo" in terms of their toxicology and use in pharmaceutical formulations.

Although the potential of cyclodextrins as solubilizing and stabilizing excipients has been the subject of numerous research papers over the last decade, the FDA has only recently approved the first commercial parenteral products containing them. Edex (alprostadil) for injection contains α-cyclodextrin at a concentration of approximately 1 mg/mL. This product is unusual, however, in that it contains an unsubstituted cyclodextrin. In general, the unsubstituted α- and β-cyclodextrins are not considered suitable for parenteral use because they can cause severe nephrotoxicity. This has led to the development of modified cyclodextrins. Hydroxypropyl-β-cyclodextrin is the most popular of the cyclodextrin family for use as a solubilizer in parenteral solutions because of its low toxicity and high inherent solubility. The first parenteral product containing this derivative (itraconazole) was approved in April 1999. This product contains 40 percent hydroxypropyl-β-cyclodextrin and is administered intravenously after a two-fold dilution with saline (Strickley 1999). Although IV grades of hydroxypropyl-β-cyclodextrin are now commercially available, its widespread use has been hampered not only because of the inherent difficulties associated with introducing a new excipient but also because it is the subject of a Janssen/National Institutes of Health (NIH) patent which does not expire in Europe for several years. Until this time, other companies wishing to incorporate this derivative into a commercial IV formulation will need to obtain a license from either NIH or Janssen. The sulphabutyl ether derivative is also suitable for parenteral use and is present in at least one formulation in clinical development, but here again, there are patent issues hampering its widespread application. Nevertheless, the use of cyclodextrin derivatives is often the only method of achieving sufficiently high aqueous concentrations of poorly soluble molecules, and they are now widely used within the pharmaceutical industry in preclinical formulations. One could speculate that the upcoming expiry of the Janssen/NIH patent, coupled with the recent approval of the itraconzole formulation, is likely to lead to their routine consideration as a first-line approach in the formulation of poorly soluble drugs.

Emulsions

Parenteral emulsions were first introduced to provide an IV source of essential fatty acids and calories. This has developed into the extensive and routine use of products such as Intraplipid, Lipofundin and Liposyn in total parenteral nutrition. There are relatively few commercially available emulsions containing active compounds; the only example on the U.S. market is Diprivan® Injectable Emulsion, the formulation of which is shown in Table 9.4. Diazepam is also available as an injectable emulsion on the UK market (Diazemuls®). For a more detailed discussion of the issues involved in developing parenteral emulsions, the reader is referred to Collins-Gold et al. (1990).

All parenteral emulsions are oil-in-water formulations, with the oil as the internal phase dispersed as fine droplets in an aqueous continuous phase. An emulsifier, usually egg or soy lecithin, is needed to lower the interfacial tension and prevent flocculation and coalescence of the dispersed oil phase. Mechanical energy, usually in the form of homogenization, is required to disperse the oil phase into droplets of a suitable size. For IV administration, the droplet size should be below 1 μm to avoid the potential for emboli formation.

Clearly, physical stability is of critical importance for emulsion formulations, and care must be taken to ensure not only that the product itself is physically stable but that any infusion solutions which may be prepared by dilution of the emulsion are also physically stable over the required period of time. In addition, parenteral emulsions should be able to withstand the stresses associated with moist heat sterilization. Alternatively, if this cannot be achieved, it may be possible to prepare an emulsion aseptically from sterile components, provided the process can be suitably validated. For a good introduction to the formulation and preparation of IV emulsions, the reader is referred to Hansrani et al. (1983).

STRATEGIES FOR FORMULATING UNSTABLE MOLECULES

Water Removal

The most common mechanism of instability in parenteral formulations is hydrolysis. Regardless of whether the formulation is a true solution, co-solvent solution, emulsion or contains a complexing agent, the largest component of the formulation is likely to be water. Frequently, the only formulation strategy which will result in adequate stability is water removal. This is usually (although not exclusively) achieved by means of lyophilization. Lyophilization has a number of advantages over other potential drying methods, such as the ability to obtain an elegant end-product with a very low moisture content, and significantly, the fact that it is amendable to being carried out in an aseptic environment.

Lyophilization is essentially a three-stage process. Following standard aseptic filling, partially stoppered vials are transferred to a steam sterilizable lyophilizer in which drying is carried out. Initially the product is frozen to a low temperature (typically, –30 to –40°C). During primary drying, a high vacuum is applied, and ice is removed via sublimation. In the secondary drying stage, the product is heated under vacuum to 20–40°C, and any remaining water is removed by desorption. Products with very low moisture contents (<2 percent) can easily be achieved. The process also allows vials to be backfilled with nitrogen, usually to slightly less than atmospheric pressure, prior to stoppering, thus creating an inert environment within the vials. At the end of the lyophilization cycle, the stoppers are fully inserted into the vials before removal of the product from the chamber.

Table 9.4
Diprivan® injectable emulsion formulation.

Component	Concentration
Propofol	10 mg/mL
Soybean oil	100 mg/mL
Glycerol	22.5 mg/mL
Egg lecithin	12 mg/mL
Disodium edetate	0.005%
Sodium hydroxide	qs
Water for Injection	to 100%

The development of lyophilized products is a specialized area and requires a detailed understanding of the thermal properties of the formulation. Subambient differential scanning calorimetry studies are required to identify the eutectic melting temperature (Te) (in the case of a crystalline solute) or the glass transition temperature of the maximally concentrated solute (Tg') (for an amorphous solute). The latter is closely related to the collapse temperature (Tc) which effectively represents the maximum allowable product temperature during the primary drying or sublimation phase of the process. Both Tc and Te can be estimated using freeze-drying microscopy, a technique in which the freeze-drying process is observed on a microscale, and the collapse or melting temperature visually determined. Lyophilized products usually contain excipients to act as bulking agents and/or improve the stability of the product. When the requirement is principally for a bulking agent, mannitol tends to be the favourite choice of formulators. Mannitol is a crystalline material with a Te of about –2°C and, as such, is easily freeze-dried to give a self-supporting cake with good aesthetic properties. On the other hand, where an increase in stability is desired, an amorphous excipient (such as sucrose) is preferred since, once dry, the unstable compound will be "dispersed" in an amorphous glass with often greatly improved stability. The downside of formulating with amorphous excipients is that their low Tg' values (approximately –32°C for sucrose) result in long lyophilization cycles. The formulator must also ensure that the product reconstitutes rapidly and that reconstitution time as well as chemical integrity are not adversely affected by storage.

For a detailed discussion of lyophilization, the reader is referred to Jennings (1999). In addition, a thorough review of the manufacturing and regulatory aspects of lyophilization is provided in *Good Pharmaceutical Freeze-Drying Practice* (Cameron 1997).

Use of Excipients

Excipients may be useful in preventing chemical and physical instability. Antioxidants are included in parenteral formulations, although their use is now in decline, and EU guidelines discourage their use unless no other alternative exists (see the section "Parenteral Products and the Regulatory Environment"). A preferred method of preventing oxidation is simply to exclude oxygen; this is usually achieved by purging the product with nitrogen and creating a nitrogen headspace within the container. Where this is insufficient, a metal chelator, such as disodium edetate, or an antioxidant compound, such as ascorbic acid or sodium metabisulphite, may be considered. These are included in marketed products typically at levels of up to 0.05, 1 and 0.3 percent, respectively.

Non-aqueous Vehicles and Emulsions

For the intramuscular and subcutaneous routes, the use of non-aqueous vehicles may be considered as a method of avoiding hydrolysis. For IV administration, the use of an oil-in-water emulsion is a possible, although little used, option. These approaches are discussed in the section "Strategies for Formulating Poorly Soluble Drugs".

STRATEGIES FOR THE FORMULATION OF MACROMOLECULES

Macromolecules present unique challenges to both the formulator and the analyst. Their large size and complex structural nature make degradation difficult to detect and sometimes difficult to prevent.

Proteins are composed of an amino acid backbone which defines their primary structure. The amino acid side chains hydrogen-bond to each other, creating areas of local order such as α helices and β-pleated sheets. These types of arrangement are known as secondary structure. The overall folding of the molecule, which defines its three-dimensional shape, is known as the tertiary structure. Finally, some proteins, such as haemoglobin, are composed of more than one subunit; the spatial arrangement of these subunits is known as the quarternary structure.

The challenge to the formulator is ensuring the preservation of both the chemical integrity of the constituent amino acids and the overall three-dimensional folding or conformation of the molecule. Several amino acids are susceptible to degradation by oxidation (e.g., methionine, cysteine, histidine) and deamidation (e.g., glutamine and asparagine). Peptide bonds in the backbone can undergo hydrolysis, and disulphide bonds between amino chains can also be disrupted and refold incorrectly (disulphide interchange). Chemical modification may be detected by high performance liquid chromatography (HPLC) techniques, but it is often extremely difficult to pinpoint where in the molecule degradation is taking place. Protein molecules frequently undergo aggregation, both covalent (through disulphide bond formation) and non-covalent. Non-covalent aggregation cannot be detected by normal HPLC methods, and techniques such as sodium dodecyl sulfate–polyacrylamide gel electrophoresis (SDS–PAGE) and size exclusion chromatography are required to detect this type of instability. In addition, protein molecules have a tendency to adsorb to surfaces such as filters.

It is clear that the formulation of a macromolecule is far from simple and requires a good understanding of protein chemistry in order that degradation pathways can be understood and degradation prevented. However, one faces the same limitation as formulators of small molecules, namely, a relatively small armoury of established excipients which can be safely used in parenteral products. Some of the excipients commonly encountered in formulations of macromolecules are listed in Table 9.5. For further guidance on the formulation of macromolecules, the reader is referred to Wang and Pearlman (1993). This text provides some excellent examples of strategies which have been used to develop commercial formulations of proteins and peptides, such as human growth hormone and alteplase.

Table 9.5
Excipients encountered in formulations of macromolecules.

Excipient	Function
Polyhydric alcohols, e.g., mannitol	Stabilisation, bulking agent
Carbohydrates, e.g., sucrose	Stabilisation
Amino acids, e.g, glycine, arginine	Stabilisation, buffer, solubilisation
Serum albumin	Prevention of adsorption
Surfactants (e.g., Tween 80, Pluronic F68)	Prevention of adsorption and aggregation
Metal ions	Stabilisation
Antioxidants	Prevention of oxidation
Chelating agents (e.g., EDTA)	Prevention of oxidation

LIPOSOMAL DELIVERY SYSTEMS

Liposomes are single or multilayer phospholipid vesicles, typically less than 300 nm in size. They are capable of entrapping both water-soluble and lipid-soluble compounds. Their use in parenteral formulations has exploited their preferential distribution to the organs of the reticuloendothelial system (RES) and their ability to accumulate preferentially at the sites of inflammation and infection. Liposome encapsulated amphotericin B is considerably less toxic than the free drug because of the altered pattern of biodistribution (Betageri and Habib 1994). A sophisticated approach has been developed (commercialised as Stealth® liposomes), in which polyethylene glycol is grafted to the surface of the lipsome, resulting in prolonged circulation of the liposomes in the bloodstream. A doxorubicin product which uses this approach (DOXIL®) is now commercially available (Martin 1999).

SUSTAINED-RELEASE PARENTERAL FORMULATIONS

The chronic administration of molecules, which have a short biological half-life and cannot be given orally, presents a difficult challenge to formulators. One strategy which might be considered is the development of a sustained-release intramuscular or subcutaneous injection. Other non-parenteral options could include the inhalation or intranasal route, both of which have their own unique challenges. Sustained-release parenteral formulations might also be required in circumstances where patient compliance is likely to be poor. This consideration has led to the development of some antipsychotics and contraceptives as sustained-release injections. Table 9.6 lists some of the sustained-release parenteral products which are available on the U.S. market and their respective formulations. The typical approaches used in the formulation of sustained-release parenterals are summarised in this section.

Table 9.6
Examples of sustained-release parenteral formulations.

Compound	Route	Formulation
Penicillin-G benzathine	IM (aqueous suspension)	0.5% Lecithin 0.6% Carboxymethylcellulose 0.6% Povidone 0.1% Methylparaben 0.01% Propylparaben in sodium citrate buffer
Haloperidol	IM (oily vehicle)	1.2% Benzyl alcohol in sesame oil
Leuprolide acetate	IM (microsphere suspension)	After reconstitution: 0.13% Gelatin 6.6% dl-Lactic and glycolic acid copolymer 13% Mannitol 0.2% Polysorbate 80 1% Carboxymethylcellulose in WFI
Dexamethasone acetate	IM/ soft tissue (aqueous suspension)	0.67% Sodium chloride 0.5% Creatinine 0.05% Disodium edetate 0.5% Sodium carboxymethylcellulose 0.075% Polysorbate 80 0.9% Benzyl alcohol 0.1% Sodium sulphite in WFI

Oily Vehicles

The use of oily vehicles as an approach for the formulation of poorly soluble molecules is discussed in the section "Non-aqueous Vehicles". For molecules which possess good oil solubility, a sustained-release profile may also be achievable. The nature of the sustained-release profile will depend to a large extent on the oil/water partition coefficient of the molecule in question. Molecules which are not oil miscible could also be formulated as oily suspensions. The latter will usually result in a longer duration of action, because the drug particles must dissolve in the oily phase prior to partitioning into the aqueous medium (Madan 1985). The use of oily vehicles would not normally be considered as a first-line approach for new formulations, however, because of concerns over allergic reactions to the oils.

Aqueous Suspensions

This approach can be used to prolong the release of compounds with limited aqueous solubility. A suspension of a compound in its saturated solution can provide both immediate-release and sustained-release components of a dose (Madan 1985). A number of water-insoluble prodrugs are also formulated as suspensions, including hydrocortisone acetate and medroxyprogesterone acetate. As with any other type of suspension, excipients will usually be required to ensure the physical stability of the formulation. Strickley's (1999) article provides a table of parenteral suspension formulations; the most popular excipient combinations are clearly polyethylene glycol/Tween 80 and carboxymethylcellulose/Tween 80.

Perhaps the most well-known example of a parenteral suspension formulation is insulin. Many insulin formulations also take advantage of the different physical forms which can be produced when insulin is complexed with zinc. Suspensions of the amorphous form of insulin zinc have a faster onset of action and shorter duration of action compared to those of the crystalline form. In order to provide both a rapid onset and a long duration of action, many formulations are composed of a mixture of amorphous and crystalline zinc insulin.

Emulsions

For a molecule with a high aqueous solubility, the use of a water-in-oil two-phase emulsion or a multiple phase water-in-oil-in-water emulsion may enable a measure of sustained-release to be achieved. In either case, the nature of the sustained-release delivery profile will be a function of the partition coefficient of the molecule between the two phases, which will define the rate at which the molecule is available for absorption.

Microspheres

Polymeric micropsheres, particularly those prepared from the biodegradable polylactide/polyglycolide polymers, have been widely investigated as a means to achieve sustained parenteral drug delivery. The advantage of formulating the polymeric matrix as microspheres is the ability to administer them via a conventional needle and syringe as a suspension formulation, rather than as an implant (see below). Lupron® depot formulations are available which can provide therapeutic blood levels of leuprolide acetate for up to four months. These products are presented as lyophilized polylactic acid microspheres which are reconstituted to form a suspension prior to administration.

Implantable Drug Delivery Systems

Implantable delivery systems extend the concept of sustained release beyond the capabilities of the strategies discussed so far in this section. Continual drug delivery lasting for months or even years has been achieved. Because these products must be administered as a solid rather than a liquid, they are usually supplied with a customised injection device.

The number of marketed implantable products is relatively limited, probably due in part to the limited market for this type of product. The most well-known example of an implantable delivery system is the Norplant® contraceptive device which can deliver levonorgestrel for up to five years. The device is composed of a number of capsules fabricated from Silastic® (dimethylsiloxane/methylvinylsiloxane copolymer)

The Norplant® device has been somewhat controversial, however, due to difficulties associated with its removal. A second example of an implantable drug delivery system is Zoladex®, which is an implantable biodegradable lactide/glycolide polymeric delivery system for the administration of goserelin acetate. It is available in one-month and three-month presentations and can be injected through a wide-bore needle.

IN VITRO AND *IN VIVO* TESTING METHODS

When developing formulations for compounds with limited solubility or stability, where extremes of pH or co-solvents might be used, it is desirable to carry out screening studies to assess their potential to cause pain or other adverse events following injection. Haemolysis and phlebitis may occur as a consequence of IV therapy, whilst pain may occur on administration of any type of injection. Several *in vitro* and *in vivo* models have been developed to evaluate the potential for adverse effects following parenteral administration; these are discussed briefly below. For a more detailed discussion of this subject, the reader is referred to the excellent review by Yalkowsky et al. (1998).

In Vitro Precipitation

Clearly, when a drug is formulated at a non-physiological pH, or using organic solvents because of low solubility, there is a real risk of precipitation immediately following injection into the bloodstream. Crude models have therefore been used in the past to assess formulations for their potential to result in *in vivo* precipitation. These have generally involved performing dilutions in a medium resembling blood and monitoring the formation of a precipitate by visual or other means. More recently, dynamic methods have been developed which more realistically simulate the *in vivo* situation. Typically, these involve a continuously circulating system of plasma or a medium representing plasma. After "injection" of the test formulation, the resulting solution passes through a flow-through cell within a spectrophotometer where light scattering associated with particle formation is monitored. Although it is obviously difficult to precisely mimic *in vivo* conditions, these models can prove useful in terms of discriminating between a number of potential formulations. In addition, they can be used to assess the effect of injection rate. Yalkowsky et al. (1983) have shown that, perhaps counterintuitively, the degree of precipitation of diazepam injection is in fact *inversely* proportional to injection rate.

Haemolysis

Haemolysis occurs when the red blood cell membrane is disrupted, resulting in release of cell contents into the plasma. Severe adverse events can occur if high levels of haemoglobin are released into plasma. Clearly, hypotonic formulations have the potential to cause haemolysis, and as discussed earlier, the administration of such formulations should be avoided. Other excipients, such as surfactants and co-solvents, can cause haemolysis, as may the drug itself. *In vitro* models to evaluate haemolytic potential typically involve exposing the formulation to blood, either in a static or a dynamic configuration, and then assessing the quantity of free haemoglobin released. The contact time between blood and the formulation is critical, as an unrealistic contact time can result in a substantial overestimation of the haemolytic potential of a given formulation (Wakerley 1999). Haemolysis can also be measured *in vivo* by the measurement of free haemoglobin in blood or urine, and Krzyzaniak (1997) has reported agreement between a dynamic *in vitro* method and *in vivo* results.

Phlebitis

Phlebitis refers to inflammation of the vein wall. It can result in clinical symptoms such as pain and oedema, and can cause thrombus formation which may have serious consequences. Particulate matter is the most widely implicated cause of phlebitis. It is not surprising, therefore, that a link has been proposed between precipitation and phlebitis. The *in vitro* precipitation models described above may therefore be a good indicator of the phlebitic potential of a formulation. Phlebitis can be tested *in vivo*, usually by means of a rabbit ear vein model in which the "test" ear is visually compared with the "control" ear.

Pain

Pain on injection is usually of greatest concern with intramuscular injections because of the long residence time of the formulation at the injection site. Not surprisingly, there are no *in vitro* models to test the potential of a formulation to cause pain! It is therefore necessary to test for the potential to cause pain by means of an *in-vivo* model. Gupta et al. (1994b) describe the use of the rat "paw lick" model for the assessment of pain in response to formulation pH and co-solvent concentration. The potential for muscle damage should also be evaluated when developing an intramuscular formulation, and the industry standard is the rabbit lesion volume model (Sutton et al. 1996).

PACKAGING OF PARENTERAL PRODUCTS

Pack Selection

The packaging of parenteral products presents unique challenges in terms of the requirements for the packaging components to withstand sterilization prior to use and the requirement for the complete primary pack to maintain sterility throughout the shelf-life of the product. Traditionally, SVPs have been packaged in ampoules which are heat sealed after filling. Because of the inherent variability in the sealing process, products packaged in ampoules must be 100 percent integrity tested after sealing, usually by means of a dye immersion test. The use of ampoules for new products is now diminishing, partly because of the desire to avoid exposing medical personnel to injury on opening. This has led to an increase in the use of glass vials sealed with rubber stoppers for the packaging of SVPs. Regardless of whether an ampoule or a vial is used, the glass quality must be type I neutral. An increasing number of simple solutions are now being filled using blow-fill-seal technology, in which the (plastic) ampoule is moulded, aseptically filled and sealed in a continuous process. These manufacturing systems operate to high levels of asepsis and are validated by media fills in the same manner as conventional filling processes.

For products packaged in vials, a suitable rubber stopper must be selected. The surface of a rubber stopper is inherently less inert than the glass of an ampoule, and it is therefore important that the formulator ensures that the product and stopper are compatible by conducting suitable testing. It is also necessary to ensure that the product does not extract an excessive quantity of leachables from the stopper. For lyophilized products, it is advisable to select a stopper with a low capacity to absorb moisture during the autoclaving process, since this can subsequently be transferred to the product during storage, which may lead to product deterioration. Various other specialized stoppers are available, such as Teflon-coated, which may be useful when a highly inert surface is required. Stoppers containing a desiccant are also under development. Stoppers cannot withstand the depyrogenation process and so are autoclaved prior to use, but the presterilization treatment should be designed to ensure a satisfactory level of endotoxin removal. Stoppers will almost always require some degree of siliconisation to allow them to be easily processed in automatic filling lines, and they can be purchased washed, presiliconised to an agreed level and packaged in ready-to-sterilize bags. Stoppers which are purchased in a ready-to-sterilize format should be tested by the supplier to a suitable endotoxin specification.

Increasingly parenteral products are being presented in more sophisticated packages, such as pre-filled syringes. These reduce the potential for needle-stick injuries by reducing the degree of manipulation required and facilitate administration in an emergency situation. A number of companies, such as Beckton-Dickinson and Vetter, specialize in this technology, and can supply purpose-designed filling equipment or can provide contract manufacturing services to fill product into their devices.

Container/Closure Integrity

Considerable emphasis is now placed on providing an assurance of container closure integrity during the shelf-life of sterile products. Historically, this has been achieved by performing sterility tests as a component of stability testing, usually initially and at 12-month intervals, but this approach alone would not now be considered sufficient to validate the integrity of a new container/closure system. Most manufacturers usually perform media immersion tests in which media-filled vials are immersed in contaminated media and subjected to repeated vacuum/overpressure cycles. This provides an assurance of the integrity of specific pack configurations under highly challenging conditions. This test should also be conducted on stored media-filled vials to provide data on the integrity of "aged" packs. FDA guidelines now allow physical tests to replace microbiological tests in demonstrating container closure integrity, but only where those physical tests are suitably validated. This is by no means straightforward because of the difficulty in correlating leakage measured by a physical method with the potential for microbial ingress. Efforts are underway to develop physical methods, however and Kirsch et al. have recently published a series of articles in which they have been able to correlate helium leak rates measured by mass spectrometry and vacuum decay methods with a probability of microbial ingress (Kirsch et al. 1999, 1997a, b, c).

MANUFACTURING OF PARENTERAL PRODUCTS

The manufacture of parenteral products is focussed at all times on the requirement for sterility of the finished product. Despite the fact that the regulators are clear in their preference for products to be terminally sterilized, the vast majority of parenterals are filtered through sterilizing grade filters and filled aseptically, primarily because stability considerations preclude the use of moist heat sterilization. The statistical limitations of sterility testing a sample from a batch are well known, and attention is now well and truly focussed on process validation. The validation program must encompass facilities, instrumentation, sterilization of container and closures, clean room garments and gowning procedures as well as including regular media simulations of aseptic processes. Guidance on the frequency and numbers of units to be filled in media simulations can be found in the publications of the Parenteral Drug Association and the Parenteral Society (see the section "Parenteral Products and the Regulatory Environment"). In a production environment, a simulation of each aseptic process will typically be carried out at six-month intervals. It is important that media fills include planned interventions, such as filter changes, so that such interventions can be permitted during a manufacture if required. In addition, holding times after filtration should be validated. Where a product is lyophilized, the media simulation must include loading into and removal from the lyophilizer and should also include pulling and releasing partial vacuums. It is obviously essential to ensure that all personnel participating in aseptic processes are adequately trained and aseptic operators are required to participate in regular media fills. Another important element of aseptic process validation is environmental monitoring and particulate monitoring; manufacturers are expected to know the organisms which may be present in their facility and to establish acceptable limits.

With the majority of parenteral products sterilized by filtration, it is not surprising that the validation of filtration processes is receiving increasing regulatory interest. The 1998 PDA Technical Report No. 26 discusses this topic in detail (see the section "Parenteral Products and the Regulatory Environment"). There is now a regulatory expectation that the bacterial retention capability of sterilizing filters is demonstrated in the presence of product rather than simply water. Fortunately, the major pharmaceutical filter companies now have specialised validation laboratories which are able to provide filter validation services. All filters used in a process, including vent filters, must also be integrity tested before and after use. Organisms have recently been identified which are capable of passing through 0.22 μm filters, and the filter companies are now starting to launch 0.1 μm filters. One might imagine that the day will come when the use of 0.1 μm filters becomes the industry "norm", although a 1997 editorial in the *Journal of the Parenteral Drug Association* advised those in the industry to resist this development. Manufacturers are required to have a knowledge of the type of organisms which may be present in the solution to be filtered; provided that these do not have the ability to pass through a 0.22 μm filter, there is no compelling scientific argument for the use of a 0.1 μm filter.

For products which can withstand sterilization in their final container, the focus of the validation exercise will clearly be the sterilization process. A detailed discussion of sterilization is beyond the scope of this chapter (for this, the reader is referred to the recent text by Nordhauser and Olson [1998]) but the premise central to all methods of sterilization is the concept of a log-reduction in viable organisms. Pharmacopoeias now require an assurance that there is less than one chance in a million that viable microorganisms are present in a sterilized article or dosage form (Hall 1994). Achieving the required sterility assurance level of 10^{-6} is of course dependent on the initial microbiological loading of the material to be sterilized, and so it is vital to have knowledge of the initial bioburden and to set limits for this. For terminally sterilized products, the focus of the validation exercise will be in providing an assurance that sterilizing conditions have been reached in all units. Thus only loads and loading patterns which have been validated, usually by means of biological indicators, can be used. The concept of validated loading patterns also applies to the sterilization of equipment and packaging components to be used in an aseptic process.

The final stage in the manufacture of a sterile product is inspection. A 100 percent inspection for particulates, cracks and defects is a regulatory requirement. The inspection may be carried out visually using suitable illumination, but in a production environment, a semi-automated or automated system is usually used.

Clearly, the manufacture of sterile products is a specialized area, and the above discussion simply serves to highlight some of the critical issues; it is by no means comprehensive. For a detailed discussion of the manufacture of sterile products, the reader is referred to Hall (1994) as well as the publications of the Parenteral Drug Association and the Parenteral Society, which are detailed in the section "Parenteral Products and the Regulatory Environment". In addition, the "Orange Guide" provides a very readable annex covering the manufacture of sterile medicinal products; this includes guidance on clean room classifications, gowning and sanitisation, as well as the manufacture and sterilization of medicinal products (MCA 1997).

ADMINISTRATION OF PARENTERAL PRODUCTS

During product development, it is essential that the formulator keeps in mind the manner in which their product will ultimately be used. This is particularly true for products intended for IV infusion, since these will require dilution with IV infusion fluids prior to administration. The formulator must ensure that the active compound is compatible with all diluents which are to be included in the product labelling and must provide stability data to demonstrate that the resultant infusion solutions are stable for the period of time specified in the labelling. During clinical trials, compatibility and stability must be assured at the maximum and minimum concentrations to be administered during the study; this data will be expected by the regulatory authorities as part of an Investigational New Drug (IND) submission. It is also important to consider other drugs which may be co-administered with the product in question. The practice of mixing more than one drug in a single infusion is diminishing rapidly, and the labelling of new IV products usually specifies that this should be avoided. One must still consider, however, the potential for incompatibilities to occur when different infusion solutions mix in the infusion line or indeed the cannula. In general, mixing prior to the cannula can be avoided by the use of a different line for each infusion, but clearly, mixing in the cannula is inevitable where patients are receiving multiple IV infusions. The labelling of some medications, notably alteplase, specifically instructs that they should be administered in a completely separate infusion line to any other medications. The nature of alteplase may justify this statement, but in practice, such restrictions should be avoided, since they will clearly cause difficulties for medical practitioners.

When compatibility or stability issues do arise, there are limited options available to the formulator. The diluent cannot usually be controlled unless the manufacturer incurs the additional cost associated with supplying a custom diluent. Leachables from infusion bags can cause degradation, particularly oxidation. In addition, the low concentrations to which drugs may be diluted for continuous infusion can result in adsorptive losses. A number of products, therefore, specify a minimum concentration to which they can be diluted, presumably to address stability or adsorption issues. The infusion set itself can also contribute to instability and/or adsorption. Some product labelling, for example, that of glyceryl trinitrate infusion, specifies that PVC infusion lines should not be used. In extreme cases, it may be necessary to add an additional excipient to the product to prevent degradation on dilution, although this approach should only be considered as a last resort.

PARENTERAL PRODUCTS AND
THE REGULATORY ENVIRONMENT

The requirement for sterility in parenteral products means that their manufacture is scrutinised perhaps more closely than that of any other product type. A number of regulatory guidelines specifically pertain to parenteral products, and these are listed below. Included in these lists are also some more general guidelines where these contain sections specifically relevant to parenteral products. European Agency for the Evaluation of Medicinal Products (EMEA) publications provide useful guidance in formulation decision making and are essential reading early on in the formulation development process. The "Decision Trees for the Selection of Sterilisation Methods" document provides clear guidance on the selection of a sterilization strategy, this is discussed in detail in Chapter 12. Similarly, the "Notes for Guidance on Inclusion of Antioxidants and Antimicrobial Preservatives in Medicinal Products" is prescriptive in terms of defining the circumstances under which antioxidants and preservatives should be used. The former, for example, should be included only where their use cannot be avoided and where the manufacturing process has been optimised to minimize the potential for oxidation.

FDA guidelines are in general directed more towards the required components of a registration dossier and do not offer much in the way of guidance to the formulator. One exception to this is the "Guide to Inspection of Lyophilization of Parenterals"; this provides a useful indication of areas of specific interest to the FDA which the formulator would be well-advised to address during the development programme.

In addition to the regulatory guidelines, more detailed advice on specific issues relating to the development and manufacture of parenteral products can be obtained from the publications of the Parenteral Drug Association. This is an American organisation representing those involved in all aspects of parenteral product development and manufacture and is very active in lobbying the FDA. The PDA produces a bimonthly journal, the *PDA Journal of Pharmaceutical Science and Technology*, which is essential reading for all those involved in the development and manufacture of parenteral products. In addition, the PDA regularly publishes technical reports which provide a detailed discussion of pertinent issues within the parenteral field. Whilst these reports are not regulatory guidelines, they do provide a good indication of the direction in which the industry and indeed the regulators, are heading and those working in the field should take their recommendations seriously. Some of the recently published technical reports are listed below. In the United Kingdom, the Parenteral Society publishes a quarterly journal in conjunction with similar bodies in France, Germany, Scandinavia and Spain. This journal covers topics similar to those in the PDA journal. The Parenteral Society also publishes a number of monographs, some of which are listed below. These monographs provide a good indication of industry "norms" in the United Kingdom.

FDA Guidelines

Inspection Guidelines

- Guide to Inspection of Lyophilization of Parenterals

Guidance for Industry

- Container Closure Systems for Packaging Human Drugs and Biologics
- Submission of Documentation for Sterilization Process Validation in Applications for Human and Veterinary Drug Products
- Container Closure Integrity Testing *in Lieu* of Sterility Testing as a Component of the Stability Protocol for Sterile Products
- Stability Testing of Drug Substances and Drug Products

EMEA Guidelines

- Note for Guidance on Maximum Shelf-Life for Sterile Products for Human Use after First Opening or Following Reconstitution
- Notes for Guidance on Development Pharmaceutics
- Development Pharmaceutics for Biotechnological and Biological Products
- Decision Trees for the Selection of Sterilisation Methods
- Notes for Guidance on Inclusion of Antioxidants and Antimicrobial Preservatives in Medicinal Products

PDA Technical Reports

- Technical Report No. 22: Process Simulation Testing for Aseptically Filled Products, 50, S1, 1996
- Technical Report No. 23: Industry Survey on Current Sterile Filtration Practices, 51, S1, 1997
- Technical Report No. 24: Current Practices in the Validation of Aseptic Processing, 51, S2, 1997
- Technical Report No. 25: Blend Uniformity Analysis: Validation and In-Process Testing, 51, S3, 1997
- Technical Report No. 26: Sterilization Filtration of Liquids, 52, S1, 1998
- Technical Report No. 27: Pharmaceutical Package Integrity, 52, S2, 1998
- Technical Report No. 28: Process Simulation Testing for Sterile Bulk Pharmaceutical Chemicals, 52, S3, 1998
- Technical Report No. 29: Points to Consider for Cleaning Validation, 52, 6, 1998
- Technical Report No. 30: Parametric Release of Sterile Pharmaceuticals Terminally Sterilized by Moist Heat, 1999
- Technical Report No. 31: Validation and Qualification of Computerized Laboratory Data Acquisition Systems, 53, 4, 1999

REFERENCES

Agalloco, J. 1997. It Just Doesn't Matter. *J. Pharm. Sci. Technol.* 149–150

Avis, K. E., H. A. Lieberman, and L. Lachman, eds. 1992. *Pharmaceutical dosage forms: Parenteral medications, volume 1*. New York: Marcel Dekker.

Betageri, G. V., and M. J. Habib. 1994. Liposomes as drug carriers. *Pharm. Eng.* 14:8, 10, 12–14.

Cameron, P., ed. 1997. *Good pharmaceutical freeze-drying practice*. Buffalo Grove, Ill; USA: Interpharm Press, Inc.

Collins-Gold, L. C., R. T. Lyons, and L. C. Bartholow. 1990. Parenteral emulsions for drug delivery. *Adv. Drug Delivery Rev.* 5:189–208.

DeLuc and Boylan. 1992. In *Pharmaceutical dosage forms: Parenteral medications, Volume 1*. edited by K. E. Avis, H. A. Lieberman, and L. Lachman. New York: Marcel Dekker.

Ford, J. L. 1988. Parenteral products. In *Pharmaceutics: The science of dosage form design*. edited by M. E. Aulton. New York: Longman.

Flynn, G. L. 1980. Buffers—pH control within pharmaceutical systems. *J. Parenteral Drug Assoc.* 34 (2):139–162.

Gupta, L. S., J. P. Patel, D. L. Jones, and R. W. Partipilo. 1994a. Parenteral formulation development of renin inhibitor Abbott-72517. *J. Pharm. Sci. Technol.* 48 (2):86–91.

Gupta, P. K., J. P. Patel, and K. R. Hahn. 1994b. Evaluation of pain and irritation following local administration of parenteral formulations using the rat paw lick model. *J. Pharm. Sci. Technol.* 48 (3):159–166.

Hall, N. A. 1994. *Achieving sterility in medical and pharmaceutical products*. New York: Marcel Dekker.

Hansrani, P. K., S. S. Davis, and M. J. Groves. 1983. The preparation and properties of sterile intravenous emulsions. *J. Parenteral Sci. Technol.* 37 (4):145–150.

Jennings, T. A. 1999. *Lyophilization: Introduction and basic principles*. Denver, Colo., USA: Interpharm Press.

Jorgensen, J. T., J. Romsing, M. Rasmussen, J. Moller-Sonnergaard, and L. Musaeus. 1996. Pain assessment of subcutaneous injections. *Ann. Pharmacother.* 30:729–732.

Kirsch, L. E., L. Nguyen, and C. S. Moeckly. 1997a. Pharmaceutical container/closure integrity I: Mass spectrometry-based helium leak rate detection for rubber-stoppered glass vials. *PDA J. Pharm. Sci. Technol.* 51 (5):187–194.

Kirsch, L. E., L. Nguyen, C. S. Moeckly, and R. Gerth. 1997b. Pharmaceutical container/closure integrity II: The relationship between microbial ingress and helium leak rates in rubber-stoppered glass vials. *PDA J. Pharm. Sci. Technol.* 51 (5):195–202.

Kirsch, L. E., L. Nguyen, and R. Gerth. 1997c. Pharmaceutical container/closure integrity III: Validation of helium leak rate method for rigid pharmaceutical containers. *PDA J. Pharm. Sci. Technol.* 51 (5):203–207.

Kirsch, L. E., L. Nguyen, A. M. Kirsch, G. Schmidt, M. Koch, T. Wertli, M. Lehmann, and G. Schramm. 1999. An evaluation of the WILCO "LFC" method for leak testing pharmaceutical glass-stoppered vials. *PDA J. Pharm. Sci. Technol.* 53 (5):235–239.

Krzyzaniak, J. F. 1997. Lysis of human red blood cells. 4. Comparison of *in vitro* and *in vivo* hemolysis data. *Amer. Chem. Soc. Amer. Pharmaceut. Assoc.* 86 (11):1215–1217.

Madan, P. 1985. Sustained-release drug delivery systems: Part V, parenteral products. *Pharm. Manu.* 2:50–57.

Martin, F. J. 1999. Stealth liposomes: A pharmaceutical perspective. In *Microspheres, microcapsules and liposomes*, edited by R. Arshady. London: Citus.

MCA. 1997. Rules and guidance for pharmaceutical manufacturers and distributors. London: Medicines Control Agency.

Nema, S., R. J. Washkuhn, and R. J. Brendel. 1997. Excipients and their use in injectable products. *PDA J. Pharm. Sci. Technol.* 51 (4):166–171.

Nordhauser, F. M. and W. P. Olson, eds. 1998. *Sterilization of drugs and devices: Technologies for the 21st century*. Buffalo Grove, Ill., USA: Interpharm Press, Inc.

Powell, M. F., T. Nguyen, and L. Baloian. 1998. Compendium of excipients for parenteral formulations. *PDA J. Pharm. Sci. Technol.* 52 (5):238–311.

Stella, V. J. and R. A. Rajewski. 1997. Cyclodextrins: Their future in drug formulation and delivery. *Pharm. Res.* 14 (5):556–567.

Strickley, R. G. 1999. Parenteral formulations of small molecule therapeutics marketed in the United States (1999)—Part I. *PDA J. Pharm. Sci. Technol.* 53:324–349.

Sutton, S. C., L. A. F. Evans, T. S. Rinaldi, and K. A. Norton. 1996. Predicting injection site muscle damage I: Evaluation of immediate release parenteral formulations in animal models. *Pharm. Res.* 13 (10):1507–1513.

Sweetang, S., and M. J. Akers. 1996. Solubility principles and practices for parental dosage form development. *PDA J. Pharm. Sci. Technol.* 50 (5):330–342.

Takada, S., T. Kurokawa, K. Miyazaki, S. Iwasa, and Y. Ogawa. 1997. Utilization of an amorphous form of a water-soluble GPIIb/IIIa antagonist for controlled release from biodegradable microspheres. *Pharm. Res.* 14 (9):1146–1150.

Thompson, D. O. 1997. Cyclodextrins—Enabling excipients: Their present and future use in pharmaceuticals. *Crit. Rev. Ther. Drug Carrier Syst.* 14 (1):1–104.

Wakerley, Z. 1999. In vitro assessment of the haemolytic potential of marketed formulations. *AAPS Pharm. Sci. Suppl.* 1 (4):S-209.

Wang, Y. J., and R. Pearlman, eds. 1993. *Stability and characterization of protein and peptide drugs, Case histories*. New York: Plenum Press.

Yalkowsky, S. H., J. F. Krzyzaniak, and G. H. Ward. 1998. Formulation-related problems associated with intravenous drug delivery. *J. Pharm. Sci.* 87 (7):787–796.

Yalkowski, S. H., S. C. Valvani, and B. W. Johnson. 1983. *In vitro* method for detecting precipitation of parenteral formulations after injection. *J. Pharm. Sci.* 72:1014–1017.

10

Inhalation Dosage Forms

Paul Wright

AstraZeneca R&D Charnwood
Loughborough, United Kingdom

Asthma and chronic obstructive pulmonary diseases (COPDs) such as bronchitis and emphysema are major and growing disease areas where the major route of administration is topically, at the site of action in the lung. Asthma is a common, chronic disease with a prevalence of more than 5 percent in adults and 15–20 percent in children, and is increasing in many parts of the world. The prevalence of COPD is even higher, and mortality rates are 10 times higher than those for asthma. At present, similar drugs are used for both diseases, with steroids and short- and long-acting β2s being the most common therapies. Anticholinergics and chromones are also employed. Inhalation allows the delivery of smaller doses directly to the lungs, with the advantage of reduced systemic side-effects. There are also other illnesses where pulmonary delivery is appropriate, such as cystic fibrosis, human immunodeficiency virus (HIV), lung cancer, pain and infections. In addition, the lung is being increasingly viewed as a route to the systemic circulation for the treatment of non-respiratory diseases, where normal oral administration is not technically possible. This is especially relevant to the delivery of peptides and proteins, of which insulin is a good example.

Unlike most other drug delivery systems, those in the respiratory area can have a major influence on physician/patient acceptance. A wide range of devices are available in the three main categories of dry powder inhalers (DPIs) and metered dose inhalers (MDIs), i.e., pressurised aerosols and nebulisers. The preferred type of inhaler varies considerably between countries (e.g., DPIs in Scandinavia and MDIs in the United States), and between patient groups (e.g., nebulisers for paediatrics).

Until the mid-1980s, the MDI was the dominant inhalation dosage form, but the Montreal Protocol lead to greatly increased activity in device development, for both existing drugs and new chemical entities. The propellants for the existing MDIs were chlorofluorocarbons

(CFCs). CFCs were implicated in the depletion of the stratospheric ozone layer, and their phase-out was agreed on internationally in the United Nations–sponsored Montreal Protocol. CFC propelled MDIs were given a time-limited essential use exemption. MDIs propelled by hydrofluoroalkanes (HFAs), also known as hydrofluorocarbons (HFCs), are being introduced to the market after extensive safety testing of the propellants. However, HFAs do have a global warming potential, and they will be regulated by another international environmental agreement, the Kyoto Protocol. This is still being developed, but it is expected that HFAs will remain available, since no other suitable propellants have been identified. The banning of CFCs has also lead to a resurgence of DPI development.

A consequence of this development activity has been corresponding patent applications for both formulations and devices. The patenting process, together with oppositions, is a lengthy operation, and some major patents published in the early 1990s are only now being decided, leading to long periods of uncertainty. Hence, a current knowledge of the patent situation is essential before commencing any practical development studies. It should also be noted that, since this area is very competitive, much of the available information is in the patent literature rather than in the scientific journals. However, it should be noted that in this chapter the references are predominately from the scientific literature, since these better illustrate points of interest.

A last general point to be made here is to emphasise the complexity of inhalation products. They all contain a high degree of engineering, and it could be argued that the device is more critical than the formulation. This engineering dimension adds considerably to development times, since an alteration to a device component can typically take 2 to 3 months, and for a MDI, there is an additional 1 month equilibration time.

While the product is in the aerosol can or nebuliser vial, the dosage form that the patient experiences is a dynamic aerosol cloud. For example, the quality of the cloud from a DPI is often dependent on the airflow through the device, and a MDI cloud rapidly evaporates as it travels through the air. These factors affect the particle size distribution in the aerosol cloud, and the particle size is the critical parameter for lung deposition.

LUNG DEPOSITION

Particles are deposited in the lung by three main mechanisms, impaction, sedimentation and diffusion. Impaction is the primary mechanism, hence the relevance of impactors in particle sizing, which is discussed later. Deposition will vary, depending on the airflow and the disease state, as smaller airways due to bronchoconstriction or inflammation will increase impaction in the upper airways. An increased airflow will also lead to increased impaction in the throat and upper airways, hence patients are instructed to breath slowly and deeply. Some DPIs may conflict with this, since a high airflow is required for powder deaggregation. Sedimentation is a secondary deposition mechanism, occurring in the low airflow region of the deep lung, hence the requirement for patients to hold their breath after inhalation. Diffusion is a relatively slow process and is not very significant in the timescales of a breathing pattern, even with breath holding.

The classic diagram of deposition versus particle size is shown in Figure 10.1, but it should be noted that this is for a normal breathing pattern at low airflows.

There is often a need to test the efficiency of a product's lung delivery, and then *in vivo* measurements must be made. Any study is complicated by the fraction (often the majority) of

Figure 10.1 Lung deposition–deposition versus aerodynamic diameter.

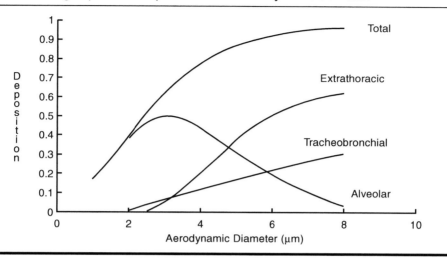

drug that is swallowed and passes into the gastro-intestinal system. The normal methods are a pharmacokinetic study or a gamma camera study. For pharmacokinetic work, the drug must either have no oral absorption or it can be negated by charcoal block absorption. This study will not give a picture of regional deposition in the lung, whereas a gamma camera study (either two- or three-dimensional) will show regional variations (Newman and Wilding 1998). A typical picture is shown in Figure 10.2 for deposition from a Turbuhaler®. Other technical approaches are urinary excretion and β2 drug challenge studies. In the challenge studies, the opening of the airways due to the β2 drug's pharmacological response can be measured by an increased ability to both inhale and exhale.

PARTICLE SIZING

The importance of particle sizing is that only small particles will reach the lung, since the nose and mouth will remove any larger particles. There is continuing debate as to what maximum size will reach the lung, but consensus is for around 5 to 7 μm. For alveoli penetration, a size of 3 μm is required, but very fine particles, below 1 μm, may be exhaled. It is the size of the droplets in the aerosol cloud that is important; for dry powders and fully evaporated liquid suspensions, this may be the original powder particle. Hence, it is essential to have powders in the micron range, and normal micronisation will usually produce a size of 1 to 3 μm. Newer techniques, such as supercritical fluid extraction, can produce smaller particles. Naturally, if the product is a solution, the particle size formed on evaporation of the solvent will depend on solution concentration.

Figure 10.2 Deposition from a Turbuhaler®.

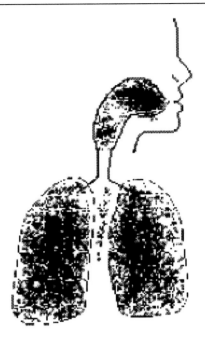

Impaction

As with most questions on particle size, the answer is very dependent on the definition used and the experimental technique. For a dynamic aerosol cloud, the correct definition is the aerodynamic particle size, which is the diameter of an equivalent sphere of unit density. An equivalent sphere is a conventional assumption in particle sizing, but for the aerodynamic size, the density is included to account for the momentum of the particle, i.e., both mass and velocity are important. The technique chosen for measurement must include these parameters, and impaction is the normally chosen technique, which also reflects the major deposition mechanism in the lung. A schematic of an impaction plate is given in Figure 10.3.

The mathematics of fluid dynamics which define the parameters are quite complex, but the critical ones are airflow, jet diameter and the jet-plate distance. A good analogy is driving a vehicle (the particle) around a sharp road bend (the change in airstream direction). A slow-moving car will navigate the bend, whilst a fast-moving car or a slow lorry will impact. In addition, impaction will measure a mass of drug on a particular plate, and hence is an unambiguous measurement.

A number of commercial impactors are built around this principle, the early ones being single stage, which have been superseded by multistage impactors, with both single and multiple jets. These are shown in Figure 10.4 for the Andersen-Graseby, Astra-Copley MSLI and the less common Marple-Miller. All of these impactors will provide a particle size distribution.

Figure 10.3 Impaction plate.

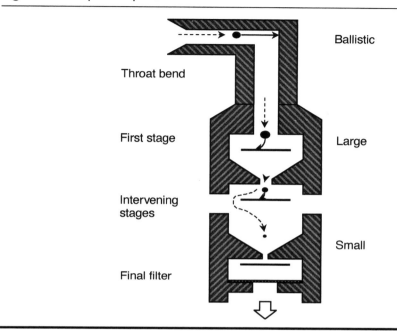

Figure 10.4 Commercial impactors.

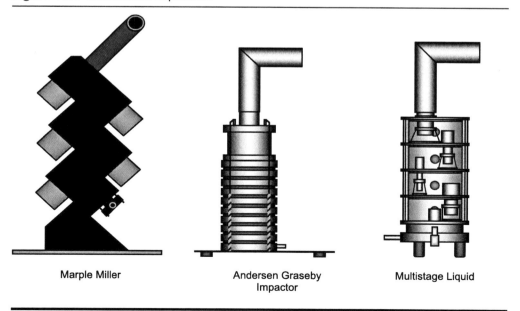

Marple Miller

Andersen Graseby
Impactor

Multistage Liquid

Depending on the dosage, different experimental criteria will be important. For MDIs, the cloud evaporates thus, the geometry of the entry port to the impactor is critical (LeBelle et al. 1997) and is well defined by the European Pharmacopoeia (EP) and the U. S. Pharmacopeia (USP). DPI performance will usually depend on the airflow through the device's aerosolisation mechanism (de Boer et al. 1997); an airflow corresponding to the device's air resistance should be chosen. The rise time to peak steady-state flow is important as well, because if it is too slow, the dose could be emitted as a bolus and not deaggregated to a fine cloud. Also the relative humidity of the air drawn through the device/impactor can have an influence, with high humidities reducing the deaggregation.

Impactor testing is very labour intensive, and some robot systems are in use for this purpose. These are often very expensive, as they mechanically take the impactor apart, wash off the drug for assay and then dry and reassemble the equipment. An industry consortium has been formed to design and develop a new multistage impactor with improved operating characteristics, which will be capable of easy automation at a reasonable price.

The discussion so far has related to the use of impactors for *in vitro* measurements used in formulation and/or device optimisation, stability testing or quality control. If the purpose of testing is to gain information on a potential *in vitro/in vivo* correlation, then modifications are sometimes made to the equipment. For MDIs, the use of an anatomical throat instead of the USP throat can improve correlation, while for DPIs, a lung machine which reproduces breathing patterns can be beneficial.

Light Scattering (Laser)

A number of commercial machines (e.g., the Malvern Mastersizer) use the light scattering technique, and for aerosol clouds, its main applicability is the sizing of essentially stationary clouds from nebuliser solutions. Here again, definitions are important, as different theories of light scattering may give different results. It is vital to distinguish between number and mass average, as the presence of relatively few large particles can give a low number particle size, but a high mass particle size, which is the important parameter.

Microscope

Microscopy is not relevant to aerodynamic particle size, since the particles are stationary on the microscope slide. The technique is, however, asked for by some regulatory agencies. It is of value during development for examining deaggregation or Ostwald ripening.

Phase Doppler Anemometry

Phase Doppler anemometry is a specialised research technique which gives information on both particle size and velocity of single particles within the cloud.

High-Speed Camera

By image analysis of single photographs, a particle size distribution can be established, but only the physical diameter is measured, not the aerodynamic component. However, it is of great value to see the establishment and decay of an aerosol cloud in slow motion. High-speed video is also possible, which gives an excellent picture of the changing aerosol cloud.

DRY POWDER INHALERS

Fisons introduced the first DPI with the capsule-based Spinhaler®. This was followed by a number of other capsule devices and then by unit dose blisters and multidose systems. DPIs are very diverse in their design and operation, since each product manufacturer has developed their own proprietary devices for their own drugs.

Formulation

The main formulation challenges come from the need to use very cohesive micronised powders, which presents problems in powder flow (Feeley et al. 1998) on filling machinery. These powders also aerosolise poorly in an airstream and give a deaggregated cloud. Unfortunately, the formulation approaches are severely limited by the very restricted number of excipients available, due to a lack of lung administration safety data. Lactose is the only excipient commonly used. Other sugars maybe considered (Naini et al. 1998), if the drug contains primary amine groups which will give the Maillard reaction, which leads to a brown discolouration with lactose (see "Compatibility" in Chapter 6 for examples).

The objective is an ordered mix of the micronised drug with larger particle size lactose (Larhrib et al. 1999), typically 60 μm, but it can be in the range of 40 to 100 μm. Mixing such a cohesive system is difficult, and often a high-energy mixer is required, together with sieving(s) to aid homogeneity (Zeng et al. 2000).

Determination of homogeneity is challenging at the level of a single dose, e.g., 5–20 mg of powder, and sampling errors with thief systems are possible (Muzzio et al. 1997). Often the best sampling system is the device itself, since further powder handling will occur during device filling. The balance of interparticle forces is very important, because a drug particle needs to be strongly attached to the lactose carrier during mixing, filling and on stability, yet becomes easily detached on aerosolisation to form a fine particle cloud (Podczeck 1998). Hence, attention must be paid to surface morphology and surface energies (Kawashima et al. 1998). If the powder mix is to go into a unit dose system, such as a capsule or blister, then the particle need not be so strongly attached as for a free-flowing reservoir system where segregation could occur.

A second approach is to spheronise the micronised particles, which gives a free-flowing powder which should break down easily on aerosolisation. The advantage is that there is no risk of poor homogeneity or segregation, but this is balanced by the difficulty of metering minute quantities of powders (spheres are typically 100–250 μg).

During unit operations, such as milling and mixing, at pilot plant or at full production scale, it is very easy to produce a powder cloud. Since the particles in this cloud can be inhaled, it is vital to protect the operator's safety by appropriate containment measures and personal protection equipment.

Devices

As stated earlier, there is little commonality between devices, although some are now available for in-licensing. This diversity makes general comment difficult, but there are three main categories:

1. Pre-metered single dose, e.g., capsule

2. Pre-metered multidose as single units, e.g., blisters on a card

3. Multidose bulk reservoir

Examples of these classes are shown in Figure 10.5.

The aerosolisation operation depends on effective turbulence being created in the airstream which lifts the powder from its metering position and carries it to the device's mouthpiece. This can be done by a number of mechanisms, such as a mesh, an orifice on a swirl chamber. All of these methods introduce turbulence to provide the energy to remove the individual drug particle from the charge carrier particle surface or the spheronised aggregate. Computational fluid dynamics (CFD) is being increasingly used to model airflows in devices, with the consequent saving in time and expense of manufacturing models, and of testing them. Each programme must be tailored to a specific device, however, and the results validated by experimental results.

Naturally, the development of the device must involve the formulation, as the engineering cannot be optimised in isolation, and close collaboration is required between formulators and design engineers.

Device design often commences with the aerosolisation mechanism, since the fine particle dose reaching the lung is the critical therapeutic dose. This is often a crude mechanism to show proof of principle. However, for regulatory constraints, the metering system is more important, and this is often given insufficient attention in the early stages of a project.

Figure 10.5 Device categories (clockwise from left): single-capsule, Spinhaler™ (Aventis), multi-dose reservoir, Pulmicort™ (AstraZeneca), multi-dose reservoir, Asmasal™ Clickhaler™ (Medeva), and multi-dose pre-metered, Flixotide™ Accuhaler™ (GlaxoWellcome).

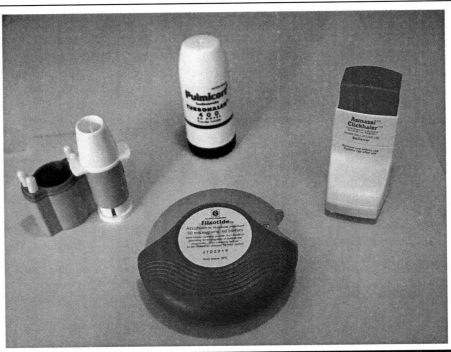

The next stage is to produce a working model which may be produced by a craftsman or, more probably, with modern technology, by soft moulds linked to a computer-aided design (CAD) system. At this stage, the project becomes complex, as almost always the engineering aspects are dealt with by an external company, even if the design work is internal.

It is essential to involve the eventual plastic moulder at this stage, since any design must be capable of production, and mould design together with plastic flow is a very specialised activity. Also, an early involvement from market research, industrial design and ergonomics is required, since the operation of the device should be heavily influenced by the user's opinion. This is the same for any consumer market product, e.g., a hair-drier. In market research, doctors, asthma nurse practitioners, patients and parents of paediatrics should all be consulted in a number of countries, since they have very different requirements for a device. Non-working models produced by stereoligography can often be used for these studies. For large quantities of working models, a single hard tool will be used.

Operation

In optimising the product, both device and formulation are modified, and the normal product release tests are evaluated. Extra investigations are also carried out, such as a standard drop test to ensure that the device is robust. Other major areas for investigation are the dependence of fine particle dose on airflow rate (Srichana et al. 1998), the effect of humidity both on storage (Naini et al. 1998), Maggi et al. 1999) and in-use, drug retention within the device, the effect of orientation and electrostatics (Carter et al. 1998).

Scale-up/Technology Transfer

For the formulation, there is a significant problem of increasing the mass of powder during blending and especially for spheronisation, since a large mass can break down fragile spheres. Powder processing is usually carried out at controlled relative humidity (RH), usually <50 percent RH.

Devices are assembled typically from 15 to 20 individual components, and each will be produced on a multicavity mould with four or eight moulds. Until this stage is reached, with devices being assembled from these production moulds, and then tested, the final variability between devices cannot be fully established. However, during development, appropriate engineering and tolerance analyses can give good confidence. The device will be delivered from the moulders with a minimum number of subassemblies and will be filled with the formulation at the pharmaceutical company. In the case of unit dose devices, the capsule or blister will usually be filled at the pharmaceutical company.

The transfer of analytical methodology is a major part of technology transfer, especially when robotics are involved.

Future Developments

At present, many DPI products are dependent on being operated by the patient. This will be reduced by the introduction of powered devices, e.g., compressed air, a fan or a hammer, and, in this way, they will be independent of airflow rate.

Such an increase in complexity, however, will probably require the introduction of a breath activation feature. Powder spaces may also be introduced.

A major question is how much market share DPIs will capture, balancing their environmental friendliness with patient acceptance, especially in the major American market.

METERED DOSE INHALERS

Riker Laboratories, now 3M Healthcare, invented the pressurised metered dose inhaler (MDI) in 1955 when they combined the atomising power of CFCs and a metering valve design. The great majority of valves still use this basic retention valve principle, and hence pressurised MDIs (pMDIs) are all similar in appearance and operation when used with a standard actuator in the normal "press and breathe" manner.

Formulation

Environment

CFC propelled pMDIs are still on the market, but as this book is being written the transition to HFAs (or HFCs) is well under way. The reason for this transition is that all CFCs are implicated in the destruction of the ozone layer due to a reaction between the ozone and the chlorine radical (see Table 10.1, Figure 10.6). Consequently the production and use of CFCs has been banned by the United Nations Montreal Protocol, but medicinal aerosols have been given an essential use exemption due to their vital performance in asthma and COPD therapy (Forte and Dibble 1999). The transition to HFAs has been slower than expected, as the change from CFCs to HFAs was not just a drop-in excipient change, as was first believed. A major development programme has been necessary involving the valve. This has taken approximately 10 years for most companies, and HFA products did not begin to reach the market in Europe until 1999.

Because CFCs are being relegated to history, this chapter will concentrate on the new HFAs. Three main factors control formulation approaches, and only one of these is pharmaceutical in nature. HFA 227 and HFA 134a are very poor solvents, hence the existing CFC surfactants/valve lubricants are not soluble in the HFAs. The second factor which is related is that any new surfactant must have adequate drug safety data, and this could mean a full New

Table 10.1
Environmental actions of propellants.

Propellant	Ozone Depletion Potential	Global Warming Potential[a]
CFC 11	1.0	4000
CFC 12	1.0	8500
CFC 114	1.0	9300
HFA 134a	0	1300
HFA 227	0	2900

[a]Carbon dioxide = 1.

Figure 10.6 Formulae of CFCs and HFAs.

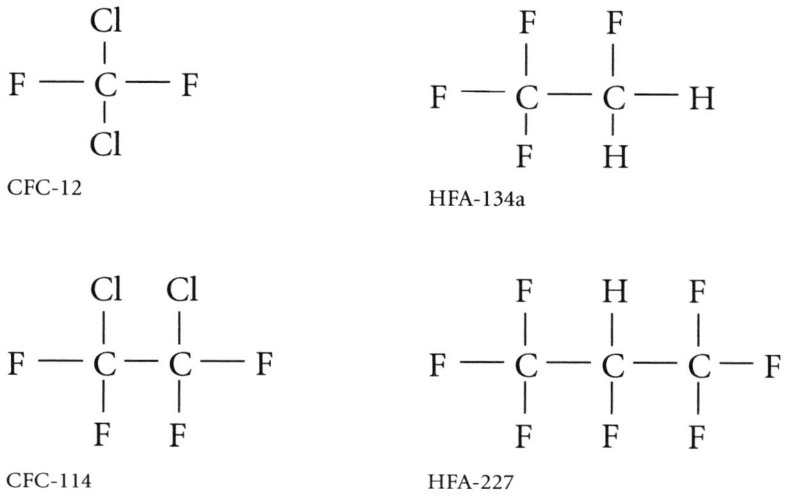

Chemical Entity (NCE) type safety testing programme. The third factor is the large number of often conflicting and overlapping patents in this area, many of which have not yet been granted or are being opposed (Bowman et al. 1999). The worldwide patent situation must be considered, since although a patent may have been revoked in Europe, it could have been granted in Australia and still be the subject of prosecution in the United States. Important examples are shown in Table 10.2, but the list is definitely not exhaustive.

Propellant Properties

The properties of the propellants are the dominant factors in formulation development for an MDI. Many formulation approaches are dictated by the fact that the HFAs are poorer solvents than the CFCs, which in absolute terms are already poor solvents, for both drugs and excipients. However, the main purpose of the propellant, as its name suggests, is to provide the energy to propel the drug from the valve in the form of droplets, which rapidly evaporate to leave the drug particles. Certain propellant properties are shown in Table 10.3.

Solution Formulations

Due to the very poor solvent properties of HFAs, only a very limited number of drugs, e.g., beclomethasone diproprionate, may dissolve completely in the propellant with or without an ethanol co-solvent (Williams et al. 1999). For a solution, the crucially important factor of suspension homogeneity is almost guaranteed, but other problems increase, relating to drug adsorption into valve rubbers and drug reactivity leading to degradation. When the valve is

Table 10.2
Important formulation patents.

Ethanol/HFA-134a	3M Healthcare
EP 0372777	Priority Date 06/12/88
HFA-227 and mixtures	Boehinger Ingelheim
EP 513099	Priority Date 03/02/90
EP 514415	
HFA Propellant only	Glaxo
WO 93/11744	Priority Date 12/12/91
PVP/PEG/HFA	Fisons (Aventis)
WO 93/05765	Priority Date 25/9/91

actuated, the propellant will evaporate leaving a precipitated particle which may well be of smaller size than that from a suspension prepared from a micronised drug. This in turn, may lead to higher fine particle fraction and increased lung deposition (Leach 1999). For a new drug, this potential increased efficiency is excellent, but it may be a problem for a generic match to an existing suspension product, as the label dose will be less, leading to possible confusion. One way of avoiding this situation is to add a non-volatile miscible liquid, e.g., polyethylene glycol, which will maintain an aerosol drop in the micrometer-size range.

Suspension Formulations

Many of the principles here are the same as for normal oral aqueous suspensions, except that the liquid is essentially non-polar, hence steric stabilisation is thought to be more important than by electrostatic means (DLVO theory). A stabilising agent is normally added to give an adequate suspension. The agent may also act as a valve lubricant, which may be necessary for

Table 10.3
Propellant properties.

Name (HFA-)	Formula	Pressure (psig @ 20°C)	Density (kg/L @ 20°C)	Water Solubility (ppm)
11	CCl_3F	−1.8	1.488	~100
114	$CClF_2CClF_2$	11.9	1.471	~100
12	CCl_2F_2	67.6	1.329	~100
12/114	60:40	49.0	1.387	
134a	CF_3CH_2F	68.0	1.226	~2000
227	CF_3CHFCF_3	41.9	1.415	~600

this mechanical device, or a second excipient may be added for this function. The potential effect of water ingress through the valve rubbers by Fickian diffusion should be investigated, since this may well destabilise the suspension.

Moisture may well be preferentially adsorbed at the particle surface, leading to a microenvironment in this region which can alter the performance of the surfactant. Another important attribute is to density match the drug particle, by blending HFA-227 and HFA-134a, where possible, since a homogeneous (Williams et al. 1998a) suspension is vital for filling uniform aliquots into the dispensing valve. Fast aggregation into loose flocs is not always a problem, since the turbulence in the aerosol stream when the valve is actuated is high, and often enough to deaggreate any such flocs.

There are three main approaches to suspension formulation. The first is to add a co-solvent to the propellant to increase its solvency power and enable the dissolution of conventional CFC surfactants such as oleic acid or sorbitan trioleate (Span) (Fedina et al. 1997). This is usually only employed with HFA 134a, since the addition of a co-solvent, usually ethanol, will lower the vapour pressure of the system and lead to larger droplets in the aerosol cloud which may then be too large to be inhaled (Steckel and Muller 1998; Williams et al. 1998b). Investigations must be made to ensure that the co-solvent for the surfactant is not also acting as a co-solvent for the drug, since even a slight solubility of the drug will lead to particle growth through Ostwald ripening.

A second approach is to use a new excipient which is soluble in the propellant only (Blondino and Byron 1998). HFA-227 is a better solvent than HFA-134a, hence most references to new surfactants (e.g., polyvinylpyrrolidone) relate to HFA-227. A third approach is not to use any excipients, the formulation here being only drug and propellant. In such a system, the suspension is expected to be more sensitive to challenges than in a more robust one containing surfactants. In these excipient-free systems, the ability of the propellant to wet the drug surface may be crucial.

Devices

The hardware for a pMDI (Figure 10.7) is as crucial as, or perhaps even more important than, the formulation. A normal "press and breathe" MDI consists of the can, valve and actuator (also sometimes called an adapter). The three components are sourced externally.

Can

The container is normally made of aluminium, and although plastic coated glass is available, it is normally only used for experimental work where direct observation of the contents is required. Stainless steel is also available, but this is too expensive for production. Drug particles in HFA suspensions have a much greater tendency to stick to the can walls than in CFC systems, and for this reason, certain formulations require the aluminium to be coated with a polymer, usually a fluoropolymer, to reduce or remove this deleterious phenomenon.

Valves

Retention valves all have a similar design and are normally bought from Valois (Figure 10.8), Bespak or 3M Neotechnic, although smaller suppliers do exist (e.g., Sprühventile). The retention valve operates in a manner analogous to canal lock gates, with an opening either to the bulk formulation in the can or to the atmosphere via the actuator.

Figure 10.7 pMDI.

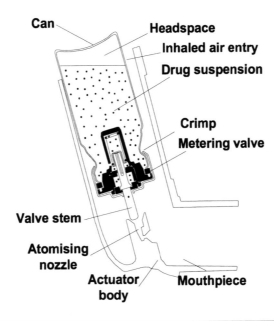

When the valve is depressed for firing, a direct pathway is opened to the atmosphere, and the vapour pressure of the propellant drives the boiling formulation out of the valve chamber to form the aerosol cloud. When the valve is released, this pathway to the atmosphere is closed; and in the "at rest" position, a small passageway of varying design is opened to the bulk formulation. This then fills the valve chamber, again driven by the propellant vapour pressure. This small passageway remains open to the can, but its narrow bore is designed to prevent emptying of the valve chamber due to surface tension.

Other valve designs exist which do not have a retention chamber, but the metering chamber is formed to collect an aliquot of bulk suspension as the valve is being operated. These designs are relatively uncommon.

Although valves appear to be standard items, each must be individually optimised for the particular formulation, in detailed design and, very importantly, with regard to the rubbers, where swell characteristics can control valve performance (Tiwari et al. 1998).

Actuator

The actuator can be obtained as a standard item or is often designed to give a company house style. The critical parameters are the expansion chamber where evaporation commences and the orifice diameter which controls the droplet particle size (Steckel and Muller 1998). If orifice diameter is too large, the droplet particle size is too great, and if too small, excessive drug deposition and blockage can occur.

Figure 10.8 Retention valve (Valois RCS).

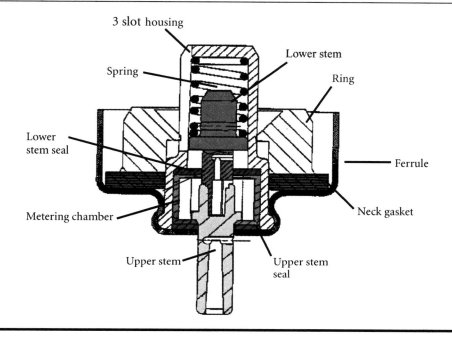

Operation

On operation, the interaction of the formulation and the valve must be considered. A major area is the performance of the valve rubbers, which can be determined only when their swelling due to propellant has reached equilibrium, which may take up to four weeks. If the rubber seals grip the valve stem too tightly, then the valve will stick, and excessive force will be required to actuate it. It may return to its rest position only under the spring force, but slowly. Alternatively, if the rubber seal to the valve stem is too loose, an alternative pathway for escape of propellant is formed, and on actuation, liquid escapes around the metering chamber (Cummings 1999). Leakage is also possible, such as gross leakage from a poorly crimped valve or low losses, on storage, from Fickian diffusion through the rubber seals. Due to its smaller molecular weight, HFA-134a has a higher loss rate than HFA-227.

There is also the possibility of loss of drug from the metering chamber on storage (Cummings 1999). This can occur if propellant drains out of the metering chamber and is known as "loss of prime", since the valve has to be primed before it is ready for use.

Another factor is that, on storage, the drug in the metering chamber may sediment, and even with shaking the can may not redisperse. Since the valve chamber is full, there is very little turbulence.

Suspension stability is very important since the valve refills after actuation, and, depending on patient use, a varying time can elapse from the can being shaken to the valve being actuated. An informative experiment is to shake the can, leave it for varying periods up to 60 sec and then actuate and collect the dose. With increasing time lapses, the drug may increase (sedimentation) or decrease (creaming). This is important for patient usage, because patients can take a considerable time to coordinate breathing, or assemble a spacer (Blondino and Byron 1998).

An alternative experiment is to use the optical suspension characterisation (OSCAR) technique, where the turbidity at the bottom and/or top of a transparent vial is measured with time to obtain a plot of sedimentation or creaming.

Scale-up

Initial formulation work, when tens of cans are required, is often carried out by cold filling, where the propellants are cooled to below their boiling point, and can then be processed as liquids without any pressure implications. This method was often used for full-scale production for CFCs, since propellant 11 has a boiling point of 23°C. However, both HFA-134a and HFA-227 have low boiling points; therefore, pressure filling is more common for the HFA propellants.

Here the formulation is made up to between a 500 and 1000 L scale in pressurised vessels and then filled into cans through the aerosol valve, precrimped onto the can. Naturally, appropriate safety precautions have to be made for working with large-scale pressurised systems. With increasing scale, there is the move to increasing automation of the filling process.

For the components, the move to hard tooling multicavity moulds for the actuator has the same implications as for DPI components, e.g., dimensions must be checked. Valves can be assembled by hand, semi-automatically or on fully automated production lines. It is important to obtain valves during development from the production line, if this is possible. A valve is constructed of 15 to 20 individual items, plastic, metal and rubber, and a number of different batches of an item may be used in a major production run. Hence, valves from a production run may well not be from the same item batches, and the definition of a production batch then becomes important.

Add-on Devices

As well as the standard actuator mouthpiece, sometimes known as "press and breathe", which describes its mode of action, there are a number of supplementary devices whose main function is to aid coordination. One of the major disadvantages of pMDIs is the need for the patient to coordinate firing the device with inhalation.

Breath-Activated Inhaler

Breath-activated inhalers (BAIs), developed by Norton and 3M Healthcare, are now relatively common. Although each has a different mechanical design, both work by a trigger threshold of airflow activating the pre-loaded can, and hence firing the pMDI. This ensures that the patient is inhaling at a medium airflow when the aerosol is fired.

Spacer

A spacer or chamber is a second way to improve co-ordination (see Figure 10.9).

The MDI is actuated as normal, but into the spacer, not the patient's mouth. The patient then inhales from the other end of the spacer, sometimes through a one-way valve. This again ensures coordination. A pMDI plus spacer is a common system used for young children,

Figure 10.9 Spacer.

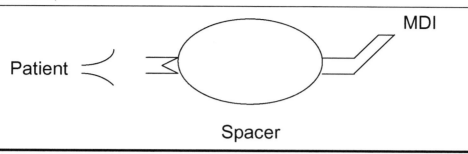

Spacer

sometimes with a face mask (Finlay 1998). Most spacers are plastic, and an electrostatic charge can build up on the plastic and attract the aerosol cloud, depositing it on the walls and significantly reducing the dose. This is especially true for unused spacers but can be reduced by washing with detergents. A metal spacer is also available which has negligible electrostatics.

A second advantage of spacers is that the large particles are deposited on the walls before finer particles, hence the dose inhaled consists of a higher percentage of fine inhalable particles. Conversely, a lower amount of non-respirable particles are deposited in the mouth and throat, where local side-effects can occur, especially for steroids.

Slowing the Cloud

The Spacehaler® slows the aerosol cloud as well as removing the larger sized particles, thereby making coordination easier.

Dose Counter

With the advent of mechanically complex BAIs, the possibility of incorporating a dose counter is more likely, and these are expected to be available in the near future. Dose counters will enable parents to check if their child has taken his medicine and will enable everyone to establish when the can is empty. Patients should not be advised to float the can in water to gauge its contents, as potential water ingress is disastrous to formulation stability.

Future

An exhaustive search for new propellants was made at the time of the switch away from CFCs, and it is unlikely that new ones will be found with the necessary physicochemical properties combined with an excellent safety profile. New surfactants are possible, but there is the major cost hurdle of drug toxicity studies to NCE standards. Particle engineering may provide benefits, e.g., production by supercritical fluid technology.

Devices are starting to appear, which contain electronics and batteries (e.g., BAI and Aradigm), and this allows the possibilities for extensive feedback to both patient and physician. (see Figure 10.10 for auxiliary devices.)

Figure 10.10 Auxiliary devices (from left to right): rear: Nebuchamber™ (AstraZeneca), Volumatic™ (Allen&Hanburys); spacers, front: Flutide™MDI (GlaxoWellcome), Qvar™ MDI (3M Health Care), Easi-breathe BAI (Baker Norton).

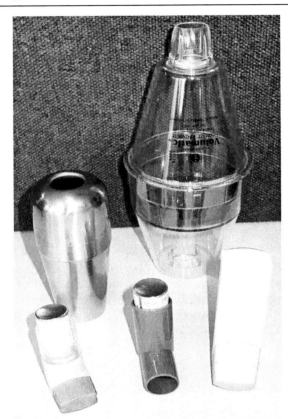

NEBULISERS

Nebuliser therapy is different, from the developer's perspective, to DPIs or pMDIs, in that nebuliser formulations and machines are developed and sold by independent companies. Hence, the formulator will take an existing commercial nebuliser machine(s) and will ensure that the formulation performs satisfactorily. Also, the target population is different, with nebulisers often being used in the hospital setting and for paediatric and geriatric patients.

Phase I Studies

It can take many months to develop an acceptable DPI or pMDI for early clinical studies, but an expeditious route is to use an extemporaneously prepared nebuliser solution of the drug and a matching placebo. This can be developed relatively quickly with only 24 h stability required (drug and microbiology) and the performance of the solution in the nebuliser established. Naturally, the drug must have suitable physicochemical properties, e.g., solubility. Sterility is not specifically required for Phase I formulation. Instead, sterile water for injection is used, and the shelf-life restricted to one working day, e.g., 8 h.

Formulation

The formulation techniques and approaches are essentially similar to those for sterile products such as parenterals or ophthalmics (chapters 9 and 12, respectively), hence the issues surrounding the production and validation of sterile solutions will not be considered here. Formulations are usually solutions, often giving a higher unit dose than the corresponding DPI or pMDI. Suspensions can also be formulated, although these are rare and usually relate to steroids. It is more difficult to get a drug particle taken up into a nebulised/aerosolised droplet; thus, a small particle size is essential (Ostrander et al. 1999), as it must naturally be significantly smaller than the droplet size, which itself has to be small to reach the lung. There are also major sterility difficulties with suspensions, since they cannot be produced asceptically using sterile filters. Because of their potential to cause bronchoconstriction, preservatives are not good practice and hence most formulations are unit dose unpreserved. Isotonicity of the solution, however, is favoured for the same reason. If the drug itself is not sufficient, normal isotonicity agents are added, e.g., sodium chloride. Naturally, if the drug solution is already hypertonic, little can be done.

The unit dose is either glass or plastic, with the use of plastic "form-fill-seal" equipment being dominant. However, glass is considered more elegant pharmaceutically in some markets, and can be terminally sterilised where this is a requirement. With "form-fill-seal" processes, a strip of ampoules is produced, with the neck being much easier to break than glass. The plastic is pervious to moisture transmission, which will occur on storage, especially in dry environments; thus an aluminium overwrap may be necessary.

In clinical practice, nebuliser solutions are mixed, and it is essential to check if the product interacts with any of the common commercial products.

Nebuliser Devices

Nebulisers are designed and supplied by medical equipment manufacturers, not by pharmaceutical companies. They range considerably in their effectiveness (Le Brun et al. 1999a), some producing droplets at around 3 μm for delivery to the deep lung, while others have such large particle sizes that they are only useful as room humidifiers. It is essential during clinical trials to ensure that all investigators are using an acceptable nebuliser, and, preferably, standardisation has occurred to a number of units. These machines should span the normal performance of nebulisers, otherwise the product may be limited to the one nebuliser used in the clinical trials by a regulatory authority. There are two types of nebulisers: pneumatic and, more recently introduced, ultrasonic (Flament et al. 1995).

Operation

The pharmaceutical company sells only the sterile ampoule, and release tests are really restricted to a sterile unit dose. Dose uniformity is for the contents of the vial, while aerosolisation is not considered for any release tests. How well the ampoule empties must be considered.

In operation, the liquid is placed into the nebuliser chamber, the machine is switched on and the aerosol cloud is produced (Dunbar and Hickey 1999). An important aspect of operation is the rate of nebulisation which controls how long the patient will take to receive the maximum dose (Le Brun et al. 1999b). A short time is preferable, since long times lead to poor compliance, with 10 to 20 min being typical. The volume of solution left in the nebuliser cup (dead volume) is also important, as this will control the dose available to the patient. Available dose is often approximately 1 mL. 50 percent of a 2 mL vial, but only 25 percent of a 4 mL vial (or 2 × 2 mL). During nebulisation, concentration can increase, and the liquid temperature can rise. For nebulisers, the aerosol cloud is produced by a power source and is almost stationary. Hence, laser diffraction (e.g., Malvern) methods can be used to size solutions where a homogeneous distribution of drug will occur. It is important to distinguish between number average and mass average, since many small drops will only carry a small percentage of the dose. Impactors can be used, but water drops will evaporate in the airstream, giving an erroneous particle size.

A face mask is often used with a nebuliser, to promote compliance over the 10–20 min of dosing, and any lengths of tubing between machine and face mask should be minimal, to prevent excessive wall losses.

STANDARDS

Regulatory and pharmacopoeial standards are always important in any development programme. Normally, they are limited to the main parameters and change only slowly. The technology available at present enables the standards to be achieved relatively easily. However, for inhalation dose forms, the regulatory and pharmacopoeial standards have been under constant revision since the late 1980s and continue to be so. In addition, they can be very extensive and are at, or perhaps sometimes beyond, the limit of current technology. These statements apply especially to U.S. Food and Drug Administration (FDA) specifications. This activity is occurring in Europe and North America (Canada is quite active), while Japan at present is dormant in this area, probably reflecting the unpopularity of DPIs and MDIs in Japan.

A brief review of the situation in early 2000 follows, but it is essential to know the present official standards and to be aware of the draft guidelines at any time in the future. Draft guidelines can be obtained from the FDA, the European Agency for the Evaluation of Medicinal Products (EMEA) and the Committee for Proprietary Medicinal Products (CPMP) Web sites and from the publications *Pharmaceutical Forum* and *Pharm. Europa*. There is relatively good harmonisation between the European Pharmacopoeia (EP), USP and CPMP, but not the FDA. Terminology is also important, with dose in the United States often expressed as ex-actuator, while in Europe it can be ex-valve. Naturally, the universal definition of dose uniformity also applies to respiratory systems, with the United States defining it around the target/label claim, while Europe defines it around the practically found mean. The former is perhaps more relevant, while the latter is more meaningful statistically. Dose and dose uniformity are always important parameters but are critical for MDIs and DPIs, since these are very challenging to achieve. Other parameters are excessively time consuming, e.g., extractives testing, or perhaps unnecessary, e.g., microscope tests for particle size.

In 1999, the Pulmonary Division of FDA issued draft guidelines for MDIs, DPIs and nebuliser systems (FDA 1998) which reflect their current thinking, and are now undergoing a review process with the Inhalation Technology Focus Group of the American Association of Pharmaceutical Scientists (AAPS) and industry groups. The CPMP stated its intention to issue update guidelines for MDIs, and there was a period of consultation during the second half of 2000. Also, the USP Aerosol Subcommittee was to reconvene in 2000, and there is a possibility of the EP Inhalanda working party also being reinstituted. The overall critical issue is one of harmonisation so that a global industry has one unified set of standards with which to work. Important issues are dose uniformity, fine particle fraction and not replicating testing for components and finished product.

There is also a parallel regulatory route for free-standing inhalation devices which are supplied without the drug, e.g., nebuliser machines, spacers and some BAIs. In this case, they are controlled by a different division of the FDA, and in Europe by a separate organisation known as the Device Directorate, although there are proposals for combining it with the pharmaceutical EMEA. It is important to recognise early in development if your product will require device authorisation, since the regulations are different following an International Organization for Standardization (ISO) pathway and not Standard Operating Procedures (SOPs) and Good Manufacturing Practice (GMP), and it is not easy to integrate the two systems.

FUTURE

Disease Types

At present, inhalation is known mainly for treating asthma, but its use in COPD, caused mainly by smoking, will gain greater recognition, since there are significantly more patients in this group. Here, delivery systems will be tailored for the elderly. Other forms of lung treatment, such as the delivery of antibiotics or drugs for cystic fibrosis, will continue, but in the medium term, oral drugs for asthma/COPD may become more important. For example, a number of leukotriene angonists have been launched.

An advancing area is the use of inhalation for systemic delivery via the alveoli in the deep lung. This avoids "first-pass" metabolism and the acid environment of the stomach, and hence is particularly suitable for bio molecules which otherwise would be delivered parenterally. A good example here is insulin, which is at present in Phase III trials by three separate companies—two DPIs and one aqueous system.

Future molecules from the biotechnology industry may be very expensive, and thus it is essential to maximise lung deposition even with the use of somewhat large devices. The cost element may also drive the device to unit dose, which is against the trend for asthma/COPD.

Delivery Systems

Technical attributes of DPIs and MDIs may converge, as BAIs become standard for MDIs, thus overcoming coordination problems, and as power sources are fitted to DPIs, they will become then independent of a patient's inspiratory ability. In addition, more information will be available to the patient and doctor, ranging from simple dose counters to sophisticated electronic recording and playback facilities for compliance, measuring peak flows or firing a device at a particular point in the inspiratory cycle to maximise lung deposition in a particular area of the lung.

Nebuliser machines are quite poorly controlled within a regulatory framework, and this will be improved. A major introduction will be the small portable multidose aqueous systems known as aqueous (aq) MDIs, or small volume nebulisers (SVNs), which are in development (Steed et al. 1997).

REFERENCES

Blondino, F. E., and P. R. Byron. 1998. Surfactant dissolution and water solubilization in chlorine-free liquified gas propellants. *Drug Dev. Ind. Pharm.* 24 (10):935–945.

Bowman, P. A., and D. Greenleaf. 1999. Non-CFC metered dose inhalers: The patent landscape. *Int. J. Pharmaceut.* 186:91–94.

Brambilla, G., D. Ganderton, R. Garzia, D. Lewis, B. Meakin, and P. Ventura. 1999. Modulation of aerosol clouds produced by pressurised inhalation aerosols. *Int. J. Pharmaceut.* 186:53–61.

Carter, P. A., G. Rowley, E. J. Fletcher, and V. Stylianopoulos. 1998. Measurement of electrostatic charge decay in pharmaceutical powders and polymer materials used in dry powder inhaler devices. *Drug Dev. Ind. Pharm.* 24 (11):1083–1088.

Cummings, R. H. 1999. Pressurized metered dose inhalers: Chlorofluorocarbon to hydrofluoroalkane transition—Valve performance. *J. Allergy Clin. Immunol.* 104 (6):S230.

de Boer, A. H., G. K. Bolhuis, D. Gjaltema, and P. Hagedoorn. 1997. Inhalation characteristics and their effects on in vitro drug delivery from dry powder inhalers. Part 3: The effect of flow increase rate (FIR) on the in vitro drug release from the Pulmicort 200 Turbohaler. *Int. J. Pharmaceut.* 153:67–77.

Dunbar, C. A., and A. J. Hickey. 1999. Selected parameters affecting characterisation of nebulized aqueous solutions by inertial impaction and comparison with phase-Doppler analysis. *Eur. J. Pharmaceut. Biopharmaceut.* 48:171–177.

FDA. 1998. *Guidance for industry: MDI and DPI drug products.* Rockville, Md., USA: Food and Drug Administration.

Fedina, L. T., R. Zelko, L. I. Fedina, Z. S. Szabados, M. Szanto, and G. Vakulya. 1997. The effect of surfactant and suspending agent concentration on the effective particle size of metered-dose inhalers. *J. Pharm. Pharmacol.* 49:1175–1177.

Feeley, J. C., P. York, B. S. Sumby, and H. Dicks. 1998. Determination of surface properties and flow characteristics of salbutamol sulphate, before and after micronisation. *Int. J. Pharmaceut.* 172:89–96.

Finlay, W. H. 1998. Inertial sizing of aerosol inhaled during pediatric tidal breathing from an MDI with attached holding chamber. *Int. J. Pharmaceut.* 168:147–152.

Flament, M-P., P. Leterme, and A. T. Gayot. 1995. Factors influencing nebulizing efficiency. *Drug Dev. Ind. Pharm.* 21 (20):2263–2285.

Forte, R., and C. Dibble. 1999. The role of international environmental agreements in metered-dose inhaler technology changes. *J. Allergy Clin. Immunol.* 104 (6):S217.

Kawashima, Y., T. Serigano, T. Hino, H. Yamamoto, and H. Takeuchi. 1998. Effect of surface morphology of carrier lactose on dry powder inhalation property of pranlukast hydrate. *Int. J. Pharmaceut.* 172:179–188.

Larhrib, H., X. M. Zeng, G. P. Martin, C. Marriot, and J. Pritchard. 1999. The use of different grades of lactose as a carrier for aerosolised salbutamol sulphate. *Int. J. Pharmaceut.* 191:1–14.

Leach, C. 1999. Effect of formulation parameters on hydrofluoroalkane-beclomethasone dipropionate drug deposition in humans. *J. Allergy Clin. Immunol.* 104 (6):S250.

LeBelle, M. J., S. J. Graham, E. D. Ormsby, R. M. Duhaime, R. C. Lawrence, and R. K. Pike. 1997. Metered-dose inhalers. II. Particle size measurement variation. *Int. J. Pharmaceut.* 151:209–221.

Le Brun, P. P. H., A. H. de Boer, D. Gjaltema, P. Hagedoorn, H. G. M. Heijerman, and H. W. Frijlink. 1999a. Inhalation of tobramycin in cystic fibrosis. Part 1: The choice of a nebuliser. *Int. J. Pharmaceut.* 189:205–214.

Le Brun, P. P. H., A. H. de Boer, D. Gjaltema, P. Hagedoorn, H. G. M. Heijerman, and H. W. Frijlink. 1999b. Inhalation of tobramycin in cystic fibrosis. Part 2: Optimization of the tobramycin solution for a jet and an ultrasonic nebulizer. *Int. J. Pharmaceut.* 189:215–225.

Maggi, L., R. Brunni, and U. Conte. 1999. Influence of the moisture on the performance of a new dry powder inhaler. *Int. J. Pharmaceut.* 177:83–91.

Muzzio, F. J., P. Robinson, C. Wightman, and D. Brone. 1997. Sampling practices in powder blending. *Int. J. Pharmaceut.* 155:153–178.

Naini, V., P. R. Byron, and E. M. Philips. 1998. Physicochemical stability of crystalline sugars and their spray-dried forms: Dependence upon relative humidity and suitability for use in powder inhalers. *Drug Dev. Ind. Pharm.* 24 (10):895–909.

Newman, S. P., and I. R. Wilding. 1998. Gamma scintigraphy: an in vivo technique for assessing the equivalence of inhaled products. *Int. J. Pharmaceut.* 170:1–9.

Ostrander, K. D., H. W. Bosch, and D. M. Bondanza. 1999. An in-vitro assessment of a NanoCrystal™ beclomethasone dipropionate colloidal dispersion via ultrasonic nebulisation. *Eur. J. Pharmaceut. Biopharmaceut.* 48:207–215.

Podczeck, F. 1998. The relationship between physical properties of lactose monohydrate and the aerodynamic behaviour of adhered drug particles. *Int. J. Pharmaceut.* 160:119–130.

Srichana, T., G. P. Martin, and C. Marriot. 1998. Dry powder inhalers: The influence of device resistance and powder formulation on drug and lactose deposition in vitro. *Eur. J. Pharmaceut. Sci.* 7:73–80.

Steckel, H., and B. W. Muller. 1998. Metered-dose inhaler formulations with beclomethasone-17,21-dipropionate using the ozone friendly propellant 134a. *Eur. J. Pharmaceut. Biopharmaceut.* 46:77–83.

Steed, K. P., L. J. Towse, B. Freund, and S. P. Newman. 1997. Lung and oropharyngeal depositions of fenoterol hydrobromide delivered from the prototype III hand-held multidose Respimat nebuliser. *Eur. J. Pharmaceut. Sci.* 5:55–61.

Tiwari, D., D. Goldman, S. Dixit, W. A. Malick, and P. L. Madan. 1998. Compatibility evaluation of metered-dose inhaler valve elastomers with Tetrafluoroethane (P134a), a non-CFC propellant. *Drug Dev. Ind. Pharm.* 24 (4):345–352.

Williams, R. O., III, M. Repka, and J. Liu. 1998a. Influence of propellant composition on drug delivery from a pressurized metered-dose inhaler. *Drug Dev. Ind. Pharm.* 24 (8):763–770.

Williams, R. O., III, and J. Liu. 1998b. Influence of formulation additives on the vapour pressure of hydrofluoroalkane propellants. *Int. J. Pharmaceut.* 166:99–103.

Williams, R. O., III, T. R. Rogers, and J. Liu. 1999. Study of solubility of steroids in hydrofluoroalkane propellants. *Drug Dev. Ind. Pharm.* 25 (12):1227–1234.

Zeng, X. M., K. H. Pandhal, and G. P. Martin. 2000. The influence of lactose carrier on the content homogeneity and dispersibility of beclomethasone dipropionate from dry powder aerosols. *Int. J. Pharmaceut.* 197:41–52.

BIBLIOGRAPHY

Byron, P. R. ed. 1990. *Respiratory drug delivery.* Boca Raton, Fla., USA: CRC Press.

D'Arcy, P. F., and J. C. McElnay, eds. 1989. *The pharmacy and pharmacology of asthma.* Ellis Horwood Series in Pharmaceutical Technology. Chichester, UK: Ellis Horwood.

Gennaro, A. R. ed. 1990. *Remington's pharmaceutical sciences*, 18th ed., Part 8, Chapter 92, "Aerosols." Easton, Penn., USA: Mack Publishing.

Hickey, A. J. ed. 1992. Inhalation aerosols: Physical and biological basis for therapy. In *Lung biology in health and diseases*, Vol. 94. New York: Marcel Dekker.

Johnsen, M. A. ed. 1983. *The aerosol handbook.* N. J., USA: Wayne Dorland Company.

Lachman, L., H. A. Lieberman, and J. L. Kanig, eds. 1986. *The theory and practice of industrial pharmacy*, 3rd ed., Chapter 20, "Pharmaceutical Aerosols". Philadelphia: Lea and Febiger.

Moren, F., M. Dolovich, S. Newman, and M. T. Newhouse. 1993. *Aerosols in medicine: Principles, diagnosis and therapy*, 2nd ed. New York: Elsevier.

Purewal, T. S., and D. J. W. Grant, eds. 1998. Metered dose inhaler technology. Buffalo Grove, Ill., USA: Interpharm Press, Inc.

11

Oral Solid Dosage Forms

Peter Davies

Roche Discovery
Welwyn, United Kingdom

In the last 15 to 20 years, there has been a huge resource in both academia and industry devoted to the development of drug delivery systems that target drugs more effectively to their therapeutic site. Much of this work has been successful and is reported within this text. In spite of this, oral solid dosage forms such as tablets and hard gelatin capsules, which have been in existence since the nineteenth century, remain the most frequently used dosage forms. This is not simply a reflection of the continued use of established products on the market, tablets and capsules still account for about half of all new medicines licensed (Table 11.1).

There are several reasons for the continued popularity of the oral solid dosage form. The oral route of delivery is perhaps the least invasive method of delivering drugs, it is a route that the patient understands and accepts. Patients are able to administer the medicine to themselves. For the manufacturer, solid oral dosage forms offer many advantages: they utilise cheap technology, are generally the most stable forms of drugs, are compact and their appearance can be modified to create brand identification.

Tablets and capsules are also very versatile. There are many different types of tablets which can be designed to fulfil specific therapeutic needs (Table 11.2). It is beyond the scope of this chapter to cover all these dosage forms, instead it will review the common principles, with more specific detail being given for those most commonly used.

For drugs that demonstrate good oral bioavailability and do not have adverse effects on the gastro-intestinal (GI) tract, there may be very little justification for attempting to design a specific drug delivery system. It is likely, therefore, that tablets and capsules will continue to remain one of the most used methods of delivering drugs to the patient in the future.

This chapter reviews the science behind the development of solid dosage forms, particularly tablets and hard gelatin capsules. Solid dosage forms are one of the most widely

Table 11.1
Number of FDA drug approvals for tablet and capsules from 1995 to 1999.

	No. of Tablets Approved	No. of Capsules Approved	No. of Other Dosage Forms Approved	Proportion of Tablets and Capsules (%)
1995	14	0	14	50
1996	69	17	101	46
1997	70	15	96	47
1998	48	9	66	46
1999	20	10	30	50

Source: Centrewatch.com, Clinical trials listing.

Table 11.2
Types of solid dosage forms.

Formulation Type	Description
Immediate release	The dosage form is designed to release the drug substance immediately after ingestion.
Delayed release	The drug substance is not released until a physical event has occurred, e.g., time elapsed, change in pH of intestinal fluids, change in gut flora.
Chewable tablets	Strong, hard tablets to give good mouth feel.
Lozenges	Strong, slowly dissolving tablets for local delivery to mouth or throat. Often prepared by a candy moulding process.
Buccal tablets	Tablets designed to be placed in buccal cavity of mouth for rapid action.
Effervescent tablets	Taken in water, the tablet forms an effervescent, often pleasant-tasting drink.
Dispersible tablets	Tablets taken in water, the tablet forms a suspension for ease of swallowing.
Soluble tablets	Tablets taken in water, the tablet forms a solution for ease of swallowing.
Hard gelatin capsules	Two-piece capsule shells which can be filled with powders, pellets, semi-solids or liquids.
Soft gelatin capsules	One-piece capsules containing a liquid or semi-solid fill.
Pastilles	Intended to dissolve in mouth slowly for the treatment of local infections. Usually composed of a base containing gelatin and glycerin.

researched areas of pharmaceutics and, given the space allowed, this chapter can only cover the science at a very basic level. It is an area that is served by a number of excellent texts, and these will be referenced at the appropriate points.

POWDER TECHNOLOGY

Virtually all solid dosage forms are manufactured from powders, and an understanding of the unique properties of powder systems is necessary for their rational formulation and manufacture. Powders consist of solid particles surrounded by spaces filled with fluid (typically air) and uniquely possess some properties of solids, liquids and gases. Powders are not solids, even though they can resist some deformation, and they are not liquids, although they can be made to flow. Still further, they are not gases, even though they can be compressed. Powder technology is concerned with solid/fluid interactions, interparticle contact and cohesion between particles. These are strongly influenced by particle size and shape and by adsorption of the fluid or other contaminants onto the surface of the particles.

While tablets and capsules, the two most common solid dosage forms, have their own unique requirements, there are similarities between them. They both require the flow of the correct weight of material into a specific volume, the behaviour of the material under pressure is important; and the wetting of the powder is critical for both granulation and subsequent disintegration and dissolution of the dosage form.

While it is not possible to deal with all aspects of powder technology in a textbook covering such a diverse range of formulations, some basic principles of powder flow, mixing and compaction and compression properties will be described. For those interested in a more in-depth treatment of the topic, there are a number of excellent texts available (Rhodes 1990; Nystrom 1995).

Particle Size and Shape

A knowledge of the particle shape and size distribution is essential to the understanding of the behaviour of powders, as it will contribute to knowledge of the secondary properties of a powder, such as flow and deformation, which influence the processability. This topic is dealt with in detail in Chapter 6.

Density

When a powder is poured into a container, the volume that it occupies depends on a number of factors, such as particle size, particle shape and surface properties. In normal circumstances, it will consist of solid particles and interparticulate air spaces (voids or pores). The particles themselves may also contain enclosed or intraparticulate pores. If the powder bed is subjected to vibration or pressure, the particles will move relative to one another to improve their packing arrangement. Ultimately, a condition is reached where further densification is not possible without particle deformation.

The density of a powder is, therefore, dependent on the handling conditions to which it has been subjected, and there are several definitions that can be applied either to the powder as a whole or to individual particles.

Particle Densities

British Standard 2955 (1958) defines three terms that apply to the particles themselves. Particle density is the mass of the particle divided by its volume. The different terms arise from the way in which the volume is defined.

1. True particle density is when the volume measured excludes both open and closed pores and is a fundamental property of a material.

2. Apparent particle density is when the volume measured includes intraparticulate pores.

3. Effective particle density is the volume "seen" by a fluid moving past the particles. It is of importance in processes such as sedimentation or fluidisation but is rarely used in solid dosage forms.

Powder Densities

The density of a powder sample is usually referred to as the bulk density, and the volume includes both the particulate volume and the pore volume. The bulk density will vary depending on the packing of the powder, and several values can be quoted

*   Minimum bulk density is when the volume of the powder is at a maximum, caused by aeration, just prior to complete breakup of the bulk.

*   Poured bulk density is when the volume is measured after pouring powder into a cylinder, creating a relatively loose structure.

*   Tapped bulk density is, in theory, the maximum bulk density that can be achieved without deformation of the particles. In practise, it is generally unrealistic to attain this theoretical tapped bulk density, and a lower value obtained after tapping the sample in a standard manner is used.

The porosity of a powder is defined as the proportion of a powder bed or compact that is occupied by pores and is a measure of the packing efficiency of a powder.

$$\text{porosity} = 1 - \left(\frac{\text{bulk density}}{\text{true density}} \right) \quad (1)$$

Relative density is the ratio of the measured bulk density divided by the true density.

$$\text{relative density} = \frac{\text{bulk density}}{\text{true density}} \quad (2)$$

POWDER FLOW

Good flow properties are a prerequisite for the successful manufacture of both tablets and powder-filled hard gelatin capsules. It is a property of all powders to resist the differential movement between particles when subjected to external stresses. This resistance is due to the cohesive forces between particles. Three principal types of interparticle force have been identified (Harnby et al. 1985): forces due to electrostatic charging, van der Waals forces and forces due to moisture.

Electrostatic forces are dependent on the nature of the particles, in particular, on their conductivity. For non-conducting particles, high cohesive stresses in the range of 10^4 to 10^7 N/m^2 have been reported.

Van der Waals forces are the most important forces for most pharmaceutical powders. The forces of attraction between two spherical particles is given by:

$$F = Ad\left(\frac{Ad}{12x^2}\right) \qquad (3)$$

where A is the Hamaker constant ($L = 10^{-19}$ J), x is the distance of separation of the particles and d is the particle diameter. The forces are inversely proportional to the square of the distance between the two particles, and hence diminish rapidly as particle size and separation increases. Powders with particles below 50 μm will generally exhibit irregular or no flow due to van der Waals forces. Particle shape is also important; for example, the force between a sphere and plane surface is about twice that between two equal sized spheres.

At low relative humidities, moisture produces a layer of adsorbed vapour on the surface of particles. Above a critical humidity, typically in the range 65–80 percent, it will form liquid bridges between particles. The attractive force due to the adsorbed layer may be about 50 times the van der Waals force for smooth surfaces, but surface roughness will reduce the effect. Where a liquid bridge forms, it will give rise to an attractive force between the particles due to surface tension or capillary forces.

The role of the formulator is to ensure that the flow properties of the powder are sufficient to enable its use on modern pharmaceutical equipment. Two types of flow present the formulator with particular challenges: flow from powder hoppers and flow through orifices.

Powder Flow in Hoppers

Tablet machines and capsule filling machines store the powder to be processed in a hopper above the machine. It is important that the powder flows from the hopper to the filling station of the machine at an appropriate rate and without segregation occurring. There are two types of flow that can occur from a powder hopper: core flow and mass flow (Figure 11.1).

The flow pattern of a core flow is shown in Figure 11.1a. When a small amount of powder is allowed to leave the hopper, there is a defined region in which downward movement takes place and the top surface begins to fall in the centre. As more material leaves the hopper, the area which moves downward begins to widen, and the upper surface becomes conical. In the areas of the hopper outside the falling region, near the walls, the material has not moved. Even when the hopper has almost emptied, there will be regions where the powder is undisturbed. A core flow hopper is characterised by the existence of dead spaces during discharge. A mass flow hopper is one in which all the material is in motion during discharge, in particular the areas adjacent to the hopper wall (Figure 11.1b). As a small amount of powder is discharged, the whole bulk of the powder will move downwards.

Core flow hoppers have two significant disadvantages. First, flow from the hopper can stop for no apparent reason. The stoppage may be due to the formation of an arch between the walls of the hopper that is strong enough to support the weight of powder above it. Alternatively, it may be the result of piping or rat holing, in which the material directly above the outlet falls out, leaving an empty cylinder. The second disadvantage is that the flow pattern is likely to encourage segregation, and there may be a considerable loss of mixing quality.

Figure 11.1 Powder flow patterns in hoppers.

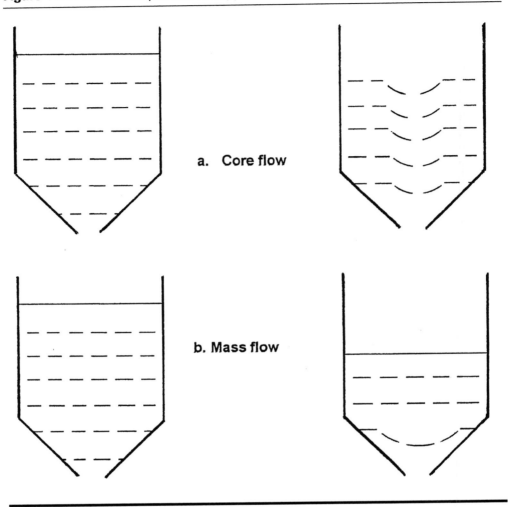

a. **Core flow**

b. **Mass flow**

Whether core flow or mass flow is achieved is dependent on the design of the hopper (geometry and wall material) and the flow properties of the powder. For most pharmaceutical applications, the hopper design for a particular machine will be fixed; thus, it is incumbent on the formulator to ensure that mass flow is achieved by modification of the powder properties.

Powder Flow into Orifices

Flow into orifices is important when filling dies in tablet machines and in certain types of capsule filling machines. For a given material, the flow into or through an orifice is dependent on the particle size, and typically, a plot of flow rate versus particle size will display the trend shown in Figure 11.2. At the lower end of the particle size range, cohesive forces will result in poor flow. As the particle size increases, the flow rate increases until a maximum is achieved, at an orifice diameter/particle diameter ratio of 20–30. As the particle size continues to increase, the rate decreases due to mechanical blocking or obstruction of the orifice. Flow will stop completely when the orifice/particle ratio falls below 6.

Measuring Powder Flow Properties

There are several different methods available for determining the flow properties of powders, and there are many literature examples demonstrating correlations between a test method and the manufacturing properties of a formulation. Listed below are some of the more commonly used tests, together with references, detailing their use in pharmaceutical applications.

Shear Cell Methods

Developed to aid silo and hopper design, shear cells provide an assessment of powder flow properties as a function of consolidation load and time. There are a number of types of shear cells available, the most common type being the Jenike shear cell (Figure 11.3).

The shear cell is filled in a standard manner to produce a powder bed with a constant bulk density. A vertical (normal) force is applied to the powder bed and a horizontal force applied to the moveable ring. As the powder bed moves due to the horizontal shear stress, it will change volume, either expanding or contracting depending on the magnitude of the vertical force. A series of tests are performed to determine the vertical load under which the bed remains at constant volume when sheared, referred to as the critical state. Once the critical state has been determined, a series of identical specimens are prepared, and each is sheared under a different vertical load, with all loads being less than the critical state.

Figure 11.2 Effect of particle size on the rate of powder flow through an orifice.

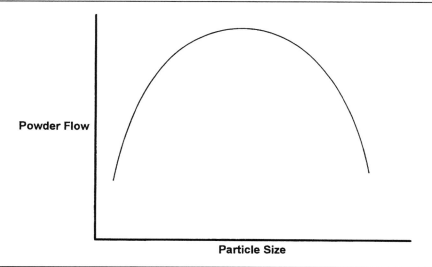

Figure 11.3 Jenike shear cell.

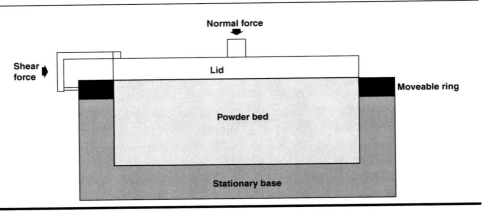

The test results are used to produce a graph referred to as a Jenike yield locus in which the shear stress required to initiate movement is plotted against the normal stress (Figure 11.4) The line gives the stress conditions needed to produce flow for the powder when compacted to a fixed bulk density. If the material is cohesive, the yield locus does not produce a straight line, and it does not pass through the origin. The intercept OT is the tensile strength of the consolidated specimen, and OC is the cohesion of the specimen, that is, the shear stress needed to initiate movement of the material when it is not subjected to normal force. The application of the yield loci to pharmaceuticals is well documented in the literature (Kocova and Pilpel 1972, 1973; Williams and Birks, 1967).

The limitations of the Jenike shear cell are that it is not very useful for measuring bulk solids with large shear deformations, e.g., plastic powders. The level of consolidation stresses required are inappropriate for pharmaceutical materials, and the quantity of material required is often beyond that available in the early stages of development. Alternative shear cells that have been used include annular shear cells (Nyquist and Brodin 1982; Irono and Pilpel 1982) and ring shear testers (Schulze 1996).

Changes in Bulk Density

The increase in bulk density of a powder is related to the cohesivity of a powder. Ratios of the poured to tapped bulk densities are expressed in two ways to give indices of flowability.

$$\text{Hausner Ratio} = \frac{\text{tapped bulk density}}{\text{poured bulk density}} \tag{4}$$

$$\text{Compressibility (Carr Index)} = \frac{100 \times (\text{tapped bulk density} - \text{poured bulk density})}{\text{poured bulk density}} \tag{5}$$

The Hausner Ratio varies from about 1.2 for a free-flowing powder to 1.6 for cohesive powders. The Carr Index classifications are listed in Table 11.3.

Figure 11.4 Jenike yield locus.

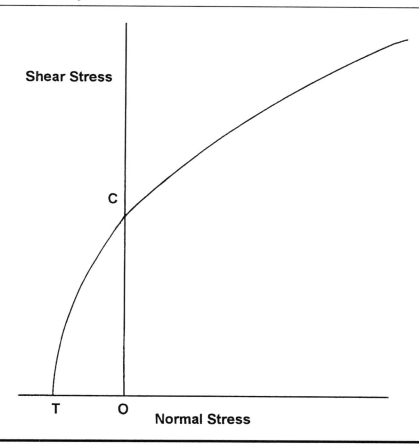

Table 11.3
Carr indices.

Carr Index (%)	Flow
5–12	Free flowing
12–16	Good
18–21	Fair
23–35	Poor
33–38	Very poor
>40	Extremely poor

Compressibility indices are a measure of the tendency for arch formation and the ease with which the arches will fail and, as such, is a useful measure of flow. A limitation of the bulk density indices is that they only measure the degree of consolidation; they do not describe how rapidly consolidation occurs.

Angle of Repose

If powder is poured from a funnel onto a horizontal surface, it will form a cone. The angle between the sides of the cone and the horizontal is referred to as the angle of repose. The angle is a measure of the cohesiveness of the powder, as it represents the point at which the interparticle attraction exceeds the gravitational pull on a particle. A free-flowing powder will form a cone with shallow sides, and hence a low angle of repose, while a cohesive powder will form a cone with steeper sides.

This method is simple in concept, but not particularly discerning. As a rough guide, angles less than 30° are usually indicative of good flow, while powders with angles greater than 40° are likely to be problematic.

Avalanching Behaviour

If a powder is rotated in a vertical disc, the cohesion between the particles and the adhesion of the powder to the surface of the disc will lead to the powder following the direction of rotation until it reaches an unstable situation where an avalanche will occur. After the avalanche, the powder will again follow the disc prior to a further avalanche. Measurement of the time between avalanches and the variability in time is a measure of the flow properties of the powder.

MIXING

The mixing of powders is a key step in the manufacture of virtually all solid dosage forms. A perfect mixture of two particles is one in which any group of particles taken from any position within a mix will contain the same proportions of each particle as the mixture as a whole (Figure 11.5). With powders, unlike liquids, this is virtually unattainable. All that is possible to achieve is a maximum degree of randomness, that is, a mixture in which the probability of finding a particle of a given component is the same at all positions in the mixture (Figure 11.6).

To determine the degree of mixing obtained in a pharmaceutical operation, it is necessary to sample the mixture and determine the variation within the mix statistically. In assessing the quality of a mixture, the method of sampling is more important than the statistical method used to describe it. Unless samples that accurately represent the system are taken, any statistical analysis is worthless. Furthermore, to provide meaningful information, the scale of scrutiny of the powder mix should be such that the weight of sample taken is similar to the weight that the powder mix contributes to the final dosage form.

A large number of statistical analyses have been applied to the mixing of powders. These tend to be indices where the variance of the actual mix is compared to the theoretical random mix. The statistics are beyond the scope of this text and can be found in a number of standard texts on powder technology (Rhodes 1990).

Figure 11.5 Perfect mix.

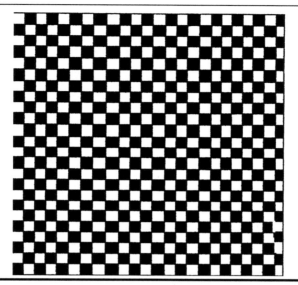

Figure 11.6 Random mix.

Segregation

If a powder consisting of two materials both having identical physical properties is mixed for sufficient time, random mixing will eventually be achieved. Unfortunately, most pharmaceutical powders consist of mixtures of materials with differing properties. This leads to segregation, where particles of similar properties tend to collect together in part of the powder. When segregating powders are mixed, as the mixing time is extended, the powders appear to unmix and equilibrium is reached between the action of the mixer introducing randomness and the resistance of the particles due to segregation.

While a number of factors can cause segregation, *differences in particle size* are far and away the most important in pharmaceutical powders. There are a number of mechanisms by which segregation of different sized particles can occur, and consideration should be given to these when designing pharmaceutical processes. *Trajectory segregation* occurs when a powder is projected horizontally in a fluid or gas; larger particles are able to travel greater horizontal distances than small particles before settling out. This could cause segregation at the end of conveyor belts or vacuum transfer lines. When a powder is discharged into a hopper or container, air is displaced upward. The upward velocity of this air may be sufficient to equal or exceed the terminal velocity of some of the smaller particles, and these will remain suspended as a cloud after the large particles have settled out. This process is known as *elutriation segregation*. The most common cause of segregation is due to *percolation* of fine particles. If a powder bed is handled in a manner that allows individual particles to move, a rearrangement in the packing of the particles will occur. As gaps between particles arise, particles from above will be able to drop into them. If the powder contains particles of different sizes there will be more opportunities for the smaller particles to drop, so there will be a tendency for these to move to the bottom of the powder, leading to segregation. This process can occur whenever movement of particles takes place, including vibration, shaking and pouring.

Ordered Mixing

As stated above, differences in particle size are the most common cause of segregation in pharmaceutical powders. One exception to this is when one component of a powder mix has a very small particle size (less than 5 μm) and the other is relatively large. In such circumstances, the fine powder may coat the surface of the larger particles, and the adhesive forces will prevent segregation. This is known as ordered mixing, and using this technique, it is possible to produce greater homogeneity than by random mixing.

COMPACTION

The manufacture of tablets, and to a lesser extent powder-filled hard gelatin capsules, involves the process of powder compaction, the purpose of which is to convert a loose incoherent mass of powder into a single solid object. Knowledge of the behaviour of powders under pressure, and the way in which bonds are formed between particles, is essential for the rational design of formulations.

A powder in a container subjected to a low compressive force will undergo particle rearrangement until it attains its tapped bulk density. Ultimately, a condition is reached where further densification is not possible without particle deformation. If, at this point, the powder bed is subjected to further compression, the particles will deform elastically to accommodate induced stresses, and the density of the bed will increase with increasing pressure at a characteristic rate. When the elastic limit is exceeded, there is a change in the rate of reduction in the bed volume as plastic deformation or brittle fracture of particles begins (Figure 11.7). Brittle materials will undergo fragmentation, and the fine particles formed will percolate through the bed to give secondary packing. Plastically deforming materials will distort to fill voids and may also exhibit void filling by percolation when the limit of plastic deformation is reached and fracture occurs. Either mechanism, therefore, consists of at least two submechanisms, and the processes could be repeated on the secondary particles produced by the fracture until the porosity is at a minimum and the internal crystalline structure supports the compressional stress.

Both processes will aid bonding to form a single compact, as plastic flow increases contact areas between particles irreversibly and fragmentation produces clean surfaces that bond strongly. The successful production of compacts depends on achieving high contact areas between uncontaminated surfaces.

To fully understand the compaction behaviour of a material, it is clear that it is necessary to be able to quantify its elasticity, plasticity and brittleness.

Figure 11.7 The behaviour of powders subjected to a compaction force: (a) brittle fracture and (b) plastic deformation.

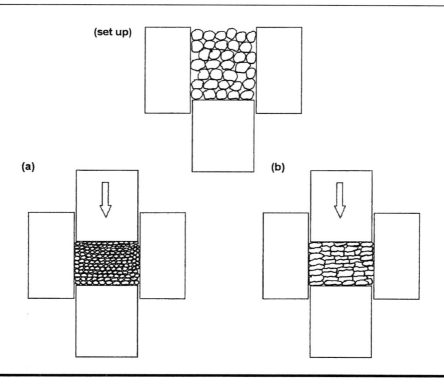

Measurement of Compaction Properties

To characterise the compaction properties of a material or formulation, it must be possible to measure the relationship between the force applied to a powder bed and the volume of the powder bed. A typical instrumentation will consist of measurement of the forces on the upper and lower punches by means of strain gauges or load cells together with a measure of the punch movement, which is performed using displacement transducers, the most common type being linear variable-differential transducers (LVDTs). The positioning and installation of the load and displacement transducers are critical to obtain meaningful information. The topic of instrumentation is comprehensively covered by Ridgway Watt (1988). There are three approaches that have been used to generate compaction information, as discussed below.

Conventional Testing Machines

Testing machines are widely used in materials science and engineering laboratories for the measurement of physical properties of various materials. Many of the basic principles of compaction and the test methodologies currently employed in pharmaceutical formulation have been developed on testing machines by the metallurgy and ceramic industries. The drawback with testing machines is that the compression speeds that can be achieved are well below those encountered on tabletting machines, so while they are of value in fundamental studies, they are not necessarily useful for predicting the behaviour of a material or formulation in the factory.

Conventional Tablet Machines

The first tablet machines to be instrumented were single punch eccentric presses. While these provide useful information, the compression profiles differ from those of rotary tablet machines used for commercial production. The profile of a single punch involves the powder bed being compressed between a moving upper punch and a stationary lower punch, while on a rotary machine, both punches move together simultaneously. Consequently, rotary machines have been instrumented, even though this is technically more challenging than single punch machines. The instrumented rotary press provides information that is directly relevant to production conditions, although it should be borne in mind that profiles do vary between machines, and any results obtained may be peculiar to that machine. A major advantage of instrumented machines is that they provide information not only on the compaction properties but also on flow and lubrication. The disadvantage of using instrumented rotary machines is the quantity of material required to perform tests, making them unsuitable for preformulation activities, when material is in short supply.

Compaction Simulators

Compaction simulators are a development of testing machines. They consist of single punch machines in which the upper and lower punches are driven individually by hydraulic rams. The movement of the hydraulic rams is controlled by computer and can be programmed either to simulate the movement of any tablet machine or to follow a simple profile similar to a testing machine. The big advantage of the compaction simulator is that it can be used to prepare a single compact using a profile that might be encountered on a production machine, so only small quantities of material are required.

Quantitative Compaction Data

There are two principal types of compaction studies used to characterise material: pressure/volume relationships and pressure/strength relationships. While ultimately it is the strength of a tablet that is important, the pressure/volume relationships provide the information about the compaction properties of a material that allows an appropriate formulation to be developed.

Heckel Plots

A large number of equations have been proposed to describe the relationship between pressure and volume reduction during the compaction process. Many of these have an empirical basis and may relate to a particular material or range of pressures, while others attempt to define the complete process of densification. The equation that has been most widely used to describe the compaction of pharmaceutical powders is the Heckel equation (Heckel 1961). This equation, originally used to describe the densification of ceramics, is essentially a curve-fitting equation that provides reasonable correlation with the observed facts over a wide range of pressures.

The equation is based on the premise that compaction is a first-order process where the rate at which pores within a powder can be eliminated is proportional to the number of pores present. As the compaction process continues, the number of pores will continue to drop, and consequently, the rate of volume reduction per unit increase in pressure will drop. This was expressed mathematically as :

$$\ln\left(\frac{1}{1-D_r}\right) = kP + A \tag{6}$$

In a system where there was no rearrangement of particles, and compaction was achieved solely by plastic deformation, a plot of $\ln(1/1 - D_r)$ versus P would yield a straight line (Figure 11.8).

Figure 11.8 Theoretical Heckel plot.

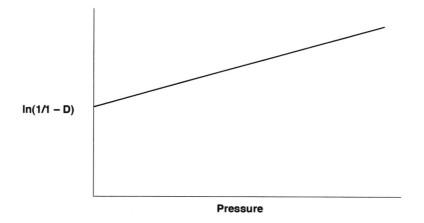

Pharmaceutical powders do not produce perfect straight lines, and the type of deviation provides information about the compaction behaviour of the material. A typical Heckel plot for a pharmaceutical powder is illustrated in Figure 11.9. A straight-line portion is obtained over a certain pressure range with a negative deviation at low pressures and a positive deviation at high pressures.

The curved portion at low pressures is due to particle rearrangement and possibly fragmentation, the deviation from a straight line (A–B) is a measure of its extent (Figure 11.9).

The gradient of the straight-line portion of the plot is related to the reciprocal of the yield pressure of the material, and as such is a measure of the plasticity of the material. While the absolute values obtained for the yield pressure will be dependent on the equipment and test conditions employed, the relative values obtained under given test conditions will provide information about the compaction properties of materials. Table 11.4 displays the values for yield pressure obtained for excipients, known to have differing compaction properties, tested using a compaction simulator.

The densification behaviour of powders has been categorised into types A, B and C (York and Pilpel 1973). Type A (plastic) exhibits parallel but distinct graphs for different size fractions, type B (fragmenting) exhibits particulate fragmentation at low pressures with graphs becoming coincident at higher pressures; and type C (extremely plastic) is characterised by a small initial curved section, a low value of mean yield pressure and a rapid approach to zero porosity at low pressure.

Figure 11.9 Heckel plots of pharmaceutical powders.

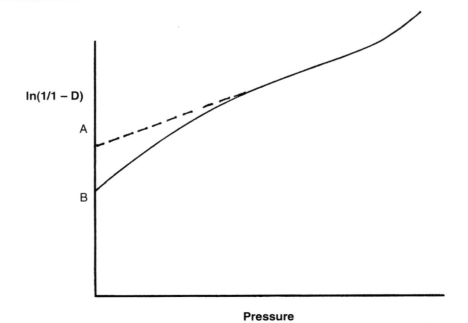

Table 11.4
Yield pressure for excipients.

Excipient	Yield Pressure (Mpa)	A–B	Deformation Mechanism
Microcrystalline cellulose	54	0.15	Plastic/deforming
Anhydrous lactose	174	0.5	
Calcium phosphate dihydrate	396	0.95	Brittle/fragmenting
Starch 1500	53	0.1	

The effect of compression speed on the yield pressure of a material has been suggested as a method of determining the time-dependent nature of materials compression properties (Roberts and Rowe 1985). Heckel plots are produced at two punch velocities, 0.03 and 300 mm sec, and the yield pressures determined. The strain rate sensitivity (SRS) is calculated as:

$$SRS = \frac{P_{y2} - P_{y1}}{P_{y1}} \times 100 \tag{7}$$

where P_{y1} = the yield pressure at 0.03 m ms and P_{y2} = the yield pressure at 300 m ms. Materials that exhibit plastic deformation have larger SRS than values fragmenting materials.

Elasticity

While Heckel plots are able to distinguish between plastic and fragmenting mechanisms, they do not readily distinguish between plastic and elastic deformation. The data presented in Table 11.4 would suggest that microcrystalline cellulose and starch 1500 have very similar properties, yet the elastic nature of starch and its derivative products is well documented in the literature. Additional methods are, therefore, required to measure elasticity.

Elasticity can be determined either by monitoring the elastic energy during the decompression phase of a compact within the die or by comparing the dimensions of the ejected compact with the dimensions of the compact within the die at peak compaction pressure.

The elastic energy is determined by plotting a force-displacement curve. If punch force is plotted against punch tip displacement or punch tip separation, a curve with a progressively increasing slope is obtained, reaching a maximum force at the point of minimum separation. As the punch begins to retract, the compact will expand due to elastic recovery and will remain in contact with the punch. This recovery is apparent from the force-displacement curve. If the material being compressed was truly elastic, the curve for the decompression phase would overlay the compression phase. For a truly plastic material the force would fall to zero immediately the punch began to retract. Pharmaceutical materials tend to show a combination of elastic and plastic deformation.

Integrating the force-displacement curves gives a measure of the energy involved in the compaction process (Figure 11.10), it being possible to calculate both the elastic energy and the net energy of compaction.

An alternative measure of elasticity is the percentage elastic recovery ($ER_\%$) (Armstrong and Haines-Nutt 1972):

$$ER_\% = \frac{H - H_c}{H_c} \times 100 \qquad (8)$$

where H = thickness of compact after ejection and recovery and H_c = minimum thickness under load.

This measure differs from the elastic energy in that it includes the viscous contribution to elastic recovery as well as the purely elastic behaviour during the unloading period of compression. Whichever method is used to calculate the elasticity, it should be borne in mind that the punches will also display a degree of elasticity, and this must be allowed for when calculating punch separations at pressure.

Indentation Hardness

An alternative method of determining the plasticity and elasticity of a material is indentation hardness testing. The principle of indentation hardness testing is that a hard indenter of specified geometry, either a sphere or square-based pyramid, is pressed onto the surface of the test

Figure 11.10 Force displacement curve for a pharmaceutical powder. The total work of compaction is represented by the area defined by OAB; elasticwork by CAB. The net work of compaction is the area defined by OAC.

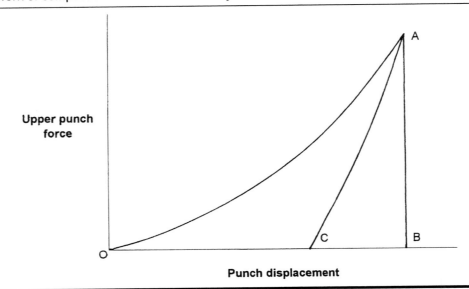

material with a measured load and the size of the indentation produced measured. The hardness of a material is the load divided by the area of the indentation, to give a measure of the contact pressure.

There are two types of hardness test: *static tests* that involve the formation of a permanent indentation on the surface of the test material and *dynamic tests* in which a pendulum is allowed to strike the test material from a known distance. Vickers and Brinell tests, two examples of static methods, are the most commonly used methods for determining the hardness of pharmaceutical materials. In the Brinell test, a steel ball of diameter D is pressed on to the surface of the material, and a load F is applied for 30 sec and then removed. The diameter d_I of the indentation produced is measured, and the Brinell Hardness Number (BHN) calculated by

$$\text{BHN} = \frac{2F}{\pi D_I \left(D_I - \sqrt{D_I^2 - d_I^2} \right)} \tag{9}$$

The Vickers Hardness test uses a square-based diamond pyramid as the indenter. The Vickers Hardness, H_v, is calculated by

$$H_v = \frac{2F \sin 68°}{d^2} \tag{10}$$

where d is the length of the diagonals of the square impression.

Traditionally, it has been necessary to perfom indentation testing on compacts due to the size of the indenters. The surface of compacts are not homogeneous, and this introduced variability. Recently, nanoindentation testers have been developed which are capable of performing indentation tests on single crystals. Such testers offer significant potential for characterising the mechanical properties of materials at an early stage of development.

Pressure/Strength Relationships

The strength of tablets has traditionally been determined in terms of the force required to fracture a specimen across its diameter, the *diametral compression test*. The fracture load obtained is usually reported as a hardness value, an unfortunate use of a term that has a specific meaning in materials science, associated with indentation. The use of the fracture load does not allow for compacts of different shapes, diameters or thicknesses to be directly compared. For flat-faced circular tablets, a complete analytical solution exists for the stress state induced during the test (Barcellos and Carneiro 1953), allowing the tensile strength to be determined from the fracture load:

$$\sigma_x = \frac{2P}{\pi Dt} \tag{11}$$

where P is the fracture load, D the tablet diameter and t the tablet thickness. The solution for tensile stresses can only be used for tablets that fail in tension, characterised by failure along the loaded diameter.

The stresses developed in convex tablets tested undergoing the diametral compression test have been examined by Pitt et al. (1989), who proposed the following equation for the calculation of the tensile strength:

$$\sigma_f = \frac{10P}{\pi D^2} \times \left(\frac{2.84t}{D} - \frac{0.126t}{C_L} + \frac{3.15C_L}{D} + 0.01 \right) \tag{12}$$

where P is the fracture load of the convex tablet, D the diameter, C_L the cylinder length and t the overall thickness of the tablet.

Typical plots of tensile strength versus compaction pressure are illustrated in Figure 11.11. Initially, most materials will demonstrate an increase in tensile strength proportional to the compaction pressure applied. As the compaction pressure increases, the tablet approaches zero porosity, and large increases in pressure are required to achieve small volume reductions, and consequently, small increases in bonding. Some materials will attain a maximum strength, and subsequent increases in pressure will produce weaker tablets.

Other materials will also display an initial increase in strength proportional to the applied pressure, but the strength reaches a maximum before falling off sharply. This is due to capping or lamination, that results in tablets failing in a characteristic manner (Figure 11.12). Capping is the partial or complete removal of the crown of a tablet from the main body, while lamination is the separation of a tablet into two or more distinct layers. The problem may be apparent on ejection of the tablet or may manifest itself when the tablet is subjected to further stress, e.g., mechanical strength testing or film coating.

Capping

Capping and lamination can affect both individual substances and formulations and constitute one of the most common problems facing the formulator. It occurs when a material is unable to relieve stresses present within a compact following compression by plastic deformation (Hiestand et al. 1984). When a material is compressed within a die by means of two opposing

Figure 11.11 Compaction pressure/tensile strength profile. Typical plot for a pharmaceutical material.

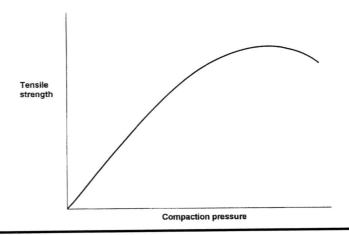

Figure 11.12 Tablet flaws: capping and lamination.

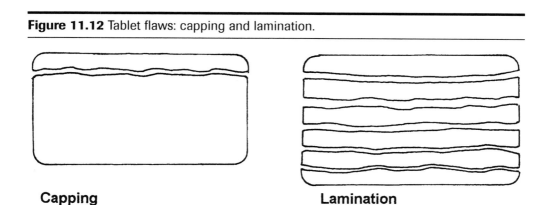

Capping   **Lamination**

punches, the axial load that is applied through the upper punch is transmitted to the die as a shearing force. In addition, force is transmitted radially to the die wall. The nature of this radial force is determined by the elastic or plastic behaviour of the compact. When an axial force is applied to a column of powder in a die, the pressures developed within the powder vary with depth. This phenomenon is attributed to the development of friction between the powder and the die wall and leads to density variations within the final compact. The nature of such variations has been the subject of a number of investigations (Train 1957; Kamm et al. 1949; Charlton and Newton 1985). These studies have been performed on a number of materials that have been compressed in dies with one moving and one stationary flat-faced punch. The results obtained in each study indicated a similar density distribution within a compact, high-density region being present on the perimeter of the compact adjacent to the moving punch and low density regions near the stationary punch. In addition, there was a second high density region remote from the moving punch (Figure 11.13). An explanation for the density distribution has been proposed that is based on the development of high-density wedges of material at the die wall adjacent to the moving punch. Figure 11.14 represents the forces developed in the compact. At equilibrium, the axial force is supported by the punch in direction *a* and by the powder in direction *b*. The radial component is supported by the die wall in direction *c* and by the powder bed in direction *d*. The resultant force acting on the mass is denoted by *k*. The pressure front can be considered as a conical surface with its focal point *B*. The region around point *B* will be exposed to the greatest pressure and will have a greater density than the surrounding areas. The wedge-shaped areas bounded by the dotted lines adjacent to the moving punch will be highly densified due to the high shearing forces that they are exposed to. The central area, *A*, will be subject to negligible shearing forces and will be protected from normal axial pressures by the vaulting effect of the high density wedges resulting in an area of low density. The area *C*, adjacent to the stationary punch, will undergo no movement relative to the die wall, and thus will not be subject to shearing forces. Density in this region will be low, as consolidation will depend solely on transmitted axial forces.

On removal of the upper punch, there will be a degree of axial elastic recovery resulting in expansion of the compact within the die. Following ejection, expansion may also occur in the radial direction. This elastic recovery is considered to be the most likely cause of capping. Train (1956) attributed capping to the strain imposed by elastic recovery of the areas of high

Figure 11.13 Regions of high density within a compact.

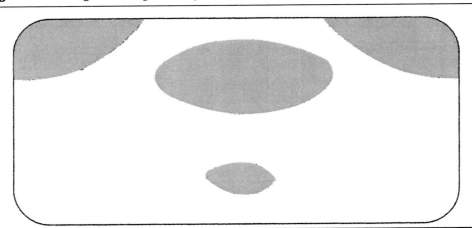

density within the compact on ejection (Figure 11.15). The elastic recovery of the dense peripheral ring would be larger than that of the adjacent, less dense, part of the tablet. The differential stress in this region is exacerbated by both axial and radial relaxation of that part of the tablet extruded from the die during the early stages of ejection.

Attempts have been made to predict the capping tendencies of materials. Malamataris et al. (1984) examined the plastoelasticity of mixtures of paracetamol and microcrystalline cellulose and showed that the tensile strengths of compacts were inversely proportional to the ratios of the samples' elastic recovery:plastic compression (as defined in Figure 11.10). Lamination and capping occurred when this ratio exceeded 9. Nystrom et al. (1978) measured the tensile strength of compacts in both the radial and axial directions and found that the values were not equal, the axial strength often decreasing at high compaction pressures. It was proposed that the ratio of axial to radial tensile strength should be close to unity for a good formulation. Krycer et al. (1982) examined the capping tendencies of three grades of paracetamol and proposed a capping index defined as the slope of the percentage elastic recovery versus residual die wall pressure (the pressure exerted on a die by a compact after removal of the upper punch). The higher the values of the capping index, the greater the tendency for capping. The residual die wall pressure relates to the irreversible deformation undergone during compaction. Low values for residual die wall pressure indicate that the compact had recovered axially and contracted radially, which would induce strain within the compact.

The methods of predicting capping discussed so far have been measures of the degree of elastic recovery occurring in the compact. For capping to occur, the stresses produced by the elastic recovery during decompression must be sufficient to disrupt the bonds that are formed during compression. Hiestand and Smith (1984) proposed a measure of the ability of a material to relieve localised stresses, called the brittle fracture index (BFI). This test involves comparing the tensile strength value obtained using the diametral compression test of a compact that contains a central, axial hole with one that does not. Under the conditions of the test, the hole acts as a stress concentrator; elasticity theory predicts that the stress concentration factor

Figure 11.14 Development of the pressure pattern within a compact (after Train 1957).

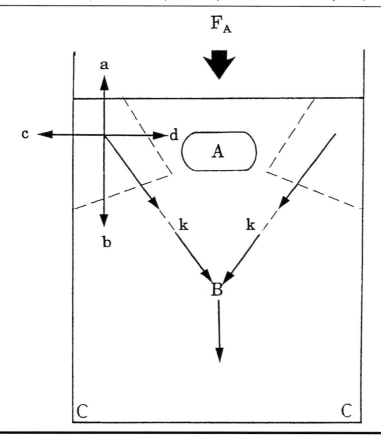

is approximately 3.2 for a hole in an isotropic solid. However, for most pharmaceutical materials, the ratio of tensile strengths obtained is less than 3 due to the relief of the highly localised stresses by plastic deformation. The BFI is defined as:

$$BFI = \frac{(\sigma_s - \sigma_0)}{2\sigma_0} \tag{13}$$

where σ_s is the tensile strength of the compact without the hole and σ_0 is the tensile strength of the tablet with the hole. A BFI of 1.0 would correspond to a purely brittle material; a value of zero would indicate that the stresses at the hole had been completely relieved by plastic deformation.

Hiestand and Smith (1984) proposed that a material with a high BFI would be less able to relieve the stresses occurring during decompression and ejection and would therefore be more susceptible to capping and lamination. Experiments showed that problems were likely

Figure 11.15 Elastic recovery of compact during ejection from die leading to capping (after Train 1956).

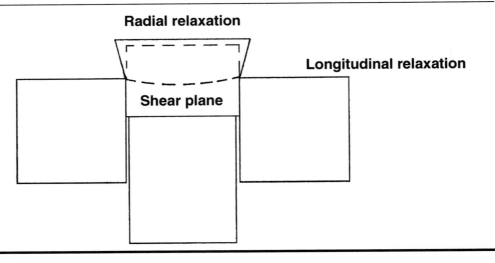

Radial relaxation

Longitudinal relaxation

Shear plane

to occur with materials having a BFI of 0.8 or more. The BFI will be dependent on the relative density of a material; at low densities, pores may act as stress concentrators in the same way as the central hole, so the measurements should be made at fixed, high relative densities. Roberts and Rowe (1986) determined the BFI of compacts produced at a range of relative densities using a range of compaction speeds. Magnesium carbonate, a brittle material, displayed increasing BFI values with increases in compaction speed and relative density, while microcrystalline cellulose showed little change.

Summary

It is clear from the preceding discussions that there is not one single technique that can be used to fully characterise the compaction properties of a powder. A number of tests have been widely applied to pharmaceutical materials, but used in isolation, they will not provide the formulator with all the data required to fully understand their behaviour when tabletted. Two sets of workers have tried to address this problem by suggesting a range of tests that, used in combination, will give a more complete picture of the materials properties.

Hiestand and Smith (1984) proposed three indices referred to as Tabletting Indices. The three indices are a strain index, bonding index and the BFI, which was described in the section on Capping. The strain index is a measure of the strain present in a material following compaction and is a measure of elastic recovery calculated by a dynamic indentation hardness test. The bonding index is a measure of the material's ability to deform plastically and form bonds and is the ratio of a compact's tensile strength and indentation hardness.

Roberts and Rowe (1987) have proposed a material classification based on a knowledge of Young's modulus of elasticity, yield stress, hardness and SRS.

Rational formulation relies on a thorough understanding of the physicochemical properties of the material. Ideally the mechanical properties should be determined at an early stage in the development process. It must, however, be borne in mind that the properties are sample dependent, and changes in particle size, morphology and so on during development will affect the compaction properties.

SOLID DOSAGE FORMS

When formulating any pharmaceutical dosage form, it is important to remember that there is an equilibrium between the bioavailability of the product, its chemical and physical stability and the technical feasibility of producing it.

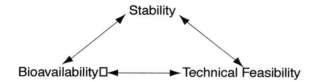

Any changes made to a formulation in an attempt to optimise one of these properties is likely to have an effect on the other two parameters that must be considered. This is especially true of immediate-release solid dosage forms. Many of the properties required to optimise the bioavailability through rapid disintegration and dissolution of the active constituent, e.g., small particle size, must be balanced with the manufacturability, where the fluidity and compactibility of a powder will often be enhanced by an increase in particle size.

Tablets and hard gelatin capsules form the vast majority of solid dosage forms on the market. While the actual processes involved of filling capsules and compressing tablets differ, the preparation of the powders to be processed are, in many cases, very similar.

TABLETS

Tablet Machines

Tablets are produced using tablet presses. While these presses vary in their output, from approximately 3,000 tablets per hour to more than 1 million per hour for the fastest machines, the principle of manufacture remains the same. Powder is filled to a specified depth in a die and compressed between two punches. The compression force is ended by removal of the upper punch, and the lower punch then moves upward in the die to eject the tablet. Presses can be divided into two types, single punch (or eccentric) presses and rotary presses.

Single Punch Presses

Single punch presses are sometimes referred to as eccentric presses because the movement of the punches is controlled by an eccentric cam. The tabletting cycle of a single punch machine is represented schematically in Figure 11.16. The powder hopper is attached to a feed shoe which oscillates horizontally.

Figure 11.16 Schematic representation of a single punch tablet machine.

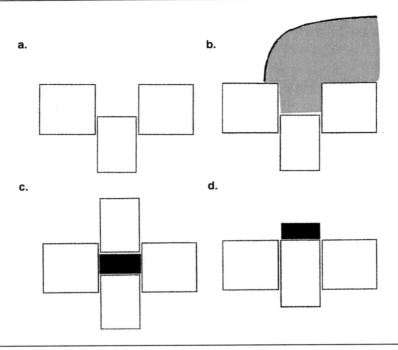

a. The upper punch is raised out of the die, and the lower punch drops to a set position.

b. The feed shoe oscillates above the die, filling it with powder.

c. The upper punch enters the die and compresses the powder.

d. The upper punch is removed, and the lower punch rises in the die to eject the tablet.

The compression cycle starts with die filling. The lower punch descends in the die. The depth of the descent can be controlled, and this determines the tablet weight. The feed shoe then passes over the die a number of times allowing the die to be filled with powder. As the die shoe moves away, it removes all excess powder away from the die table leaving the die filled to an even level.

The upper punch then descends into the die, compressing the powder. The depth to which the punch descends into the die is adjustable, and this controls the compaction pressure applied. The lower punch remains stationary during the compression phase.

As the upper punch moves upward at the end of the compression phase, the lower punch will rise in the die until it is level with the die table. The feed shoe will then begin its oscillatory phase and knocks the tablet off the lower punch and down a collection chute. The lower punch then descends to its filling position as a second cycle commences.

Single punch presses are rarely seen in production environments due to their relatively slow production rates, although there are still a number of old products that can only be successfully produced on this type of machine. They are still used in development laboratories because they require only relatively small amounts of material to produce tablets compared to most rotary machines.

Rotary Tablet Machines

Commercial manufacture of tablets is performed almost exclusively on rotary tablet machines due to their higher output. On a rotary machine, the punch and dies are positioned on a rotating turret, and output will depend on the number of stations positioned around the turret and the speed of rotation. Machines are available with anything from 4 stations for a development machine to 79 stations for the largest production machines. All such machines operate using virtually identical principles that are represented in Figure 11.17.

The powder hopper is positioned above a feed frame, a frame that retains a powder bed above the dies when the lower punch is in the filling position. As the lower punches pass below the feed frame, they descend within the die to their lowest possible position so the whole die cavity can be filled with powder. The powder is filled into the dies by the suction effect caused by their descent and gravity from the feed frame above. To optimise filling, the feed frame is designed so that the powder in contact with the die table and following the rotary action of the table is directed in a manner that makes it pass to and fro across the dies. Some machines

Figure 11.17 Schematic representation of a rotary tablet machine.

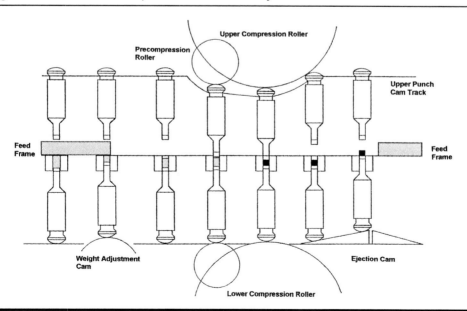

also have mechanical paddles in the feed frame. As the lower punches approach the end of the feed frame, they pass over a weight control cam, this causes the punch to rise, ejecting some of the powder which is scraped off by the edge of the feed frame. Adjusting the height of the cam controls the amount of material remaining in the die as the punch moves toward the compression stage.

Compression takes place when the upper and lower punches pass between compression rollers. During compression, the upper and lower punches move together, in contrast to the single punch machine, where only the upper punch moves. The compression force is controlled by moving the lower compression roller up or down, thus adjusting the distance between the punches at the point of maximum compaction. Some machines are fitted with two sets of rollers, a small roller being positioned between the feed frame, and the main compression roller allowing a small degree of compression to take place. This is termed *precompression*, and was introduced to minimise capping and lamination by removing air from the powder bed and effectively increasing the dwell time of the compression phase.

Following compression, the upper punches are removed by the upper punch cam track, and the lower punches pass over an ejection cam, a gentle ramp that moves the lower punches vertically within the die until the tablet is fully ejected. The tablets are removed from the punch tip by a scraper blade positioned on the edge of the feed frame, and the punch then descends to allow die filling to occur for the next cycle.

When developing formulations, it is usual for the early batches to be manufactured on either single punch machines or small rotary machines, due to the batch sizes being produced and the limited availability of new drug substances. It should be borne in mind that the formulations that are being developed may ultimately be required to run on larger rotary machines, and there are great differences in the rate of compression between the machines generally found in formulation laboratories and those found in production. These differences are summarised in Table 11.5.

The differences in punch speed at initial contact and dwell times, the period at which the compact is held at maximum compression, are likely to affect the nature of any tablets which have any viscoelastic components. Compaction simulators that are able to reproduce the punch speeds of production machines, yet only require small quantities of powder for testing, can have a valuable role to play in formulation development.

Tablet Formulation

A tablet formulation should possess the following properties to optimise the technical feasibility, stability and bioavailability of the formulation.

- Compatibility of drug substance with excipients

- Flowability

- Compactibility

- Lubricity

- Appearance

- Disintegration

- Dissolution

Table 11.5
Speed-related data for a number of commonly used tablet presses
operating at maximum output (adapted from Armstrong 1989).

Tablet Press	Production Rate per Die (tablets/min)	Time for Punch to Descend Last 5 mm (msec)	Punch Speed at First Contact with Powder (mm/sec)	Dwell Time (msec)
Manesty				
F3 (Single Punch)	85	68.6	139	0
B3B	44	61.4	163	10.84
Express	100	26.7	416	3.94
Unipress	121	19.1	485	3.16
Novapress	100	10.0	720	2.14
Kilian				
Tx	105	19.0	494	2.96
F1000	55	36.4	232	6.60
F1000	75	26.6	317	4.84
F2000	75	23.1	402	3.68
F2000	100	17.3	526	2.76
Korsch				
300	80	21.7	419	3.44
300	100	17.3	526	2.76

Compatibility

Compatibility studies have been discussed in detail in Chapter 6. The solid-state compatibility is of particular importance in tablets, due to the compaction process increasing the contact area between particles, and hence the potential for reactivity.

Flowability

The importance of powder flow was emphasised in the section on Powder Flow. The formulation should have sufficient flowability to ensure that the appropriate quantity of powder flows into the dies of the tablet machine on a consistent basis. While the tests described for powder flow are useful development tools, the ultimate test of a formulation is the uniformity of weight of tablets manufactured on a production tablet machine.

There is bound to be some variability in tablet weight during manufacture due to variation in the particle size of the material being compacted, flow property variation and machine parameters (e.g., small differences in the lengths of the lower punches). To allow for such variability, Pharmacopoeias set tolerances to ensure adequate control without providing a specification that is impossible to achieve in production. The European Pharmacopoeia (EP) test is to weigh 20 individual tablets and calculate the mean. The individual tablet weights are then compared to the mean. The sample is acceptable if no more than two tablets are outside the stated percentage limit and no tablet is outside twice the stated limit (Table 11.6). The pharmacopoeial limits are generous, and typically much more stringent limits will be applied as in-process controls. The in-process controls will also apply strict limits for the value of the mean tablet weight.

Uniformity of weight does not guarantee that there is uniformity of active ingredient throughout a batch of tablets. If there is segregation of the active ingredient occurring, the weights may remain uniform while the potency varies. For this reason, the U.S. Pharmacopeia (USP) only allows a uniformity of weight test for tablets containing 50 mg or more of an active ingredient comprising 50 percent or more, by weight, of the tablet. In all other instances, a content uniformity test must be performed.

Uniformity of weight is also important in achieving consistency of tablet strength, as there is a relationship between the quantity of powder in the die and the compaction pressure required to compress it to a given thickness, which is what the tablet machine is effectively doing. If the quantity of powder in the die is reduced to a lower compaction, pressure will be applied producing a weaker tablet. Variation in tablet strength may in turn lead to variability in the disintegration and dissolution properties of the product.

With low dose drugs, it may be possible to influence the flow properties by combining the drug substance with excipients possessing good flow properties. Where a formulation is prepared by simply dry mixing the drug with excipients prior to compaction, the process is referred to as direct compression. With high dose drugs, the quantity of such excipients that would be needed to achieve suitable flow and compaction properties may result in the final weight of the dosage form being unrealistically high. In such cases, the usual formulation approach is to granulate, a process that imparts two primary requisites to formulations: compactibility and flowability. Granulation is a process of size enlargement, whereby small particles are gathered into larger, permanent aggregates in which the original particles can still be identified. The direct compression and granulation processes and their relative merits are discussed in greater detail in the section "Processing of Formulations".

The flow properties of a powder can be enhanced by the inclusion of a glidant. These are added to overcome powder cohesiveness by interposing between particles to reduce surface rugosity, thus preventing interlocking of particles and lowering the interparticulate friction. Commonly used glidants are listed in Table 11.7.

Table 11.6
European Pharmacopoeia uniformity of weight limits.

Average Tablet Weight (mg)	Percentage Deviation
80 mg or less	10
More than 80 mg and less than 250 mg	7.5
250 mg or more	5

Table 11.7
Commonly used glidants.

Glidant	Typical Percentage
Talc	1–5
Fumed silicon dioxide	0.1–0.5
Aerosil	
Cab-O-Sil	
Syloid	
Starch	1–10
Calcium silicate	0.5–2
Magnesium carbonate (heavy)	1–3
Magnesium oxide (heavy)	1–3
Magnesium lauryl sulphate	0.2–2
Sodium lauryl sulphate	0.2–2

Talc is traditionally one of the most commonly used glidants, having the additional benefit of being an excellent antiadherent. The level of talc that can be added to a formulation is restricted by its hydophobic nature, too high levels resulting in decreased wetting of the tablet and a subsequent reduction in the rate of dissolution.

The *fumed silicon dioxides* are perhaps the most effective glidants. These are materials with very small (10 nm) spherical particles that may achieve their glidant properties by rolling over each other under shear stress. They are available in a number of grades with a range of hydrophobic and hydrophillic forms.

Starch has been used as a glidant, though relatively large amounts are required. The use of large amounts of starch has also aided the disintegration properties.

Compactibility

The aim of the formulator is to design a formulation that will reliably compact to form a strong tablet. The production manager wants a formulation that achieves the appropriate strength at a low compaction pressure, to reduce wear and tear on the tablet machine and increase the life of the punches.

The compaction properties of a formulation will largely be governed by its major components. For a high dose drug, the active ingredient will strongly influence the compaction, while for low dose drugs, it will be necessary for the tablet to be bulked out with an inactive material termed a diluent. High dose formulations may also use a diluent to overcome compaction problems experienced with an active substance. The selection of the diluent will depend to an extent on the type of processing to be used. A direct compression formulation will require a diluent with good flow and compaction properties. While a granulated formulation can be more forgiving, some degree of compactibility is desirable.

There are a number of general rules for selecting a diluent. The compaction properties of the active ingredient should be considered. If the material is extremely plastic, it is appropriate to add a diluent that compacts by brittle fracture; similarly, a brittle drug substance should be combined with a plastic filler. The solubility of the drug substance should also be considered. A soluble drug is normally formulated with an insoluble filler to optimise the disintegration process.

Apart from their flow and compaction properties, all diluents, and indeed other tablet excipients, should have the following properties:

- They should be inert and physically and chemically compatible with the active substance and the other excipients being used in the formulation.

- They should be physiologically inert.

- They should not have an unacceptable microbiological burden.

- They should not have a deleterious effect on the bioavailability.

- They should have regulatory acceptability in all countries where the product is to be marketed.

There will also be commercial factors in the selection of the diluent. There are hundreds of different brands and grades of diluents available, but it would be unrealistic for the formulator to expect to have a totally free choice. Most manufacturing companies wish to limit the inventory that they carry and will try to rationalise the excipients used in the factory. This inventory will have been selected on the basis of cost, availability and performance and will provide the formulator with a starting point.

Table 11.8 lists the more commonly used diluents. These have been listed in terms of their chemical nature. For each of the substances listed, there will be several suppliers offering branded goods that may or may not be equivalent. Most products will be available with a range of particle sizes.

As can be seen from the table, the excipients all have pharmacopoeial monographs, but it is important to understand that compliance with a monograph does not indicate equivalence between different grades or suppliers. The monographs confirm the chemical identity and purity of the excipients but do not measure the performance of the materials as diluents. To establish the equivalency of excipients obtained from different sources, it is necessary to perform some kind of functionality testing. The *Handbook of Pharmaceutical Excipients*, a joint publication between the Pharmaceutical Press and the American Pharmaceutical Association, contains some details of functional tests carried out on a wide range of excipients, but the onus on establishing equivalency of excipients still remains with the user.

Lubricity

The section on flowability discussed the role of glidants in tablet formulation. Glidants are one of three interrelated types of lubricant employed in solid dosage form manufacture. The two other classes of lubricant are antiadherent excipients, which reduce the friction between the tablet punch faces and tablet punches, and die-wall lubricant excipients, which reduce the friction between the tablet surface and the die wall during and after compaction to enable easy ejection of the tablet.

When two contacting solids are displaced relative to each other and parallel to the plane of contact, the resistance to the movement is termed friction. Contacting surfaces initially

Table 11.8
Common tablet diluents.

Diluent	Pharmacopoeia	Comments
Lactose	USP, Ph. Eur., JP	Available as anhydrous and monohydrate. Anhydrous material used for direct compression due to superior compressibility.
Microcrystalline cellulose	USP, Ph. Eur., JP	Originally a direct compression excipient, now often included in granulations due to its excellent compressibility.
Dextrose, glucose	USP, Ph. Eur., JP	Direct compression diluent, often used in chewable tablets.
Sucrose	USP, Ph. Eur., JP	Was widely used as a sweetener/filler in effervescent tablets and chewable tablets. Less popular nowadays due to cariogenicity.
Starch and derivatives	USP, Ph. Eur., JP	Versatile material, can be used as diluent binder and disintegrant.
Calcium carbonate	USP, Ph. Eur., JP	Brittle material
Dicalcium phosphate	USP, Ph. Eur., JP	Excellent flow properties. Brittle material.
Magnesium carbonate	USP, Ph. Eur., JP	Direct compression diluent.

touch at points on the asperities of the two surfaces. If a force is applied, these asperities will deform to form a contact area. For relative movement of the materials to occur parallel to the contact area, the materials must be sheared. The higher the shear strength of the materials in contact, the greater the force that will be required to produce movement. Die-wall lubricants work by reducing the shear force necessary to promote movement.

The level of a lubricant required in a tablet is formulation dependent and can be optimised using an instrumented tablet machine. On a single punch machine, strain gauges or load cells on the lower punch can directly measure the force required to eject the tablet. An alternative method of measuring lubrication is to measure the ratio of the maximum forces on the upper and lower punches during the compaction cycle (Hölzer and Sjøgren 1978). On a single punch machine, the lower punch remains stationary during the compaction phase, and the compaction pressure is exerted by the movement of the upper punch. If there were no resistance to the movement of particles in the die, the force transmitted through the powder bed to the lower punch would be the same as the force applied by the upper punch. In practise, the interparticle friction and friction between the particles and the die wall result in a lower force being transmitted to the lower punch. The ratio of the upper to lower punch forces, termed the R-value, has been used as a measure of the lubricant efficacy. The R-value cannot be used on a rotary machine because the compaction pressure is applied from both the upper and lower punches simultaneously. The ejection force can be measured either by instrumenting the punch tips or by positioning load cells or strain gauges below the ejection cam. If an instrumented machine is not available, the signs of inadequate lubricity are the presence of scoring around the tablet circumference and screeching during ejection. While these problems can be overcome by increasing the level of lubricant added, the aim should be to use the minimum level of lubricant required to produce acceptable product, for reasons discussed later.

Die-wall lubricants can be divided into two classes, fluid and boundary lubricants. *Fluid lubricants* work by separating moving surfaces completely with a layer of lubricant. These are typically mineral oils or vegetable oils, and they may be either added to the mix or applied directly to the die wall by means of wicked punches. Tablets containing oily lubricants may have a mottled appearance due to uneven distribution. When added to the mix, they have an adverse effect on powder flow due to their tacky nature and have been reported to reduce tablet strength (Asker et al. 1973). Low melting point lipophilic solids can also act as fluid lubricants because the heat generated at the die wall is sufficient to cause them to melt, forming a fluid layer which solidifies on ejection. Fluid lubricants include stearic acid, mineral oils, hydrogenated vegetable oils, glyceryl behenate, paraffins and waxes. Low melting point lubricants should be used with caution in tablets that are to be film coated. Lubricants can melt on the tablet surface during the film coating process, resulting in tablets with a pitted appearance (Rowe and Forse, 1983). Their use tends to be restricted to applications where a suitable boundary lubricant cannot be identified.

Boundary lubricants work by forming a thin solid film at the interface of the die and the tablet. Metallic stearates are the most widely used boundary lubricants, and their activity has been attributed to adherence of polar molecular portions on their surface to the surfaces of one particle species and of non-polar surface components to the other species' surface. Such lubricants should have a low shear strength of their own and form interparticulate films that resist wear and reduce surface wear. A list of lubricants with typical ranges for their usage is given in Table 11.9.

Magnesium stearate is the most widely used lubricant; it forms dense, high melting point films between the powder and the die wall to reduce friction and has low shear strength between its own surfaces. Despite its popularity, which is a reflection of its excellent lubricant properties, the material is far from ideal and has had problems associated with product consistency, its effect on tablet strength and its hydrophobicity.

The magnesium stearate used in the pharmaceutical industry is not a pure substance but a mixture of magnesium salts of fatty acids though predominantly magnesium stearate and magnesium palmitate. The USP requires that the stearate content should account for not less than 40 percent of the fatty acid content of the material, and the stearate and palmitate combined should account for not less than 90 percent. Within this definition, there is clearly scope for a range of materials to be supplied as magnesium stearate. Furthermore, there is no pharmacopoeial particle size specification for the material. As the lubrication activity of the material is related to its surface area, substantial decreases in ejection force are noted when using sources of magnesium stearate with larger surface areas. For a given formulation, it is important that a single source of magnesium stearate is used for all batches. A new supplier should not be used until the effect on the compaction properties and dissolution rates have been assessed.

The lubricant activity of magnesium stearate is related to its readiness to form films on the die wall surface. When it is mixed in a tablet formulation, it will display the same film forming propensity on the surfaces of the drug and excipient particles, which can have two consequences: a reduction in the ability of the powder to form strong compacts and, due to its hydrophobicity, a deleterious effect on the dissolution rate of the tablets. Figure 11.18 illustrates the effect of mixing time on the mechanical strength of compacts produced using a range of excipients. While the strength decreases with increasing mixing time for all the materials tested, the effect is far more marked for materials that deform plastically. When plastic deforming materials are compressed, the film of magnesium stearate around the particles remains relatively intact, so the interparticulate bonds are primarily between

Table 11.9
Lubricants and their usage.

Lubricant	Level Required (%)	Comments
Boundary Lubricants		
Magnesium stearate	0.2–2.0	Hydrophobic, variable properties between suppliers.
Calcium stearate	0.5–4	Hydrophobic.
Sodium stearyl fumarate	0.5–2	Less hydrophobic than metallic stearates, partially soluble.
Polyethylene glycol 4000 and 6000	2–10	Soluble, poorer lubricant activity than fatty acid ester salts.
Sodium lauryl sulphate	1–3	Soluble, also acts as wetting agent.
Magnesium lauryl sulphate	1–3	Acts as wetting agent.
Sodium benzoate	2–5	Soluble.
Fluid Lubricants		
Light mineral oil	1–3	Hydrophobic, can be applied to either formulation or tooling.
Hydrogenated vegetable oils	1–5	Hydrophobic, used at higher concentrations as controlled release agents.
Stearic acid	0.25–2	Hydrophobic.
Glyceryl behenate	0.5%–4	Hydrophobic also used as controlled release agent.

Figure 11.18 Effect of magnesium stearate mixing time on the strength of compacts.

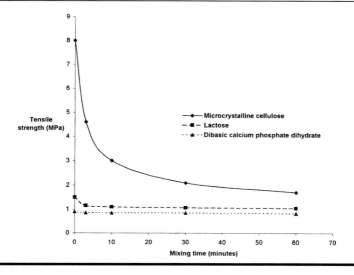

magnesium stearate particles which, by virtue of its lubricant properties, are inherently weak. Materials that compact by fragmentation are less sensitive to the lubricant because the fragmentation process produces a number of clean, uncontaminated surfaces that are able to form strong bonds.

The hydrophobic surfaces created by magnesium stearate have been shown to reduce the rate of dissolution and bioavailability of several tablet formulations. To minimise this effect, the manufacturing process should be designed to ensure that the lubricant is the last excipient to be added. When both lubricant and disintegrant are being added to a granulated formulation, the disintegrant should be blended with the granules prior to the addition of the lubricant to minimise the risk of forming a hydrophobic film around the disintegrant. The mixing time for the lubricant should be set as the minimum time required to produce the desired effect.

The third class of lubricant activity is the antiadherent. Some materials have adhesive properties and can adhere to the punch surfaces during compression. This will initially manifest itself as sticking, with a film forming on the surface of the tablets, leading to dull tablet surfaces. A more extreme version of sticking is picking, where solid particles from the tablet stick to the punch surface. This will often be evident in the intagliations on the tablet surface, resulting in poor definition of the surface markings.

Attempts have been made to assess picking tendencies using instrumented tablet machines. Load cells have been fitted to the edge of feed frames of rotary machines to monitor the force required to knock tablets off the lower punch following ejection. Shah et al. (1986) postulated that the magnitude of the residual force remaining on the lower punch of a single punch machine following removal of the upper punch was inversely related to the degree of adherence to the upper punch. In practise, sticking tends to be monitored during extended runs on tablet machines.

Most die-wall lubricants have antiadherent actions, and in many formulations, the addition of a specific antiadherent will not be required. Materials that can be added include talc, maize starch and microcrystalline cellulose.

Appearance

The appearance of a tablet is of great importance to the way that it is perceived by the patient. The macroscopic appearance of a tablet, its shape, size, colour and markings can all contribute to the patients' expectations of a medicine, while the microscopic appearance, such as surface roughness and colour homogeneity, are easily perceived as measures of quality. It is now the norm to be able to identify new products because of their unique appearance achieved by a combination of shape, size, colour and surface markings.

The size of a tablet is very often governed by the dose being administered. The compression weight of a high-dose drug will usually be determined by the level of filler required to impart the appropriate compatibility on the formulation, the aim being to produce the smallest possible tablet for ease of swallowing. For low-dose drugs, the quantity of filler added is determined by the minimum acceptable size for a tablet. The actual minimum acceptable size for a tablet will vary between pharmaceutical companies but is generally in the region of 6 or 7 mm diameter for a circular tablet, which would equate with a compression weight of 80 to 100 mg. Tablets below this range tend to be difficult for the patients to handle.

Early tablets were produced in cylindrical dies with flat-faced, flat bevel-edged or concave punches. While the majority of tablets are still circular, over the last 20 years, there has been an increasing shift away from circular to shaped tablets for new products. The tablet identification section of the *Chemist and Druggist Directory* (2000) describes 274 non-circular tablet products that are on the market in Britain, while the *Physicians' Desk Reference* (PDR) (1998) contains illustrations of 502 non-circular tablets that are available in the United States. After round tablets, the most common presentation is the capsule-shaped tablet, sometimes referred to as a caplet. This shape is particularly popular for high dose products where the compression weight is necessarily high, as the elongated shape makes the tablet easier to swallow than round tablets of equal weight. A survey performed on the reaction of patients to the appearance of tablets has indicated thet the tablet shape can influence patients' expectations of a medicine in terms of its potency, side-effects and suitability for a particular ailment (Anon. 1989). The studies found that tablets with highly angular appearances were universally disliked on the basis that they would be hard to swallow. Less predictable was the finding that other elements of tablet design, such as the number and depth of scorelines, the degree of rounding of corners and the hardness of the finish indicated by surface shine, appeared to play a role in determining how easy or hard to swallow a tablet might be. When designing a tablet shape, consideration should also be given to the processes following compression, such as coating and packaging. These processes depend on tablets being able to move relative to each other, and if the tablet shape allows tablets to form "structures" (e.g., due to straight sides), it may be problematic.

The colouring of tablets can be achieved either by incorporating a dye or pigment into the powder prior to compression or by applying a coloured coat to the tablet following compression. Coating methods, which are dealt with in the section "Tablet Coating", tend to provide a more uniform colour than inclusion of pigments in the compression mix but have the disadvantage of requiring an additional manufacturing process.

Colourants come in three forms: soluble dyes, insoluble pigments and lakes. Lakes are formed by adsorbing dyes onto the surface of an inert substrate, usually aluminium hydroxide. If the colourant is being added to a granulate, soluble dyes can be dissolved in the granulating fluid to ensure a uniform mix. When adding colourants as solids, the mixing process needs to be very efficient to achieve a uniform colour with no mottling. The usual method of inclusion is to form a premix with a portion of the powder mix and to mill this prior to incorporating the remaining ingredients. The problem can be reduced by the appropriate selection of colours, mottling being less evident with pastel shades. The insoluble pigments tend to be more light stable and less prone to fading than the soluble dyes.

The choice of colour is severely restricted by the number of regulatory acceptable dyes and pigments available to the formulator. This is particularly true when trying to achieve a globally acceptable formulation, due to the lack of international harmonisation of permitted colourants. Table 11.10 lists the commonly used pigments and dyes together with their international acceptability. It can be seen that for an international formulation the choice of colourants is restricted to the iron oxide pigments and indigo carmine, and as a result there are large numbers of tablets with varying shades of red, yellow, orange and brown being introduced onto the market.

The easiest way to give a tablet a unique identity is to mark the surface with a code or unique identifier. This can be achieved by applying a printed logo to the surface of the tablet or by compressing the powder with punches that are embossed with the code, producing tablets with intagliations. Printing is performed with ink jet printers applying approved inks to the surface of tablets. The advantage of printing is that it is possible to fit more information on to the surface than is possible with embossed punches, but it is an additional process and not all tablet surfaces are suitable for printing. The use of embossed punches does not increase the manufacturing time, but it does stress a formulation. The embossing of the punches

Table 11.10
Pharmaceutical colourants and their regulatory acceptability.

Colour	Other Names	Regulatory Acceptability		
		UK	USA	Japan
Azorubine	Carmoisine	+	–	–
FD&C Red 40	Allura Red	–	+[a]	–
FD&C Red 2	Amaranth Bordeaux S	+	–	+[b]
Ponceau 4R	Cochineal Red A Brilliant Scarlet 4R	+	–	+[b]
FD&C Red 33	Acid Fuchsin D Naphtalone Red B	–	+ ADI 0–0.75 mg	–
Canthaxanthin	Food Orange 8	+	+	–
Red 2G	Food Red 10	–	–	–
FD&C Red 22	Eosin Y	–	+[a]	–
FD&C Red 28	Phloxine B	–	+[a]	+ AL-lake only
FD&C Red 3	Erythrosine	+	+[a] lakes are prohibited	+
Cochineal Extract	Natural Red 4 Carmine	+	+	+
Iron Oxide–Red		+	+ ADI 0–0.5 mg elemental iron	+
Anthocyanin		+	–	–
Beetroot Red	Betanin	+	–	–
Fast Yellow	Acid Yellow G	–	–	–
FD&C Yellow 6	Sunset Yellow FCF Yellow Orange S	+	+	+
Yellow 2G		–	–	–
FD&C Yellow 5	Tartrazine	+[c]	+[a,c]	+
FD&C Yellow 10	Quinoline Yellow WS	+	+[a]	–
β-Carotene		+	+	+
Turmeric	Curcumin Natural Yellow 3 Indian Saffron	+	–	–
Iron Oxide– Yellow		+	+ ADI 0–0.5 mg elemental iron	+
Riboflavin	Lactoflavin Vitamin B_2	+	–	+

Table 11.10 continued on next page

Table 11.10 continued from previous page

Colour	Other Names	Regulatory Acceptability		
		UK	USA	Japan
Patent Blue V		+	−	−
FD&C Blue 1	Brilliant Blue FCF	−	+[a]	+
FD&C Blue 2	Indigotine Indigo Carmine	+	+	+
FD&C Green 3	Fast Green FCF	−	+[a]	+
Acid Brilliant Green BS	Green S Lissamine Green	+	−	−
Chlorophyllin		+	−	+
Brilliant Black BN	Food Black 1	+	−	−
Carbon Black	Medicinal Vegetable Charcoal	+	−	+
Iron Oxide–Black		+	+ ADI 0–0.5 mg elemental iron	−
Caramel	Burnt Sugar	+	+	+
Titanium dioxide		+	+	+

+ Permitted
− Not permitted
[a]Requires FDA certification on each lot of dye.
[b]Manufacturers have imposed a voluntary ban on this colour.
[c]Requires label declaration.

will exacerbate any tendency for punch adherence, and this should be considered when selecting the levels of lubricant and antiadherent in the tablet. The intagliations will also highlight the presence of any abrasion on the crown of the tablet, and care must be taken to ensure that the surfaces are sufficiently robust, particularly if they are to be subsequently film coated.

Disintegration

The chapter to date has concentrated on ensuring that it is possible to produce a tablet of sufficient strength that it can withstand the stresses of subsequent manufacturing operations, such as coating and packaging, and will reach the patient in an acceptable condition. However, once an immediate-release tablet is taken by the patient, it is important that it breaks up rapidly to ensure rapid dissolution of the active ingredient.

To maximise the dissolution rate of a drug substance from a tablet, it is necessary to overcome the cohesive strength produced by the compression process and break the tablet into the primary particles as rapidly as possible (Figure 11.19). This is achieved by adding disintegrants which will induce this process.

Starch was the first disintegrant used in tablet manufacture and is still used, although it has largely been superseded by the so-called super disintegrants, croscarmellose sodium,

Figure 11.19 Dissolution of drugs from tablets.

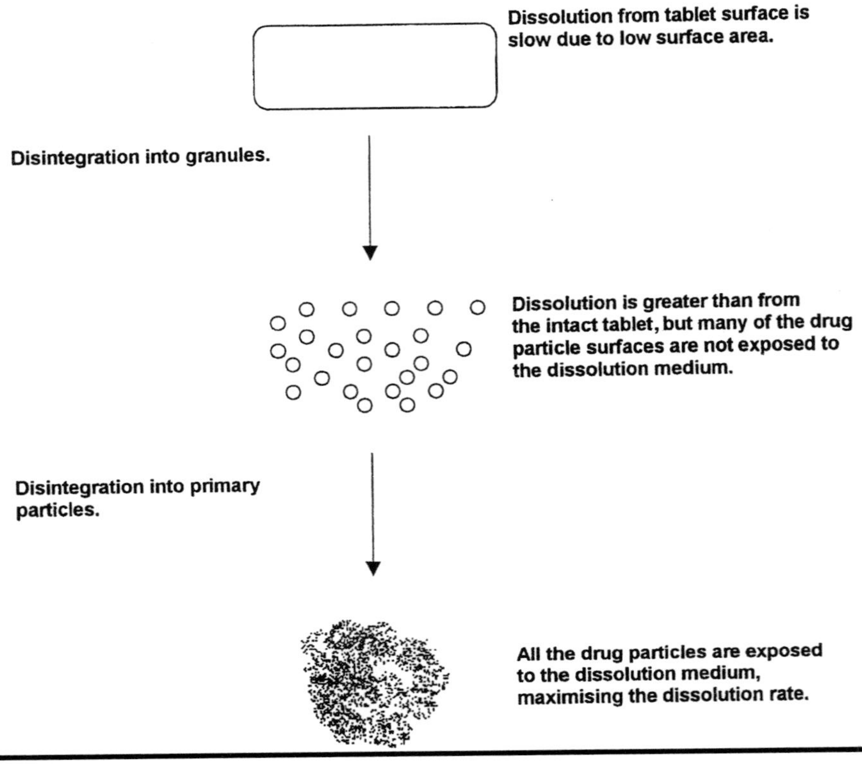

Dissolution from tablet surface is
slow due to low surface area.

Disintegration into granules.

Dissolution is greater than from
the intact tablet, but many of the drug
particle surfaces are not exposed to
the dissolution medium.

Disintegration into primary
particles.

All the drug particles are exposed
to the dissolution medium,
maximising the dissolution rate.

sodium starch glycolate and crospovidone, which display excellent disintegrant activity at low concentrations and possess better compression properties than starches.

Traditionally, swelling and rate of swelling have been regarded as the most important characteristics of disintegrants. Rudnic et al. (1982) quantified the rate of swelling and force generated by the swelling of disintegrants and found no simple relationship between the maximum disintegrating force and disintegration time. It was the ability to develop a significant swelling force rapidly that appeared to be more important. The other important factor in a formulation is that as the swelling develops, it should not be accommodated within the tablet, which prevents a significant disruptive force from being generated. If the tablet displays elasticity to the swelling, the force will be expended on the system, and disintegration will not take place. Similarly, if the tablet is composed entirely of soluble components, their dissolution will deprive the disintegrant of a matrix to push against. As a general rule, soluble drugs are formulated with insoluble fillers to maximise the effect of disintegrants.

The positioning of disintegrants within the intragranular and extragranular portions of granulated formulations can affect their efficacy. Placing the disintegrant in the extragranular portion results in rapid disintegration to granular particles, while the disintegrant present in the granule will promote further disintegration to the primary particles thus aiding dissolution. Studies performed to determine the optimum location of disintegrant (Shotton and

Leonard 1972; Rubenstein and Bodey 1974) suggest that dividing it between the two portions, with between 20 and 50 percent being in the extragranular portion, produces the best results.

Optimising the level of disintegrant in a formulation is a good example of a situation where there are a number of opposing factors to consider, and the final formulation needs to be a compromise. To optimise the biopharmaceutical properties of the formulation, the tablet should disintegrate rapidly, which can be achieved by increasing the level of disintegrant. The particle size of most disintegrants is small to maximise the surface area, and thus increase the rate of water uptake. The addition of large quantities of such materials could have an adverse effect on the flow properties of the formulation. The compaction properties of many disintegrants, including starch, are less than ideal, and high concentrations could also reduce the strength of tablets produced. By their nature, disintegrants are hygroscopic materials and will absorb moisture from the atmosphere, which could negatively affect the stability of water sensitive drugs. The super disintegrants, if used at excessive concentrations, can actually absorb sufficient moisture from the atmosphere to initiate disintegration on storage, if the packaging does not provide adequate protection from the environment. Disintegrant activity can be affected by mixing with hydrophobic lubricants, so care needs to be taken to optimise the manufacturing process as well as the formulation. The commonly used disintegrants are listed in Table 11.11.

For a disintegrant to be able to function properly, the tablet surface must be amenable to wetting. If the tablet contains a high proportion of a hydrophobic drug that has a high contact angle, it may be wise to include a wetting agent or surfactant in the formulation, which will aid not only the disintegration time of the tablet but also the subsequent dissolution of the drug substance. The most commonly used wetting agents are sodium lauryl sulphate and the polysorbates.

An alternative mechanism of disintegration is used in effervescent tablets, which utilises a gas-liberating chemical reaction to effect rapid disintegration. These tablets contain an organic acid and an alkali metal carbonate which, when added to water prior to administration, react to produce carbon dioxide, e.g.,

$$RCOOH + NaHCO_3 \rightarrow RCOONa + CO_2 + H_2O \qquad (14)$$

Most pharmacopoeias include a disintegration test which can be applied to tablets and capsules. The USP test consists of six glass tubes, 3 in. long and open at the top, with a 10-mesh screen at the bottom and immersed in a beaker of disintegration fluid that is maintained at 37°C. The tubes are raised and lowered 5–6 cm at 30 cycles per minute such that the bottom of the tubes remain 2–5 cm below the liquid surface at the top of the stroke and are no closer than 2–5 cm from the base of the beaker at the lowest point. One tablet is placed in each tube, and the disintegration time is the time taken for all six tablets to break up sufficiently for all material to pass through the mesh at the bottom of the tube. If the dosage form floats, it is permitted to place perforated plastic discs in the tubes to ensure that they remain submerged during the test. Pharmacopoeial tests use water as the disintegration fluid for non-enteric coated tablets, but during development, it is prudent to test the tablets over a range of pH values.

Disintegration testing is an important part of in-process control testing during production to ensure batch-to-batch uniformity, but its role in end-product testing has largely been superseded by dissolution testing.

Table 11.11
Commonly used disintegrants.

Disintegrant	Normal Usage Concentration (%)	Comments
Starch	5–10	Probably work by wicking; swelling is minimal at body temperature.
Microcrystalline cellulose		Strong wicking action. Loses disintegrant action when highly compressed.
Insoluble ion exchange resins		Strong wicking tendencies with some swelling action.
Sodium starch glycolate	2–8	Free-flowing powder that swells rapidly on contact with water.
Croscarmellose sodium	1–5	Swells on contact with water.
Gums—agar, guar, xanthan	< 5	Swell on contact with water; form viscous gels that can retard dissolution, thus limiting concentration that can be used.
Alginic acid, sodium alginate	4–6	Swell like the gums but form less viscous gels.
Crospovidone	1–5	High wicking activity.

Dissolution

Drug materials administered orally are required to dissolve in the GI fluids before absorption can take place. Dissolution occurs most rapidly from the primary particles of the drug substance, hence the importance of rapid disintegration to this state. However, disintegration studies only demonstrate that a tablet will break up when immersed in fluid; there are many other factors that can influence the dissolution of a material. A carefully designed dissolution test will, therefore, be a better indication of the performance of a dosage form. The design of dissolution tests and the correlation between *in vitro* dissolution and *in vivo* performance is discussed in Chapter 7, "Biopharmaceutical Support in Formulation Development". The optimisation of the dissolution of a substance is discussed in Chapter 8.

Processing of Formulations

The performance requirements of a tablet were discussed in the previous section, and it is clear that most tablets will contain several ingredients. The drug substance, probably a filler, a disintegrant and a lubricant will be common to most formulations, while glidants, colourants and wetting agents may also be included. The quality of the final product will be as dependent on the way in which the components are combined as it is on the components selected. Traditionally, tablet formulations have been prepared by one of two methods: direct compression or granulation.

Direct compression is the term used to define the process where powder blends of the drug substance and excipients are compressed on a tablet machine. There is no mechanical treatment of the powder apart from a mixing process. Granulation is a generic term for particle enlargement, whereby powders are formed into permanent aggregates. The purpose of granulating tablet formulations is to improve the flow and compaction properties prior to compression. There are a number of different methods that can be used to granulate a powder blend but the most common one for pharmaceuticals is wet granulation, where a liquid is added to aid agglomeration and then removed by drying prior to compression. Even from this short description, it is obvious that direct compression is a much simpler process; yet it is not universally adopted. This section will review the advantages and disadvantages of the two techniques in an attempt to explain why granulation still plays an important role in tablet manufacture.

Direct Compression

The term *direct compression* was initially applied to the formation of compacts from materials that required no pretreatment and the addition of no additives or excipients. As such, it was only used for inorganic materials such as potassium bromide. Today, within the pharmaceutical industry, the term is used for tablet manufacture that does not involve the pretreatment of the drug substance apart from blending with excipients.

Advantages of Direct Compression. The most obvious advantage of direct compression is its simplicity and subsequent economy. The manufacture requires fewer operations, and the omission of a drying step results in lower energy consumption. If a new production line is being built for a product, there will be considerable savings in the plant required, equipment such as granulators and dryers being unnecessary. The reduced processing times will produce savings in labour costs, and the simplicity of the process should make process validation simpler. Some of these savings will, however, be offset by the need to use specialised, more expensive, excipients.

Direct compression can provide technical, as well as economic, benefits. Stability of certain drugs can be improved, and the elimination of a wetting and drying process can be beneficial when formulating drugs that are thermolabile or moisture sensitive.

For certain drugs, the dissolution rate can be improved by utilising direct compression. In the section on Disintegration, it was stated that for optimal dissolution, the tablet must disintegrate into its primary particles as quickly as possible. With no agglomeration stage involved in direct compression, the tablets will disintegrate directly to the primary particles.

Disadvantages of Direct Compression. The main limitation of direct compression is that it cannot be used for all drug substances; the technique depends on the major components of the formulation having appropriate flow and compaction properties. While it is possible to modify the properties of drug substances by particle engineering, this is usually outside the scope of the formulator, and the formulation must be designed to accommodate the limitations imposed by the drug substance. For low dose drugs, it is usually possible to overcome such limitations through careful selection of excipients, but there will be a dose level at which it becomes impractical to produce a tablet of acceptable size.

The challenges facing the formulator of low dose drugs by direct compression are related to achieving and maintaining a homogeneous mix. Very low dose drugs can be formulated to form ordered mixes that reduce the risk of segregation. Consideration must be given to the entire manufacturing process to minimise the possibility of segregation.

Direct compression places greater demands on the excipients, particularly the fillers. This has resulted in the introduction of a number of excipients that have been designed specifically for use in direct compression formulations, although they tend to be expensive.

Armstrong (1998) described the following requirements for direct compression fillers:

- Have good flow properties

- Possess good compaction properties

- Have high capacity (defined as the ability to retain their compaction properties when mixed with drugs substances)

- Have appropriate particle size distribution to minimize the segregation potential

- Have high bulk density

- Be capable of being manufactured reproducibly to minimise batch-to-batch variation

Jivraj et al. (2000) have classified the direct compression fillers in terms of their disintegration and flow properties (Table 11.12).

In addition to these excipients, there are also a number of proprietary preparations that combine two or more materials to optimise the flow and compaction properties. Examples of such excipients include the following:

- Ludipress—a combination of a-lactose monohydrate, polyvinylpyrrolidone and crospovidone

- Cellactose—microcrystalline cellulose and lactose

- Cel-O-Cal—co-processed microcrystalline cellulose and calcium sulphate

- Silicified microcrystalline cellulose—co-processed microcrystalline cellulose that has been silicified with colloidal silicon dioxide

A number of active drug substances are also available in co-processed forms for use in direct compression formulations. While such materials might not be considered direct compression in its purest form, they do pass on the advantages of direct compression technology to the tablet manufacturers.

Granulation

Granulation is the most widely used technique to prepare powders for compaction. The term *granulation* is a generic description for a process of particle enlargement in which particles are agglomerated while retaining the integrity of the original particles. A number of methods can be used to achieve the agglomeration; these are normally classified as either wet granulation, where a liquid is used to aid the agglomeration process, or dry granulation, where no liquid is used.

The purpose of granulating is to transform the powdered starting materials, which would otherwise be unsuitable for tabletting, into a form that will run smoothly on a tablet machine. This is achieved in a number of ways. The most obvious benefit of granulation is the improved flow properties resulting from the increase in particle size.

In forming granules, individual particles of the starting ingredients are agglomerated together. If a homogeneous powder mix is achieved before commencing agglomeration, the granules will consist of a homgeneous mix of those ingredients. More importantly, the

Table 11.12
Direct compression fillers.

Classification	Examples	Comments
Materials that act as disintegration agents with poor flow characteristics	Microcrystalline cellulose	Probably the most widely used direct compression excipients. Excellent compactibility at low pressures, high dilution capacity.
	Directly compressible starch	
Free-flowing materials that do not disintegrate	Dibasic calcium phosphate dihydrate	Excellent flow properties. Very brittle material, and is best used in combination with microcrystalline cellulose or directly compressible starch.
Free-flowing powders that disintegrate by dissolution	Lactose	Anhydrous β-lactose possesses excellent compaction properties. Picks up moisture at elevated humidities and may be less compatible with moisture-sensitive compounds than the monohydrate form (Jain et al. 1998).
	Sorbitol	Good compactibility. Popular in chewable tablets due to its cool mouth feel.
	Mannitol	Hygroscopic.

particles of drug substance will be bound to the particles of the excipients, thus reducing the potential for segregation and improving the chances of content uniformity.

The granulation process usually involves the addition of a polymeric binder that sticks the individual particles together. It has been demonstrated with paracetamol (Armstrong and Morton 1977) that this process can reduce the elasticity of starting materials, thus improving the compactibility.

The polymers used as binders are usually hydrophillic in nature. This can have a beneficial effect on the dissolution of hydrophobic drugs. During the granulation process, a film of hydrophilic polymer will form over the surface of hydrophobic drug particles, which will aid wetting.

One of the advantages of granulation is that it results in the densification and subsequent volume reduction of the starting material. This is particularly useful in the case of voluminous starting materials. A further benefit is that the densified, coarse material will reduce the amount of air entrapment.

A number of methods are routinely used within the pharmaceutical industry to produce granulations. These are traditionally classified as dry granulation and wet granulation, depending on whether a liquid is used to aid the agglomeration.

Wet Granulation. Wet granulation methods are the most commonly used in tablet manufacture. These methods involve the addition of a liquid and, usually, a polymeric binder to the powdered starting materials, and a form of agitation to promote agglomeration followed by a drying process. In most cases, the liquid used is water, although in certain circumstances organic solvents such as ethanol or ethanol/water mixes are used. Non-aqueous granulation will be considered when the active substance is particularly unstable in the presence of water, when water will not wet the powder or, possibly, if the drug substance forms a significant portion of the granulate and demonstrates extreme solubility in aqueous media and control of the granulation process becomes difficult due to the occurrence of significant dissolution. While there are a number of approaches to wet granulation used in the pharmaceutical industry, they all share the following basic principles.

- Dry mixing—The starting materials are mixed together. Prior to mixing, the ingredients may be deagglomerated by a milling or sieving process. If the granulate has a low drug content, the active substance may be premixed with one of the ingredients prior to being added to the granulation vessel to ensure good content uniformity

- Addition of granulating liquid—The granulating fluid is added to the dry ingredients and mixed to form a wet mass. The mixing of the fluid with the dry ingredients leads to agglomeration of the powder. This agglomeration can be controlled by altering the amount of fluid added, the intensity of the mixing and the duration of the mixing. Depending on the state of agglomeration achieved, this stage may be followed by a wet sieving process to break up the larger agglomerates

- Drying—The fluid is removed by a drying process

- Milling—The dried granulate undergoes a sieving or milling operation to obtain the desired particle size distribution

To understand the granulation process, it is necessary to consider what is occurring at the particulate level during the process. The aim of granulation is to increase the particle size of a powder mix, and this is achieved in wet granulation by the formation of liquid bridges between the powder particles. If a liquid that is able to wet the powder is added, the system will minimise its surface free energy by forming liquid bridges between the particles. The nature and extent of these bridges will be dependent on the amount of liquid added.

At low liquid levels, it is assumed that the liquid will distribute itself evenly through the bed, forming discrete liquid bridges at points of contact between particles (Figure 11.20). This is known as the pendular state. The strength of an individual pendular bond, σ, between two spherical particles can be calculated:

$$\sigma = \frac{2\pi rT}{1 + \tan\frac{1}{2}\phi} \tag{15}$$

where r is the radius of the spherical particle, T is the surface tension of the liquid and ϕ is the angle formed between the line joining the centre of the spheres and the edge of the pendular bond (Figure 11.21) (Eaves and Jones 1972). This equation predicts that the bond strength will increase as the surface tension of the liquid increases and as the liquid content decreases. In practise, the strength of agglomerates tends to zero at very low liquid contents, and this has

Figure 11.20 Stages involved in granulation.

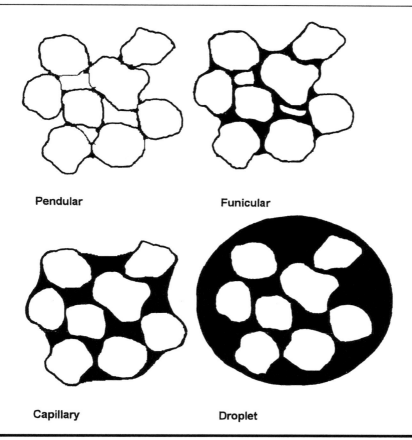

Pendular   Funicular

Capillary   Droplet

been attributed to the presence of dry joints occurring between particles, due to uneven distribution of the liquid throughout the powder bed.

As the liquid content is increased, the pendular state will remain until the pendular bonds start to coalesce and liquid bridges form between non-touching points. This is known as the funicular state (Figure 11.20). The state depends on the degree of liquid saturation or voidage saturation, which is defined as the ratio of the liquid volume to the total volume of pores in the powder bed. Typically, a powder bed will remain in the pendular state until the liquid saturation reaches around 25 percent, and in the funicular state between 25 and 80 percent.

As the liquid saturation rises above 80 percent, the powder reaches the capillary state, and the granule is held together by capillary suction as the liquid air interfaces on the granule surface. While the tensile strength of the granule is greater in the capillary state, the granulate is starting to assume a paste-like consistency which is unsuitable for wet sieving.

The theoretical tensile strength of agglomerates in the funicular and capillary states has been derived by Rumpf et al. (1974):

Figure 11.21 Calculation of the strength of a pendular liquid bridge.

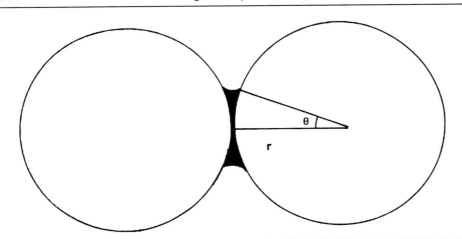

$$\sigma = SC\left(\frac{1-\varepsilon}{\varepsilon}\right)\left(\frac{\gamma}{d}\right)\cos\theta \tag{16}$$

This equation applies to the strength of agglomerates formed from monosize spheres with diameter d that are packed to porosity ε. The degrees of liquid saturation is S, and the liquid has surface tension γ and a contact angle θ with the solid. C is a material constant. Note that in these states, the strength of agglomerates now increases with decreasing particle size. The porosity of the powder also affects the strength; if the material is densified, the agglomerate strength will increase. Addition of further liquid converts the capillary state into the droplet state where the particles are enclosed in a water droplet, and the mass takes on the properties of a slurry.

The gradual transition from pendular through funicular to capillary bonding assumes that there is always a uniform distribution of liquid throughout a powder bed. In practise, this is obviously not always the case because the dispersion of liquid through the powder is achieved by mechanical agitation which will take a finite time. What actually happens in a powder bed during a typical granulation process will be the creation of small areas of high saturation that will lead to the formation of agglomerates which, through mechanical agitation, are dispersed throughout the powder bed. The fate of the agglomerates will change as the degree of liquid saturation increases.

Three phases of agglomeration are recognised, and these will to an extent be occurring simultaneously within a powder bed as the liquid becomes distributed by agitation. The first stage of particle growth is nucleation, which occurs whenever a powder is wetted, particles being held together by liquid bridges. In practise, the liquid addition will lead to overwet agglomerates being formed, to which further powder adheres until the number of liquid bridges is saturated. At low saturation levels, interactions such as friction will also contribute to the strength of the agglomerates. The theoretical strength of the agglomerates is proportional to the degree of liquid saturation, so the initial agglomerates will tend to be weak, and in an agitated environment, agglomerates will be constantly being formed and destroyed. The survival of the agglomerates will increase during the granulation process as the liquid saturation increases and as densification occurs, reducing the porosity of the powder bed.

The powder then undergoes a transition state as it takes up sufficient liquid for the effects of particle interactions to diminish, and the strength becomes controlled by the liquid bridges. The agglomerates become less brittle and more plastic in nature. At this stage, coalescence between colliding particles occurs, and particle growth takes place.

The final stage of granulation is ball growth, a period characterised by rapid growth in particle size. The large granules are formed by smaller granules being fractured, and the resulting fragments build up in layers on the surface of the larger agglomerates.

The above description of the granulation process illustrates that the formulator is dealing with a complex system and the quality of the final product will be influenced by a large number of factors, from the selection of the raw materials to the processing conditions employed.

While one of the stated advantages of granulation over direct compression is that the technique is better able to cope with variations in raw material, the agglomeration process will be affected by significant changes in the raw materials used. The particle size of the starting materials will affect the strength of granules produced, as predicted in equation 16. The quantity of granulating fluid required to achieve granulation is dependent on the particle size and shape. This additional requirement is partly related to the increase in surface area but also relates to the material packing properties that affect the granule porosity and the degree of liquid saturation achieved. Granulation is essentially a wetting process and, as such, is dependent on the surface chemistry of the particles. It is well established that powder handling processes such as milling and drying can significantly affect the surface properties of powders. Small areas of amorphous material on the particle surface produced by particle attrition, too small to be detected by techniques such as X-ray powder diffraction, can have dramatic effects on the wetting characteristics.

Granulating Agents (Binders). It is possible to granulate a powder simply by adding water or an organic solvent to a powder. Provided that the liquid is able to wet the powder surface, it will form liquid bridges. When the granulate dries, the crystallisation of any solids that had dissolved in the liquid will form solid bonds between the particles. These bonds will usually be fairly weak, and friable granulates will be formed; often the granules will not be sufficiently robust to withstand the drying process. It is usual, therefore, to include granulating agents or binders to granulations to increase the granule strength. Granulating agents are usually hydrophillic polymers that have cohesive properties that both aid the granulation process and impart strength on the dried granulate.

For a granulating agent to be effective, it is vital that it is able to form a film on the particle surface. Rowe (1989) has suggested that binders should be selected on the basis of their spreading coefficients, where the spreading coefficient is defined as the difference between the "work of adhesion" of the binder and the substrate and the "work of cohesion" of the binder. The commonly used granulating agents are listed in Table 11.13.

The synthetic polymers such as polyvinyl pyrrolidine (PVP) and hydroxypropyl methylcellulose (HPMC) have almost totally superseded the use of natural products such as starch, acacia and tragacanth in modern formulations. The most common method of adding binders is as a solution in the granulating fluid. It is possible to add some of the synthetic polymers such as PVP and HPMC as powders and use water as the granulating agent. This approach, which has the advantage of not requiring a solution manufacturing step in production, is likely to result in incomplete hydration of the polymers during processing, which will affect the quality of the final granulate.

Table 11.13
Commonly used granulating agents.

Granulating agent	Normal Usage Concentration (%)	Comments
Starch	5–25	Was once the most commonly used binder. The starch has to be prepared as a paste, which is time consuming.
Pre-gelatinised starch	5–10	Cold water-soluble, so easier to prepare than starch.
Acacia	1–5	Requires preparation of paste prior to use. Can lead to prolonged disintegration times if used at too high a concentration.
Polyvinylpyrrolidone (PVP)	2–8	Available in range of molecular weights/ viscosities. Can be added either dry or in solution. Soluble in water and ethanol.
Hydroxypropyl methylcellulose (HPMC)	2–8	Available in range of molecular weight/ viscosities. Soluble in water and ethanol.
Methylcellulose (MC)	1–5	Low-viscosity grades most widely used.

The level of binder used needs to be a balance between the level required to produce a robust, compressible granulate and the biopharmaceutical properties. As the granule strength increases, there is often an adverse effect on disintegration and dissolution. The binders form hydophillic films on the surface of the granules, which can aid the wetting of hydrophobic drugs; but if added in too great concentrations, the films can form viscous gels on the granule surface, which will retard dissolution. To optimise the dissolution of a drug from a granulated product, it is important that the granule should disintegrate into its primary particles as rapidly as possible, and it is usual to position at least a portion of any disintegrant inside the granules.

Wet Granulation Methods. A number of processing methods are commonly used within the pharmaceutical industry. Each method will impart particular characteristics and, as such, granulates produced by each method may not be equivalent in terms of either their physical properties (which will influence subsequent performance on tablet machines) or their biopharmaceutical properties. This latter point is well recognised by regulatory authorities who regard changes in the granulation method as potentially having a significant effect on the bioavailability of poorly soluble, poorly permeable compounds. The U.S. Food and Drug Administration (FDA) and industry representatives have outlined their expectations regarding the testing required when changing the method of granulation in *SUPAC-IR: Immediate-Release Solid Oral Dosage Forms: Scale-Up and Post-Approval Changes: Chemistry, Manufacturing and Controls, In Vitro Dissolution Testing, and In Vivo Bioequivalence Documentation.* This document concludes that changing the type of granulation process used can, for some drug substances, result in the need to perform a bioequivalence study prior to the change being granted regulatory approval.

The three main methods of producing pharmaceutical granulates are low-shear granulation, high-shear granulation and fluid bed granulation. *Low-shear mixers* encompass machines such as Z-blade mixers and planetary mixers which, as their name suggests, impart relatively low shear stresses onto the granulate. Widely used in the past, this approach has largely been superseded by high-shear mixers. The low level of shear applied is often insufficient to ensure good powder mixing, so a premix is often required. The process is forgiving in terms of the amount of liquid added, although it does result in long granulation times. The degree of ball growth tends to be uncontrolled because there is insufficient shear to break up the plastic agglomerates, so a wet screening stage is almost always necessary prior to drying to reduce the larger agglomerates.

High-shear granulators are closed vessels that normally have two agitators; an impeller which normally covers the diameter of the mixing vessel and a small chopper positioned perpendicular to the impeller. The powders are dry mixed using the impeller, and then the granulating fluid is added. Wet massing takes place using the impeller and the chopper, and granulation is usually completed in a number of minutes. The granulation process can be controlled using an appropriate combination of impeller and chopper speeds and time. The ability of the chopper to limit the size of the agglomerates can negate the need for a wet screening stage for many granulates. High-shear mixers provide a greater degree of densification than the low-shear mixers. This, combined with the relatively short processing times, can lead to the process being very sensitive to the amount of granulating liquid added.

In both high-shear and low-shear mixers, the mode of liquid addition can affect the quality of the final product. The liquid can either be added in one go or slowly sprayed onto the powders. Slow spraying leads to the most uniform distribution of liquid but can increase the overall processing time. Pouring the liquid onto the powder will result initially in large over-wet granulates being formed. The mixer needs to impart sufficient energy to the system to break up the agglomerates to achieve uniform distribution of liquid.

Fluid bed granulation involves spraying the dry powder with a granulating fluid inside a fluid bed drier. The powder is fluidised in heated air and then sprayed with the granulating fluid. When all the granulating liquid has been added, the fluidisation of the powder continues until the granules are dry. Advantages of this technique are that the granulation and drying are performed in a continuous manner in the same vessel, and there is no need for a wet screening operation. Nucleation occurs by random collisions between the droplets of granulating fluid and particles until all the individual particles have been incorporated into agglomerates. Densification of materials is limited due to the lack of shear forces.

Seager et al. (1985) produced a detailed analysis on the influence of manufacturing method on the tabletting performance of paracetamol granulated with hydrolysed gelatin. The main difference in the granules produced by different methods was their final density, high shear mixers producing denser granules than low shear granulators, which in turn produced denser granules than fluid bed granulations. Disintegration times were greater for tablets produced from the denser granules.

Extrusion/Spheronisation

One specialised method of particle agglomeration is extrusion and spheronisation, to produce spherical or near-spherical particles. Such particles are suitable for coating with release modifying coats to produce controlled release formulations. The particles are usually filled into hard gelatin capsules for administration to patients. The process of extrusion/spheronisation is depicted in Figure 11.22.

Figure 11.22 Schematic description of extrusion/spheronisation.

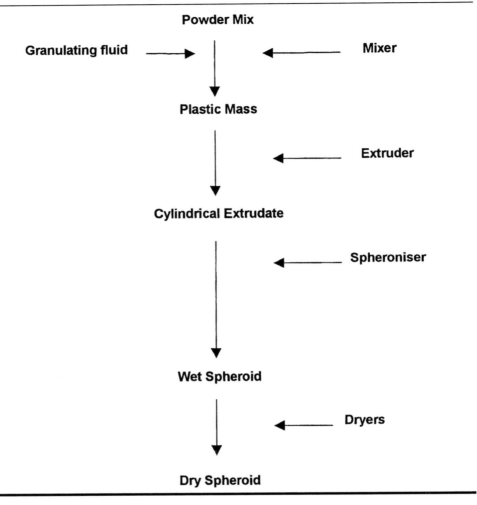

The drug and filler are mixed with water to form a wet mass. This step will be performed using equipment similar to that of conventional wet granulation, though the quantity of water added will be greater, resulting in a plastic mass rather than granules. The mass is then extruded, that is, forced through a screen containing circular holes, to form a spaghetti-like extrudate. The extrudate is cut into lengths roughly twice the diameter of the holes and rolled by frictional and centrifugal forces on a rotating grooved plate known as a marumeriser or spheroniser. The rolling action compresses the cylinder along the length and rounds the ends, forming dumbells which become further compressed along their length to form spheres. The spheroids are discharged from the spheroniser and dried, usually by fluid bed drying.

The basic ingredients of most spheroids are the drug substance, microcrystalline cellulose and water. Microcrystalline cellulose appears to be unique in its ability to form spheroids by this method, due perhaps to its ability to hold onto the water during extrusion. The squeezing of the wet mass through a screen during extrusion forces most materials to lose water, and the resulting extrudates do not have the necessary plasticity to form spheroids.

The robustness of microcrystalline cellulose means that for most low dose drugs it is possible to make spheroids, certainly if the drug loading is below 10 percent. As the drug loading increases, the process becomes more difficult. Two factors appear to be required for success, the mass must retain the water during the extrusion process, and the extrudate must have the appropriate rheological properties.

There are many types of extruders available, with very different shear forces. The different shear forces will have an effect on the water distribution in the extrudates. As the water level is critical for optimising the spheronisation process, it is clear that the formulation development and process development need to be considered as one for this type of process.

Dry Granulation

It is possible to form granulates without the addition of a granulating fluid, by techniques generically referred to as dry granulation. These methods are useful for materials that are sensitive to heat and moisture but which may not be suitable for direct compression.

Dry granulation involves the aggregation of particles by high pressure to form bonds between particles by virtue of their close proximity. Two approaches to dry granulation are used in the pharmaceutical industry: slugging and roller compaction. In either method, the material can be compacted with a binder to improve the bonding strength.

Slugging. Granulation by slugging is, in effect, the manufacture of large compacts by direct compression. The slugs produced are larger than tablets and are often poorly formed tablets exhibiting cracking and lamination. As with tablets, it may be necessay to add a lubricant to prevent the compacts sticking to the punches and dies. The compressed material is broken up and sieved to form granules of the appropriate size. The granules are then blended with disintegrant and lubricant and compressed on a normal tablet machine.

Roller Compaction. In roller compaction, the powder is compacted by means of pressure rollers (Figure 11.23). The powder is fed between two cylindrical rollers, rotating in opposite directions. The rollers may be flat, which will produce sheets of compacted material, or they may be dimpled, in which case, briquettes in the shape of the dimples will be formed. If sheets are produced, they are milled and screened to the required size. Roller compaction requires less lubricant to be added than does slugging.

Selection of the Appropriate Process

The methods of formulating and manufacturing tablets have been described in the preceding sections. Each method has certain unique benefits and advantages as well as drawbacks, and these are summarised in Table 11.14.

For any given compound there will normally be more than one approach that is technically feasible, so how does one choose which approach to take? For most formulators, the choice is strongly influenced by the philosophy of the production department of the company in which they work. Different companies can have very different philosophies; some believe that the cost savings of direct compression are such that attempts should be made to

Figure 11.23 Principles of roller compaction.

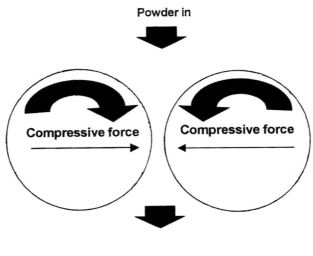

Table 11.14
Manufacturing and formulating tablets—advantages and disadvantages.

Method	Advantages	Disadvantages
Direct compression	Simple, cheap process. No heat or moisture, so good for unstable compounds. Prime particle dissolution.	Not suitable for all drugs, generally limited to low dose compounds. Segregation potential. Expensive excipients.
Wet granulation (aqueous)	Robust process suitable for most compounds. Imparts flowability to a formulation. Can reduce elasticity problems. Coating surface with hydrophillic polymer can improve wettability. Binds drug with excipient, thus reducing segregation potential.	Expensive: time and energy consuming process. Specialised equipment required. Stability issues for moisture sensitive and thermolabile drugs with aqueous granulation.
Wet granulation (non-aqueous)	Suitable for moisture sensitive drugs. Vacuum drying techniques can remove/reduce need for heat.	Expensive equipment; explosion proof; solvent recovery.
Dry granulation (slugging)	Eliminates exposure to moisture and drying.	Dusty procedure. Not suitable for all compounds. Slow process.
Dry granulation (roller compaction)	Eliminates exposure to moisture and drying.	Slow process.

formulate all tablets by this route, other companies feel that wet granulation is a more robust process and should be used even when a compound looks amenable to the direct compression route.

Tablet Coating

For some tablets, compression marks the final stage of the production process, but many formulations involve coating the compressed tablet. There are several reasons for applying a coat:

- Protection of the drug from the environment (moisture, air, light) for stability reasons

- Taste masking

- Minimising patient/operator contact with drug substance, particularly for skin sensitisers

- Improving product identity and appearance

- Improving ease of swallowing

- Improving mechanical resistance; reducing abrasion and attrition during handling

- Modifing release properties

There are three main methods used to coat pharmaceutical tablets: sugar coating, film coating and compression coating. Sugar coating was the most commonly used method until the 1970s, when it was largely superseded by film coating.

Sugar Coating

Sugar coating, as its name suggests, involves coating tablets with sucrose. This is a highly skilled, multistep process that is very labour intensive. The process involves applying a number of aqueous solutions of sucrose, together with additional components, which gradually build up into a smooth, aesthetically pleasing coat. The final coat can account for up to 50 percent of the final tablet weight and will result in a significant increase in the tablet size. Traditionally, sugar coating has been performed in coating pans in which the tablets are tumbled. With the appropriate tablet load and rotation speed, the tablets are tumbled in a three-dimensional direction. The pan is supplied with a source of warm air for drying and an extraction system to remove moist air and dust.

The coating solution is ladled onto the tablet bed and is distributed around the tablets by their tumbling action. The tablets are then tumbled for a period of time to allow the coating to dry before a further quantity of solution is added. A dusting powder may be sprinkled onto the surface of the tablets during the drying phase to prevent the tablets sticking together. One of the skills of sugar coating is adding an appropriate quantity of solution. If too little is added, then not all tablets will pick up some of the coating and an uneven distribution will result. If too much solution is added, the tablets will stick together. The cycle of wetting and drying is continued until the desired amount of coating has been applied to the tablets. Typically, a sugar coating will consist of three types of coat: a sealing coat, a subcoat and a smoothing coat (Figure 11.24).

Figure 11.24 Stages of sugar coating.

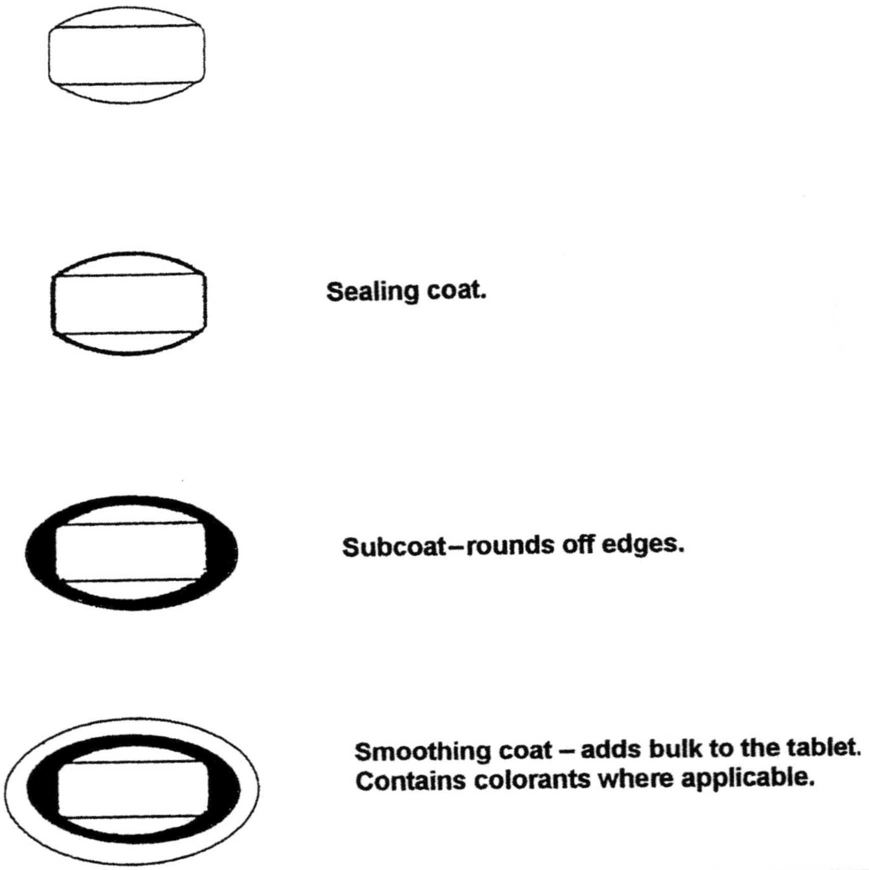

Sealing coat.

Subcoat–rounds off edges.

Smoothing coat – adds bulk to the tablet.
Contains colorants where applicable.

One of the reasons for coating tablets is to protect the drug substance from environmental factors such as moisture, so it is important that the coating solution does not penetrate into the core. This is achieved by applying a sealing coat. Traditionally, a coating of shellac dissolved in ethanol was applied, but this has largely been replaced by the use of synthetic water-resistant polymers such as cellulose acetate phthalate or polyvinylacetate phthalate. The challenge for the formulator is to optimise the quantity of subcoat applied to ensure the core is protected while minimising the effect on drug release.

The subcoat is an adhesive coat on which the smoothing coat can be built. A second purpose of the subcoat is to round off the sharp corners of the tablet to produce a smooth surface. The subcoat is a mixture of a sucrose solution and an adhesive gum, such as acacia or gelatin, which rapidly distributes over the tablet surface. A dusting follows each application of solution with a subcoat powder containing materials such as calcium carbonate, calcium sulphate, acacia, talc and kaolin that help to produce a hard coat. The application of the subcoat continues until the tablets have a rounded appearance and the edges are well covered.

The smoothing coat consists of the majority of the tablet bulk and provides the tablet with a smooth finish. The coat consists of a sucrose syrup which may contain starch or calcium carbonate. Each application is dried, and layers are added until the required bulk has been achieved. The last few coatings will consist of sucrose solution and colourants, where required. The colourants may be either soluble dyes or lakes, lakes often being preferred because a uniform colour is easier to achieve with them.

The coated tablets are usually transferred to a polishing pan and coated with a beeswax-carnauba wax mixture to provide a glossy finish to the surface.

Film Coating

Film coating involves the application of a polymer film to the surface of the tablet and, in contrast to sugar coating, only adds up to 5 percent weight to the final tablet, with a negligible increase in tablet size. It is a technique which, while used mainly to coat tablets, can also be applied to hard gelatin capsules, soft gelatin capsules and multiparticulate systems such as spheroids.

The method of application of the coat differs from sugar coating in that the coating suspension is sprayed directly onto the surface of the tablets, and drying occurs as soon as the coat hits the tablet surface. To achieve this, the tablet only receives a small quantity of coat at a time and the coat is built up in an intermittent manner. While the coating can be applied using a number of methods, all share the following properties: a method of atomising the coating suspension, the ability to heat large volumes of air (which heat the tablets and facilitate the rapid drying of the applied coat) and a method of moving the tablets that ensures all tablets are evenly sprayed. The main methods of coating are modified conventional coating pans, side-vented pans and fluid bed coating.

When the technique of film coating was first applied to tablets, the coatings were suspended in organic solvents, and conventional coating pans were used. Additional air handling was required to provide the volume of air necessary to dry the tablets and to extract the vapours from drying. The nature of the pans is such that the drying air is only present on the surface of the tablet bed; there is no mechanism for it to percolate through it. Providing the volume of air required for such drying was difficult, and a number of modifications have been made to the pans. The limitation in drying efficiency, however, remains a constraint, particularly as most coating now uses aqueous suspensions which impose even greater energy demands. A further limitation to the use of conventional coating pans is their poor mixing efficiency that results in dead spots in the tablet bed.

The side-vented pan, which is now the most commonly used equipment for film coating, was designed to maximise the interaction between the tablet bed and the drying air. In such apparatus, the coating pan is made of perforated metal. The drying air is introduced into the centre of the pan but exhausted through the perforations in the pan beneath the tablet bed (Figure 11.25). Mixing efficiency is achieved by the use of appropriately designed baffles on the pan surface.

Fluid bed coating offers an alternative to pan coating and is particularly popular for coating multiparticulate systems. In fluid bed systems, the objects being coated are suspended in an upward stream of air, maximising the surface available for coating. The coating is applied by an atomiser, and this is dried by the fluidising air. There are three methods by which the coating can be applied (Figure 11.26):

1. Top spraying involves the spray being applied from the top of the fluid bed chamber into the fluidising air using equipment similar to that used for spray granulation.

Figure 11.25 Schematic of the side-vented coating pan.

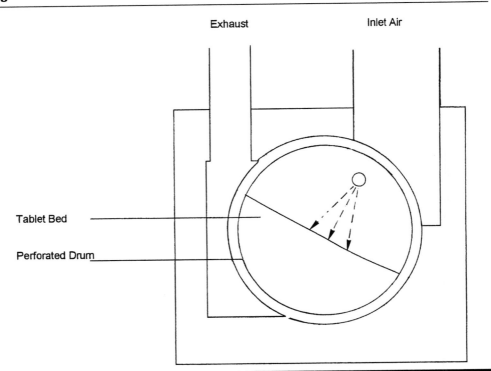

Exhaust

Inlet Air

Tablet Bed

Perforated Drum

2. *Bottom spraying*, sometimes referred to as the Wurster process, involves the spraying of the tablets at the bottom of the fluid bed. In this setup, there is a column introduced into the fluid bed chamber, which ensures that tablets in the centre of the chamber are directed upward. At the top of the column, the tablets descend the chamber at the edge of the chamber from where they will be redirected to the spraying region.

3. The third method of coating is tangential coating which is restricted to the coating of spheroids.

A polymer for film coating will ideally meet the following criteria.

*   Solubility in the solvent selected for application. These days, the solvent will usually be water, although certain types of film coat may require organic solvents to be used. Commonly used solvents include alcohols (methanol, ethanol and isopropanol), esters (ethyl acetate and ethyl lactate), ketones (acetone) and chlorinated hydrocarbons (dichloromethane and trichloroethane). The polymer should not only be soluble in the chosen solvent but should adopt a conformation in solution that yields the maximum polymer extension, which will result in films with the greatest cohesion strength. If mixed solvents are used, consideration should be given to the effect of the solvent ratios changing during the drying process. If the polymer is most soluble in

Figure 11.26 Fluid bed coating of tablets.

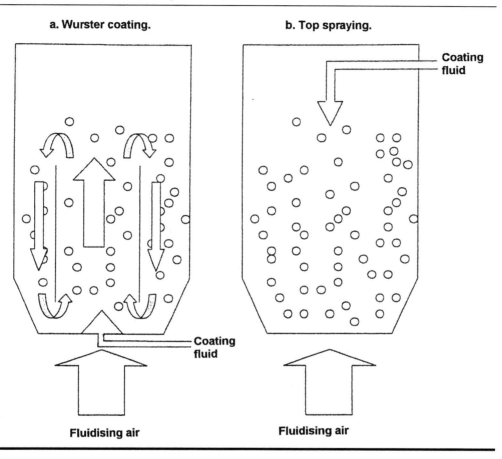

a. Wurster coating.   **b. Top spraying.**

the most volatile component, it may precipitate out during the spraying before reaching the tablet surface.

- Solubility in GI fluids. Unless the coating is being applied for enteric coating or taste masking purposes, it should ideally be soluble across the range of pH values encountered in the GI tract.

- Capacity to produce an elegant film even in the presence of additives such as pigments and opacifiers

- Compatibility with film coating additives and the tablet being coated

- Stability in the environment under normal storage conditions

- Free from undesirable taste or odour

- Lack of toxicity

Table 11.15 lists the most commonly used polymers. With the exception of HPMC, the polymers are rarely used alone but are combined with other polymers to optimise the film-forming properties.

The actual film coating process is described schematically in Figure 11.27. There are two important stages: droplet formation and film formation. The film formation is itself a multi-stage process involving the wetting of the tablet surface followed by spreading of the film and eventually coalescence of the individual film particles into a continuous film. In order for such coalescence to be able to occur, it is necessary for the polymer to be in a plasticised state, that is, above its glass transition temperature, the point at which a polymer goes from being a rigid, brittle material to a flexible material. Most film forming polymers have glass transition temperatures in excess of the temperatures reached during the coating process (typically 40–50°C), so it is necessary to add plasticisers to the formulations, which act by reducing the glass transition temperature. The choice of plasticiser is dependent on the particular polymer(s) being used. The main factors to consider in selection are permanence and compatibility. Permanence is the duration of the plasticiser effect; the plasticiser should remain within the polymer film to retain its effect, so it should have a low vapour pressure and diffusion rate. Compatibility requires the plasticiser to be miscible with the polymer. Commonly used plasticisers include phthalate esters, citrate esters, triacetin, propylene glycol, polyethylene glycols and glycerol.

Film coating provides an opportunity to colour tablets, and most film coats will contain pigments or opacifiers. Insoluble pigments are normally preferred to soluble dyes for a number of reasons. Solid pigments produce a more opaque coat than dyes, protecting the tablet

Table 11.15
Commonly used polymers.

Polymer	Comments
Methylcellulose (MC)	Soluble in cold water, GI fluids and a range of organic solvents.
Ethylcellulose (EC)	Soluble in organic solvents, insoluble in water and GI fluids. Used alone in modified release formulations and in combination with water-soluble celluloses for immediate-release formulations.
Hydroxyethylcellulose (HEC)	Soluble in water and GI fluids.
Methyl hydroxyethylcellulose (MHEC)	Soluble in water and GI fluids. Has similar film forming properties to HPMC but is less soluble in organic solvents, which limited its popularity when solvent coating was the norm.
Hydroxypropyl cellulose (HPC)	Soluble in cold water, GI fluids and polar solvents. Becomes tacky when dried, so is unsuitable for use alone, often used in combination with other polymers to optimise adhesion of coat.
Hydroxypropyl methylcellulose (HPMC)	Soluble in cold water, GI fluids, alcohols and halogenated hydrocarbons. Excellent film former, and the most widely used polymer. Can be used with lactose to improve adhesiveness.
Sodium carboxymethylcellulose (NaCMC)	Soluble in water and polar solvents.

Figure 11.27 Mechanism of film formation on the tablet surface.

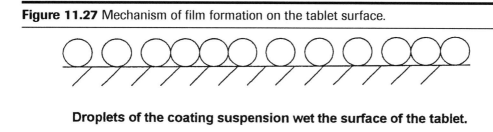

Droplets of the coating suspension wet the surface of the tablet.

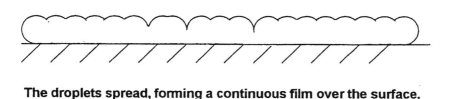

The droplets spread, forming a continuous film over the surface.

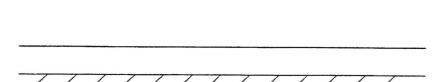

Eventually the droplets completely coalesce to form a smooth film.

from light. The presence of insoluble particles in the suspension allows the rate of solid application to the tablet to be increased without having an adverse effect on the viscosity of the coating suspension, improving productivity. The pigments also tend to exhibit better colour stability than dyes.

Film coating of tablets requires both the process and the formulation to be optimised if a uniform intact coating is to be achieved. The most common flaws, their cause and possible remedies are described in Table 11.16.

It has been emphasised to this point that the coat should not delay the release of the drug substance from the tablet. It is possible to design a coat that will modify the release of a drug substance for a beneficial effect.

The most common type of modified release coating is the enteric coat that is designed to prevent release of the drug substance in the stomach because the drug is either irritant to the gastric mucosa or it is unstable in gastric juice. The most common method of achieving an enteric coating is to apply a polymer that contains acidic substitutions, thus giving it a pH-dependent solubility profile. Examples of such polymers are listed in Table 11.17.

Table 11.16
Film-coating defects.

Flaw	Cause	Remedy
Wrinkling or blistering Film detaches from tablet surface causing blister which can burst to form wrinkles.	Gases forming on tablet surface during coating; exacerbated by poor adhesion of film to tablet surface.	Reduce drying air temperature.
Picking Areas of tablet surface are not covered by film coat.	Overwet tablets stick together and pull film off surface as they move apart.	Decrease spraying rate. Increase drying temperature.
Pitting Holes appear on tablet surface.	Melting of lubricant on tablet surface. Most common with stearic acid.	Decrease coating temperature to below melting point of lubricant. Substitute lubricant.
Blooming Dulling of surface, normally after prolonged storage.	Migration of low molecular weight components of film to tablet surface.	Decrease temperature and length of drying process. Increase molecular weight of plasticiser.
Mottling Uneven colour distribution in film.	Inadequate pigment dispersion. Colour migration, a problem with dyes and lakes rather than pigments.	Alter suspension prepartion to ensure pigment aggregates are dispersed. Replace dyes with pigments.
Orange Peel Film surface has a rough finish resembling orange peel.	Film coat droplets are too dry or too viscous to spread on tablet surface.	Reduce solids content of coating suspension. Reduce drying temperature. Reduce viscosity of polymer.
Bridging Film forms a bridge over intagliations, leaving them indistinct.	High internal stresses in film relieved by pulling the film off the surface of the intagliation.	Increase adhesion of coat to tablet by changing core formulation. Add plasticiser or increase plasticiser concentration. Alter geometry of intagliations.
Cracking, splitting, peeling The film cracks on the crown of the surface or splits on the tablet edge. Can be differentiated from picking by presence of loose film around the flaw.	High stresses in the film that cannot be relieved due to the strong adhesion of the film to the tablet surface.	Increase plasticiser concentration. Use stronger polymer.

Table 11.17
Commonly used enteric coating polymers.

Polymer	Solubility Profile	Comments
Shellac	Above pH 7	The original enteric coating material, originally used in sugar-coated tablets. The high pH required for dissolution may delay drug release. Natural product which exhibits batch-to-batch variability.
Cellulose acetate phthalate (CAP)	Above pH 6	The high pH required for dissolution is a disadvantage. Forms brittle films, so must be combined with other polymers.
Polyvinylacetate phthalate (PVAP)	Above pH 5	
Hydroxypropyl methylcellulose phthalate (HPMCP)	Above pH 4.5	Optimal dissolution profile for enteric coating.
Polymers of methacrylic acid and its esters	Various grades available with dissolution occurring above pH 6	

Film coating can also be used to delay the release of drugs. This is normally applied to multiparticulate systems where particles will be coated with differing thicknesses of water-insoluble polymers such as ethylcellulose

Compression Coating

The third type of tablet coating used in pharmaceuticals is compression coating. This technique involves producing a relatively soft tablet core containing the drug substance and compressing a coating around it (Figure 11.28). This is achieved by placing the core in a large die that already contains some of the coating formulation. Further coating material is then added to the die and the contents compressed. The three types of coating have now been described, and the relative merits of each approach are summarised in Table 11.18.

HARD GELATIN CAPSULES

After tablets, hard gelatin capsules are the most common solid dosage form. Hard gelatin capsules are rigid two-piece capsules made from gelatin, water and colourants. The capsules are produced as empty shells consisting of a cap and body, which during the manufacture of the finished product are separated, filled with the formulation and then rejoined.

Hard gelatin capsules are generally considered to be more forgiving than tablets, from a formulator's perspective. While many of the challenges facing the formulator of tablets are still present, the need for a free-flowing material, powder homogeneity, lubricity and optimising the biopharmaceutical properties, the challenges of forming a robust compact have been

Figure 11.28 Schematic of the compression coating process.

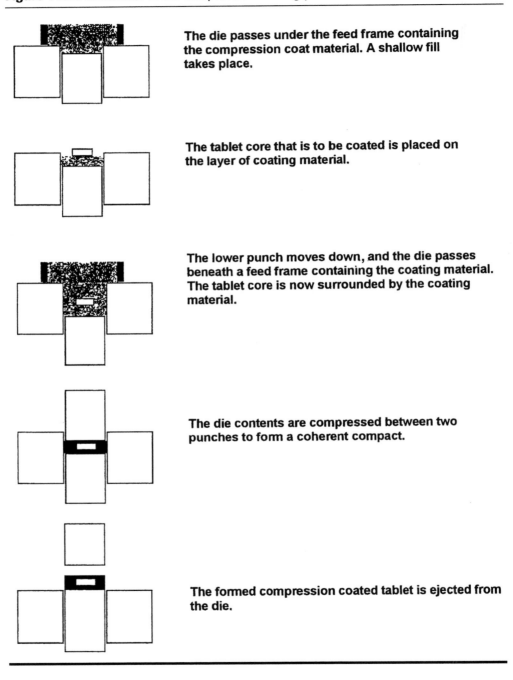

The die passes under the feed frame containing the compression coat material. A shallow fill takes place.

The tablet core that is to be coated is placed on the layer of coating material.

The lower punch moves down, and the die passes beneath a feed frame containing the coating material. The tablet core is now surrounded by the coating material.

The die contents are compressed between two punches to form a coherent compact.

The formed compression coated tablet is ejected from the die.

Table 11.18
Coating methods.

Coating Method	Advantages	Disadvantages
Sugar coating	Elegant final product. Tablets can be printed for identification purposes. Cheap, readily available starting materials. Simple equipment requirements. Excellent protection from environment.	Long process time. Traditional manufacture more an art than a science; high operator dependency. Significantly increases tablet size.
Film coating	Quick process, easy to automate. Negligible increase in tablet size. Tablets can be identified either by printing or through intagliations. Minimal effect on drug release. Enteric coating feasible.	Finish not as elegant as sugar coating. Coating process stresses tablet formulation, cores must be robust to resist abrasion and edge chipping during coating.
Compression coating	It is a dry process, so suitable for moisture-sensitive compounds. Can be used for combination products where the active substances are incompatible.	Significant increase in tablet weight. Possible to produce tablets with no inner core.

removed. Capsules have traditionally been filled with solid formulations such as powder mixes and granulations, but increasingly, multiparticulate formulations, liquid and semi-solid fills are being developed.

Hard gelatin capsules have some disadvantages compared with tablets. The filling speeds of capsule machines are lower than the speeds of the fastest tablet presses, and the cost of the capsule shells makes them a more expensive dosage form. Certain materials are unsuitable for inclusion in capsule shells due to incompatibility with gelatin or because of their affinity for water. One advantage sometimes claimed for capsules is ease of swallowing due to their elongated shape, but this may be countered by the fact that capsules are often larger than corresponding tablets due to the reduced compression of the powder and incomplete filling of the shells. Furthermore, there are concerns that capsules are more prone to sticking in the oesophagus than tablets following swallowing.

The manufacture and formulation of hard gelatin capsules has not been the subject of as much research as tabletting, partly because encapsulation unlike compression is not a science shared by many other disciplines. Nevertheless, there has been important work performed on this dosage form, and much of it is captured in *Hard Capsules Development and Technology* (Ridgway 1987).

Manufacture of Empty Capsule Shells

Gelatin is a heterogeneous product prepared by the hydrolysis of collagen, the principal constituent of connective tissue. The suitability of gelatin for capsule manufacture is due to the following properties:

- It is commonly used in foods and has global regulatory acceptability. However, because it can be derived from a number of animal sources, not all gelatin is acceptable in all markets, and capsule manufacturers will produce capsules from different animal sources to allow for local religious restrictions. All pharmaceutical capsule manufacturers now use gelatin produced in accordance with current requirements relating to bovine spongiform encephalopathy.

- It is a good film former, producing a strong flexible film.

- It is readily soluble in water and in GI fluids at body temperature, so will not retard the release of drugs.

- It changes state at low temperatures enabling a homogeneous film to be formed at ambient temperature.

The properties of a given batch of gelatin are determined by a number of factors: the source of the parent collagen, method of extraction, the pH of the hydrolytic process and its electrolyte content. The properties of most interest to capsule manufacturers are the bloom strength and the viscosity.

The bloom strength is a standard, but arbitary, test of the rigidity of gel produced by a sample of gelatin. The test measures the force required to depress the surface of a 6.67 percent w/w gel, matured at 10°C for 16–18 h, by a distance of 4 mm using a flat-bottomed plunger 12.7 mm in diameter. The force is applied in the form of a stream of lead shot, and the weight, in grammes, is termed the bloom strength. Bloom strengths in the region of 230 to 275 are used for the manufacture of hard gelatin capsule shells. The standard viscosity is measured using a U-tube viscometer with a 6.67 percent w/w solution, and values in the range of 3.3 to 4.7 mPas being used for capsule shells.

Capsule shells are manufactured by dipping moulds into a gelatin solution, drying the gelatin to form a film, removing the dried film from the mould and trimming the film to the right size. The moulds are made of stainless steel and are referred to as pins. The cap and body of the capsule shells are made on separate pins with the body pins being longer than the cap. The external diameter of the body at its open end is slightly larger than the internal diameter of the cap at its closed end to ensure a snug fit when closed.

The empty capsule shells contain 13–15 percent water, a level that is important for optimum performance on capsule filling machines. If the level falls below 13 percent, the capsules become brittle, while if they take up too much water, the gelatin becomes soft and there are problems with capsule separation. The dimensions of the capsule shell will also change with variations in water content, typically increasing by 0.5 percent for every 1 percent increase in moisture content. It is important that capsule shells are both stored and filled in areas where the relative humidity is controlled between 30–50 percent.

It is also important that the capsule fill not adversely affect the moisture content of the shell. This is not a suitable dosage form either for deliquescent materials, which will dry the capsules making them brittle, causing cracking or splitting, or for efflorescent materials, which will soften the shells and may lead to capsules sticking together. Similarly, the presence of moisture in the capsule shells makes them an unsuitable delivery form for drugs that are highly moisture sensitive.

Any fill materials must be chemically compatible with gelatin. Cross-linking of gelatin can be catalysed by trace quantities of formaldehyde, rendering the gelatin insoluble in gastric fluids. Formaldehyde is sometimes present at trace levels in a number of excipients.

Capsules manufactured for use on automatic filling machines, which covers almost all pharmaceutical capsules, have locking devices moulded into the side of the capsule (Figure 11.29). There are two locking positions, a pre-lock to prevent premature opening prior to the

Figure 11.29 Locking mechanism of a hard gelatin capsule shell.

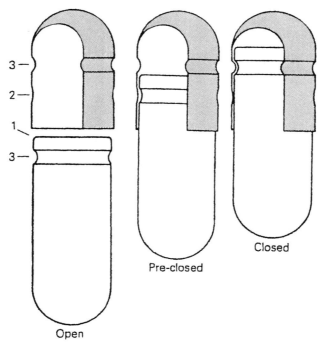

Open

Pre-closed

Closed

1. The tapered rim prevents faulty joins.

2. These indentations prevent the pre-closed capsules from opening too early.

3. These grooves lock the two halves together after filling.

filling process and a locked position which forms an interference seal to prevent the capsule coming apart after filling.

There are a number of companies manufacturing capsule shells for use in the pharmaceutical industry, and all produce capsules to standard sizes, which enables them to be filled on standard filling machines. There are eight sizes of capsules commercially available, listed in Table 11.19. The largest capsule size normally considered for oral administration is size 0, with the 00 and 000 capsules being difficult to swallow due to their size.

Capsule Filling

Before considering how to formulate products for filling into hard gelatin capsules, it is necessary to understand the capsule-filling mechanisms available. All capsule filling machines perform three basic operations: the orientation and separation of the empty capsule shell, the filling of the material into the shell and finally rejoining the cap and the body. From the formulator's perspective, the important stage is the filling, as this will determine the properties

Table 11.19
Capsule sizes.

Capsule Size	000	00	0	1	2	3	4	5
Fill Volume (mL)	1.37	0.95	0.68	0.50	0.37	0.30	0.21	0.13

required of the formulation. The requirements imposed by the filling mechanism will include factors such as powder flow, lubricity and compressibility, and as discussed in the section on tablets, the optimisation of these factors needs to take into consideration the effects on drug release from the formulation.

Drug release from capsules involves an additional step compared to tablets, the dissolution of the capsule shell. When placed in a dissolution medium at 37°C, the gelatin will begin to dissolve, initially retaining its integrity. Eventually, the capsule shell will rupture at its thinnest points, the shoulders of the cap and body, allowing the dissolution medium to penetrate into the capsule contents. The rate of penetration and, where appropriate, the disintegration of the capsule fill will be determined by a combination of the formulation and the processing method, including the filling mechanism.

Powder and Granulate Filling

The requirements of capsule formulations are very similar to those of tablets, and the general formulation principles described earlier apply equally to capsules. As with tablets, most capsules will contain a combination of ingredients including some or all of the following: the active drug substance, filler(s), disintegrant, binder, glidant and lubricant. The main difference in the requirements is the demands placed on the compressibility of the formulation. With tablets, it is necessary to produce a compact capable of withstanding the rigours of subsequent handling. For capsules, it is often necessary to form a plug for ejection into the capsule body, but it is not necessary for the plug to retain its integrity beyond the filling stage. While good flow is necessary for the successful manufacture of both tablets and capsules, the filling mechanisms on certain production capsule machines tend to be more forgiving than tablet machines.

Powder fills for capsules can be either simple blends of starting materials, analogous to direct compression formulations, or granulations. The reduced demands on compressibility and flow increase the options for powder mixes, making capsules a potential dosage form for active substances that do not possess the compression properties required for direct compression tablets and are not amenable to granulation.

Powders account for the majority of capsule fills and a number of quite disparate filling mechanisms have been developed unlike tabletting, where the principle of manufacture, compression between two punches in a die, is the same for all machines. The mechanisms can be divided into two broad groups, those that rely on the volume of the capsule shell to control the dose, known as capsule dependent, and those methods where the quantity of powder to be filled is measured away from the capsule, known as capsule independent. The dependent mechanisms require the capsule shell to be well filled to achieve weight uniformity and are less flexible than the independent methods.

Dependent Methods

The simplest method of dependent capsule filling is levelling, in which the capsule bodies are held flush with a dosing table, and powder is filled into the bodies by gravity. The powder within the capsule bodies may be consolidated by vibration or tamping, and additional powder added to fill the space generated. The final fill weight will depend on the bulk density of the powder and the degree of tamping applied. This method is popular in hand filling devices such as the Tevopharm, Feton, Bonaface and Zuma, which are amenable to most powder mixes. Poor flowing powders will take longer to fill, but with skilled operators, should be feasible. The major formulation challenge is to prepare a blend that will provide an appropriate fill for a standard size capsule.

Osaka Automatic Machine Co. produce a fluidisation machine which is an automatic dependent filling machine. The capsule body in its holder passes below the powder hopper. The powder is fluidised by a vibrating plate to aid flow into the capsule body. The capsule body can be held below the hopper base so that it becomes overfilled, and the fill can be compressed into the capsule by raising the body against a flat surface prior to the capsule closing. This technique has not been the subject of published formulation studies, but appropriate flow properties and lubrication are likely to be required.

Independent Methods

Auger or Screw Method. This was the first mechanism used in industrial-scale machines, although the dosator and piston tamp mechanisms have now largely superseded it. The capsule body in its holder passes beneath the powder hopper on a turntable. The powder is fed into the capsule body by a revolving archimedian screw. The auger rotates at a constant rate so the fill weight is related to the duration of filling that is related to the speed of rotation of the turntable.

Fomulation studies on auger machines have tended to concentrate on the optimisation of fill weight uniformity. Reier et al. (1968) demonstrated that the variation in the capsule fill weight was influenced by the machine speed, capsule size, powder density, powder flow and the presence of a glidant. Ito et al. (1969) determined that there was an optimum level of glidant for minimum weight variation. Powders still account for the majority of capsule fills, and a number of quite disparate filling mechanisms have been developed. Powders should be adequately lubricated to prevent build up of densified material on the auger.

Piston Tamp Method. In piston tamp machines, the powder passes over a dosing plate containing cavities slightly smaller than the internal diameter of the capsule. The powder falls into the holes by gravity and is then tamped by a pin to form a soft plug. This procedure is repeated several times until the cavity is full. Excess powder is removed from above the cavity by a deflector plate. The cavity is then positioned over the capsule body and the plug ejected (Figure 11.30). The dose is controlled by the thickness of the dosing plate, the degree of tamping applied and the height of the powder bed above the dosing plate.

The uniformity of fill weight for the piston tamp machines has been shown to correlate well with the angle of repose of the powders (Kurihara and Ichikawa 1978) and the angle of internal flow (Podczech et al. 1999). Lubrication of formulations is important to prevent build up of material on the tamping pins and to ensure smooth ejection of the plugs from the dosing plate. The ability of the material to compress into a plug, is important; if a formulation does not form a plug, the ejection will not be as clean and can lead to increased weight

Figure 11.30 Schematic of a tamping pin type capsule filling machine.

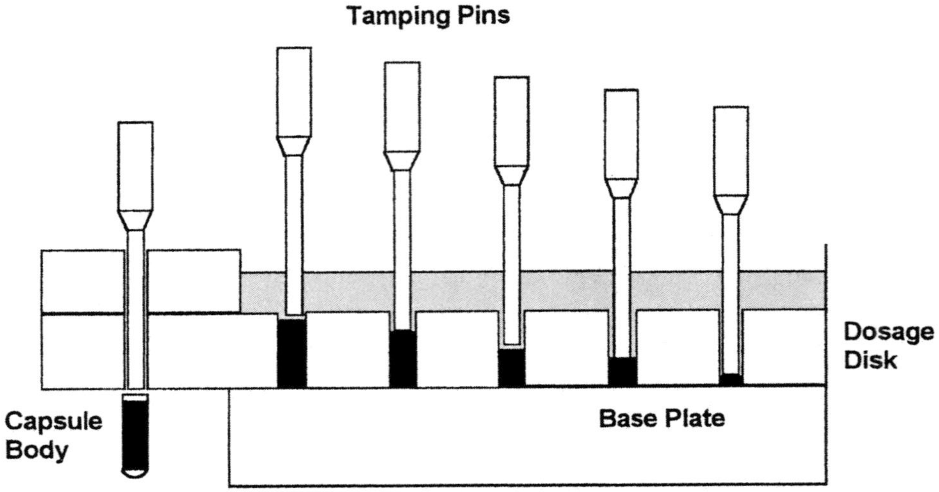

variation. Studies have shown that for certain formulations, the tamping pressure applied by the pins can affect the dissolution rate of the final product (Shah et al. 1983). The minimum tamping force necessary to obtain a plug that will fit inside the body of the capsule shell should be aimed for.

Dosator Method. A dosator, consisting of a stainless steel cylinder containing a spring-loaded stainless steel piston, is lowered, open end first, into a flat powder bed. As the cylinder passes into the bed, powder is forced up into the cylinder until it reaches the piston, forming a plug. Additional compression of the plug can be obtained by applying a downward pressure on the piston. The dosator is lifted from the powder bed and, if a suitable plug has formed, the powder will remain within. The dosator is positioned above a capsule body and the plug ejected by lowering the piston. The dose is controlled by the dimensions of the dosator, the position of the piston within the dosator as it enters the powder bed and the height of the powder bed (Figure 11.31).

This mechanism is the most widely used mechanism and can be found on small pilot scale machines using an intermittent action similar to rotary machines capable of production rates in excess of 120,000 capsules per hour. As a result of its popularity, there have been considerable studies into the formulation of powder for filling on these types of machines and instrumentation of the dosators.

The fundamental requirements of a formulation to be filled on a dosator type machine are good flow properties, compressibility and lubricity. *Flow* is important in the powder bed: when the dosator dips into the powder, it leaves a void which must be closed with material of the same bulk density prior to the next dosator entering that area of the hopper. Irwin et al. (1970) investigated the effect of powder flow on the uniformity of weight achieved on a Zanasi filling machine and concluded that the better the rate of flow the better the uniformity of fill.

Figure 11.31 Schematic of a dosator type capsule filling machine.

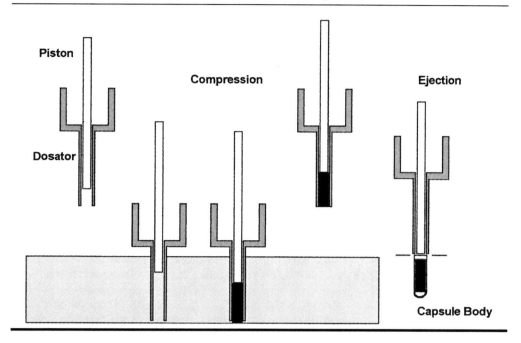

Compressibility is necessary to form a plug of sufficient strength that powder does not escape from the dosator as it leaves the powder hopper and positions itself above the capsule body. Jolliffe and Newton (1982a,b) considered the theoretical aspects of powder retention using powder hopper design theory to calculate the forces required to hold a free powder surface in an open-end cylinder. The powder retention relies on the formation of a stable powder arch which is dependent on the shear developed at the dosator walls and the unconfined yield strength. It was demonstrated that the angle of wall friction between the powder and dosator could have an important influence on powder retention. This was explored experimentally (Jolliffe and Newton 1982a,b) by showing that the internal friction changed during manufacture as the powder fill coated the internal wall of the dosator. Furthermore, these authors proposed that the optimum design for a dosator would have two types of surface finish, a smooth finish with a low value of wall friction for the main body of the cylinder together with a higher value of wall friction at the outlet to promote arch formation. The dosator mechanism does permit high compressive forces to be applied to powder beds. The objective of a capsule formulation is not to make a mini tablet that can be filled into a capsule, the compression force should be restricted to the minimum level necessary to form a coherent plug. Whenever powders are compressed, there is the possibility of elastic recovery when the compressive stress is removed. The tolerance between the internal diameter of the dosators and the internal diameter of capsule shells is fairly tight, and any elasticity in capsule formulations can lead to the plugs not sitting properly in the capsule shells, resulting in powder loss as the cap is reunited with the body. In such circumstances, the pragmatic approach is to use dosators designed for the next smallest capsule size.

The *lubricity* requirements of formulations being filled with dosators has been examined by Small and Augsburer (1978) using a Zanasi machine on which strain gauges had been attached to the dosator pistons. The magnitude of the force required to eject the powder plug from the piston was shown to be dependent on the identity and level of lubricant, the height of the initial powder bed, the piston height and the compression force applied.

Filling Capsules with Pellets

The use of multiparticulate systems to provide modified release formulations is ever increasing, and hard gelatin capsules provide an ideal way of delivering unit doses of such formulations. The two most common approaches to pellet formulation are extrusion/spheronisation (discussed in an earlier section) and the coating of non-pareil seeds. Non-pareil seeds are sucrose beads which can be film coated with a solution/suspension of the drug substance followed by layers of modified-release coatings to obtain the release profile required. The capsule filling method has to be gentle enough on the pellets to retain the integrity of the coating.

As with powder filling, the filling of pellets into capsules can be dependent or independent. A dependent method often performed uses a modified augur type machine, in which the pellets are simply poured by gravity into the capsule shells. The critical formulation aspect of this approach is ensuring that the required dosage of active substance is present in the volume of pellets taken to fill the capsule body.

An independent method uses a volumetric fill by a modified dosator method. The piston inside the dosator is narrower than those used for powder filling, and this allows air to flow between the piston and the dosator wall. The dosator is lowered into the pellet bed, but in this case, there is no compression applied. A vacuum source is applied from above the piston to retain the pellets as the dosator is moved above the capsule body. Once over the capsule body, the vacuum is removed, and the ejection of the pellets is aided by an air jet.

Tablets

Capsules can also be filled with tablets, which can be of use when preparing blinded clinical trial materials. Tablets are fed from a hopper into a chamber that simply releases one or more tablets into the capsule body as it passes underneath. The optimum formulation for capsule filling is a biconvex film-coated tablet, the film coating reducing abrasion and material loss.

Capsugel produce a range of specially sized opaque capsules specifically for the encapsulation of tablets for double blind clinical trial supplies. The capsules are wider than standard-sized capsules to allow larger diameter tablets to be filled but have shorter bodies to retain patient acceptability/tolerability.

Liquids and Semi-Solids

Two types of liquid formulations can be filled into hard gelatin capsules, those which are liquid at room temperature and those which are solid at room temperature. Such solid formulations can be liquefied either by heating to temperatures up to 70°C (the maximum temperature the gelatin shell can withstand) or by the application of shear stress. In the case of liquids that are mobile at room temperature, the capsules need to be sealed after filling to prevent leakage of the contents.

The filling of such formulations requires machines fitted with hoppers that can provide a heating and stirring system. For most formulations, the capsules are filled using a volumetric pump, although certain viscous preparations may require an extrusion pump. The pump must be designed to be non-drip, and the capsule handling needs to be modified to control product spillage. A sensing system is required to detect the presence or absence of caps or bodies so that the pump can be stopped and the bushes not contaminated with fill material. With powder fills, contamination of the exterior of capsules can be removed by vacuum dedusting. With liquids, if one capsule is covered with liquid it can lead to major problems with capsules sticking together.

There are a number of applications for liquid/semi-solid filled capsules:

- Improvement of bioavailabilty

- Safety—minimising operator exposure to dusty processes

- Content uniformity—it is easier to achieve and maintain content uniformity in a solution system than a powder system

- Stability

These advantages are similar to those of soft gelatin capsules and are dealt with in greater depth in a following section.

With soft gelatin capsule technology being so well established, what advantages does liquid filling of hard gelatin capsules provide the formulator? The major advantage is that it is a technology that can be installed in-house relatively simply, unlike soft gelatin capsule manufacture which remains in the hands of a limited number of contract suppliers. This has been made possible by the development of techniques for sealing the capsules.

The approach taken to formulate a liquid-filled capsule will depend on the reason for selecting such a dosage form. The most important aspect of the formulation is to ensure that the fill is compatible with the gelatin shell. It is well known that the gelatin shell is sensitive to changes in moisture levels, and hence liquids that readily take up moisture such as the low-molecular-weight polyethylene glycols will be unsuitable. Capsugel, one of the main suppliers of capsule shells, performed extensive compatibility testing of liquid vehicles and has published a list of those deemed to be compatible (Stegemann 1999) (Table 11.20).

Capsule Sealing

The filling of liquids into hard gelatin capsules has been thought about for many years but was not commercially feasible until reliable methods for capsule sealing were available. The incidents involving the tampering of paracetamol capsules in the United States in the mid-1980s forced capsule manufacturers to develop a method of making capsules tamper evident. This, in turn, led to the development of the Quali-Seal capsule banding machine. This machine applies a narrow band of gelatin around the joint of the cap and body of filled capsules, which can be dried without the application of heat. Heat would cause air expansion within the capsule, disrupting the seal.

A recent development in sealing technology has been liquid encapsulation microspray sealing (LEMS) in which a sealing fluid of approximately 50 percent water and 50 percent

Table 11.20
Liquid excipients compatible with hard gelatin capsule shells.

Lipophilic Excipients	Hydrophilic Excipients	Amphiphilic Excipients
Vegetable Oils	Polyethylene glycol (PEG) 3000–6000 molecular weight	Poloxamers
Peanut oil		Lecithin
Castor oil		PEG Esters (e.g., Gelucir 44/14; 50/13; Labrafil)
Olive oil		
Fractionated coconut oil		
Corn oil		
Sesame oil		
Hydrogenated vegetable oils		
Soybean oil		
Esters		
Glycerol stearate		
Glycol stearate		
Isopropyl myristate		
Ethyl oleate		
Fatty Acids		
Stearic acid		
Lauric acid		
Palmitic acid		
Oleic acid		
Fatty Alcohols		
Cetyl alcohol		
Stearyl alcohol		

ethanol is sprayed onto the joint between the cap and body. This fluid penetrates the cap/body joint by capillary action and lowers the melting point of the gelatin; the capsule is then exposed to a short cycle of warm air which melts and fuses the gelatin at the joint. This technique is an elegant method of sealing, as the seal is not visible to the user.

Alternatives to Gelatin Capsules

There have been a number of attempts to make capsules from materials other than gelatin. Initially, the attempts were aimed at overcoming the original patents filed by Mothe in the nineteenth century and used materials such as starch, gluten and animal membranes. However, the only material with the correct film-forming properties was gelatin.

More recently, the attention has moved to synthetic polymers with the aim being to produce capsules that will overcome the shortcomings of gelatin, particularly its moisture content. Two alternative materials have been offered by capsule manufacturers, starch and hydroxypropyl methylcellulose (HPMC).

The starch capsules are produced by an injection moulding process using potato starch, and are produced in five sizes, all of the same diameter but with different lengths (Vilivalam et al. 2000). While the fill volumes are similar to gelatin capsules, the different dimensions necessitate specialised filling equipment. The capsule surface is less smooth than gelatin capsules, and the injection moulding allows a smooth join between cap and body to be obtained. These properties make the capsules amenable to film coating processes. The moisture content of the capsules is 14 percent.

HPMC capsules are made by the pin-dipping process used for gelatin capsules and are made to the same size specifications, allowing them to be filled on conventional capsule filling equipment. These capsules have a lower moisture content than gelatin capsules, and the moisture is tighter bound, making them more suitable for moisture sensitive drugs and hygroscopic excipients. The capsule surfaces have rougher finishes than gelatin capsules, and colouring the capsules is more difficult. The rough coat leads to better adhesion with coating materials, so they could have applications for enteric coating.

SOFT GELATIN CAPSULES

Soft gelatin capsules are included in this chapter on oral solid dosage forms, although there is debate as to whether or not they are solid or liquid dosage forms. The drug is presented in a liquid encapsulated in a solid thus combining advantages of liquid dosage forms with the unit dosage convenience of solid forms.

Manufacture

Unlike hard gelatin capsule shells which are manufactured empty and subsequently filled in a separate operation, soft gelatin capsules are manufactured and filled in one operation. This is a specialised process and tends to be performed by a limited number of companies. One consequence, therefore, of selecting a soft gelatin capsule formulation is that the product will probably be manufactured by a contract manufacturer. A desire to keep all manufacturing in-house is one of the reasons for companies considering the use of liquid-filled hard gelatin capsules as an alternative.

The shell ingredients of a soft gelatin capsule are gelatin, glycerol, which acts as a plasticiser, and potentially other ingredients which could include additional plasticisers such as sorbitol or propylene glycol, dies or pigments, preservatives and flavours. The glycero-gelatin mix is dissolved in water, then heated and pumped onto two cooling drums to form two gelatin ribbons which are fed into the filling machine. The liquid fill is pumped between the gelatin ribbons as they pass between the two die rolls of the filling machine, forcing the gelatin to adopt the shape of the die. The two ribbons are sealed together by heat and pressure and the capsules are cut from the ribbon (Figure 11.32). They then pass through a tumble dryer to remove the bulk of the water and conditioned at 20 percent relative humidity (RH).

The fill can be either a solution or a suspension, liquid or semi-solid. The main limitation is that the fill must be compatible with the shell. The main incompatibilities are: high

Figure 11.32 Schematic of the soft gelatin capsule manufacturing process.

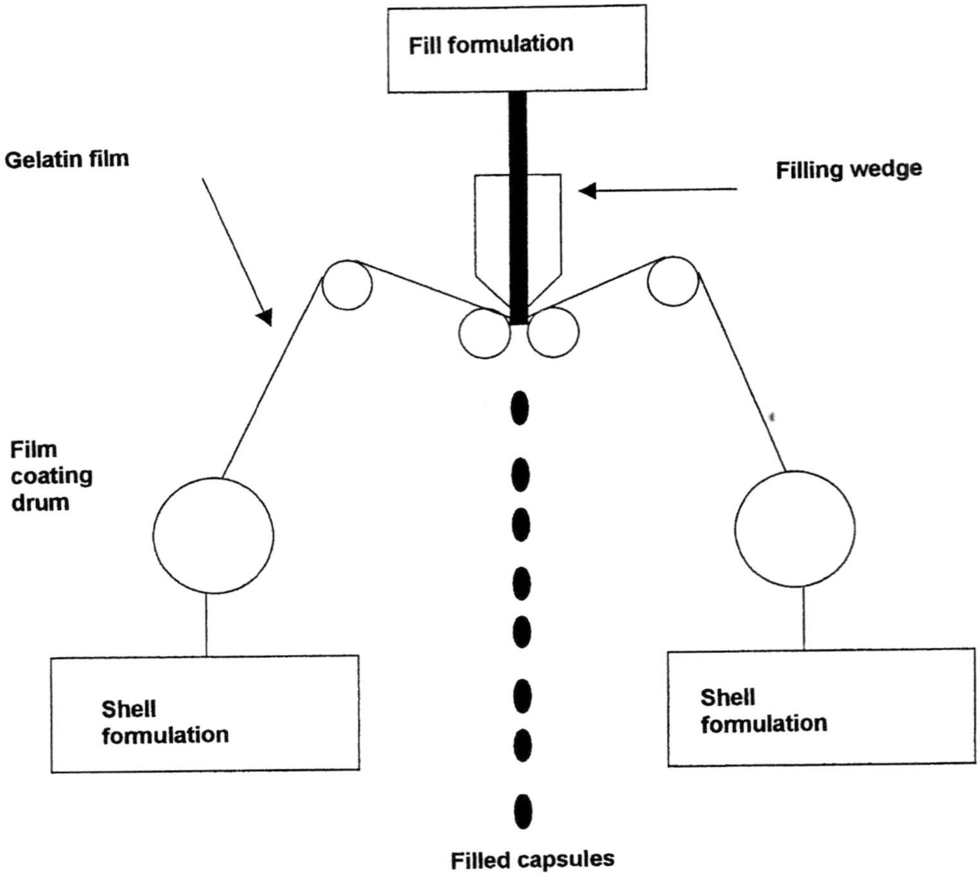

Filled capsules

concentrations of water or other solvents that will dissolve the shell, high pH (>7.5) solutions which will cause cross-linking of the gelatin which will retard dissolution of the shell, low pH solutions which may hydrolyse the gelatin and aldehydes which promote cross-linking. The types of vehicles that can be used in soft gelatin capsules are similar to those used for liquid-filled hard gelatin capsule shells listed in Table 11.20.

Benefits of Soft Gelatin Capsule Formulations

Soft gelatin capsules are a more expensive dosage form than either tablets or capsules, so they tend to be considered when they can offer a major benefit to the formulator. Justifications for their use include improved content uniformity, safety, improved stability and improved bioavailability.

Improved Content Uniformity

Because soft gelatin capsules are filled with liquids or suspensions, excellent content uniformity can be achieved with even the most potent of drugs. The accuracy of the filling mechanism enables the dose to be filled to a tolerance of ± 1 percent for solutions and ± 3 percent for pastes.

Safety

Dissolving potent drugs in a liquid vehicle reduces the risk of operator exposure to dusts that is present with tablet and hard gelatin capsule manufacturing operations.

Improved Stability

Varying the level of glycerol in the shell formulation will alter the permeability of the shell to oxygen. The filling process can be performed under nitrogen, so by appropriate selection of shell composition, this technology can provide excellent protection for oxygen sensitive drugs.

Improved Bioavailability

Presenting the drug to the GI tract in a solubilised form overcomes the processes of disintegration and dissolution that are required from hard gelatin capsules and tablets before the drug substance is available for absorption. This has been utilised to improve the bioavailability of drugs with a range of solubilities.

Acid soluble drugs can be dissolved or dispersed in water miscible vehicles that rapidly distribute the drug throughout the stomach following administration. Acid insoluble drugs can be dissolved in water miscible vehicles, which results in the drug precipitating as a fine suspension in the stomach. The surface area of the solid in suspension is high, resulting in rapid dissolution.

Formulation of compounds that have very low aqueous solubility in lipid vehicles is an area that has seen the most growth in recent years. Two approaches can be used, depending on the solubility characteristics of the drug substance. For compounds with log P values in the region of 2 to 4, the preferred approach is to form self-emulsifying systems. These formulations comprise a lipid vehicle, typically a medium-chain triglyceride together with a surfactant which, on contact with an aquaeous environment, spontaneously form micelles. The drug remains solubilised in the micelles. Drugs with higher log P values can be dissolved in a digestible oil such as medium-chain monoglycerides that is immiscible with water. On release from the capsule the drug remains solubilised in the immiscible oil. The precise mechanism by which the drug is absorbed from the oil is not fully understood but there are a number of compounds on the market which have successfully demonstrated improved bioavailability by this route.

SUMMARY

This chapter has summarised some of the key aspects of powder technology that are important to the development of the principal solid dosage forms, tablets and capsules. Space restrictions have prevented this being a very detailed review, and there are many specific types of tablets that have not been discussed at all. The area of solid dosage forms is very well served by the literature, and those interested in studying the subject area further are encouraged to consult the texts listed in the reference section.

REFERENCES

Alderborn, G., and C. Nystrom. 1995. Pharmaceutical powder compaction technology. *Drugs and the pharmaceutical sciences*, vol. 71. New York: Marcel Dekker.

Anon. 1989. Can the appearance of medication improve compliance? *Pharm. J.* 281:88.

Armstrong, N. A. 1987. Time dependent factors involved in powder compression and tablet manufacture. *Int. J. Pharm.* 48:173–177.

Armstrong, N. A., and F. S. S. Morton. 1977. The effect of granulating agents on the elasticity and plasticity of powders. *J. Powder Bulk Solids Technol.* 1:32.

Armstrong, N. A. 1998. Direct compression characteristics of granulated Lactitol. *Pharm. Technol.* 22:84–92.

Armstrong, N. A., and R. F. Haines-Nutt. 1972. Elastic recovery and surface area changes in compacted powder systems. *J. Pharm. Pharmacol.* 26:135P.

Asker, A., M. el-Nakeeb, M. Motawi, and N. el-Gindy. 1973. Effect of certain tablet formulation factors on the antimicrobial activity of tetracycline hydrochloride and chloramphenicol. 3. Effect of lubricants. *Pharmazie.* 28:476–478.

Barcellos, F. L. L. B., and A. Carneiro. 1953. Concrete tensile strength. *R.I.L.E.M. Bulletin.* 13:97–123.

Charlton, B., and J. M. Newton. 1985. Application of gamma-ray attenuation to the determination of density distributions within compacted powders. *Powder Technol.* 41:123–134.

Chemist and druggist directory and tablet and capsule identification guide. 2000. London: Benn Publications Ltd.

Eaves, T., and T. M. Jones. 1972. Effect of moisture on tensile strength of bulk solids. 1. Sodium chloride and effect of particle size. *J. Pharm. Sci.* 61:256–261.

FDA. 1995. *Guidance for industry. Immediate release solid oral dosage forms. Scale-up and postapproval changes: Chemistry, manufacturing, and controls, in vitro dissolution testing, and in vivo bioequivalence documentation.* Rockville, Md., USA: Food and Drug Administration, Center for Drug Evaluation and Research.

Handbook of pharmaceutical excipients, 3rd ed. 2000. London: Pharmaceutical Press and the American Pharmaceutical Association.

Harnby, N., M. F. Edwards, and A. W. Nienow. 1985. *Butterworths series in chemical engineering: Mixing in the process industries.*

Heckel, R. W. 1961. Density-pressure relationships in powder compaction. *Trans. Metall. Soc., A.I.M.E.* 221:671–675.

Hiestand, E. N., and D. P. Smith. 1984. Three indexes for characterizing the tabletting performance of materials. *Adv. Ceram.* 9:47–57.

Hölzer, A. W., and J. Sjøgren. 1978. The influence of the tablet thickness on measurements of friction during tabletting. *Acta Pharm. Suec.* 5:59–66.

Irono, C. I. and N. Pilpel. 1982. Effects of paraffin coatings on the shearing properties of lactose. *J. Pharm. Pharmacol.* 34:480–485.

Irwin, G. M., G. J. Dodson, and L. J. Ravin. 1970. Encapsulation of clomacron phosphate. 1. Effect of flowability of powder blends, lot-to-lot variability, and concentration of active ingredient on weight variation of capsules filled on an automatic filling machine. *J. Pharm. Sci.* 59:547.

Ito, K., S-I. Kaga, and Y. Takeya. 1969. Studies on hard gelatin capsules. II. The capsule filling of powders and effects of glidant by ring filling method. *Chem. Pharm. Bull.* 17:1138.

Jain, R., A. S. Railkar, A. W. Malick, C. T. Rhodes, and N. H. Shah. 1998. Stability of a hydrophobic drug in the presence of hydrous and anhydrous lactose. *Eur. J. Pharm. Biopharm.* 46:177–182.

Jivraj, M., L. G. Martini, and C. M. Thomson. 2000. An overview of the different excipients useful for the direct compression of tablets. *Pharm. Sci. Technol. Today* 3 (2):58–63.

Jolliffe, I. G., and J. M. Newton. 1982a. Practical implications of theoretical consideration of capsule filling by the dosator nozzle system. *J. Pharm. Pharmacol.* 34:293–298.

Jolliffe, I. G., and J. M. Newton. 1982b. An investigation of the relationship between particle size and compression during capsule filling with an automated mG2 simulator. *J. Pharm. Pharmacol.* 34:415–419.

Kamm, R., M. A. Steinberg, and J. Wulff. 1949. Lead-grid study of metal powder compaction. *Trans. A.I.M. (Met) E.* 180:694–706.

Kocova, S., and N. Pilpel. 1972. Failure properties of lactose and calcium carbonate powders. *Powder Technol.* 5:329–343.

Kocova, S., and N. Pilpel. 1973. Failure properties of some simple and complex powders and the significance of their yield locus parameters. *Powder Technol.* 8:33–35.

Krycer, I., D. G. Pope, and J. A. Hersey. 1982. The prediction of paracetamol capping tendencies. *J. Pharm. Pharmacol.* 34:802–804.

Kurihara, K., and I. Ichikawa. 1978. Effect of powder flowability on capsule-filling—weight—variation. *Chem. Pharm. Bull.* 26:1250–1256.

Malamataris, S., S. Bin Baie, and N. Pilpel. 1984. Plasto-elasticity and tabletting of paracetamol, Avicel and other powders. *J. Pharm. Phamacol.* 36:616–617.

Nyquist, H., and A. Brodin. 1982. Ring shear cell measurements of granule flowability and the correlation to weight variations at tabletting. *Acta Pharm. Suec.* 19:81–90.

Nyström, C., K. Malmquist, J. Mazur, W. Alex, and A. W. Hölzer. 1978. Measurement of axial and radial tensile strength of tablets and their relation to capping. *Acta Pharm. Suec.* 15:226–232.

Physicians' Desk Reference, 52nd ed. 1998. New York: Medical Economics Co.

Pitt, K. G., J. M. Newton, R. Richardson, and P. Stanley. 1989. The material tensile strength of convex-faced aspirin tablets. *J. Pharm. Pharmacol.* 41:289–292.

Podczechk, F., S. Blackwell, M. Gold, and J. M. Newton. 1999. The filling of granules into hard gelatine capsules. *Int. J. Pharm.* 188:49–59.

Reier, G., R. Cohn, S. Rock, and F. Wagenblast. 1968. Evaluation of factors affecting the encapsulation of powders in hard gelatin capsules. I. Semi-automatic machines. *J. Pharm. Sci.* 57:660–666.

Rhodes, M. 1990. *Principles in powder technology.* New York: Wiley.

Ridgway, K. 1987. *Hard capsules development and technology.* London: Pharmaceutical Press.

Ridgway, K., and P. Watt. *Tablet machine instrumentation in pharmaceutics: Principles and practise.* 1988. Chichester, UK: Ellis Horwood Ltd.

Roberts, R. J., and R. C. Rowe. 1985. The effect of punch velocity on the compaction of a variety of materials. *J. Pharm. Pharmacol.* 37:377–384.

Roberts, R. J., and R. C. Rowe. 1986. Brittle fracture propensity measurements on "tablet-sized" compacts. *J. Pharm. Pharmacol.* 38:526–528.

Roberts, R. J., and R. C. Rowe. 1987. The compaction of pharmaceutical and other model materials—a pragmatic approach. *Chem. Eng. Sci.* 42:903–911.

Rowe, R. C. 1989. Binder-substrate interactions in granulation: A theoretical approach based on surface free energy and polarity. *Int. J. Pharm.* 38:149–154.

Rowe, R. C., and S. F. Forse. 1983. Pitting—A defect on film coated tablets. *Int. J. Pharm.* 17:343.

Rubenstein, M. H., and D. M. Bodey. 1974. Disaggregation of compressed tablets. *J. Pharm. Pharmacol.* 26:104P.

Rudnic, E. M., C. T. Rhodes, S. Welch, and P. Bernardo. 1982. Evaluations of the mechanism of disintegrant action. *Drug Dev. Ind. Pharm.* 8:87–110.

Rumpf, H. 1974. *Chem. Ing. Tech.* 46:1.

Schulze, D. 1996. Comparison of the flow behaviour of easily flowing bulk materials. *Schuettgut.* 2:347–356.

Seager, H., P. J. Rue, I. Burt, J. Ryder, N. K. Warrack, and M. J. Gamlen. 1985. Choice of method for the manufacture of tablets suitable for film coating. *Int. J. Pharm. Tech. Prod. Mfr.* 6:1–20.

Shah, K. B., L. L. Augsburger, L. E. Small, and G. P. Polli. 1983. Instrumentation of a dosing disc automatic capsule filling machine. *Pharm. Technol.* 7:42–54.

Shah, N. H., D. Stiel, M. Weiss, M. H. Infeld, and A. W. Malick. 1986. Evaluation of two new tablet lubricants—sodium stearyl fumarate and glyceryl behenate. Measurement of physical parameters (compaction, ejection and residual forces) in the tabletting process and effect of the dissolution rate. *Drug Dev. Ind. Pharm.* 12:1329–1346.

Shotton, E., and G. S. Leonard. 1972. The effect of intra- and extragranular maize starch on the disintegration of compressed tablets. *J. Pharm. Pharmacol.* 24:798–803.

Small, L. E., and L. L. Augsburger. 1978. Aspects of the lubrication requirements for an automatic capsule-filing machine. *Drug Dev. Ind. Pharm.* 4:345–372.

Stegemann, S. 1999. Liquid and semi-solid formulaion in hard gelatin capsules. *Swiss Pharma.* 21 (6):21–28.

Train, D. 1956. An investigation into the compaction of powders. *J. Pharm. Pharmacol.* 8:745–761.

Train, D. 1957. Agglomeration of solids by compaction. *Trans. Ins. Chem. Engrs.* 35:258–262.

Vilivalam, V. D., L. Illum, and K. Iqbal. 2000. Starch capsules: An alternative system for oral drug delivery. *Pharm. Sci. Technol. Today* 3 (2):64–69.

Williams, J. C., and A. H. Birks. 1967. The comparison of the failure measurements of powders with theory. *Powder Technol.* 1:199–206.

York, P. and N. Pilpel. 1973. The tensile strength and compression behaviour of lactose, four fatty acids and their mixtures in relation to tabletting. *J. Pharm. Pharmacol.* 25:Suppl. 1P–11P.

12

Ophthalmic Dosage Forms

Mark Gibson

AstraZeneca R&D Charnwood
Loughborough, United Kingdom

There are many diseases affecting the eye that are treated with various types of drugs and drug delivery systems. Table 12.1 lists some of the main therapeutic classes of drugs currently used to treat eye diseases and types of dosage forms commercially available.

Drugs such as antibiotics and corticosteroids can be administered systemically to treat certain eye conditions, but this route of administration is not often favoured because of the poor drug penetration into the eye from the systemic circulation. Subsequently, high doses have to be administered, leading to systemic side-effects and toxicity. Periocular injections are also used to administer anti-infective drugs, mydriatics or corticosteroids. However, injections tend to be reserved for serious conditions affecting the anterior portion of the eye where topical therapy is ineffective. By far, the most popular route of administration for drug treatment in ocular diseases and diagnostics is the topical route, and this route is therefore the main focus of this chapter.

In recent years, there have been increased efforts to find safer and effective drugs to treat various ocular conditions and diseases that are poorly controlled now, as well as to develop novel dosage forms and delivery systems to improve the topical delivery of existing drugs. Table 12.2 shows some potentially new drugs in clinical development at the time of writing, which promise to alter traditional lines of therapy for a variety of disorders. There is an unmet demand for new products in some markets, such as antiglaucoma products for patients that do not respond to currently available marketed products. Carbonic anhydrase inhibitors, which were formally only available as oral products, are being developed as topical products for glaucoma treatment. Table 12.3 lists some examples of the newer ocular drugs and delivery systems that have been introduced into the market in recent years. The data show the dramatic increase in conventional new drugs to treat infections, glaucoma, anti-inflammatory and antiallergic conditions, as well as the emergence of peptides and proteins.

Table 12.1
Examples of therapeutic classes of drugs currently used to treat ocular diseases.

Class	Drugs	Action	Clinical use	Dosage forms
Antibacterial	Chloramphenicol framycetin	Bacteriostatic or bacteriocidal	Eye infections	Eye-drop solution, viscous drops, eye ointment, liquid gel
Antiviral	Acyclovir	Antiviral	Control of viral infections	Eye ointment
Anti-inflammatory	Dexamethasone, sodium cromoglycate	Inhibition of inflammatory response	Inflammation, allergic conjunctivitis	Eye-drop solution, suspension, eye ointment
Mydriatics and Cycloplegics	Tropicamide, cyclopentolate	Dilation of pupil Examine the fundus of eye	Examination of	Eye-drop solution, eye ointment
Beta-blockers	Timolol, betaxolol	Reduce aqueous humour production	Treatment of glaucoma	Eye-drop solution, suspension, gel-forming solution
Miotics	Pilocarpine, carbachol	Constriction of pupil	Treatment of glaucoma	Eye-drop solution, viscous eye drops, ocular insert, gel
Local anaesthetics	Oxybuprocaine amethocaine	Irreversibly blocks pain sensation	Tonometry and prior to minor surgery	Eye-drop solution
Diagnostics	Fluorescein sodium	Colours the eye	Locating damaged areas of cornea	Eye-drops
Artificial tear preparations	Hypromellose polyacrylic acid	Eye lubrication	Tear deficiency	Liquid gel, viscous eye-drops

The development of new ocular drug-products, and more sophisticated delivery systems for the effective administration to the patient, pose several technical challenges for the formulator. These are discussed in more detail later in this chapter.

OCULAR TOPICAL DRUG DELIVERY ISSUES AND CHALLENGES

Ocular topical drug delivery is particularly challenging because of the inherent difficulties associated with absorption of topically applied drugs into the eye. Ophthalmic dosage forms are administered via the topical route to treat both surface and intraocular conditions. Consideration of the anatomical and physiological features of the eye, as well as the physicochemical properties of the drug, are all important when developing a topical ophthalmic delivery system.

Table 12.2
Examples of ocular drugs in clinical development.

Agent	Company	Indication	Stage
Diclofenac	Ciba Vision/ Pharmacia and Upjohn	Glaucoma	Phase I
Lactoferrin	Gist-Brocades/ Santen Japan	Anti-infective	Phase I
ADL-2-1294 (opioid mu receptor agonist)	Adolor USA	Conjunctivitis	Phase II
DWP-401 (epidermal growth factor)	Daewoong	Corneal wounds	Phase II
CT-112 (aldose reductase inhibitor)	Senju Japan	Diabetic keratopathy	Phase II
Proparacaine	InSite Vision	Local anaesthetic	Phase II
Zenarestat	Fujisawa/Warner-Lambert	Diabetic neuropathy	Phase III
WP-934	Wakamoto Japan	Glaucoma	Preregistration
Nipradilol	KowaPharmaceuticals	Glaucoma	Preregistration
Fluorometholone	InSite Vision/Ciba Vision	Inflammation	Preregistration
Acitazanolast	Wakamoto Japan	Conjunctivitis	Preregistration

Physiological Barriers

A good overview of the physiological features of the eye and the implications for ophthalmic drug delivery is presented in a review by Jarvinen et al. (1995). The most salient points are summarised briefly here.

Figure 12.1 shows the structure of the outside of the eye and a cross-section of the anterior segment of the eye. The front part of the globe of the eye is clear and colourless and is called the cornea. It contains no blood vessels, but is rich in nerve endings. The cornea consists of three major layers: the outer epithelium, middle stroma and inner endothelium. When topically applied products are administered to the eye, they first encounter the cornea and conjunctiva, representing the primary barriers to drug penetration. The epithelium and endothelium of the cornea are rich in lipid content, making them barriers to the permeation of polar, water-soluble compounds. The stroma, on the other hand, is a hydrophilic layer containing 70 to 80 percent water, presenting a barrier to the permeation of non-polar, lipid-soluble compounds.

The other part of the boundary layer to the front of the eye is the sclera. This is white in colour and opaque, and contains most of the blood vessels supplying the anterior tissues of the eye. The outer surface of the schlera is loosely covered by the conjunctival membrane, which is continuous with the inner surface of the eyelids, and also presents a significant

Table 12.3
Examples of ocular drugs launched in recent years.

Drug	Company	Indication	First Year of Launch
Loteprednol	Pharmos/Bausch & Lomb	Uveitis/conjunctivitis	Registered USA 1999
Brinzolamide	Alcon USA	Glaucoma	Registered USA 1999
Ibopamine	Angelini Italy	Surgery adjunct glaucoma	Registered Italy 1999
Olopatadine	Kyowa Hakko/ Alcon USA	Allergic conjunctivitis	USA 1998
Dexamethasone	Chauvin France	Ocular inflammation	UK 1998
Cromoglicic acid	Transphyto France	Conjunctivitis	France 1998
Latanoprost	Pharmacia & Upjohn/ Transphyto France	Glaucoma	US 1996
Ketorolac	Roche/Allergan USA	Inflammation/ conjunctivitis	Europe and Canada 1992
Hyaluronic acid	Fidia Italy	Dry eye	Italy 1993
Isopropyl unoprostone	Fujisawa/Ciba Vision	Glaucoma	Japan 1994
Brimonidine	Allergan USA	Glaucoma	USA 1996
Nedocromil	Fisons/RPR	Allergic conjunctivitis	Europe 1995
Dorzolamide	Merck & Co. USA	Glaucoma	Europe/USA 1995
Levocabastine	Chauvin/J & J USA/ Kyowa Hakko Japan	Allergic conjunctivitis	Europe 1991

Source: Pharmaprojects.

permeability barrier to most drugs. For drugs that permeate the vascular systems of the schlera and conjunctiva, transport tends to be away from the eye into the general circulation.

Other major physiological barrier mechanisms are due to tear production and the blink reflex. The conjunctival and corneal surfaces of the eye are continuously lubricated by a film of fluid secreted by the conjunctival and lachrymal glands. The lachrymal glands secrete a watery fluid called tears, and the sebaceous glands on the margins of the eyelids secrete an oily fluid which spreads over the tear film. The latter reduces the rate of evaporation of the tear film from the exposed surface of the eyes. Blinking assists to evenly spread the tear film over the surface of the eye and to drain the tears via the nasolachrymal duct into the nose, and ultimately down the back of the throat into the gastro-intestinal (GI) tract.

Upon administration of topically applied eye-drops [possessing a volume typically of 25 to 56 μL (Lederer and Harold 1986)], removal from the eye is rapid due to tear production and the blinking processes occurring simultaneously. The precorneal volume is about 7 μL, but volumes of up to 20 to 30 μL can be held in this area before spillage occurs. Instillation of volumes greater than this will simply spill out onto the cheek or will be rapidly lost with the

Figure 12.1 Structure of anterior segment of the eye (Glasspool 1984).

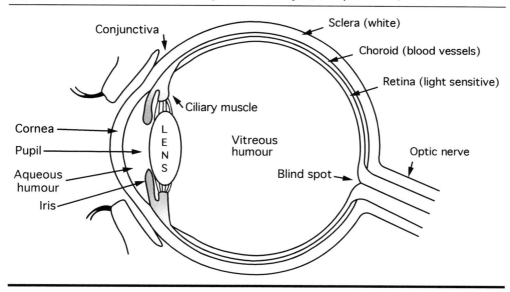

tears through drainage into the nasolachrymal duct. Also, the instilled product is diluted by normal tear production, with tear production rates in man reported as 1 μL per minute under resting conditions (Maurice and Mishima 1984). In practice, the introduction of any eye-drop product, but particularly products causing irritation, are likely to stimulate the tear production rate and increase the rate of drug removal from the eye. The removal of material by dilution is also aided by the blink reflex where each blink pumps approximately 2 μL of tear fluid into the nasolachrymal duct. It is estimated that the turnover for material instilled into the eye is approximately 16 percent per minute of the total volume, indicating a rapid removal from the precorneal area (Schell 1982). The net result is that less than 10 percent, and typically 1 percent or less, of the topically instilled dose into the eye actually permeates the cornea and is absorbed into the eye (Burstein and Anderson 1985).

Other physiological factors affecting ocular delivery of topical drugs are protein binding and drug metabolism. Protein accounts for up to 2 percent of the total content of normal tears and can be higher under certain pathological conditions such as uveitis. The increased size of the protein-drug complex will render the bound drug molecules unavailable for absorption, and lachrymal drainage will rapidly remove them from the eye. Tears are known to contain a range of enzymes, such as esterases, monoamine oxidases and aminopeptidases, among others. Consequently, many ocularly applied drugs are metabolised during or after absorption in the eye. This can be detrimental if the enzyme is responsible for inactivating the topically applied drug, for example, pilocarpine being inactivated with esterases (Bundgaard et al. 1985). Alternatively, there are several examples, such as dipivalyl epinephrine, where metabolism by esterases is advantageously used to bioactivate a topically applied prodrug administered to the eye (Tammara and Crider 1996).

Patient Compliance

Another factor that can affect the ocular bioavailability of a topically applied product is patient compliance and how the patient is using the medication. Patient compliance could be related to the acceptability of the product. Adverse effects such as irritation, burning, stinging or blurring of vision may provide a reason for patients to stop their medication. Local irritation is very common with many ophthalmic products, especially when high drug concentrations are involved. The design of the formulation and selection of excipients can influence the degree of irritation. For example, the use of cyclodextrins in eye drops has been shown to reduce ocular irritation by pilocarpine prodrugs (Suhonen et al. 1995). Formulation design can also be important in minimising the amount of systemic absorption of the instilled drug and possible systemic side-effects that may affect patient compliance. A variety of modified drug delivery systems have been developed to reduce systemic absorption and increase absorption into the eye. Some of these are discussed later in this chapter.

Finally, how the patient uses the product can affect ocular bioavailability. For example, applying more than one drop, or a larger drop by squeezing the dropper bottle harder, is not likely to be beneficial. The drug administered in the first drop is dramatically reduced when a second drop is instilled straight afterwards. Also, it has been shown that increasing the instilled solution volume actually reduces the fraction of dose absorbed because of a resultant increase in the drainage rate (Patton 1980). The ideal volume of instilled drug is 5 to 10 μL, but this is not likely to be achievable with a conventional eye-drop pack. There are, however, new pack devices that are able to accurately deliver such small quantities (see "Packaging Design Considerations" later in this chapter).

DRUG CANDIDATE SELECTION

Physicochemical drug properties, such as solubility, lipophilicity, molecular size and shape, charge and degree of ionisation, will affect the rate and route of permeation into the cornea.

For most topically applied drugs, passive diffusion along the concentration gradient, either transcellularly or paracellularly, is the main permeation mechanism across the cornea. Occasionally, a carrier-mediated active transport mechanism is indicated (Liaw et al. 1992). Lipophilic drugs tend to favour the transcellular route, whereas hydrophilic drugs usually permeate via the paracellular route through intercellular spaces (Borchardt 1990).

Since the cornea is a membrane barrier containing both lipophilic and hydrophilic layers, drugs possessing both lipophilic and hydrophilic properties permeate it most effectively. The optimal range for the octanol/buffer pH 7.4 distribution coefficient (log P) for corneal permeation is 2 to 3 (Schoenwald and Ward 1978), observed for a wide variety of drugs.

Drugs capable of existing in both the ionised and unionised form (weak acids and bases) tend to permeate the cornea the best. The unionised form usually permeates the lipid membranes more easily than the ionised form. The ratio of ionised to unionised drug in the eye will depend on the pK_a of the drug and the pH of both the eye-drop and the lachrymal fluid. Therefore, drugs formulated at a pH providing a higher concentration of unionised drug usually provide the best corneal absorption.

For ionisable drugs, the nature of the charge, as well as the degree of ionisation, will affect corneal permeability. The corneal epithelium is negatively charged above its isoelectric point (pI 3.2). As a result, charged cationic drugs permeate more easily through the cornea than do anionic species. Below the isoelectric point, the cornea is selective to negatively charged drugs, but in practice, the pH would be too acidic and irritating to use (Rojanasakul et al. 1992).

The molecular size of the drug does not seem to be a major factor for corneal permeability, providing the molecular weight is less than 500. Larger compounds than this are usually poorly absorbed when instilled into the eye.

The chemical form of the drug can be very important for ocular bioavailability. Changing the salt can affect the solubility and lipophilicity of the drug. For example, dexamethasone acetate ester has the preferred solubility and partition coefficient properties for corneal permeation compared to the very water-soluble phosphate salt or very lipophilic freebase.

During the candidate drug selection stage, preformulation studies should be performed to establish measurements of the physicochemical properties of potential compounds for development. Ideally, the compound with the preferred properties is selected. In cases where the physicochemical properties of the drug are not considered optimum to reach the site of action in the eye, it may be possible to design a suitable inactive bioreversible derivative (or prodrug) of the drug. The prodrug is then converted enzymatically or chemically to the parent drug in the eye in order to elicit a pharmacological effect.

The prodrug approach has been used in ocular drug delivery to not only improve drug bioavailability but to increase solubility, stability and potency and to decrease systemic side-effects. The aim of the prodrug approach is to modify the physicochemical properties, such as solubility or lipophilicity, by making prodrug derivatives (Lee and Li 1989). Some examples of prodrugs used in ophthalmic drug delivery are given in Table 12.4.

If the most appropriate physicochemical properties are not built into the candidate drug during candidate selection, the formulator faces a challenge in trying to overcome these deficiencies during formulation development. In practice, this is usually the case. Some of the formulation and drug delivery options that may be considered are discussed later in this chapter.

PRODUCT DESIGN CONSIDERATIONS

Formulation Design Options

Traditionally, topical ophthalmic dosage forms have been available as aqueous and oily solutions or suspensions, and administered as drops, gels, ointments or solid devices. The selection of formulation type will be largely dependent on the properties of the drug such as its aqueous drug solubility. Other factors will be the target concentration of drug required in the dose to be delivered and the eye condition to be treated. In recent years, there has been a lot of research and development of novel ophthalmic delivery systems to try and improve corneal retention time, reduce the frequency of administration and improve compliance. The scope and limitations of various ophthalmic dosage forms are discussed briefly below with the implications for formulation and pack design.

Solutions

Fortunately, many therapeutic agents used in eye products are water-soluble compounds or can be formulated as water-soluble salts, and a sufficiently high solution concentration can be achieved in the administered dose. In comparison with more sophisticated multiphase

Table 12.4
Examples of prodrugs used in ophthalmic drug delivery.

Parent Compound	Prodrug Moiety	Comments
Acyclovir	2′ –O–Glycyl ester	Prodrug developed to increase solubility (30 times enhancement)
Pilocarpine	Acid diesters	Prodrug developed to increase aqueous stability
		Prodrugs developed to increase efficacy:
Terbutaline	Diisobutyl ester (ibuterol)	100 times more potent to reduce intraocular pressure
Timolol	Aliphatic and aromatic amines, (acycloxy) alkyl carbomates	Increased corneal penetration and efficacy to treat glaucoma
		Prodrug developed to reduce systemic side-effects:
5-Fluorouracil	1-Alkoxycarbonyl, 3-acyl, and 1-acyloxymethyl.	Significant enhancemen in corneal penetration, resulting in reduction in dose and toxicity

systems, solution products are preferred because they are generally easier to manufacture and potentially provide better dose uniformity and ocular bioavailability.

However, solution eye-drops do have the disadvantage of being rapidly drained from the eye, with corresponding loss of drug. The inclusion of viscosity-increasing agents in the formulation, such as hypromellose, hydroxyethylcellulose, polyvinyl alcohol, povidone or dextran, can be used to increase the tear viscosity, which decreases drainage, thereby prolonging precorneal retention of the drops in the eye. Various studies have shown that an increase in product viscosity increases residence time in the eye (Li and Robinson 1989, Chrai and Robinson 1974), but there is a danger that high viscosity products may not be well tolerated in the eye. For this reason, most ophthalmic products are formulated within the range of 10 to 25 cP by the addition of viscosity-increasing agents. Certain viscosity-increasing materials, such as hyaluronic acid and its derivatives, or carbomer, have been shown to be more effective in achieving precorneal retention because of their mucoadhesive properties (Seattone et al. 1991; Vulovic et al. 1989).

Water-Based Gels

Ophthalmic delivery systems can be developed containing polymers that undergo a phase change from liquid to semi-solid as a result of changes in temperature (e.g., poloxamers), changes in pH (e.g., cellulose acetate hydrogen phthalate latex) or changes in ionic strength in the tear film (e.g., low-acetyl gellan gum, Gelrite™) (Rozier et al. 1989). These formulations are liquid formulations upon administration, but gel on contact with the eye to provide extended retention times. *In situ* gel formers also have the advantage of ease of administration, and improved patient compliance, because they can be instilled as a liquid drop (Robinson and Mlynek 1995). Many drugs already in commercial use have been reformulated in longer-acting liquid dosage form for once-daily application such as an *in situ* gelling preparation of timolol (Timoptic XE, Merck and Co., Inc.)

Semi-solid gel type preparations have also been developed for ophthalmic delivery as an alternative to traditional ointments, based on the effect of increasing the viscosity to prolong the retention of drug in the eye (for example, Pilopine HS gel, Alcon Laboratories, Inc.). Several types of gelling agents have been used, such as polyacrylic acid derivatives, carbomer and hypromellose.

Suspensions

Aqueous or oily suspension eye-drop formulations may be considered for drugs that are poorly water soluble, or because of poor aqueous drug stability. The drug particle size must be reduced to less than 10 μm levels to avoid irritation of the eye surface, leading to blinking and excessive lachrymation. One possible advantage of ophthalmic suspensions is that they should prolong the residence time of drug particles in the eye, allowing time for dissolution in the tears and an increase in ocular bioavailability (Sieg and Robinson 1975). This is only true if the dissolution rate of the particles and the rate of ocular absorption are faster than the rate of clearance of the drug from the eye. In practice, it is more likely that particles acceptable for ophthalmic suspensions, smaller than 10 μm, are removed from the eye as rapidly as drugs in solution.

Suspensions may also be used to overcome chemical instability of the drug, but at the same time may pose physical instability problems. For example, there may be an increase in particle size with time (Ostwald ripening), or difficulties in resuspension after periods of storage. The latter may result in problems with homogeneity and dose uniformity. The selection of a suitable salt with a low aqueous solubility can be employed to minimise the risk of Ostwald ripening, but it is also important that the suspended particles dissolve reasonably quickly in the eye, or else bioavailability will be reduced.

Suspension products may pose challenges to the formulator in manufacturing to achieve a sterile product. The possibilities of either degradation or morphological changes occurring during the sterilisation process exist and must be prevented.

Ointments

Eye ointments are sterile semi-solid preparations intended for application to the conjunctiva. They are attractive because of their increased contact time and better bioavailability compared to solutions. They can be very useful for night-time application, However, they are not always well accepted by patients because upon application they often cause blurred vision. A wide variety of ointments are available commercially.

The majority of water-free oleaginous eye ointment bases are composed of white petrolatum and liquid petrolatum (mineral oil), or a modification of the petrolatum base formula. They are designed to melt at body temperature. Other types of lipophilic ointment bases can also be used. An anhydrous vehicle can be advantageous for moisture sensitive drugs. Alternatively, semi-solid, anhydrous, water-soluble bases for ophthalmic use have been formulated from non-aqueous organogels, such as carbomer gelled with polyethylene glycols, and a suitable amine, providing good spreadability in the eye and low irritation potential. The drug can be incorporated in the vehicle as a solution or as a finely divided powder. For multidose products, a suitable antimicrobial preservative is required, such as chlorbutol, phenylethyl alcohol or parabens.

Like suspensions, ointments can be more difficult to manufacture in sterile form. They can be terminally sterilised; alternatively, they must be manufactured from sterile ingredients in an aseptic environment. Filtration through a suitable membrane or dry heat sterilisation is often used.

Ocular Inserts

Solid erodible (soluble) or non-erodible (insoluble) inserts have been commercially available for some time as a means of prolonging the release of drugs in to the eye. The Ocusert™ non-erodible system developed by Alza Corporation was first marketed in the United States in 1974. It is a membrane-controlled reservoir insert containing pilocarpine alginate, enclosed above and below by thin ethylene vinyl acetate (EVA) membranes. Ocusert™ is used in contact with the surface of the eye and is capable of releasing the drug at a reproducible and constant rate over 1 week. Other non-erodible therapeutic systems are based on hydrogel contact lenses filled with drug. Merkli et al. (1995) have written a comprehensive review of the various erodible polymers currently available, and particularly on the use of biodegradable polymers for ophthalmic drug delivery. The authors discuss the different possible erosion mechanisms which depend on the polymer type, and the type of drugs best suited for a particular polymer type. Only a few of these biodegradable polymers have so far led to commercial products. This could be because large inserts can be difficult to administer and sometimes even more difficult to remove, especially in elderly patients. However, they do appear to have a promising future for the treatment of various ocular diseases.

Soluble insert products have also been developed in which the drug is bound to an erodible matrix such as hydroxypropyl cellulose (HPC), hyaluronic acid, carbomer or polyacrylic acids. They are placed in the lower cul-de-sac and generally dissolve within 12 to 24 h. The advantage over non-erodible systems is that the erodible polymeric device undergoes gradual dissolution while releasing the drug, and so the patient does not have to remove it following use.

An example of a commercially available erodible insert is the Soluble Ophthalmic Drug Insert (SODI™), a soluble copolymer of acrylamide, N-vinylpyrrolidone and ethyl acrylate, designated as ABE. It is in the form of sterile thin film of oval shape, which is introduced to the upper conjunctival sac. Following application, it softens in 10 to 15 sec, conforming to the shape of the eyeball, and then in the next 10–15 min, the film turns to a clot which gradually dissolves while releasing the drug. SODI™ was developed as a result of a vast collaborative effort between Russian chemists and ophthalmologists in the 1970s (Khromow et al. 1976).

Saettone and Salminen (1995) provide a good review of the advantages, disadvantages and requirements for success of ocular inserts, and examine the few inserts which are available on the market or are in development including Ocusert™, SODI™, Collagen Shields, Ocufit, Minidisc and Nods. They conclude that it is surprising that insert devices, in spite of the advantages demonstrated by extensive investigations and clinical tests, have not gained a wider acceptance. The commercial failure has been attributed to psychological factors, such as the reluctance of ophthalmologists and patients to abandon the traditional liquid and semi-solid medications. Commercial failure may also be attributed to the relatively high cost of treatment compared to conventional liquid products, and to occasional therapeutic failures.

Novel Ophthalmic Drug Delivery Systems

The shortfalls of conventional topical liquid eye-drops, discussed earlier, particularly the relatively short precorneal half-life, have resulted in several new ophthalmic drug delivery approaches being investigated in recent years. Promising systems have been evaluated employing small colloidal carrier particles such as liposomes, microspheres, microcapsules, nanoparticles or nanocapsules. These systems have the advantage that they may be applied in liquid form, just like eye-drop solutions, because of their low viscosity. Thus they avoid the discomfort often associated with viscous gels and ointments but still provide a reservoir from which the drug can be delivered slowly.

Liposomes may increase the ocular bioavailability of certain drugs by increasing the association of the drug with the cornea by means of an increased lipophilic liposomal bilayer interaction with the corneal epithelium. Several other potential advantages of using liposomes as drug carriers for ophthalmic drug delivery have been reported (Meisner and Mezei 1995). They can accommodate both hydrophilic and lipophilic drugs, they are biocompatible and biodegradable, they can protect the encapsulated drug from metabolic degradation; and they can act as a depot, releasing the drug slowly. Liposomes, however, have the disadvantages of reduced physical stability and difficulties in sterilising the product. Temperatures required for autoclaving can cause irreversible damage to vesicles, while filtration is only applicable to vesicles less than 0.2 μm. Consequently, the use of liposomes is still in an experimental stage.

Microparticles and nanoparticles are colloidal drug carriers in the micrometer and submicrometer range. Microspheres are monolithic particles possessing a porous or solid polymer matrix, whereas microcapsules consist of a polymeric membrane surrounding a solid or liquid drug reservoir. Nanoparticles, including nanospheres or nanocapsules, have a particle size in the nanometer size range from 10 to 1000 nm. Drugs can be incorporated into the core of the carrier, either dissolved in the polymer matrix in the form of a solid solution or suspended in the form of a solid dispersion. Alternatively, the drug may be adsorbed on the particle surface. Release of drug can be attributed to degradation of the polymer, drug desorption from the polymer surface or diffusion through the polymeric matrix. Various synthetic and natural biocompatible polymers have been used to prepare microparticles and nanoparticles, particularly poly(alkyl)cyanoacrylate derivatives with various lengths of alkyl chain. The ocular bioavailability of a number of drugs has been demonstrated in animal models, compared to conventional aqueous eye-drops (Zimmer and Kreuter 1995). In addition, nanoparticles have been shown to adhere preferentially to inflamed precorneal tissues of the eye. Although there are currently no commercial formulations on the market using novel polymers, these carrier systems show a lot of promise for the future. The challenge will be to demonstrate safety and tolerability, and gain acceptance by the regulatory authorities.

Other attempts to improve ocular bioavailability have focussed on overcoming poor corneal permeability with penetration enhancers, or by improving the lipophilicity of the drug through ion-pair formation. Also, proposals have been made to improve packaging and device design to deliver the dosage form in a more precise manner. Ophthalmic packaging is discussed in more detail in the next section.

Packaging Design Considerations

The choice of packaging for ophthalmic products will depend on the type of dosage form, such as whether it is a liquid solution/suspension or semi-solid gel or ointment. Also, choice will depend on how the product is to be used by the patient, such as whether it is intended to be a unit-dose or multidose application. For any formulation type, the packaging design acceptance criteria must ensure that the

- materials are compatible with the formulation and ensure product stability,

- sterility of the product can be achieved and assured for the entire shelf-life,

- materials meet pharmacopoeial and regulatory standard requirements,

- containers should be tamper-evident and

- pack design offers ease of administration to the patient.

Liquid Drops (Solutions/Suspensions)

Traditionally, ophthalmic liquid products were packed in glass containers fitted with rubber teats for the eye dropper. Glass containers have (limited) use today when there are product stability or compatibility issues which exclude the use of flexible plastic containers made of polyethylene or polypropylene. Most liquid eye products on the market are plastic containers fitted with nozzles from which, by gentle squeezing, the contents may be expressed as drops.

Plastic containers have several advantages over the glass-dropper combination such as minimising the risk of the contents being contaminated with micro-organisms by the replacement of a pipette which may have become contaminated by touching the infected eye. Also, plastic containers are cheap, light in weight, more robust to handle and easier to use than glass-dropper-type containers. Multidose plastic bottles can be conventional dropper bottles or a form-fill-seal bottle where the dropper tip is an integral part of the bottle.

However, there are some disadvantages of plastic eye-drop containers. Some plastic materials such as polyethylene can absorb some antimicrobrial preservatives [e.g., benzalkonium chloride (BKC)], or some drugs. They may also leach plasticizers into the product or printing inks from the label through the plastic into the product. It is necessary to conduct compatibility and stability studies to ascertain whether this is likely to be a problem. For ophthalmic solutions that require the addition of a preservative because the drug product itself has no adequate antimicrobial properties, it may be necessary to use glass. Alternatively, a preservative-free product could be considered. The challenge is to develop a packaging system for preservative-free products, which maintains the sterility of the product throughout its shelf-life and during use.

Unit-dose systems offer the easiest technical solution to this problem, but have the disadvantages of higher cost of manufacture and of not being as compact as a multidose product containing equivalent doses. Unit-dose products are usually made of low-density polyethylene (LDPE), with the formulated sterile solution being without a preservative, and sealed using the form-fill-seal process.

An alternative approach is to develop a multidose preservative-free system. The container is required to be collapsible, and the suck-back of air, which could contain bacteria, has to be avoided. Containers are being developed that contain a valve mechanism to achieve this.

Due to the safety and regulatory concerns raised by preservatives used in ophthalmic products, there have been efforts to develop new eye-drop packaging systems which can remove the preservative from the formulation during administration. BKC is the most common preservative used in commercial eye-drops, and yet there are reports of side-effects such as allergic reactions, irritation, decreased lacrimation and damage to the corneal endothelium caused by its multiple use in eye products (Fraunfelder and Meyer 1989). Also, BKC can accumulate in soft contact lenses and is therefore not recommended for these patients. A French pharmaceutical research company, Transphyto, have patented a multidose preserved ophthalmic product with an adsorbant membrane in the neck of the bottle to remove the preservative during administration. It also contains a 0.2 μm bacteriological membrane to prevent the ingress of bacteria into the bottle during use (ABAK device).

Plastic containers can also be permeable to water vapour and oxygen over prolonged periods of storage. This can lead to gradual loss of liquid product or oxidation of an unstable drug over time.

Polyethylene containers are not able to withstand autoclaving and are usually sterilised by ethylene oxide or by irradiation before being filled aseptically with pre-sterilised product. Polypropylene containers can be autoclaved, but are not as flexible as polyethylene for eye-dropper use. Guidance recently available on the manufacture of sterile medicinal products from a number of regulatory sources suggests that there is a changing attitude to the use of manufacturing processes other than terminal sterilisation (Matthews 1999). The implication is that the type of container is not a satisfactory reason for not autoclaving the product, and the manufacturer should use a package which is currently available as a heat-stable alternative (such as polypropylene) and use standard terminal sterilisation by heat as recommended in the European Pharmocopoeia (EP). If a non-heat stable container is progressed, and terminal sterilisation is not possible, a full justification will be required for this approach. This may put manufacturers off investing in novel packaging concepts which offer advantages to the patient.

A variety of novel ophthalmic liquid pack design features are in development or have been developed recently. For example, the "Optidyne system" being developed by Scherer DDS is an atomised spray which delivers a tiny volume (about 5 μL) directly to the front of the eyeball so fast that it beats the blink reflex. The volume is similar to the capacity of the precorneal volume in the eye. Unlike the traditional eye-drops, the spray product can be directed more easily and should reduce the wastage associated with conventional eye-drops, which have a typical volume of 40 μL.

Another device to aid administration is an eyecup fitted to a metered dose pump to help the patient position the product correctly over the eye during administration. Novel devices have been developed to accommodate moisture and/or oxygen sensitive drugs, such as a dual chamber container that can hold drug, or freeze-dried drug, and diluent separately in a single package. The drug, or lyophilised drug, is contained in a glass bottle, and the reconstitution liquid is contained in a plastic bottle. Prior to use, the liquid contents are transferred into the glass bottle by rupturing a membrane, and a drug solution is produced by mixing ready for administration.

Semi-Solid Gels and Ointments

Semi-solid products have been traditionally packed in collapsible tin tubes. Metal tubes are a potential source of metal particles in ophthalmic products, and so the tubes have to be cleaned carefully prior to sterilisation. Also, the final product must meet limits for the number of metal particles found. Plastic tubes are not suitable because of their non-collapsible nature, which causes air to enter the tube after withdrawal of each dose. However, collapsible tubes made from laminates of plastic, aluminium foil and paper are a good alternative to tin tubes. Laminated tubes fitted with polypropylene caps can be sterilised by autoclaving, whereas tubes fitted with polyethylene caps are sterilised by gamma irradiation. The tubes are usually filled aseptically, sealed with an adhesive and then crimped.

Design Specifications and Critical Quality Parameters

In addition to the design selection criteria, there are some other design specification criteria and critical quality parameters that should be emphasised.

Ophthalmic products should comply with compendial requirements specified for the territory in which the product is to be registered. Reference to the major pharmacopoeias (European, U.S. and Japanese) should highlight the majority of requirements. The British and European Pharmacopoeias offer the most detailed guidance for the different types of preparations, eye drops, eye lotions, semi-solid preparations or ophthalmic inserts. There are also pharmacopoeial requirements relating to the container to be used, which have already been discussed in the previous section on pack design considerations. One very important design requirement worth stressing is that the container/delivery system be easy to use. Glaucoma is a common eye condition affecting many elderly patients who may have poor eyesight and manual dexterity, and thus are not capable of administering a complex delivery system. Design of a new delivery system should include consumer trials and customer feedback to ensure the new device is acceptable.

All ophthalmic products are required to be sterile up to the point of use and must comply with the pharmacopoeial tests for sterility. Terminal sterilisation is the preferred method from a regulatory point of view, as opposed to aseptic manufacture. If terminal sterilisation is not used, for example, because the drug substance cannot withstand the processing conditions, good supporting documentation will be required to gain regulatory approval (also see a later section on ophthalmic processing).

The advantage of using established excipients which have been used previously in registered ophthalmic products has been emphasised previously in this book (see Chapter 5). A list of excipients used previously in registered ophthalmic products is available from various reference sources (e.g., those listed in Table 8.1, Chapter 8, Product Optimisation). Another advantage of using established excipients in a topically applied formulation is to improve the chance of patient tolerability and patient compliance. An essential product design requirement is to minimise ocular side-effects such as irritation, burning, stinging and blurring of vision, any of which may provide a reason for patients to stop their medication.

Typical finished product specification and control tests for an ophthalmic multidose (preserved) solution product, required to demonstrate that the product is of a quality suitable for the intended use, may include the following:

- Appearance: description, e.g., clear, coloured, absence of foreign particles

- Identification test(s) for drug

- Quantitative drug assay/impurities and degradation products: limits based on analytical capability and stability data

- Quantitative preservative assay: limits based on analytical capability and levels required for antimicrobial preservative efficacy

- pH: limits based on stability, solubility and physiological acceptability

- Osmolality: limits based on physiological acceptability

- Volume/weight of contents: to ensure that label claim number of doses can be dispensed, but not more than 10 μL, unless otherwise justified

- Sterility

Additional tests would be required for an ophthalmic suspension or other type of dosage form. Such tests might be one for particle size and one to show whether the suspension sediments can be readily dispersed on shaking to enable the correct dose to be delivered.

Finally, as for any pharmaceutical product, ophthalmic products have to be designed to be stable. Ideally, the product should be stable at room temperature over a shelf-life period of 2–3 years. Multidose products must also be stable, after opening the pack, over the period of use. If antimicrobial preservatives are included to maintain sterility over this period, the effectiveness of the chosen preservative has to be demonstrated. There must be a discard statement on the label of multidose products indicating that the contents must not be used after a stated period. Normally, this does not exceed 28 days after opening the pack, unless there is a good justification.

PRODUCT OPTIMISATION CONSIDERATIONS

The exact product optimisation studies to be conducted will depend on the type of ophthalmic dosage form to be developed (liquid drops, semi-solid gel/ointment or solid device). However, the dosage form type should be clearly defined from the product design evaluation and supporting preformulation studies, to enable the formulator to focus on the most relevant product optimisation studies.

The physicochemical properties of the drug gained from preformulation studies are often the most significant determinant of the dosage form type to be developed. Preformulation data on drug solubility, lipophilicity, charge, degree of ionisation, compatibility with other excipients and packaging components will all be relevant.

Depending on the basic physicochemical properties of the drug, a variety of different components may have to be included in the formulation to achieve the target pharmaceutical product profile required. An important recommendation for any formulation developed is to keep it as simple as possible, adding only components which are required to serve a clear function in the product. This is also true for ophthalmic products, but because of the wide-ranging design requirements, it can be difficult to achieve in practice. The complexity of ophthalmic formulation development is illustrated in Table 12.5, which shows typical components included in different types of conventional ophthalmic dosage forms, taken from a review by Lang (1995). Some components will always be included in the formulation, indicated by a Y in Table 12.5. Other components are optional, indicated by an O.

Further discussion about the considerations for formulation development of conventional ophthalmic dosage is given below.

Ocular Solutions

Solubility

The advantages of solution ophthalmic products over multiphase systems have been emphasised in the "Product Design Considerations" section. If the tear-film concentration of drug is too low because of poor drug solubility, the rate of absorption may not be sufficient to achieve adequate tissue levels of drug in the eye.

For compounds possessing a low aqueous solubility, there are several approaches that can be used to enhance the concentration of drug in solution. Many drugs are weak bases or acids and can be formulated as water-soluble, pharmaceutically acceptable salts. Ideally, salt

Table 12.5
Formulation components used in common ophthalmic dosage forms.

Component	Solution	Suspension	Gel	Ointment	Insert
Drug	Y	Y	Y	Y	Y
Drug carrier	O	O	O	O	O
Water	Y	Y	Y		O
Buffering agent	Y	Y	Y		
Tonicity agent	O	O	O		
Antimicrobial preservative	Y	Y	Y	Y	
Viscosity modifier	O	O			
Solubilizer	O		O		
Salts	O	O	O		
Bioadhesive agent	O	O	O		O
Suspending agent		Y			
Phase modifier			Y		
Permeation enhancer	O	O	O		O
Cross-linked polymer					Y
Wax/oil/petrolatum				Y	

Note. (Y) Component is included, (O) Component optional.

Reprinted from *Advanced Drug Delivery Reviews*, Vol. 16, John C. Lang, Ocular drug delivery conventional ocular formulations, Pages 39–43, 1995, with permission from Elsevier Science.

selection should be fixed during preclinical candidate selection. It is not a good idea to change the salt form during clinical development because it could result in significant changes to the drug absorption and bioavailibility profiles and may result in the need to do additional human bioavailability studies. For more information about salt selection, refer to Chapter 3 on preformulation.

Manipulation of Formulation pH. Generally, the eye can tolerate eye preparations formulated over a range of pH values as low as 3.5 and as high as pH 9. However, it is preferable to formulate as close to physiological pH values as possible (pH 7.4), or at slightly alkaline pH values, to minimise the potential for pH induced lacrimation, eye irritation and discomfort (Meyer and McCulley 1992). If it is necessary to formulate at the extremes of the above pH range, for example, to maintain stability of the drug or to achieve optimum antimicrobial preservative efficacy, the buffer strength should be kept to a minimum to reduce buffer irritation effects (Allergan Pharmaceuticals 1969). The majority of drugs exhibit a pH-solubility profile, and the pH of optimum solubility is determined from preformulation studies. However, a greater degree of corneal permeation is observed when drugs are formulated at a pH providing a higher concentration of unionized drug, which may be away from the pH-solubility optimum.

Another important consideration when selecting the optimum formulation pH is the drug stability for pH sensitive drugs, such as peptides and proteins. Also, pH might affect the function of other components in the formulation. For example, the antimicrobial preservative, parabens (parahydroxybenzoic acid derivatives), is inactive at alkaline pH and more active as the pH becomes more acid. Another example is the viscosity of aqueous ophthalmic gels formulated with acrylic acid polymers (carbomer), Carbopol™ resins (BFGoodrich), which are particularly sensitive to pH changes. To maintain a low viscosity in the dosing solutions, the pH is typically in the 4 to 5 range. When placed in the eye, the immediate increase in pH causes a rapid gellation, which results in an increase residence time and bioavailability.

A variety of regulatory approved buffers are available covering the useful pH range. For acidic pH adjustment, acetic acid/sodium acetate or citric acid/sodium citrate are often employed. For alkaline-buffered solutions, phosphate or borate buffers are frequently used.

If pH manipulation fails to increase the drug solubility sufficiently, the next logical step is to try adding solubility-enhancing materials to the formulation. The choice of approved materials for use in ophthalmic products is somewhat limited because of the irritation potential of many adjuvants. Co-solvents, for example, are not generally acceptable. Materials approved and typically used include polyethylene glycols, propylene glycol, polyvinyl alcohol, poloxamers, glycerin, cellulose derivatives and surfactants. For a complete list of adjuvants approved for use in ophthalmic products the formulator should refer to one of the inactive ingredients guides listed in Table 8.1, in the Product Optimisation chapter.

Cyclodextrins and their derivatives, which can form inclusion complexes with some drugs, have shown promising results in rabbit studies. Both drug solubility and/or ocular bioavailability are increased, and sometimes tolerability is improved. However, the properties of cyclodextrins in ophthalmic drug delivery are poorly understood, and their benefits are still to be proven in the clinic (Jarvinen et al. 1995).

If the desired aqueous solubility is not achievable by any means, then alternatively, an oily solution or emulsion formulation could be considered. These systems rely on the drug partitioning out of the oily phase available in the eye, and are generally not as well tolerated as aqueous based delivery systems. For these reasons, aqueous suspension formulations are probably preferred to oily vehicles, employing very small drug particles to encourage dissolution and drug availability in the eye.

Osmolarity

Ophthalmic products instilled into the eye may be tolerated over a fairly wide range of tonicity (0.5–1.5 percent NaCl equivalents; Hind and Goyan 1950). However, to minimise irritation and discomfort, ophthalmic solutions should ideally be isotonic with the tears, equivalent to 0.9 percent w/v solution of sodium chloride.

Hypotonic ophthalmic solutions or suspensions can be rendered isotonic by the addition of tonicity agents such as sodium chloride, potassium chloride, dextrose, glycerol and buffering salts. As with other adjuvants, the formulator should give due consideration to possible interactions between the tonicity agent and other components of the formulation, including the drug itself.

Vehicle Viscosity

It is generally agreed that an increase in vehicle viscosity increases the residence time in the eye, although there are conflicting reports in the literature to support the optimal viscosity for ocular bioavailability (Seattone et al. 1991). Products formulated with a high viscosity are not well tolerated in the eye, causing lacrimation and blinking until the original viscosity of the tears is regained. Drug diffusion out of the formulation into the eye may also be inhibited due to high product viscosity. Finally, administration of high viscosity liquid products tends to be more difficult. Therefore, most commercial liquid eye drop products are adjusted to within the range of 10 to 25 cP, using an appropriate viscosity-enhancing agent.

Ophthalmic ointments are designed to be of very high viscosity to prolong the residence time in the eye, compared to solutions and suspensions. However, ointments are the least tolerated and so tend to be restricted to application at night when the patient is asleep.

A list of regulatory approved synthetic viscosity-enhancing agents, with typical concentrations used in aqueous ophthalmic formulations, is given in Table 12.6. There are also a variety of naturally occurring viscosity enhancers such as xanthan gum, alginates and gelatin, but these are not as popular as the synthetic alternatives because they are good mediums for microbial growth. Some viscosity-enhancing agents, such as carbomer 940 and hydroxyethylcellulose, also possess mucoadhesive properties which will contribute to increasing the residence time in the eye. Cellulose derivatives may also provide the product with lubrication properties by reducing the friction between the cornea and the eyelids. The reversible thermosetting properties of poloxamers (particularly poloxamer 407) can be exploited to provide a low viscosity free-flowing liquid at room temperature suitable for easier administration to the eye. On contact with the eye, a viscous gel is produced which prolongs the residence time of the drug in the eye.

Stabilisers

For drugs that are susceptible to oxidative degradation, stabilisers such as antioxidants and/or chelating agents can be included in the formulation to improve the product shelf-life. The use of plastic bottles, which allow gases to permeate through the container, will be particularly susceptible to oxidative degradation. Oxidation reactions are often catalysed in the presence of heavy metal ions, and so chelating agents such as disodium edetate are often included to complex with any metal ions.

There are a variety of regulatory approved antioxidants commonly used in liquid ophthalmic products, such as sodium metabisulphite, sodium sulphite, ascorbic acid acetylcysteine, 8-hydroxyquinoline and antipyrine.

Antimicrobial Preservatives

Ophthalmic products have to be manufactured sterile and be free from micro-organisms. Once opened, the sterility of a multidose product must be maintained during its period of use. This is usually required for at least 4 weeks, after which the product is discarded. If the drug itself does not possess antimicrobial properties, then an antimicrobial preservative must be included in the formulation to ensure that any micro-organisms accidentally introduced during use are destroyed.

There are a limited number of regulatory approved antimicrobial preservatives which can be used in ophthalmic products, and some of these are becoming less favoured because of increasing awareness of ocular toxicity concerns. Therefore, it can be a challenging exercise for the formulator to find a preservative to use with the following attributes:

•   Effective at the optimal formulation pH

•   Stable to processing, possibly heat sterilisation

•   Stable over the product shelf-life

Table 12.6
FDA approved ophthalmic viscosity-enhancing agents.

Viscosity Enhancer	Typical Concentration Range (%)
Methylcellulose	0.2–2.5
Hydroxypropyl cellulose	0.2–2.5
Hydroxypropyl methylcellulose	0.2–2.5
Hydroxyethylcellulose	0.2–2.5
Carboxymethylcellulose sodium	0.2–2.5
Polyvinyl alcohol	0.1–5.0
Povidone	0.1–2.0
Polyethylene glycol 400	0.2–1.0
Carbomer 940/934P	0.05–2.5[a]
Poloxamer 407	0.2–5.0

[a] Capable of forming a very stiff gel depending on concentration of polymer and pH.

- Does not physically interact with other components in the formulation

- Does not interact with the pack components

A list of regulatory approved antimicrobial preservatives used in ophthalmic formulations with recommended concentration ranges is shown in Table 12.7. The use of methyl- and propylparabens, thimerosal and other mercurial preservatives has decreased in recent years due to adverse reactions associated with their use (Wade and Weller 1994).

By far, the most widely used antimicrobial preservative used in ophthalmics is BKC (70 percent of all commercial products). It is often used in combination with disodium edetate because of the synergistic effects, allowing lower concentrations of BKC to be used. Even the use of BKC has been questioned because of some evidence of eye toxicity in rabbits (Dormans and van Logten 1982), and some people have developed hypersensitivity to this preservative. However, BKC does possess good pharmaceutical properties, being stable in solution, stable to autoclaving, and at the usual concentration of 0.01 percent, is an effective preservative over the range of pH values typically used in ophthalmic formulations.

BKC is a mixture of alkylbenzyl dimethylammonium chlorides of different alkyl chain lengths, containing even carbon numbers from C8 to C18, mostly C12 and C14. Being cationic in nature, it is not compatible with anionic drugs, and its activity is reduced in the presence of some materials, such as multivalent metal ions and anionic and non-ionic surfactants. It may still be possible to use a preservative even if there is a known drug interaction. The best-known examples of commercial ophthalmic formulations are sodium cromoglycate and nedocromil sodium interacting with BKC. Both of these drugs will form an insoluble emulsion complex with BKC, due to ion-pair formation between the drug anions and the benzalkonium cation. This is acceptable, because the insoluble complex can be removed by filtration during processing in a controlled and reproducible fashion. An excess of preservative is added during manufacture, leaving 0.01 percent BKC in the final solution, which effectively preserves the product.

Table 12.7
Regulatory approved ophthalmic antimicrobial preservatives.

Antimicrobial preservative	Typical Concentration Range (%)
Benzalkonium chloride	0.01–0.02
Benzethonium chloride	0.01–0.02
Chlorhexidine	0.002–0.01
Chlorobutanol	Up to 0.5
Methylparaben	0.015–0.05
Phenylethyl alcohol	Up to 0.5
Phenylmercuric acetate	0.001–0.002
Phenylmercuric borate	0.002–0.004
Phenylmercuric nitrate	0.002–0.004
Propylparaben	0.005–0.01
Thimerosal	0.001–0.15

Chlorhexidine is also cationic like BKC and exhibits similar incompatibilities. It is not as stable as BKC to autoclaving and may irritate the eyes. It tends to be more favoured in Europe than in the United States, and is particularly used in contact lens products. Chlorobutanol and phenylethyl aclohol are also widely used in ophthalmic products. However, chlorobutanol will hydrolyse in solution, and autoclaving is not usually possible without loss of preservative activity. It is also volatile and may be lost through the walls of plastic containers.

The effectiveness of any antimicrobial preservative in a formulation must be demonstrated by using specified test procedures described in relevant pharmacopoeias. Unfortunately, the preservative challenge test procedures and acceptance criteria are different in the major pharmacopoeias of Europe, United States and Japan, in spite of attempts to harmonise them. All the tests involve mixing the preserved formulation with standard cultures of gram-positive and gram-negative bacteria, yeasts and moulds, and counting the number of viable micro-organisms remaining at different time points after inoculation. The preservative is effective in the formulation if the concentration of each test micro-organism remains at or below stipulated levels during the test period.

To effectively preserve a formulation, the preservative system must have a broad spectrum of activity against a range of micro-organisms. Each type of micro-organism used in the preservative challenge test presents a particular challenge. Pharmacopoeial challenge tests have been designed to do this, and to demonstrate that any test micro-organisms inoculated are totally cleared from the formulation over the period of the test. In this respect, the USP limits must be considered to be inadequate for ophthalmic products, allowing 2 weeks to reduce a bacterial count by 99.9 percent. This is recognised in the EP test which is far more stringent, stipulating that bacteria should be reduced by 99.9 percent within 6 h and cleared within 24 h, and fungi should be reduced by 99 percent in 7 days with no subsequent growth thereafter.

Therefore, if the product will pass the EP test, it should pass any other pharmacopoeial challenge tests.

Standard pharmacopoeial tests are time consuming, taking up to 28 days to conduct the test and a further few days to analyse the data. During formulation optimisation, when several trial formulations may have to be evaluated, *D*-value testing is a faster way of generating data quickly to select the preservative and optimise the concentration. The *D*-value (the decimal reduction time) is the time required for a reduction of one logarithm in the concentration of a test micro-organism. Typically, the time taken for the concentration of a bacteria to fall to one-tenth of its starting concentration can be achieved over a few hours or so if the preservative is effective. The rate of kill (*D*-values) for different preservative systems can be determined to provide a rank order and to aid final selection. However, it will then be necessary to demonstrate that the final formulation is effectively preserved, using the standard type pharmacopoeial challenge tests. Testing should be performed after processing, and over time, at different storage conditions. It is also good practice to test the product at and below the lower limit of the proposed specification range for preservative label claim to demonstrate that the product will retain its preservative efficacy over its shelf-life. This is particularly important if there is likely to be any loss of preservative into the pack, or through the pack, over time.

It is also useful to conduct a simulated use test in which the product is opened each day and drops administered according to the dosing instructions for 28 days. The remaining formulation should pass the preservative efficacy test at the end of this period.

Ophthalmic Suspensions

For ophthalmic suspension products, the drug particle size must be reduced to less than 10 μm to prevent irritation of the eye. The product should comply with pharmacopoeial limits for the number of particles greater than the stated size permitted in ophthalmic products. The EP includes a microscopic test with the following limits: not more than 20 particles per 10 μg of the solid phase have a maximum dimension greater than 25 μm, not more than 2 of these particles have a maximum dimension greater than 50 μm and no particles are greater than 90 μm. During formulation optimisation, the potential for any changes in particle size due to Ostwald ripening or particle agglomeration need to be evaluated through stability testing. Excipients such as povidone can be included in the formulation to inhibit crystal growth.

Surfactants may be included in an ophthalmic suspension to disperse the drug effectively during manufacture and in the product during use. Non-ionic surfactants are generally preferred because they tend to be less toxic. The level of surfactant included in the formulation should be carefully evaluated, as excessive amounts can lead to irritation in the eye, foaming during manufacture and upon shaking the product, or interactions with other excipients. The most likely interaction is with the preservative. For example, polysorbate 80 interacts with chlorobutanol, benzyl alcohol, parabens and phenyl ethanol and may result in a reduced preservative effectiveness in the product.

Consideration must be given to establishing good physical stability of a suspension. If the particles settle and eventually produce a cake at the bottom of the container, they must redisperse readily to achieve dosage uniformity. Viscosity-enhancing agents can be used to keep the particles suspended. Preparation of flocculated suspensions is not recommended because the larger flocs may irritate the eye.

Drug and Excipient Interactions

The consequences of having several components in an ophthalmic formulation are the increased possibility of physical or chemical incompatibilities occurring, resulting in an unstable product, or one component not functioning in the presence of another. Several examples of potential interactions have been mentioned throughout this chapter. The presence of an interaction between the drug, excipients or pack does not necessarily mean that they cannot be used together. However, the formulator will be required to determine the extent and nature of such an interaction, and conduct sufficient testing to develop an effective formulation.

A systematic approach to formulation development of an ophthalmic product is therefore recommended. The product design requirements should be evaluated systematically to try and achieve the targets and limits for specification tests, such as appearance, drug solubility, pH, viscosity, osmolarity and preservative effectiveness. By experimentation, and iteration, the selection and quantity of each type of component can be established, until the acceptance criteria are met for each product design requirement. For example, in the first stage of experimentation, the requirement might be to achieve the target drug solubility. If solubility in an aqueous vehicle is insufficient, pH manipulation or the addition of various solubility enhancers can be evaluated over a range of concentrations, to establish the optimum combination which meets the design criteria. In the next stages of experimentation, viscosity enhancers and tonicity agents can be evaluated to meet the specification test limits for viscosity and osmolality. Finally, a variety of antimicrobial preservatives are evaluated, but at the same time, the formulator checks to ensure that drug solubility, viscosity and osmolality are not significantly affected. Further experimentation and testing is continued until all of the various components have been added in this iterative manner, and the product design requirements have been met.

Alternatively, an experimental design approach could be attempted to reduce the number of experiments, but this can be very complex if a large number of components are involved.

Accelerated stress stability testing of the final product, with all the components added, should establish whether there are any compatibility problems between the drug, excipients and packaging. Stability data from accelerated studies can be used to predict shelf-lives at ambient conditions (see the section "Stability Testing" in Chapter 8, "Product Optimisation," for more details). It is worthwhile including temperature cycling from low (4°C) to high (40°C) temperatures in the stability programme, particularly if solubility enhancers have been used. For example, an experimental formulation of the antiglaucoma drug, acetazolamide, was formulated with povidone to enhance its solubility. The product was perfectly stable when stored at constant temperatures of 4, 25 and 45°C. However, when the product was stored in a warehouse with no control of temperature, the drug precipitated out of solution because of the repeated wide fluctuations in temperature.

Administration and Use

As part of the optimisation programme, it is important to evaluate the ocular irritation potential of formulation prototypes. The Draize test, established in the 1940s, is the most widely used method for the identification of primary irritants. There have been modifications to the original test, but they all involve instilling a drop of the formulation into the conjunctival sac of one eye of an albino rabbit, the other eye acting as a control. The condition of both eyes is then evaluated after stipulated time periods and scored relative to the control eye. A high score indicates that the formulation is likely to be an irritant and would not be recommended for progression.

More recently, there has been much effort to replace animal tests with *in vitro* test models, such as isolated tissues and cell cultures (Hutak and Jacaruso 1996). These have some advantages in that they are less costly than *in vivo* tests, use relatively simple methodology and can be used to identify primary changes at the cellular level. The disadvantages are that they do not mimic the eye response, they cannot be used to evaluate insoluble materials (e.g., suspensions), and the various methods differ widely in their ability to predict irritancy potential. It is conceivable that *in vitro* methods could be used for primary screening tests, while more standard *in vivo* methods are used to verify the result.

Compatibility tests with contact lenses can also be carried out *in vitro*. Contact lenses are manufactured from a range of materials and may be broadly classified as rigid, soft and scleral lenses, based on differences in purpose and material used. The potential for interaction between the drug or excipients and a contact lens depends largely on the material of the lens. It is most likely that highly water-soluble and charged materials will interact with a soft, hydrophilic contact lens. There are several consequences of this happening, including a reduction in available drug, potential alterations to aesthetics of the contact lens (especially if the drug is coloured) and possible deformation of the lens polymer affecting patient vision.

The uptake and release of ophthalmic drugs into contact lenses can be evaluated with *in vitro* models designed to simulate the human eye. This involves soaking the contact lens in buffered saline containing drug product and continuously diluting the system with buffered saline to simulate tear turnover in the eye. Fresh drug product is instilled at the times of dosing during the day. The lens is removed for cleaning at the end of a day according to routine wear, and left to soak overnight. This can be continued over several days and the soaking solutions analysed for drug at intervals to determine the build-up of drug in the lens.

Alternatively, a simpler *in vitro* study can be conducted to determine the uptake/release profile of drug, based on the FDA procedure for the assessment of uptake/release of antimicrobial preservatives that might be included in soft contact lens solutions (FDA 1989). This test involves subjecting a range of contact lenses to incubation in a series of dilutions of drug product. The potential for build-up of drug on the lens over time is determined by analytical techniques such as high performance liquid chromatography (HPLC), atomic absorption spectroscopy, laser fluorescence spectroscopy or ^{14}C-labelled drug. If the uptake of drug into the lens appears to be problematic, the use of the drug product with contact lens wearers may be contraindicated, or, alternatively, a specific cleaning/soaking programme may be recommended.

It should be noted that any eye product containing BKC preservative is contraindicated in patients wearing soft contact lenses. Wherever possible, wearers of such lenses should remove them before administration and allow time for the medication to be removed by the tears. Otherwise, the use of a unit-dose preparation is another option.

Finally, compatibility tests can be carried out to demonstrate that the drug product is compatible with other commercially available eye products which may be co-administered. Each mixture is examined for signs of chemical and physical compatibility over a short period of time. These *in vitro* results should be validated by the successful use of the drug product with concomitant therapy in clinical studies.

PROCESSING CONSIDERATIONS

The objectives of the process design and optimisation stages of product development have been discussed in chapter 8, "Product Optimisation". For ophthalmic products, like parenterals, process development can be quite challenging because the formulation must be manufactured sterile. Quite often, it is discovered that some formulations cannot withstand a stressful sterile process such as autoclaving. Chemical degradation or changes to the formulation properties of multiphase systems, such as suspensions and gels, can occur. In all cases, the compendial sterility test requirements described in the various pharmacopoeias must be complied with.

There are certain expectations and requirements for "acceptable" sterile products from the regulatory agencies, particularly in Europe (Matthews 1999) and also the United States. The Committee for Proprietary Medicinal Products (CPMP) has recently published a "Note for Guidance on Development Pharmaceutics" (January 1998), and its Annex, "Decision Trees for the Selection of Sterilisation Methods" (February 1999), advising that, for products intended to be sterile (including ophthalmic products), an appropriate method of sterilisation should be chosen and the choice justified. Whenever possible, all such products should be terminally sterilised in their final container, using a fully validated terminal sterilisation method using steam, dry heat or ionising radiation, as described in the EP. The guidance emphasises that heat lability of a packaging material should not itself be considered adequate justification for not utilising terminal sterilisation, for otherwise heat-stable products. Alternative packaging material should be thoroughly investigated before making any decision to use a non-terminal sterilisation process. However, it could be that the drug candidate, or one or more of the formulation excipients, are not stable to heat.

For ophthalmic products, there is a dilemma because recent market trends show that flexible LDPE plastic dropper bottles are popular with users because they offer several advantages, including ease of administration, better control of drop delivery and lower risk of contamination during patient use; plastic dropper bottles are lightweight, yet more robust than glass. However, one disadvantage of LDPE containers is that they cannot withstand terminal heat sterilisation using pharmacopoeial recommended heat cycles.

According to the decision trees, where it is not possible to carry out terminal sterilisation by heating due to formulation instability, a decision should be made to utilise an alternative method of terminal sterilisation, filtration and/or aseptic processing. If this alternative route is taken, then a clear scientific justification for not using terminal heat sterilisation will be required in the NDA/MAA dossier. Commercial reasons will not be acceptable because terminal sterilisation offers the highest possible level of sterility assurance.

If using non-terminal sterilisation methods, it is important to ensure that a low level of pre-sterilisation bioburden is achieved prior to and during manufacture. For example, the raw materials used for aseptic manufacture by sterile filtration should be sterile if possible, or should meet a low specified bioburden control limit, e.g., <100 CFU/mL. Also, there should be a pre-sterilisation bioburden limit for the bulk product that is within the validated capacity of the filters used to remove micro-organisms. The FDA guidance on *Sterile Drug Products Produced by Aseptic Processing* (1987) and the recently revised Annex 1 of the EC GMP Guide *Manufacture of Sterile Medicinal Products* (1998) should both be referred to for further guidance.

It will be necessary to conduct preliminary feasibility studies to establish an acceptable and effective method for sterilisation of the product. There is a clear responsibility with the manufacturer to provide evidence to the regulatory agencies that the product can or cannot be terminally sterilised. Preformulation studies will indicate whether the candidate drug and proposed formulation can withstand the sterilisation process using small samples of product.

There are several comprehensive texts on the sterile processing of pharmaceutical products. A book edited by Groves and Murty (1995) is particularly recommended.

Process design and optimisation for ophthalmic products is discussed further below with the aid of three examples of manufacturing processes for different types of ophthalmic products, based on the author's experience.

Ophthalmic Solution Eye-Drops

The first example of novel packaging design approaches is a multidose eye-drop pack containing an aqueous solution of a drug used for the treatment of allergic conjunctivitis. The drug is a polar, ionic compound, available as the sodium salt, which is highly water-soluble and has a low lipophilicity. Formulation details are as follows:

Formulation	Rationale
Drug (2.0%)	Active
Disodium edetate	Ion sequester
Sodium chloride	Tonicity adjustment
Benzalkonium chloride	Preservative
Purified water	Vehicle

Solubility of the drug in the aqueous vehicle, even at 2 percent, was not an issue. Disodium edetate was included to prevent the drug from forming insoluble salts with metal ions such as calcium, zinc and magnesium. The tonicity of the solution was adjusted to within acceptable physiological limits by the addition of sodium chloride.

Microbiological preservation was achieved by the inclusion of BKC, the only preservative found to be safe and effective. It was selected in spite of a known interaction between the drug anion and the benzalkonium cation, producing an insoluble emulsion complex of a yellow-brown colour, removed by filtration during manufacture. However, to compensate for the loss of BKC resulting from the filtration process, an excess was added during manufacture, so that 0.01 percent w/v remains in solution after removal of the complex.

The critical parameters potentially affecting quality or performance of the proposed process were evaluated to ensure the consistency of the interaction between the drug and BKC and assurance of product sterility.

It was demonstrated that the drug in the formulation could not withstand terminal heat sterilisation. Furthermore, the product was poured into LDPE bottles fitted with an LDPE dropper plug and polypropylene cap, which could not withstand heat sterilisation either. It was therefore necessary to develop a process to sterilise the solution by aseptic filtration followed by aseptic filling into pre-sterilised packaging components. This process was accomplished by exposure of the drug, the LDPE bottles, the dropper plug and the polypropylene cap to ethylene oxide.

The optimised process entailed the addition of a solution of BKC to a solution containing the remainder of the ingredients. The solution temperature was maintained between 15 and 25°C, and the mixture stirred for at least 30 min, to ensure that the ion-pair reaction between the drug and BKC consistently goes to completion before clarification by filtration. Mixing speed was evaluated and determined not to be a critical parameter over a wide range of speeds tested. During the clarification filtration evaluation, it was found that a reduced flow rate of solution passing through the filters was important for retaining the drug-benzalkonium emulsion complex, and for avoiding excessive foaming on the surface of the filtered solution.

The clarified bulk solution was sterilised by passing through a 0.22 μm sterilising grade cartridge filter fitted in-line and after the clarification filter. Samples taken from the sterile filtered solution showed that the BKC levels were low in the first few litres collected. This was due to physical adsorption of BKC onto the sterilising grade filter surface. Once the filter surface was saturated, the preservative level rose to the target level. To ensure that the final level of BKC was within the specification limits, the initial quantity of filtered solution had to be discarded prior to filling the dropper bottles.

In-process controls included tests on the integrity of the sterilising filter before and after filtration, a microbial count before filtration and monitoring of fill volume and cap torque during the filling operation. These controls helped to ensure that the product met the required standard for sterility, that an adequate volume was dispensed into each container and that leakage of product from the container was prevented.

Viscous Ophthalmic Solutions

A second example of a manufacturing process for ophthalmic topical drug delivery involves the cromone drug, sodium cromoglycate, used for the treatment of allergic conjunctivitis. This particular aqueous formulation was made viscous by the addition of carbomer, to increase the residence time in the eye and to reduce the dose regimen from four applications daily to once or twice daily. It was filled into a LDPE unit-dose pack using a form-filled seal process. The formula and rationale are given below:

Formulation	Rationale
Sodium cromoglycate	Active
Glycerol	Tonicity adjuster
Carbomer 940 (0.5%)	Viscosity modifier
Sodium hydroxide (to pH 6.0)	pH adjustment
Water for Injection (WFI)	Vehicle

Glycerol was used to adjust the tonicity of solution to physiological limits, in preference to sodium chloride, because the latter was shown to reduce the viscosity of carbomer solution to unacceptable levels. The formulation did not include a preservative because it was intended for single-dose application once the pack was opened.

Unlike the previous example, sodium cromoglycate was able to withstand terminal heat sterilisation. However, the final product was too viscous to be autoclaved, not allowing effective heat transfer, and so a combination of heat sterilisation and aseptic manufacture was developed. The drug and carbomer were dispersed by homogenisation in the majority of the Water for Injection contained in a large stainless steel mixing vessel. A thin watery dispersion that resulted was sealed in the vessel and autoclaved at 121°C for 15 min. The bulk dispersion was then cooled to ambient temperature (18–22°C). Filter-sterilised sodium hydroxide was added aseptically to pH 6.0 to increase the viscosity by neutralising the carbomer. After making up to weight with the remaining WFI and thoroughly mixing, the liquid formulation was aseptically filled into sterile LDPE unit-dose dropper packs using a form-filled seal process.

A number of process parameters were found to critically affect the quality or performance of the final product. Obviously, the order of addition of the materials was important for successful manufacture. It was necessary to autoclave the carbomer dispersion before pH adjustment, otherwise the product would have been too viscous to allow effective heat transfer.

Even prior to pH adjustment, it was important to stir the watery dispersion continuously during the heating cycle to ensure even temperatures were obtained throughout the bulk, thus avoiding cold and hot spots. It was also necessary to stir the bulk product during the cooling phase, and to use a vessel with a cooling jacket, to reduce the cooling time to an acceptable limit. Finally, the pH target of 6.0 was critical; below pH 6 the drug was unstable and above pH 6 produced a too viscous product for drug delivery to the eye. However, it could be demonstrated that this narrow pH window could be achieved during repeated manufacture.

Semi-Solid Gel Suspension

The final example of a novel process development formulation involves a semi-solid ophthalmic gel containing a carbonic anhydrase inhibitor drug for the treatment of glaucoma. It is administered to the patient by extruding the gel from an ophthalmic tube into the conjunctival sac of the eye. The drug had a very low aqueous solubility. It was necessary to reduce the particle size of the drug to less than 10 μm and suspend it in a very thick carbomer gel vehicle, to increase the residence time of the gel and maximise corneal permeation. The formulation details are given below:

Formula	Rationale
Antiglaucoma drug	Active
Carbomer 934P (2.5%)	Viscosity enhancer
Chlorbutol (0.5%)	Preservative
Sodium hydroxide (to pH 4.5)	pH adjustment
Water for Injection	Vehicle

The pH was adjusted to 4.5 with sodium hydroxide solution to ensure drug stability and an acceptable product shelf-life, in addition to neutralising the carbomer and producing a thick gel. Chlorbutol was included as an antimicrobial preservative because of its activity in this pH range.

Process development studies showed that terminal sterilisation of the gel was not possible. Heat sterilisation and gamma irradiation methods both caused unacceptable physical degradation of the gel and also caused chlorbutol hydrolysis. Aseptic filtration was not possible because the drug was suspended in the gel vehicle and viscosity would also have been a problem. The process described below was therefore developed with consideration of the sterilisation of the product components and the maintenance of asepsis throughout manufacture.

The drug was sterilised by gamma irradiation prior to aseptic dispersion in the gel. The chlorbutol was dissolved in a portion of the WFI and sterile filtered through a 0.2 μm cartridge filter. Attempts to use heat sterilisation methods caused an unacceptable loss of chlorbutol potency and also caused volatilisation. The carbomer was sterilised by autoclaving a "concentrate" of carbomer in water, contained in the manufacturing vessel, whereas an aqueous sodium hydroxide solution was sterilised by autoclaving, but then added to the other components in the manufacturing vessel by aseptic filtration. The ophthalmic tubes were sterilised by gamma irradiation.

Careful selection of the processing equipment and design features were important for successful manufacture. Stainless steel mixing vessels fitted with a paddle stirrer for general mixing, and a homogeniser head for high-speed mixing of the drug and carbomer, were required, respectively. One vessel was jacketed for heating and cooling, pressure-rated to allow *in situ* sterilization of the contents and fitted with ports to allow the aseptic addition of liquid and powders.

The process was constrained by the limited aqueous solubility of chlorbutol such that half of the available water was required to produce a chlorbutol solution. Also, a higher temperature of the chlorbutol solution had to be maintained. The remainder of the available water was used for the preparation of an intermediate carbomer gel concentrate (approximately 6 percent carbomer concentration) and the sodium hydroxide solution. Initially, the carbomer concentrate was prepared clean, but not sterile, by the slow addition of carbomer to the water in the stainless steel vessel fitted with a homogeniser head. A heavy-duty diaphragm pump was then used to transfer the carbomer concentrate (by weight) to the second steam-sterilised jacketed stainless steel mixing vessel fitted with paddle stirrer, situated in the Class 100 sterile area. The filter-sterilised aqueous-chlorbutol solution was aseptically transferred and mixed with the carbomer dispersion, followed by the drug powder and then the filter-sterilised sodium hydroxide solution. Finally, the total contents were mixed continuously using the paddle stirrer whilst filling the product into sterilised ophthalmic tubes. A schematic diagram showing the process steps is given in Figure 12.2.

CONCLUDING REMARKS

In the introduction to this chapter the current status of ophthalmic drug delivery was discussed. The abundance of compounds in clinical development, and the recent introduction of new ophthalmic products to the market, indicates the importance of this area. The next section discussed the challenges and issues associated with ophthalmic topical drug delivery, which need to be understood if a new drug delivery system is to be successfully developed. Some novel formulation and packaging design approaches were discussed to show the progress being made to overcome these challenges.

Due to the wide variety of ophthalmic formulation types available, it was not possible to cover all aspects of every formulation type in detail. However, there should be sufficient guidance and practical examples in this chapter to give the preformulation or formulation scientist a good understanding of the subject, and to provide some direction in their endeavours to develop a new ophthalmic product. It is hoped that some of the possible pitfalls mentioned will be avoided along the way.

Figure 12.2 Steps in the process for the manufacture of a semi-solid ophthalmic gel suspension.

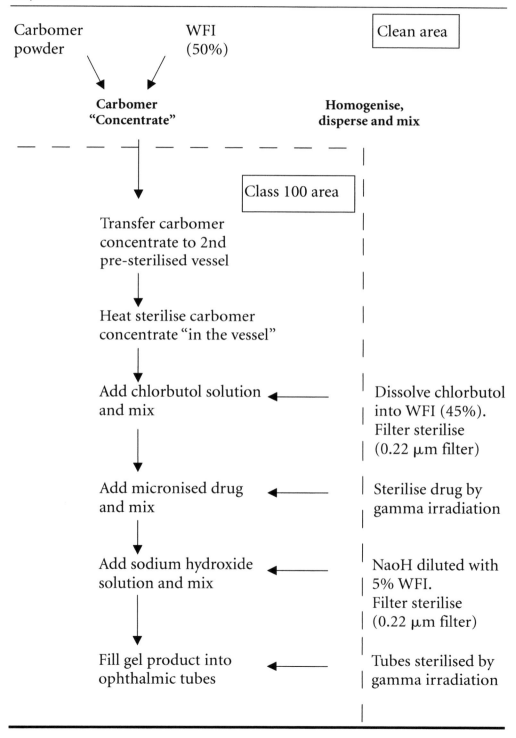

REFERENCES

Allergan Pharmaceuticals. 1969. The effects of pH on contact lens wearing. *J. Amer. Optom. Assoc.* 40 (7):719–722.

Borchardt, R. T. 1990. Assessment of transport barriers using cell and tissue culture systems. *Drug. Dev. Ind. Pharm.* 16 (8):2595–2612.

Bundgaard, H., E. Falch, C. Larsen, G. L. Mosher, and T. J. Mikkelson. 1985. Pilocarpic and estrers as novel sequentially labile pilocarpine prodrugs for improved ocular delivery. *J. Med. Chem.* 28 (8): 979–981.

Burnstein, N. L., and J. A. Anderson. 1985. Review: Corneal penetration and ocular availability of drugs. *J. Ocular Pharmacol.* 1:309–326.

Chrai, S. S., and J. R. Robinson. 1974. Ocular evaluation of methylcenulose vehicle in albino rabbits. *J. Pharm. Sci.* 63:1218–1223.

CPMP. 1998. *Note for guidance on development pharmaceutics and annex (1999) decision trees for the selection of sterilisation methods.* Brussels, Belgium: Committee for Proprietary Medicinal Products.

Dormans, J. A. M. A., and van Logten. 1982. The effects of ophthalmic preservatives on cornmeal epitheliusm of the rabbit: a scanning electron microscopical study. *Toxicol. Appl. Pharmacol.* 62:251–261.

European Commission. 1998. EC GMP guide to good manufacturing practice. Revised Annex 1: Manufacture of sterile medicinal products. In *The rules governing medicinal products in the EU.* Vol. 4: *Good Manufacturing Practices.* Luxembourg: European Commission.

FDA. 1989. *Guidelines to contact lens manufacturers: Preservative uptake/release procedures.* Chem. Appendix B. Rockville, Md., USA: Food and Drug Administration.

Fraunfelder, F. T., and S. M. Meyer. 1989. In *Drug-induced ocular side effects and drug interactions,* 3rd ed. Portland, Ore., USA: Oregon Health Sciences University, pp. 476–480.

Glasspool, M., ed. 1984. *Eyes: Their problems and treatments.* London: Martin Dunitz, p. 11.

Groves, M. J., and R. Murty, eds. 1995. *Aseptic pharmaceutical manufacturing II: Applications for the 1990s,* vol. 2. Buffalo Grove, Ill., USA: Interpharm Press, Inc.

Hind, H., and F. Goyan. 1950. Contact lens solutions. *J. Amer. Pharm. Assoc.* 11:732.

Hutak, C. M., and R. B. Jacaruso. 1996. Evaluation of primary ocular irritation: Alternatives to the Draize test. In *Ocular therapeutics and drug delivery,* edited by I. K. Reddy. Lancaster, Penn., USA: Technomic Publishing Company, pp. 489–525.

Jarvinen, K., T. Jarvinen, and A. Urtti. 1995. Ocular absorption following topical delivery. Adv. *Drug Delivery Rev.* 16:3–19.

Khromow, G. L., A. B. Davydov, Y. F. Maychuk, and I. F. Tishina. 1976. Base for ophthalmological medicinal preparations and an opththalmological medicinal film. U.S. Patent #3,935,303.

Lang, J. C. 1995. Ocular drug delivery conventional ocular formulations. *Adv. Drug Delivery Rev.* 16:39–43.

Lederer, C. M. Jr., and R. E. Harold. 1986. Dropsize of commercial glaucoma medications. *Amer. J. Ophthamol.* 101:691–694.

Lee, V. H. L., and V. H. K. Li. 1989. Prodrugs for improved ocular drug delivery. *Adv. Drug Delivery Rev.* 3:1–38.

Li, V. H. K., and J. R. Robinson. 1989. Solution viscosity effects on the ocular disposition of cromolyn sodium in the albino rabbit. *Int. J. Pharmaceutics* 53 (3):219–225.

Liaw, J., Y. Rojanasakul, and J. R. Robinson. 1992. The effect of drug charge type and charge density on corneal transport. *Int. J. Pharm.* 88:111–124.

Matthews, B. R. 1999. Recent developments in the European regulation of ophthalmic, parenteral and other sterile products. *Eur. J. Parenteral Sci.* 4 (3):103–109.

Maurice, D. M., and S. Mishima. 1984. Ocular pharmacokinetics. In *Pharmacology of the eye, Handbook of experimental pharmacology*, Vol. 69, edited by M. L. Sears. Berlin-Heidelberg: Springer-Verlag, pp. 19–116.

Meisner, D., and M. Mezei. 1995. Liposomal ocular delivery systems. *Adv. Drug Delivery Rev.* 16:75–93.

Merkli, A., C. Tabatabay, and R. Gurny. 1995. Use of insoluble biodegradable polymers in ophthalmic systems for the sustained release of drugs. *Eur. J. Pharm. Biopharm.* 41 (5):271–283.

Meyer, D. R., and J. P. McCulley. 1992. pH tolerance of rabbit corneal epithelium in tissue culture. *J. Toxicol. Cut. Ocular Toxicol.* 11 (1):15–30.

Patton, T. F. 1980. *Ophthalmic drug delivery systems.* Washington, D. C.: American Pharmaceutical Association.

Robinson, J. R., and G. M. Mylnek. 1995. Bioadhesive and phase-change polymers for ocular drug delivery. *Adv. Drug Delivery Rev.* 16:45–50.

Rojanasakul, Y., L-Y. Wang, M. Bhat, D. D. Glover, C. J. Malanga, and J. K. H. Ma. 1992. The transport barrier of epimelia: A comparative study on membrane permeability and charge selectivity in the rabbit. *Pharm. Res.* 9:1029–1034.

Rozier, A., C. Mazuel, J. Grove, and B. Plazonnet. 1989. Gelrite: A novel, ion-activated, in-situ gelling polymer for opthalmic vehicles. Effect on bioavailability of timolol. *Int. J. Pharm.* 57:163–168.

Schell, J. W. 1982. *Survey Ophthalmol.* 27:217–218.

Schoenwald, R. D. and R. Ward. 1978. Relationship between steroid permeability across excised rabbit cornea and octanol-water partition coefficients. *J. Pharm. Sci.* 67:786–788.

Seattone, M. F., P. Giannaccini, P. Chetoni, M. T. Toracca, and D. Monti. 1991. *Int. J. Pharmaceut.* 72:131–139.

Saettone, M. F., and L. Salminen. 1995. Ocular inserts for topical delivery. *Adv. Drug Delivery Rev.* 16:95–106.

Sieg, J. W. and J. R. Robinson. 1975. *J. Pharm. Sci.* 64:931.

Suhonen, P., T. Jarvinen, K. Lehmussaari, T. Reunamaki, and A. Urtti. 1995. Ocular absorption and irritation of pilocarpine prodrug is modified with buffer, polymer, and cyclodextrin in the eyedrop. *Pharm. Res.* 12 (4):529–530.

Tammara, V. K. and M. A. Crider. 1996. Prodrugs: A chemical approach to ocular drug delivery. *Ocular therapeutics and drug delivery*, edited by I. K. Reddy. Lancaster, Penn., USA. Technomic Publishing Company, pp. 285–334.

Vulovic, N., M. Primorac, M. Stupar, J. L. Ford. 1989. Some studies into the properties of indomethacin Suspensions intended for ophthalmic use. *Int. J. Pharmaceut.* 55:123–128.

Wade, A., and P. J. Weller. (eds.) 1994. *Handbook of pharmaceutical excipients*, 2nd ed. Washington DC: American Pharmaceutical Association, and London: The Pharmaceutical Press.

Zimmer, A., and J. Kreuter. 1995. Microspheres and nanoparticles used in ocular delivery systems. *Adv. Drug Delivery Rev.* 16:61–73.

13

Aqueous Nasal Dosage Forms

Nigel Day

AstraZeneca R&D Charnwood
Loughborough, United Kingdom

> Nasal spray products contain therapeutically active ingredients (drug substances) dissolved or suspended in solutions or mixtures of excipients (e.g., preservatives, viscosity modifiers, emulsifiers, buffering agents) in nonpressurised dispensers that use metering spray pumps. (FDA 1999)

The nasal route of drug delivery is convenient for administering active pharmaceutical agents. These agents can be for *local* therapy (e.g., established treatments such as corticosteroids for rhinitis) or for *systemic* therapy (e.g., new-generation migraine therapies such as Imigran™/ Imitrex™ [UK/U.S.]). Table 13.1 summarises a range of aqueous nasal products marketed in the United States and the United Kingdom. The number of active ingredients are relatively small and comprise both simple low molecular mass molecules and newer peptide molecules.

For local therapy, the advantages of nasal delivery are clear. For systemic therapy, the advantages can only be realised for certain categories of drugs. Typically, those agents metabolised in the gastro-intestinal (GI) tract, or by first-pass metabolism, are candidates for evaluation in nasal delivery systems. The opportunity for delivering peptide drugs by this route has stimulated much research interest in recent years. There are many factors to consider, such as the physicochemical properties of the drug and the dose required for clinical effect. The rate of absorption from the nasal cavity can be quite rapid. Whilst still slower and less dose-efficient than intravenous (IV) delivery, nasal delivery is likely in most cases to be

Table 13.1
Marketed aqueous nasal products in the United States and the United Kingdom.

Product/ Manufacturer	Active Ingredient	Excipients Listed	Pack/Pump Information
AFRIN (DURATION) Schering-Plough (U.S.)	Oxymetazoline 0.05% Nasal decongestant	BKC, Na$_2$edta, PEG1450, pov, PG, NaP	Plastic squeeze bottle Spray pump bottle
AFRIN SINUS Schering-Plough (U.S.)	Oxymetazoline 0.05%	BKC, BA, Na$_2$edta, NaP, camphor, eucalyptol, menthol, Tw80, PG	Plastic squeeze bottle
AFRIN 4 hour Schering-Plough (U.S.)	Phenylephrine HCl 0.5% Nasal decongestant	BKC, Na$_2$edta, PEG1450, pov, PG, NaP, glycerine	Plastic squeeze bottle
ASTELIN, Wallace (U.S.) RHINOLAST Asta Medica (UK)	Azelastine HCl 0.1% Antihistamine, $M_r = 418$	BKC (125 μg/mL), Na$_2$edta, HPMC, cit, NaP, NaCl, (pH 6.8)	Metered spray HDPE bottle 0.137 μL dose
ATROVENT 0.03/0.06% Boehringer Ingelheim (U.S.) RINATEC 0.03% B.Ing (UK)	Ipatropium bromide 0.03% Anticholinergic, $M_r = 430$	BKC, Na$_2$edta, NaCl, NaOH, HCl, (pH 4.7) isotonic	Metered spray HDPE bottle 70 μl dose each
BECONASE GlaxoSmithKline (U.S./UK)	Beclomethasone dipropionate 0.042% (micronised) SAI, $M_r = 521$	BKC, MCC, NaCMC, dex, Tw80, PE-OH (0.25% w/v), HCl, (pH 4.5–7.0)	Amber neutral glass bottle with metering atomising pump and nasal adapter
DDAVP Aventis (U.S.) DESMOSPRAY Ferring (UK)	Desmopressin acetate 0.01% Antidiuretic hormone, $M_r = 1183$	BKC (50%) (0.2 mg/mL), NaCl, cit, NaP	Spray pump bottle delivering 50 × 10 μg sprays
FLONASE/FLIXONASE GlaxoSmithKline (U.S./UK)	Fluticasone propionate 0.05% w/w, SAI, $M_r = 501$	BKC (0.02% w/w), dex, MCC, NaCMC, Tw80, PE-OH (0.25% w/w)	Amber glass bottle, actuations of 100 mg suspension
MIACALCIN nasal spray Novartis (U.S.)	Calcitonin-salmon 32 amino acids, $M_r = 3527$	BKC 0.1 mg/mL, NaCl 8.5 mg/mL, HCl, N$_2$	Glass bottles, screw-on pump 90 μL per actuation
NASACORT AQ Aventis (U.S.)	Triamcinolone acetonide Corticosteroid, $M_r = 435$	BKC, MCC, NaCMC, Tw80, dex, HCl, Na$_2$edta, (pH 4.5–6.0)	HDPE bottle with metered-dose pump spray
NASAREL Dura (U.S.) SYNTARIS Roche (U.S./UK)	Flunisolide 0.025% SAI, $M_r = 444$	BKC, BHT, cit, Na$_2$edta, PEG 400, Tw20, PG, NaCit, sorbitol, NaOH, HCl, (pH 5.2)	Spray bottle fitted with metered pump
NASCOBAL Schwarz (U.S.)	Cyanocobalamin $M_r = 1355$	BKC, MeC, NaCit, cit, glycerine, (pH 4.5–5.5)	Glass bottle dosing 500 μg/100 μL gel
NEO-SYNEPHRINE Bayer (U.S.)	Phenylephrine HCl	BKC, thimerosal (0.001%), NaCl, cit, NaCit	0.25%, 0.5% bottles as drops and spray; 1% bottle as spray
NEO-SYNEPHRINE 12 h Bayer (U.S.)	Oxymetazoline HCl 0.05%	BKC, phenylmercuric acetate (0.002%), glycine, sorbitol	Nasal spray bottle

Table 13.1 continued on the next page

Table 13.1 continued from the previous page

Product/ Manufacturer	Active Ingredient	Excipients Listed	Pack/Pump Information
NICOTROL NS McNeil (U.S.)	Nicotine $M_r = 162$	NaP, citric acid, MePB, PrPB, NaCl, Na$_2$edta, Tw80 (isotonic, pH 7)	Glass bottle, 50 μL actuation (droplet size > 8 μm)
NOSTRILLA 12 h Novartis (U.S.)	Oxymetazoline HCl 0.05%	BKC, glycine, sorbitol	White plastic bottle
OTRIVIN Novartis (U.S./UK)	Xylometazoline HCl 0.05/0.1%	BKC, NaP, Na$_2$edta, NaCl	Spray or dropper bottle
PRIVINE Novartis (U.S.)	Naphazoline HCl	BKC, NaP, Na$_2$edta, NaCl	Bottle
RHINOCORT AQUA AstraZeneca (U.S./UK)	Budesonide, micronised SAI, $M_r = 430$	Na$_2$edta, potassium sorbate, dex, MCC, NaCMC, Tw80, HCl (pH 4.5)	Glass bottle, nasal spray 100 μg actuations
STADOL NS BMS (U.S.)	Butorphanol tartrate	NaCl, cit, BzCl, NaOH, HCl (pH 5)	10 mg/mL active solution
SYNAREL Searle (U.S./UK)	Nafarelin acetate, $M_r = 1113$	BKC, acetic acid, NaOH, HCl, sorbitol	Bottle delivering 100 μL spray containing 200 μg nafarelin
VANCENASE AQ Schering (U.S.)	Beclomethasone dipropionate $M_r = 521$	BKC, MCC, dex, Tw80, PE-OH (0.25% v/w), HCl, (pH 4.5–7.0)	HDPE nasal spray bottle
DEXA-RHINASPRAY Boehringer Ingelheim (UK)	Tramazoline hydrochloride 120 μg decongestant	BKC, NaCl, Tw80, glycerol, NaOH	Amber Type I bottle with 70 μL metering pump
IMIGRAN/IMITREX GlaxoSmithKline (UK/U.S.)	Sumitriptan 20 mg 5HT$_1$ receptor antagonist	KP, NaP, H$_2$SO$_4$, NaOH	100 μL unit dose vial with rubber stopper and applicator
LIVOSTIN Novartis (UK)	Levocabistine hydrochloride selective H$_1$ antagonist	BKC, Na$_2$edta, PG, Tw80, NaP, hypromellose, (pH 6–8)	Plastic bottle, spray pump containing microsuspension
LOCABIOTAL Servier (UK)	Fusfungine antibiotic	EtOH, saccharin, IPM, flavour	Type III glass bottle (plasticised with PVC)
NASONEX Schering-Plough (UK)	Mometasone furoate 50 μg glucocorticosteroid	BKC, MCC, CCS, glycerol, NaCit, cit, Tw80, PE-OH	White HDPE bottle and metered-dose pump
SUPRECUR SUPREFACT Shire (UK) (from HMR)	Buserelin acetate (100/150 μg buserelin) LHRH analogue, $M_r = 1300$	BKC, NaCl, NaCit, cit	Bottle

References: ABPI (1999); PDR (1999). All products in UPPERCASE are registered trademarks of the named manufacturer.

Abbreviations: BA: benzyl alcohol; BHT: butylated hydroxytoluene; BKC: benzalkonium chloride; BzCl: benethonium chloride; CCS: croscarmellose sodium; cit: citric acid; dex: dextrose; IPM: isopropyl myristate; KP: potassium phosphates; MCC: microcrystalline cellulose; MeC: methyl cellulose; MePB: methyl parabens; M_r: relative molecular mass; NaCit: Na citrate; NaCMC: Na carboxymethylcellulose; Na$_2$edta: disodium edetate; NaP: sodium phosphate; PEG: polyethylene glycol; PE-OH: phenylethyl alcohol; PG: propylene glycol; pov: povidone; PrPB: propyl parabens; SAI: steroidal anti-inflammatory; Tw: Tween (polysorbate) more rapid than oral dosing. A good example is the migraine therapy Imigran™ (sumatriptan). The oral dose is 50 or 100 mg. By contrast, the nasal dose is 20 mg, with a clinical response said to be within 15 min of dosing (GlaxoWellcome 1999). The subcutaneous dose is 6 mg; in this example, nasal delivery offers an improved bioavailability over oral delivery without the trauma of a subcutaneous injection.

Absorption of drugs from the nasal mucosa is also influenced by the contact time between drug and epithelial tissue. This contact time is dependent upon the clearance of the drug formulation from the nasal cavity. The mean $t_{1/2}$ (clearance) is about 25 min (90 percent within the range 5 to 40 min). The short half-life is caused by rapid clearance from the nose to the throat by ciliary movement. A typical dose volume for a nasal spray is up to about 200 μL. Larger volumes are lost from the absorptive region; they are either swallowed or run out of the nose. It is preferable to test formulation prototypes in man, rather than using *in vitro* or animal models, because the latter do not mimic the human nasal mucociliary clearance system and may give misleading absorption data. Additionally, only a human study will confirm whether drug metabolism is a critical factor in the nose. The physiological condition of the nose vascularity, the speed of mucus flow, and the presence of infection and atmospheric conditions (e.g., relative humidity [RH]) will affect the efficacy of nasal absorption. In the formulation, the concentration, viscosity, surface tension, tonicity, pH and excipients will have an effect. Finally, the delivery device volume, droplet size, spray characteristics and site of deposition will be relevant.

In summary, the advantages of nasal drug delivery are as follows:

- Avoidance of parenteral administration/non-invasive

- Rapid absorption, peaking generally within 15–30 min

- Avoidance of first-pass effect

- Apparent permeability to some peptides

- Ease of self-administration/patient compliance good

If the route is technically feasible, the disadvantages are few:

- Environmental conditions, infection and intersubject variability can lead to inconsistent absorption.

- Short time span available for absorption due to rapid clearance.

- Local metabolism in the nose and instability of compound (especially for peptide drugs).

NASAL ANATOMY AND PHYSIOLOGY

The respiratory tract is divided into regions: the nasopharyngeal airway (upper respiratory tract) and the tracheobronchial and pulmonary airways (lower respiratory tract). The anterior one-third of the nasal cavity viewed in cross-section reveals a central septum dividing the two cavities. This region, including the proximal portion of the inferior and middle turbinates, is non-ciliated (Figure 13.1). The meatuses are spaces formed by the folds of the two inferior and middle turbinates. In the posterior two-thirds of the nasal cavity, clearance of deposited par-

Figure 13.1 The upper airways seen from the midline with cross-sections at three points (A, B, C). NV1, Nasal valve; IT1, Inferior turbinate; MT1, Middle turbinate; ST1, Superior turbinate (from Mygind 1979; reproduced by permission).

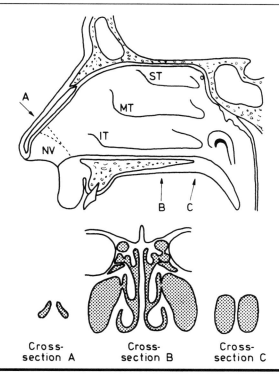

Cross-
section A   Cross-
section B   Cross-
section C

ticles occurs by slow spreading of the mucus layer into the ciliated regions along the inferior and middle meatuses, followed by a more rapid mucociliary clearance into the nasopharynx from where they are swallowed (Mygind 1979).

The nose functions both as a passageway for the movement of air into the respiratory tract and as an "air-conditioner" by filtering environmental pollutants and warming and humidifying the air. Large particles trapped in the nasal filter undergo a relatively rapid clearance (minutes compared to hours or weeks for the bronchi and alveoli, respectively). In the anterior region of the nose (about 1.5 cm in from the nares), the airways are constricted on each side to a cross-sectional area of only about 30 to 40 mm^2 at the location of the nasal valve (Proctor 1982). Subsequently, the airstream undergoes a sharp turbulent change in the direction of nearly 90° upon entry to the turbinates. *In vitro* studies using molds of the human nose, and *in vivo* studies in humans using gamma scintigraphy under conditions of natural breathing, have shown that particles delivered by intranasal spray devices are deposited in the anterior regions of the nasal cavity primarily between the nasal valve and the ciliated epithelium (frontal turbinates) (Kim et al. 1985; Hallworth and Padfield 1986; Newman et al. 1987a). Particles impact onto a layer of mucus covering the surface, underlying which there is a layer of ciliated epithelial cells beating towards the pharynx. The site of particle deposition and the rate of clearance are of primary importance for nasally administered drugs that act locally. Particles > 5–10 μm in diameter (typical of intranasal sprays) do not penetrate the pulmonary airways, but tend to deposit at their impaction sites within the upper respiratory tract. Particles <5 μm are regarded as respirable and are deposited within the lung. Particles <1 μm are inhaled deeply into the pulmonary airways, but undergo little gravitational settling and are likely to be exhaled without deposition during normal tidal breathing (Bates et al. 1966; Brain and Valberg 1979). For good nasal absorption of drug to occur, dosing must be achieved in the region above the level of the nasal palate. The region below this (effectively the "anterior" visible area of the outer nasal cavity) shows poor absorption. This knowledge of nasal anatomy and the importance of particle size on deposition has enabled nasal device manufacturers to design their delivery systems accordingly. This is discussed further in the section "Device Selection Considerations".

FORMULATION SELECTION CONSIDERATIONS

There are many factors to be considered in the successful "product design" and development of an aqueous nasal formulation. A typical development programme should consider the technical challenges of the molecule and balance these against the clinical and marketing requirements for the product. Several issues need to be addressed. For example, is the drug to be administered to one or two nostrils, is the drug sufficiently soluble to permit administration as a solution, and is the dose feasible (e.g., are there existing formulations for similar molecules)? If the dose levels are limited, solubility enhancement may be possible with permitted excipients, or permeability enhancers may be required. If solubility is limited, a suspension product is the only alternative, but there are more technical challenges than are present for solution products.

Preformulation and Bulk Drug Properties

A preformulation package provides essential information on the physicochemical properties of the drug, such as pK_a, aqueous solubility, aqueous stability, light stability, and lipophilicity (this may predict potential for binding to plastic/rubber pump components). The pK_as of any ionisable groups are particularly important as they affect stability, solubility and lipophilicity and should indicate the optimum pH for the nasal solution. For physiological reasons, formulated products are usually in the range of pH 4.0–7.4.

If the drug is insufficiently soluble to allow delivery of the required dose as a solution (the maximum delivered dose for each nostril is 200 μL), then a suspension formulation will be required. There are additional issues for suspension products, for example crystal growth, physical stability, resuspension, homogeneity and dose uniformity. Suspension products will also require information on density, particle size distribution, particle morphology, solvates and hydrates, polymorphs, amorphous forms, moisture and/or residual solvent content and microbial quality (sterile filtration of the bulk liquid during manufacture is not feasible).

Selection of Excipients

Aqueous nasal products are listed as marketed in the United States and the United Kingdom (Table 13.1) (PDR 1999; ABPI 1999). This table shows a relatively limited range of excipients used and accepted by the regulatory authorities. Excipients featured in marketed nasal products in the United States are listed in Table 13.2 (Weiner and Bernstein 1989; FDA 1996). According to the pH chosen and the ionisation properties of the drug, an appropriate buffer system is usually incorporated, often a mixed phosphate buffer system. However, if it is appropriate to choose the pK_a of the drug itself, then this becomes a self-buffered system. If it is feasible, there are advantages in choosing a pH equal to the pK_a; during manufacturing, it is easier to titrate to the target pH in the region of maximum buffer capacity (pK_a). Aqueous nasal preparations are usually isotonic to ensure physiological acceptability. A choice needs to be made between ionic tonicity (e.g., saline) or non-ionic tonicity (e.g., dextrose). Counter-ion effects may influence the decision on pH-adjustment and buffers. Flavours or sweetening agents are sometimes added to a formulation to mask the taste, a small proportion of which may be swallowed following nasal delivery (Batts et al. 1991). Perceptions of taste do vary with age, and therefore paediatric formulations may have to be slightly different from adult formulations. Sometimes a metal-chelating agent (e.g., disodium edetate) is included. This may also enhance preservative efficacy. Oxygen is sometimes excluded by means of a nitrogen purge, and antioxidants may also be included to improve stability. Suspension systems usually require an appropriate surfactant and viscosity adjuster.

Penetration Enhancers

For many years, penetration (or permeation) enhancers have been used in experimental studies to overcome the resistance of peptide and protein drugs to nasal absorption (refer to "Special Considerations for Peptide Nasal Delivery"). Aqueous nasal products using permeation enhancers are not currently available in the United States or the United Kingdom. Examples of enhancers used in animal studies are: chitosan (Aspden et al. 1997a, b), cyclodextrins (Marttin et al. 1998; Merkus et al. 1999), bile salts (sodium cholate, deoxycholate and taurodihydrofusidate) (Illum and Fisher 1997), bioadhesive degradable starch microspheres, glycyrrhizin and liposomes. Their modes of action vary between bioadhesion (thereby retaining the drug at the absorption site for longer) and interference with the "tight" epithelial cell junctions. The slow introduction of enhancers into clinical products may be largely attributed to concerns over histological damage which has been observed under certain circumstances in experimental systems (Chandler et al. 1991).

Preservatives

If a traditional multidose nasal spray is used, then a preservative will have to be included in the formulation, and preservative challenge testing will be required (e.g., in accordance with U.S. Pharmacopeia (USP) <51> Antimicrobial Effectiveness Testing). The test is usually performed over 4 weeks using 50 mL of formulation, covering five organisms. Testing is required at zero time (initial) and at the 1, 2 and 3 year time-point of the stability programme. This work must also cover concentration ranges of preservative at the limits of specification. It is important to consider the effect of pH on preservative efficacy. The most common preservatives in aqueous nasal formulations are benzalkonium chloride (BKC) and phenylethyl alcohol. BKC is often chosen because it is a good preservative, but it does have two known complications. The benzalkonium cation can react with anionic actives and can lead to a reduction in either active potency or preservative efficacy. In addition to this, it is reported that BKC can have a long-term adverse effect on nasal mucosa (Hallén and Graf 1995). Clinically, this was exhibited by increased nasal stuffiness from symptom scores and swelling of the nasal mucosa. This may be related to the observed experimental effect of BKC on nasal cilia (Batts et al. 1989, 1990; Deitmer and Scheffler 1993; Bernstein 2000). Preservative efficacy testing can

Table 13.2
Excipients used in aqueous nasal products.

Excipient	Function	Typical Concentration
Acetic and citric acids	pH adjustment/buffer	0.12%/0.10%
Sodium hydroxide/ hydrochloric acid	pH adjustment	No range
Sodium acetate, citrate, and phosphates (mixed), potassium phosphate (mixed)	Buffer	No range
Edetate disodium	Metal chelator/preservative enhancer	0.01%
Benzalkonium chloride	Preservative (known effect on cilia)	0.01–0.02% w/v
Benzethonium chloride	Preservative	No range
Benzyl alcohol	Preservative	Not listed by FDA
Chlorobutanol	Preservative (known effect on cilia)	0.05–0.1%
Methylparaben	Preservative (known effect on cilia)	0.033%
Phenylethyl alcohol	Preservative	0.25%
Phenylmercuric acetate	Preservative (known effect on cilia)	Not listed by FDA
Propylparaben	Preservative (known effect on cilia)	0.017%
Thimerosal	Preservative (**no** effect on cilia at 0.01%)	Not listed by FDA
Potassium chloride	Tonicity adjustment	Not listed by FDA
Sodium chloride	Tonicity adjustment	0.5–0.9%
Me-OH-Pr cellulose	Viscosity adjustment	<1%
Na CMC	Viscosity adjustment	<1%
Microcrystalline cellulose	Viscosity adjustment	<1%
Ethanol	Solvent	No range
Glycerol	Solvent/tonicity adjustment	1.0–2.5%
Glycine	Solvent/tonicity adjustment	No range
PEG (mixed)	Solvent	<5%
PG	Solvent	<10%
Glyceryl dioleate	Solvent	<10%
Glyceryl monoleate	Surfactant	<7%
Lecithin	Surfactant	<5%
Polysorbate 20 & 80	Surfactant	<2%
Triglycerides		<2%
Menthol	Flavouring agent	No range
Saccharin sodium	Flavouring agent (sweetener)	No range
Sorbitol	Flavouring agent (sweetener)	<10% (2.5%)

produce variable results, and it is important to evaluate several alternatives during formulation development (Hodges et al. 1996). Some traditional preservatives have now become less popular (e.g., the mercury-based preservatives thiomersal and phenylmercuric nitrate) because of toxicological concern with chronic use. It is vital that the international acceptability of a preservative is checked.

Stability and Compatibility

Both the formulation and the delivery device together need to be considered in the stability testing programme. The active must be compatible with the excipients, but in addition, *both* must be compatible with the delivery device. Stability testing must be conducted according to International Conference on Harmonisation (ICH) guidelines, depending on the intended territories. Specific considerations relevant to the pack are the type of plastic bottle (e.g., high density polyethylene [HDPE]) or glass bottle (e.g., amber), binding of active to the bottle or pump components, and the appearance of leachables and extractables from the plastics and elastomers used in the delivery device.

Processing Issues

It is essential to look forward to the manufacturing and processing issues which will be encountered during development of a nasal product, particularly the effect of scaling-up from the laboratory (e.g., 5 L scale) to stability and small-scale clinical trial (e.g., 50 L) through to production scale (e.g., 500 L). For solution products, it is important to consider the rate of dissolution and mixing time required. Filter (membrane) compatibility data should be generated, if possible using a filtration system that can be appropriately scaled-up from laboratory to production. A membrane system based upon polyvinylidene fluoride (PVDF), polysulphone or polycarbonate is often chosen. The availability of this information is especially important for peptide drugs, for which there are often issues of stability and adsorption.

For suspension products, there are particular issues already mentioned in the section "Preformulation and Bulk Drug Properties". In general, there are more issues in scaling-up suspension products than there are for solution products. Such issues are the need to "wet" larger quantities of drug, the possibility of foaming and homogeneity during the extended time of filling.

DEVICE SELECTION CONSIDERATIONS

Following the discussion in the section on "Nasal Anatomy and Physiology", it is apparent that data on droplet size and spray angle from a nasal device are important for the regulatory authorities. This section reviews the types of nasal devices available, discusses clinical studies on spray angle and droplet size and reviews device testing.

Types of Nasal Devices

The three key requirements of the nasal delivery device are

1.   Stability with the formulated product

2.   User-friendly design for patient compliance

3.   Reliability in use.

The longest-established systems typically dispense nasal drops or a crude spray via a flexible plastic squeeze bottle. These systems are often described as "open", since they readily allow contaminated air back into the bottle after discharge. Bacteria can thus enter the system and, whilst the use of preservatives can minimise the risk of growth, these systems are now regarded as the least satisfactory design. In addition, the instillation of drops per se into the nasal cavity is inefficient because the drug solution is inevitably cleared along the floor of the nasal cavity, with a correspondingly short residence time. Squeeze-bottle systems that dispense a spray (as opposed to drops) have better distribution within the nasal cavity, but these suffer from imprecise dosing. Key dosing parameters such as spray angle, droplet size and delivered dose (volume or weight) are all subject to variability due to (a) the squeeze pressure applied to the bottle and (b) the ratio of liquid to air in the squeeze bottle (which changes significantly during the life of the bottle).

The more sophisticated devices are capable of overcoming all the typical problems associated with squeeze-bottle systems. These devices are multiple- or unit-dose systems based on a mechanical pump dispenser mounted on a glass or rigid plastic bottle. There are several manufacturers of specialist nasal pumps, most notably Becton-Dickinson, Pfeiffer, Sofab and Valois. Many of these companies have manufacturing facilities physically separated (often on different sites) from their other pump business interests (e.g., cosmetic applications). This is particularly important to ensure the highest standards are current Good Manufacturing Practice (cGMP) expected by the pharmaceutical regulatory authorities. A summary of some of the devices available from the major manufacturers is in Table 13.3. There are examples of unit-dose and multiple-dose devices. All the manufacturers offer a range of designs to cover both the adult and paediatric market. Dose-counting systems are now available to allow the patient to monitor the actuation life of the product.

There are two key elements in the design of nasal spray pumps. First, it is essential the suppliers fully understand the complex nature of the plastic, elastomer and metallic components that comprise the pump mechanism. Injection moulding and the tooling dimensions must be tightly controlled to ensure consistency of component product from plastic and elastomer components. These components will often require the addition of additives such as plasticisers and lubricants during manufacture, either to ensure a smooth manufacturing process or to optimise the properties of the component in the fully assembled pump unit. Ideally, the number of different polymers will be minimised; this reduces the number of potential interactions with other components and (more importantly) the formulation. It also reduces the problems of supply-chain management. The pump manufacturers usually source all their raw materials from third parties. Once a design is established and committed to commercial production, it is essential for the pump manufacturer to have an assured level of stockpile of all the components for several years of production. It is advisable for the pump manufacturer to dual-source all raw material supplies. This is because the pump customer (the pharmaceutical industry) will have invested considerable time and money in extensive

Table 13.3
Examples of commercially available nasal delivery systems.

Company	Device	Features	Performance
Becton-Dickinson	AccuSpray™	Based upon Hypak™ syringe system. Adaptable to aseptic use. 0.1–0.2 mL dose per nostril. Dose divider available to deliver one dose per nostril. Type I borosilicate glass/elastomeric stopper contact.	Spray angle: 60° ± 10° Droplet size: 5% < 14 μm 85% = 14–150 μm 10% > 150 μm
Pfeiffer (AptarGroup Inc.)	Unit-dose system	Comprises plastic body, glass ampoule and West Company elastomeric plunger.	
	Nasal spray (multi-dose)	Available with screw or crimp closure. 0.05–0.14 mL per actuation. Also available as a preservative-free system	
Sofab	SP5 pump	Pump for small capacity bottles (minimum 0.6 mL). No elastomer gasket in design. Acetal (non-contact). Polyethylene and stainless steel (contact). Integrated dip tube.	Typical dose 50, 70 μL; for 50 μL dose (example): volume = 56 μL ± 10% (98% ethanol)
	SP27 pump	Traditional pump design, compatible with wide range of nasal applicators for paediatric, adult or geriatric use. Airless/preservative-free systems also available. Acetal, polyethylene, polypropylene, elastomer, stainless steel (contact)	Typical dose 50, 70, 100, 130 μL; For 200 × 100 μL doses (example): volume = 102.8 μL ± 4.2% (distilled water)
	SP270 pump	Improved version of SP27. With M17 ring, avoids use of aluminium ferrules and elastomer gaskets by plastic/plastic design. Components polyethylene, polypropylene, stainless steel. Integrated dip tube.	Better performance than SP27 at 45°C (±5% dose consistency)
Valois (AptarGroup Inc.)	Monospray	Single-dose system	
	Bidose	Two-dose system	
	VP3 Pump	Classic multiple dose	Spray angle typically 43.2 ± 1.8°
	VP7 Pump	Airless multiple dose	Droplet size typically 56.8 ± 1.8 μm

Data from manufacturers' literature.

stability tests of their formulations with the specific pump and bottle system. To repeat these studies may take 2–3 years to generate sufficient data to satisfy a pack change to a regulatory authority. In addition to the complexities of pump and bottle manufacture and supply, testing the pack system for interactions with the formulation is also required. Testing is not restricted to the relatively simple issue of adsorption of active ingredients onto the container; it also involves the adsorption of excipients, particularly preservatives such as BKC, which are notorious for binding to elastomeric and polymeric surfaces. The regulatory authorities (particularly the FDA) have also shown great interest in the leaching and extraction of elastomeric and polymeric components into the formulation itself. Sophisticated modern analytical techniques will not always detect these; so perhaps the best remedy is to provide data showing the levels are low and consistent from batch to batch. Precise identification of the leachables and extractables may not always be possible, but certain classes of compounds are now almost always to be avoided, e.g., polynuclear aromatic hydrocarbons found in the carbon black used in black rubber gaskets; these are now not acceptable for any new product applications because they are proven carcinogens.

In the basic mechanical pump, the dispensed volume (or weight) is controlled by the volume of the metering chamber. The spray angle and droplet size are controlled by the dimensions and geometry of the orifice, as well as by the pressure build-up in the metering chamber prior to dispensing (influenced by the spring characteristics). It is usually more convenient to document the effect of varying dimension, geometry and spring on the subsequent spray angle and droplet size, and then to place relevant specification controls on the component, rather than to routinely test the product for spray angle and droplet size for the purpose of release.

Recent innovations in pump design have allowed preservative-free formulations to be developed. Such designs have obvious advantages in the avoidance of the use of preservatives, some of which can affect mucociliary clearance, and some of which can interact with active ingredients. Another advantage is that a new formulation with no preservative will usually achieve a patent extension over the existing product. These systems can only exist if the contents of the nasal spray bottle are sealed to ingress from the environment. Two of the companies that have developed a preservative-free system are Pfeiffer and Valois. The Pfeiffer system uses a sealing mechanism in the nasal actuator to prevent air from entering the container upon actuation; air is allowed to enter the container and equalise with atmospheric pressure through a microbiological filter. A second approach is to use a collapsible bag (containing the formulation) inside the rigid bottle. The bag remains sealed and clean and the displaced solution is compensated for by ingress of air into the space between the bag and the bottle. A third approach is to adopt a sliding piston (analogous to the displacement of a syringe); this has the advantage of allowing the device to be used at any angle (Bommer 1999). Valois has adopted a fourth alternative, whereby the bottle is filled only to about half capacity. The Valois VP7-D nasal pack has a special closure (exclusive to AstraZeneca and used in Nezeril™) that does not require a preservative. The product is prepared under aseptic conditions as a partial fill, for dose delivery without allowing air to pass back into the bottle. This has the significant benefit of reducing the amount of solution required for stability testing (determined in this case by the number of bottles). The unique feature of the VP7-D pump is the special polymeric foam pad arrangement to dry the nozzle after dosing, thus keeping the area dry and resistant to bacterial growth. Other preservative-free packs are available or are in development from Sofab (see Table 13.3). Typical multidose and unit-dose nasal devices are illustrated in Figures 13.2 and 13.3.

Figure 13.2 Cross-section of a traditional multidose nasal device.

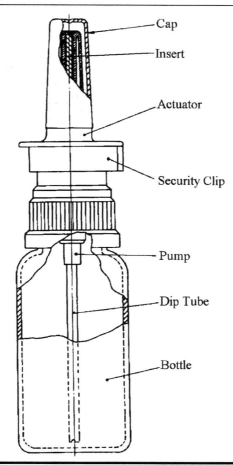

Spray Angle/Droplet Size Studies in Man

Various studies (Bond et al. 1984; Newman et al. 1987a) have found droplet size distributions of aqueous nasal spray products to have mass mean (median) diameter values between 44 and 62 μm. These studies showed that the majority of the dose was deposited locally in the anterior one-third of the nose. The relationship between retention time and viscosity has shown that the addition of various concentrations of methylcellulose (MC) to a metered spray pump containing desmopressin resulted in a dose-related increase in mean particle size from 51 μm (0 percent MC) to 81 μm (0.25 percent MC) to 200 μm (0.5 percent MC), without a change in mean spray weight. The longest retention time was observed for the 0.25 percent MC solution, which was attributed to its particle size (81 μm) and not to an increase in viscosity, since a decrease in retention time was observed for the highest viscosity (0.5 percent MC) solution

Figure 13.3 A typical unit-dose nasal device.

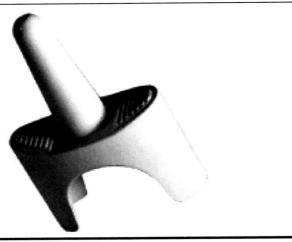

(Harris et al. 1988). Bond et al. (1984) have shown that there is a curvilinear relationship between the percentages remaining in the nasal cavity versus time, with no significant dependence on the spray angle delivered to the patient over the range 30 to 60°. This is not surprising, since any effect of spray angle on dispersion within the nasal cavity is mitigated by the short distance (a few millimeters) between the nasal actuator tip and the site of impaction. Newman and co-workers (1987a) simulated the suspension of budesonide crystals found in Rhinocort™ Nasal Spray with radiolabelled Teflon™ particles (mean diameter 2 μm). The droplet mass median diameter was 62 μm for this aqueous nasal pump with a spray cone of 60°. Particle deposition was chiefly confined to the anterior region of the nose, with 44 percent clearance after 30 min via the nasopharynx (Newman et al. 1987a). Aoki and Crawley (1976) compared nasal drops (administered in the supine position) with a nasal pump spray (administered in the seated position) and found a more uniform deposition pattern for the nasal drops. However, retention time in the nasal cavity was not affected by differences in initial deposition pattern, volume administered (0.1 mL for spray, 0.75 mL for drops), mode of administration (spray vs drops) or concentration (3–30 percent radiolabelled human serum albumin) (Aoki and Crawley 1976). Clearance of nasally administered drug has been shown to be biphasic, with an initial rapid phase representing removal of product from the ciliated regions, followed by a slower phase representing removal of product retained in the nonciliated anterior region of the nose (Lee et al. 1984).

Testing of Nasal Devices

Spray Weight, Droplet Size and Spray Angle

It is important for data on nasal sprays to include the following: (a) *spray weight* variation (important to measure the amount of drug reaching the patient), (b) *droplet size* distribution and (c) *spray angle*. Spray weight is volume dependent and is effectively a measure of the amount of drug reaching the patient for a solution formulation. The spray pump controls spray weight, and any variation should be limited by the dimensional tolerances of the pump chamber (expected to be very small). The dimensions of the orifice in the nasal actuator are considered critical to produce the droplet size distribution and spray angle. Control of these parameters is therefore best achieved by controlling the dimensions during manufacture. Once the specifications for the actuator orifice dimensions (diameter, length) are established, samples at each extreme can be manufactured (i.e., four populations at minimum/maximum orifice diameter/length). It is then feasible to test these parameters to record the effect on spray angle and droplet size. Spray angle is usually measured by a high-speed video camera, and droplet size can be measured by laser light scattering (e.g., Malvern). Testing should be done at the beginning, middle and end of the pack life, ideally using an automated actuating machine to eliminate operator variability. Of the three parameters measured, spray weight is the most clinically relevant, since it determines the nominal dose-to-patient relationship. Methods normally used for evaluating aerosols designed for pulmonary use, such as assessments of spray plume patterns and droplet size distribution, are not generally considered useful for evaluating the clinical performance of intranasal products because they do not take into account the unique morphology of the nasal passages. Nonetheless, for regulatory purposes, the provision of these data is *essential*.

In addition to the fundamental testing of spray weight, droplet size and spray angle, there are a variety of additional tests to be performed as part of the development process.

Dose Accuracy

Dose accuracy over time should be recorded; this is done at the beginning, middle and end of *delivery* life for the product. This test is usually performed during the stability test programme to check dose accuracy at the end of *shelf* life.

Pump Priming

This is tested by reference to the number of shots required to initially prime the pump, and the loss of prime during a typical user test (i.e., the pump should not require repriming during normal daily use). If the product is only used intermittently, then repriming may be required.

Weight Loss

Weight loss from the bottle is important in two respects. First, loss of water vapour will affect the concentration of all the formulation ingredients, and second, the fill volume will need adjustment to ensure there are sufficient initial contents to guarantee delivery of the stated number of shots during the whole of the shelf life of the product.

Fill Volume

This is calculated taking into account the label claim (number of doses), the upper limit of dose delivered for each actuation, the number of shots required to prime the pump, the moisture loss through the pack life and the residual volume (ullage) remaining in the bottle at the end of life (affected, for example, by the positioning of the dip tube relative to the bottom of the bottle).

Cap Removal Torque

This test is designed to measure the potential for leakage during product life. Cap *on-* and *off-* torques are measured at zero time and also during the period of the stability testing programme.

Supplier Issues

It should be assumed that the regulatory authorities will question as much, if not more, the nasal delivery device, rather than the formulation per se. They will critically examine for equivalence between the nasal device used in clinical trials and that proposed for the market. As the nasal device is usually more complicated in design than the formulation, and is manufactured by a third party, it is absolutely essential to work closely with the device provider. Among the key questions to ask of the supplier are the following:

- What is the composition of *every* component of the device (formulation contact and non-contact)?

- Is dual-sourcing in place for all the components?

- What is the component stockpile?

- What are the dimensional tolerances of all the components?

- Is microscopic surface analysis (i.e., low power electron microscopy) performed routinely?

- Is a legally binding supply contract in place to control *all* of the above?

- Does the supplier have a Drug Master File (DMF)?

- Is this a new device, never before released on the market (i.e., are you developing both a new pharmaceutical formulation and a new delivery device simultaneously)?

REGULATORY ASPECTS

Many of the points raised in this section have been mentioned in the earlier sections on formulation and device. A "Guidance for Industry" document in draft form was issued by the FDA during 1999, *Nasal Spray and Inhalation Solution, Suspension, and Spray Drug Products: Chemistry, Manufacturing and Controls Documentation* (FDA 1999). This document provides a plethora of information on issues the FDA will consider in submitted documentation supporting the approval of nasal products. There are over 1,600 lines in the document, and industry comments have been invited. Whilst the final document has yet to be issued, the draft is still an important reference. A brief review of the content of this draft document follows.

It is stated that nasal sprays have unique characteristics with respect to formulation, container closure system, manufacturing, in-process and final controls and stability. The product must deliver reproducible doses during the whole life of the product. Excipient controls are discussed in the FDA draft guidance; in many respects, the chemistry, manufacturing and controls (CMC) standards expected of excipients are starting to approach those required of the active pharmaceutical ingredient (API).

Test parameters are discussed in the FDA draft guidance. These include appearance, colour, clarity, identification, drug content (assay), impurities and degradation products and preservatives and stabilising excipients assay. For the device, the parameters include pump delivery, spray content uniformity through container life, spray pattern and plume geometry, droplet size distribution, particle size distribution (suspensions), microscopic evaluation (suspensions), foreign particles, microbial limits, preservative effectiveness, net content and weight loss (stability), leachables (stability), pH and osmolality.

The section on the container closure system is an important area for the FDA. They comment:

> The clinical efficacy of nasal and inhalation spray drug products is directly dependent on the design, reproducibility, and performance characteristics of the container closure system.

Also mentioned is the selection of a pump suitable for the formulation, and

> compatibility of the pump, container, and closure with formulation components, should be thoroughly investigated and established before initiating critical clinical, bioequivalence, and primary stability studies.

Thus, it is no longer acceptable for the formulator to delay this compatibility testing until later in the development programme. The key message is for the formulator to test early and ensure equivalence of the whole product throughout the development cycle. Leachables are specifically mentioned; data on their identity and concentration in the product and placebo are required through the shelf life and also under accelerated stability test conditions. Information should be submitted on source, chemical composition and physical dimensions of the container closure system, together with control and routine extraction tests. Acceptance criteria are also required.

The section on drug product stability provides clear guidance for the formulator. Considerations are the content of the stability protocol, test parameters, acceptance criteria and procedures, test intervals (long term, accelerated, intermediate), container storage (upright, inverted, horizontal) and test storage conditions (40°C/75 percent RH, 30°C/60 percent RH, 25°C/60 percent RH). For products packaged in semipermeable containers, the storage conditions are 40°C/15 percent RH, 30°C/40 percent RH and 25°C/40 percent RH; the reason for this is to provide a challenging environment to test the moisture permeability of the container. Moisture vapour loss will change the concentrations of all formulation ingredients (and hence the delivered dose), and may even result in precipitation of the active ingredient. The FDA requires stability data from three batches as the minimum to evaluate batch-to-batch variability, and also requires the expiry date to be based on data from full shelf-life stability studies of at least three batches of drug product.

Another section states that drug product characterisation studies are required to "characterise the optimum performance properties of the drug product and to support appropriate labelling statements". These include studies on priming and repriming of the pump in various orientations, and studies on non-use after different periods. Also, the number of sprays required to prime the device should be determined. Resting time and temperature cycling are also discussed.

Table 13.4 summarises the major testing requirements of the European Pharmacopoeia and the FDA guidelines/USP. The manufacturers of nasal sprays try to design their products to perform within the requirements of the PharmEur/FDA/USP; for example, Valois aims to produce pumps which deliver a mean dose ±10 percent of target, with all doses ±15 percent of target.

In summary, it is apparent there are no short-cuts to attaining regulatory approval. A formulator who dismisses the requirements of the draft guidelines without strong scientific justification will give the FDA an unequivocal opportunity to delay the approval whilst the outstanding questions are answered.

SPECIAL CONSIDERATIONS FOR PEPTIDE NASAL DELIVERY

Peptide and protein nasal drug delivery have challenges related to their unique physical and chemical properties and comprise issues of chemical stability, loss due to physical absorption (especially for low-dose/high-potency molecules) and self-aggregation. The two key factors for nasal delivery of peptides are molecular mass and lipophilicity. The transitional area between a predicted "good absorption" and a predicted "increasing difficulty" of absorption is a molecular mass of about 1,000 (McMartin et al. 1987). Complete absorption of a peptide, by

Table 13.4
Regulatory requirements for nasal devices

	PharmEur	FDA Guidelines/USP
Materials, safety	Chapters 3.1, 3.2	21 CFR: food additive regulations USP tests: physicochemical <661> biological reactivity <87>, <88>
Uniformity of delivered dose	8/10 ± 25% 10/10 ± 35%	
Weight loss, container closure	No requirements	Characterise weight loss Check bacterial resistance Measure light or gas contamination
Priming	< 5 strokes	Measure priming
Droplet (particle) size	Suitable for nasal deposition	Measure droplet size distribution
Spray characteristics	No requirements	Measure spray pattern and plume geometry
Extractables	No requirements	Measure extractables from polymeric and elastomeric systems
Actuators	No requirements	Dimensional controls

After Williams (1998)

any non-parenteral route, is unlikely. The maximum absorption expected is usually about 30 percent. However, there are isolated examples of more complete peptide absorption, often with the assistance of chemical enhancement. Chemical enhancers can, however, have a pathophysiological effect on the nasal mucosa. As this "effect" on the mucosa is fundamental in their mode of action, the key to success will be to seek the optimum balance in the "enhancement" vs. "pathology" equation.

A further difficulty with peptide delivery is the risk of metabolism during the absorption phase. This can only be assessed in a complete system; metabolic studies using homogenised cell fractions are not representative of the intact membrane(s).

Penetration enhancers are often used to improve peptide bioavailability in nasal formulations. A variety of different enhancers have been tried, and they work by one or several combined mechanisms. Some act by increasing the membrane fluidity and reducing the viscosity of the mucus layer, thereby increasing membrane permeability. Others act by transient loosening of the tight junctions between epithelial cells. The types of penetration enhancers discussed in the research literature include the following.

- Bile salts (sodium glycocholate, deoxycholate, cholate)

- Surfactants (polyoxyethylene lauryl ether-[laureth-9])

- Chelating agents (ethylenediaminetetraacetic acid [EDTA], salicylates)

- Fatty acids (sodium caprylate, laurate, caprate, oleic acid, monoolein)

- Glycosides (saponin)

- Glycyrrhetinic acid derivatives (sodium and dipotassium glycyrrhetinates)

- Fusidic acid derivatives (sodium taurodihydrofusidate, sodium dihydrofusidate)

- Phospholipids (lysophosphatidylcholine and palmitoyl and stearoyl derivatives)

See, e.g., Donovan et al. (1990a, b) and Yamamoto et al. (1993). Of these penetration enhancers, the steroidal surfactants have been the subject of most study and have been examined in clinical trials. However, in most cases, there are adverse reactions of a stinging or burning sensation, discomfort, or a certain degree of pain, indicative of irritation potential. In experimental studies, the use of penetration enhancers is often accompanied by pathohistological changes to the nasal mucosa (Chandler et al. 1991).

One reason for poor absorption by the nasal route may be the rapid removal of the drug from the site of absorption by mucociliary clearance (Dondeti et al. 1996; Quraishi et al. 1997). Bioadhesive gels adhere to the mucous and can reduce clearance and improve bioavailability. Microcrystalline cellulose, hydroxypropyl cellulose and neutralised Carbopol 934 have all shown different degrees of enhancement of nasal absorption of insulin in dogs. Bioadhesive starch microspheres have also shown enhanced absorption of desmopressin in sheep (Critchley et al. 1994). Gamma scintigraphy has been used to study microsphere clearance in man, and great differences have been observed. Starch microspheres have been used for nasal delivery of insulin in the rat with a bioavailability of about 30 percent (Björk and Edman 1988). The use of cyclodextrins to improve the nasal absorption of insulin has been demonstrated in rats (Merkus et al. 1991). Combinations of an absorption enhancer and a bioadhesive agent have been shown to provide a synergistic improvement in bioavailability (Dondeti et al. 1996).

Freeze-dried preparations are generating a lot of interest for peptides because of potentially improved stability, the avoidance of preservatives, which can have a damaging effect on nasal mucosa during chronic treatment, and improved bioavailability. There are devices to deliver the powder, but this concept is still at the research stage and is likely to be expensive to market.

Successful nasal delivery of peptide compounds has led to a number of peptide drugs being marketed for systematic absorption. These peptide drugs include buserelin (Suprefact™, Hoechst), gonadorelin (Kryptocur™, Hoechst), protirelin (Relefact™ TRH nasal, Hoechst), calcitonin (Miacalcic™, Sandoz), nafarelin (Synarel™, Syntex) and desmopressin (Minirin™, Ferring). Table 13.5 summarises the characteristics of some peptides studied in the nose.

Table 13.5
Peptides studied in the nose.

Peptide/Protein	Approx M_r	Species	Bioavailability
Protirelin* (TRH: thyrotropin-releasing hormone)	362	Human	20–30%
Metkephamid	600	Rat/human	70–90%
Vasopressin analogues	1,000	Human	10%
Nafarelin*	1,113	Monkey/human	5–10% 20–30% with 2% sodium glycocholate
GRF 1–29-NH$_2$	3,600	Human	<2%
Human pancreatic GHRH	5,000	Human	<2%
Ovine corticotrophin-releasing hormone	5,000	Human	<1%
Insulin	5,700	Dog/human	10–30% with bile salts
β-Interferon	20,000	Rabbit	<2% with 3% sodium glycochlolate
Buserelin*	1,300	Human	Not available
Gonadorelin*	1,182	Human	Not available
Calcitonin*	3,527	Human	Not available
Desmopressin*	1,069	Human	Not available

*Currently marketed products.

REFERENCES

Association of the British Pharmaceutical Industry (ABPI). 1999. *Data sheet compendium*. London: Association of the British Pharmaceutical Industry.

Aoki, F. Y., and J. C. W. Crawley. 1976. Distribution and removal of human serum albumin-technetium-99m instilled intranasally. *Brit. J. Clin. Pharmacal.* 3:869–878.

Aspden, T., L. Illum and O. Skaugrud. 1997a. The effect of chronic nasal application of chitosan solutions on cilia beat frequency in guinea pigs. *Int. J. Pharm.* 153:137–146.

Aspden, T., J. T. D. Mason, N. S. Jones, J. Lowe, O. Skaugrud, and L. Illum. 1997b. Chitosan as a nasal delivery system: The effect of chitosan solutions on *in vitro* and *in vivo* mucociliary transport rates in human turbinates and volunteers. *J. Pharm. Sci.* 86:509–513.

Bates, D.V., B. R. Fish, T. F. Hatch, T. T. Mercer, and P. E. Morrow. 1966. Deposition and retention models for internal dosimetry of the human respiratory tract. Task group on lung dynamics. *Health Phys.* 12:173–207.

Batts, A. H., C. Marriott, G. P. Martin, and S. W. Bond. 1989. The effect of some preservatives used in nasal preparations on mucociliary clearance. *J. Pharm. Pharmacol.* 41:156–159.

Batts, A. H., C. Marriott, G. P. Martin, C. F. Wood, and S. W. Bond. 1990. The effect of some preservatives used in nasal preparations on the mucus and ciliary components of mucociliary clearance. *J. Pharm. Pharmacol.* 42:145–151.

Batts, A. H., C. Marriott, G. P. Martin, S. W. Bond, J. L. Greaves, and C. G. Wilson. 1991. The use of radiolabelled saccharin to monitor the effect of the preservatives thiomersal, benzalkonium chloride and EDTA on human nasal clearance. *J. Pharm. Pharmacol.* 43:180–185.

Bernstein, I. L. 2000. Is the use of benzalkonium chloride as a preservative for nasal formulations a safety concern? A cautionary note based on compromised mucociliary transport. *J. Allergy Clin. Immunol.* 105:39–44.

Björk, E., and P. Edman. 1988. Degradable starch microspheres as a nasal delivery system for insulin. *Int. J. Pharm.* 47:233–236.

Bommer, R. 1999. Advances in nasal drug delivery technology. *Pharm. Tech. Eur.* September:26–33.

Bond, S. W., J. G. Hardy, and C. G. Wilson. 1984. Deposition and clearance of nasal sprays. In *Proceedings of the Second European Congress of Biopharmaceutics and Pharmacokinetics*, edited by J. M. Aiache and J. Hirtz, Salamanca, April 1984, pp. 93–98.

Brain, J. D., and P. A. Valberg. 1979. Deposition of aerosol in the respiratory tract. *Amer. Rev. Respir. Dis.* 120:1325–1373.

Chandler, S. G., L. Illum, and N. W. Thomas. 1991. Nasal absorption in the rat. I: A method to demonstrate the histological effects of nasal formulations. *Int. J. Pharm.* 70:19–27.

Critchley, H., S. S. Davies, N. Farraj, and L. Illum. Nasal absorption of desmopressin in rats and sheep. Effect of a bioadhesive microsphere delivery system. *J. Pharm. Pharmacol.* 46:651–656.

Deitmer, T., and R. Scheffler. 1993. The effect of different preparations of nasal decongestants on ciliary beat frequency *in vitro*. *Rhinology* 31:151–153.

Dondeti, P., H. Zia, and T. E. Needham. 1996. Bioadhesive and formulation parameters affecting nasal absorption. *Int. J. Pharm.* 127:115–133.

Donovan, M. D., G. Flynn, and G. Amidon. 1990a. The molecular weight dependence of nasal absorption: The effect of absorption enhancers. *Pharm. Res.* 7:808–814.

Donovan, M. D., G. Flynn, and G. Amidon. 1990b. Absorption of polyethylene glycols 600 through 2000: The molecular weight dependence of gastrointestinal and nasal absorption. *Pharm. Res.* 7:863–868.

Edman, P., and E. Björk. 1992. Nasal delivery of peptide drugs. *Advanced Drug Delivery Rev.* 8:165–177.

FDA. 1996. *Inactive ingredient guide.* Rockville, Md., USA: Food and Drug Administration.

FDA. 1999. *Nasal spray and inhalation solution, suspension and spray drug products: Chemistry Manufacturing and Controls Documentation*, Draft Guidance for Industry. Rockville, Md., USA: Food and Drug Administration.

GlaxoWellcome. 1999. *Patient information leaflet for Imigran™.* Uxbridge, Middx, UK: GlaxoWellcome.

Hallén, H., and P. Graf. 1995. Benzalkonium chloride in nasal decongestive sprays has a long-lasting adverse effect on the nasal mucosa of healthy volunteers. *Clin. Exp. Allergy* 25:401–405.

Hallworth, G. W., and J. M. Padfield. 1986. A comparison of the regional deposition in a model nose of a drug discharged from metered aerosol and metered-pump nasal delivery systems. *J. Allergy Clin. Immunol.* 77:348–353.

Harris, A. S., E. Svensson, Z. G. Wagner, S. Lethagen, and I. M. Nilsson. 1988. Effect of viscosity on particle size, deposition, and clearance of nasal delivery systems containing desmopressin. *J. Pharm. Sci.* 77:405–408.

Hodges, N. A., S. P. Denyer, G. W. Hanlon, and J. P. Reynolds. 1996. Preservative efficacy tests in formulated nasal products: reproducibility and factors affecting preservative efficacy. *J. Pharm. Pharmacol.* 48:1237–1242.

Illum, L., and A. N. Fisher. 1997. Intranasal delivery of peptides and proteins. *Inhalation delivery of therapeutic peptides and proteins*, edited by A. L. Adjei and P. K. Gupta. New York. Marcel Dekker, pp. 135–184.

Kim, C. S., M. A. Eldridge, M. A. Sackner, and D. L. Swift. 1985. Deposition of aerosol particles in the human nose. *Amer. Rev. Respir. Dis.* 131:A370.

Lee, S. W., J. G. Hardy, C. G. Wilson, and G. J. C. Smelt. 1984. Nasal sprays and polyps. *Nucl. Med. Commun.* 5:697–703.

McMartin, C., L. E. F. Hutchinson, R. Hyde, and C. E. Peters. 1987. Analysis of structural requirements for the absorption of drugs and macromolecules from the nasal cavity. *J. Pharm. Sci.* 76:535–540.

Marttin, E., J. C. Verhoef, and F. W. H. M. Merkus. 1998. Efficacy, safety and mechanism of cyclodextrins as absorption enhancers in nasal delivery of peptide protein drugs. *J. Drug Targeting* 6:17–36.

Merkus, F. W. H. M., J. C. Verhoef, S. G. Romeijn, and N. G. M. Schipper. 1991. Absorption enhancing effect of cyclodextrins on intranasally administered insulin in rats. *Pharm. Res.* 8:588–592.

Merkus, F. W. H. M., J. C. Verhoef, E. Marttin, S. G. Romeijn, P. H. M. van der Kuy, and N. G. M. Schipper. 1999. Cyclodextrins in nasal drug delivery. *Adv. Drug Delivery Rev.* 36:41–57.

Mygind, N. 1979. *Nasal allergy.* Oxford: Blackwell Scientific.

Newman, S. P., F. Morén and S. W. Clarke. 1987a. Deposition pattern from a nasal pump spray. *Rhinology* 25:77–82.

Newman, S. P., F. Morén and S. W. Clarke. 1987b. Deposition pattern of nasal sprays in man. *Rhinology* 25:111–120.

Physicians' Desk Reference (PDR). 1999. *Physicians' desk reference.* Oradell, N.J., USA: Medical Economics Company.

Proctor, D. F. 1982. The upper airway. In *The nose: Upper airway physiology and the atmospheric environment*, edited by D. F. Proctor and I. B. Andersen. Amsterdam: Elsevier Biomedical Press, pp. 23–43.

Quraishi, M. S., N. S. Jones, and J. D. T. Mason. 1997. The nasal delivery of drugs. *Clin. Otolaryngol.* 22:289–301.

Weiner, M., and I. L. Bernstein. 1989. *Adverse reactions to drug formulation agents*. New York: Marcel Dekker.

Williams, G. 1998. *Nasal drug delivery devices, performance and regulatory requirements—The manufacturer's view*. London: Management Forum.

Yamamoto, A., T. Morita, M. Hashida, and H. Sezaki. 1992. Effect of absorption promoters on the nasal absorption of drugs with various molecular weights. *Int. J. Pharm.* 93:91–99.

ADDITIONAL READING

Advanced Drug Delivery Reviews. 1998. (Various papers related to nasal drug delivery.) 29:1–194.

Chien, Y. W. (Ed.) 1985. *Transnasal systemic medications*. Amsterdam: Elsevier.

Chien, Y. W., K. S. E. Su, and S. F. Chang. 1989. *Nasal systemic drug delivery*. New York: Marcel Dekker.

Illum, L. 1996. Nasal delivery. The use of animal models to predict performance in man. *J. Drug Targeting* 3:427–442.

14

Topical and Transdermal Delivery

Kenneth A. Walters and Keith R. Brain

An-eX Analytical Services Ltd.
Cardiff, United Kingdom

> Our primitive forebears had little difficulty in recognizing a disorder of the skin ... [but] ... when a single remedy ... [was] ... of no avail, it ... [was] ... easy and tempting to add others ad infinitum. There can be no other ready explanation for the complexities of dermatological therapy of the past and, indeed, of the present day.

These words, written by Frazier and Blank in 1954, suggested that the external treatment of skin disorders in the mid-twentieth century was probably as haphazard as it was in ancient times. Now, some 40-plus years later, we have to ask ourselves, "Have things changed that much?" There have certainly been considerable advances in our understanding of the physicochemical properties of formulation systems and their ingredients, resulting in the ability to develop physically, chemically and biologically stable products which, after two or three years on the shelf, are as potent as they were when they were first manufactured. There have also been considerable advances in our knowledge of the skin and the processes which control the passage of chemicals across this unique biological stratum. In this instance, the ground rules were laid down by Scheuplein and Blank in the late 1960s and early 1970s (Scheuplein and Blank 1971), and these have been updated on a reasonably regular basis (Idson 1975; Barry 1983; Shah and Maibach 1993; Schaefer and Redelmeier 1996; Roberts and Walters 1998).

Thus we know, for example, that permeation of compounds across the skin is, in most cases, controlled by the stratum corneum, and that it is the chemical composition and morphology of this layer that usually determines the rate and extent of absorption (Elias 1981; Raykar et al. 1988). We also know how to modify this barrier, by chemical or physical means, to alter the rate of diffusion of many permeating molecules (Walters and Hadgraft 1993; Smith and Maibach 1995).

A basic flaw, however, in the application of our understanding of the barrier properties of the skin to dermatological and transdermal therapy is that this knowledge has largely been generated by investigations on normal rather than pathological skin. The relevance of such information to diseased skin, where permeation characteristics are likely to be significantly altered, has yet to be fully established. There are some data on transport across skin which has been artificially damaged (Behl et al. 1981; Flynn et al. 1982; Bronaugh and Stewart 1985b; Scott et al. 1986; Scott 1991; Bond and Barry 1988). However, the limited information available on permeation through diseased skin has been obtained in the clinic (van der Valk et al. 1985; Turpeinen et al. 1986; Turpeinen 1991; Fartasch and Diepgen 1992) and, for obvious reasons, has not been systematically evaluated.

With these limitations in mind, this chapter concentrates on the specific considerations which are fundamental to the development of pharmaceutical dosage forms designed for application to the skin. Many of the early pharmaceutical development stages for these dosage forms, such as preformulation and drug substance stability, are common to dosage forms designed for other routes of delivery. These have been fully discussed elsewhere in this volume and will not be discussed in depth here.

In modern-day pharmaceutical practice, therapeutic compounds are applied to the skin for dermatological (within the skin) or local (regional) action, or for transdermal (systemic) delivery. Whatever the target site or organ, it will usually be necessary for the drug compound to cross the outermost layer of the skin, the stratum corneum. It is a major function of the stratum corneum to provide a protective barrier to the ingress of xenobiotics and to control the rate of water loss from the body. Evolution has generated a robust and durable membrane which fulfils its biological function throughout the lifespan. A basic, yet thorough, understanding of the structure and transport properties of this membrane is essential to the rational development of topical dosage forms.

THE SKIN AND PERCUTANEOUS ABSORPTION

Skin Structure

The skin is the body's largest organ, accounting for more than 10 percent of body mass, and the one which enables the body to interact most intimately with its environment. The skin consists of four layers: the stratum corneum (nonviable epidermis), the remaining layers of the epidermis (viable epidermis), dermis and subcutaneous tissues. There are also a number of associated appendages: hair follicles, sweat ducts, apocrine glands and nails. Many of the functions of the skin are essential to survival of humans in a terrestrial environment. These functions, which are both integrated and overlapping, are usually classified as either protective, homeostatic or sensing.

The stratum corneum is a 10–20 μm thick non-viable epidermis, consisting of 15 to 25 flattened and stacked cornified cells. Each stratum corneum cell is composed mainly of insoluble bundled keratins (~70 percent) and lipids (~20 percent) encased in a cell envelope. The intercellular region consists mainly of lipids together with desmosomes which provide corneocyte cohesion, as described later. There is continuous desquamation of the outermost layer of the stratum corneum, with a total turnover occurring once every two to three weeks. The most important function of the viable epidermis is the generation of the stratum corneum, which is described in detail below. Other functions include metabolism and the synthesis of melanin from melanocytes for skin pigmentation and sun protection.

The dermis provides support for the epidermis and also plays a role in regulating temperature, pressure and pain. The dermis mainly consists of collagen fibres, which provide the support, and elastic connective tissue, which provides elasticity, in a semi-gel matrix of mucopolysaccharides. The dermis contains an extensive vascular network with many arteriovenous anastomoses which are critical to the functions of heat regulation and blood vessel control.

Epidermal Cell Composition

It is the nature of the stratum corneum, the outermost skin layer, that is responsible for the ability of terrestrial animals to exist in a non-aquatic environment without desiccation. The ability to control both the loss of water and the influx of potentially harmful chemicals and micro-organisms is the result of the evolution of a unique mixture of protein and lipid materials which collectively form this coherent membrane composed of distinct domains. These domains are principally protein, associated with the keratinocytes, and lipid, largely contained within the intercellular spaces.

The cells of the stratum corneum originate in the viable epidermis and undergo many changes before desquamation. Thus, the epidermis consists of several cell strata at varying levels of differentiation. The germinative cells of the epidermis lie in the basal lamina between the dermis and viable epidermis. In this layer, there are other cells such as melanocytes, Langerhans cells and Merkel cells. The cells of the basal lamina are attached to the basement membrane by hemidesmosomes. The cohesiveness of, and communication between, the viable epidermal cells is maintained in a fashion similar to the cell-matrix connection, except that desmosomes replace hemidesmosomes. In the epidermis, the desmosomes are responsible for interconnecting individual cell keratin cytoskeletal structures and thereby create a tissue very resistant to shearing forces.

The Langerhans cells are the prominent antigen-presenting cells of the skin's immune system, and their main function appears to be to pick up contact allergens in the skin and present these agents to T lymphocytes in the skin-draining lymph nodes; that is, they play an important role in contact sensitisation. Melanocytes are a further functional cell type of the epidermal basal layer whose main activity is to produce melanin, which results in pigmentation of the skin. The final type of cell found in the basal layer of the stratum corneum is the Merkel cell. Merkel cells are closely associated with nerve endings, present on the other side of the basement membrane, which suggests they function as sensory receptors of the nervous system.

Differentiation in the Epidermis

Development of the stratum corneum from the keratinocytes of the basal layer involves several steps of cell differentiation which has resulted in a structure based classification of the layers above the basal layer (the stratum basale). Thus the cells progress through the stratum spinosum, the stratum granulosum and, the stratum lucidium to the stratum corneum. Cell turnover, from stratum basale to stratum corneum, is estimated to be about 21 days. The stratum spinosum (prickle cell layer), which lies immediately above the basal layer, consists of several layers of cells which are connected by desmosomes and contain prominent keratin tonofilaments. In the outer cell layers of the stratum spinosum, membrane-coating granules appear, and this reflects the border between this stratum and the overlying stratum granulosum. The most characteristic feature of the stratum granulosum is the presence of many intracellular membrane-coating granules. Within these granules, lamellar subunits arranged in parallel stacks are observed. These are believed to be the precursors of the intercellular lipid lamellae of the stratum corneum (Wertz and Downing 1982). In the outermost layers of the stratum granulosum, the lamellar granules migrate to the cell surface where they fuse and eventually extrude their contents into the intercellular space. At this stage in the differentiation process, the keratinocytes lose their nuclei and other cytoplasmic organelles and become flattened and compacted to form the stratum lucidum, which eventually forms the stratum corneum. The extrusion of the contents of lamellar granules is a fundamental requirement for the formation of the epidermal permeability barrier.

The majority of the protein in the stratum corneum is composed of intracellular keratin filaments which are cross-linked by intermolecular disulphide bridges (Baden 1979). In the terminal stages of differentiation, the keratinocytes contain keratin intermediate filaments together with two other proteins, loricrin and profilaggrin. Loricrin is a major component of the cornified cell envelope, whereas profilaggrin is implicated both in the alignment of the keratin filaments and in epidermal flexibility. The cornified cell envelope of the stratum corneum appears to be composed of a cross-linked protein complex which lies adjacent to the interior surface of the plasma membrane. The cross-linked protein complex of the corneocyte envelope is very insoluble and chemically resistant. The corneocyte protein envelope appears to play an important role in the structural assembly of the intercellular lipid lamellae of the stratum corneum. The work of Downing, Wertz and colleagues (Lazo et al. 1995) has demonstrated that the corneocyte possesses a chemically bound lipid envelope comprised of N-(ω-hydroxyacyl) sphingosines which are covalently linked to glutamate side chains of the envelope protein. This lipid envelop may provide the framework for the generation of the intercellular lipid lamellae, the composition of which is unique in biological systems (Table 14.1). A remarkable feature is the lack of phospholipids and preponderance of cholesterol and ceramides. Overall, the intercellular lipid lamellae appear to be highly structured and very stable and constitute a highly effective barrier to chemical penetration and permeation.

Skin Permeability

The Relationship Between Stratum Corneum Microstructure and Barrier Function—Absorption Pathways

It has been known for some time that the intercellular lipids of the stratum corneum play a very important role in the skin barrier function. This knowledge has been accumulated from systematic studies on skin permeability of compounds of varying lipophilicity (Scheuplein 1965; Roberts et al. 1977; Durrheim et al. 1980; Surber et al. 1993) and investigations of alterations in transepidermal water loss (Elias and Feingold 1992; Aszterbaum et al. 1992). Because the major route of permeation across the stratum corneum is via the intercellular lipid, the rate at which permeation occurs is largely dependent on the physicochemical characteristics of the penetrant, the most important of which is the relative ability to partition into the intercellular lamellae.

Three major variables account for differences in the rate at which different compounds permeate the skin: the concentration of permeant applied, the partition coefficient of the permeant between the stratum corneum lipids and the vehicle and the diffusivity of the compound within the stratum corneum. For a homologous series of chemicals, such as the alkanols, in which lipid/water partition coefficients increase exponentially with increasing alkyl chain length (Flynn and Yalkowski 1972) and for permeation through a lipid membrane of fixed or normalized thickness, the permeability coefficients will directly reflect partitioning

Table 14.1
Composition of human stratum corneum lipids.

Lipid	% (w/w)	mol %
Cholesterol esters	10.0	7.5[a]
Cholesterol	26.9	33.4
Cholesterol sulphate	1.9	2.0
Total cholesterol derivatives	38.8	42.9
Ceramide 1	3.2	1.6
Ceramide 2	8.9	6.6
Ceramide 3	4.9	3.5
Ceramide 4	6.1	4.2
Ceramide 5	5.7	5.0
Ceramide 6	12.3	8.6
Total ceramides	41.1	29.5
Fatty acids	9.1	17.0[a]
Others	11.1	10.6[b]

[a]Based on C16 alkyl chain.
[b]Based on MW of 500.
Source: Wertz and Downing (1989).

tendencies and increase exponentially. This relationship will hold as long as the rate-determining step in crossing the membrane is passage through a lipid region and indicates that, for a pure lipid membrane, a plot of the logarithm of the permeability coefficient versus the alkyl chain length of the permeant will be a straight line. However, as the stratum corneum is not a pure lipid membrane, a plot of the log of the permeability rate versus permeant lipophilicity is sigmoidal (Figure 14.1), which reflects the existence of barriers of a more hydrophilic nature. Relatively polar permeants would preferentially partition into and diffuse through these hydrophilic regions, and there is, therefore, no lipid partitioning dependency in the initial part of the curve. There is a further loss of direct lipid partitioning sensitivity in the mass transfer process at higher permeant lipophilicity (Figure 14.1, region C). This is often attributed to a barrier of hydrophilic nature, known as the aqueous boundary layer, but may also represent a reduction in mobility due to an increase in molecular size. In skin, the most obvious hydrophilic boundary layer is the viable epidermis (the layers between the stratum granulosum and stratum basale). Overall, compounds with partition coefficients which indicate an ability to dissolve in both oil and water (i.e., log P of 1–3) permeate the skin relatively rapidly.

Physicochemistry of Skin Permeation

There are three basic steps in the process of percutaneous absorption, and the first two are governed by the physicochemical properties of the permeating molecule. Initially the permeant has to escape from the vehicle and penetrate into the stratum corneum (step 1), which is largely a function of partition and solubility characteristics. Diffusion across the stratum

Figure 14.1 Effect of permeant lipophilicity on the rate of skin permeation. Average permeability coefficient data for aqueous alcohol solutions through human stratum corneum as a function of alcohol chain length (data from Scheuplein and Blank 1973). Note: the y-axis is a log scale.

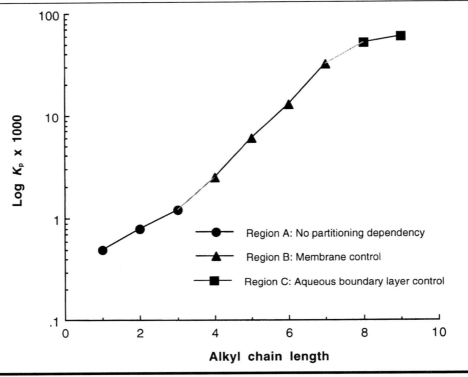

corneum (step 2) is related to binding characteristics and, to a lesser extent, molecular size of the diffusing molecule. On the other hand, clearance from the epidermis/dermis (step 3) is governed mainly by physiological factors such as blood flow.

The most important factor in step 1 is the ability to partition from the application vehicle into the intercellular lamellae of the stratum corneum. The partition coefficient (K) of a drug between the skin and vehicle can be written as C_{sc}/C_v, where C_v is the concentration of drug in the vehicle. Thus, the steady-state flux (J_S) across the skin can be expressed as:

$$J_s = \frac{ADKC_v}{h} \tag{1}$$

In this equation, A is the area of application, D is the apparent diffusion coefficient and h is the diffusional path length (often taken as the thickness of the membrane). The permeability coefficient (k_p) is the steady-state flux per unit area divided by the concentration of drug applied in solution and may be calculated from:

$$k_p = \frac{J_s}{AC_v} = K\left(\frac{D}{h}\right) \tag{2}$$

In the consideration of therapeutic activity following dermal application, emphasis is placed on quantifying the extent of absorption of a drug through the skin or some relevant pharmacodynamic response. The amount absorbed (Q) may be expressed in terms of the area of application and the exposure time (T). The amount absorbed will be determined by the permeability coefficient of the drug, the diffusional lag time across the barrier (*lag*) and the concentration of the drug in the vehicle:

$$Q = k_p AC_v(T - lag) \tag{3}$$

In reality, the overall amount absorbed should simply be $k_p AC_v T$. Equation 3 is based on steady-state conditions and assumes that there is no appreciable accumulation of the drug on the distal side of the barrier or depletion of the drug on the application side.

It is evident, therefore, that a number of principles apply in dermal absorption. These include the fact that the amount of a drug absorbed will depend on the area of application, the concentration applied, the duration of application and the permeability coefficient, which, as shown above, is defined by the physicochemical properties of the solute and the vehicle.

Permeability Coefficients and Diffusivity

In order to understand more fully the role of drug structure and applied vehicle on the amount of drug absorbed through the skin, the steady-state flux J_s of the drug across the stratum corneum barrier may be deconvoluted into its fundamental components of drug diffusivity (D), the path length for diffusion (h) and the concentrations of drug immediately below the outside $C_{sc(o)}$ and the inside $C_{sc(i)}$ of the stratum corneum.

$$J_s = \frac{Q}{(T - lag)} = \frac{DA}{h}\left(C_{sc(o)} - C_{sc(i)}\right) \tag{4}$$

If the drug stratum corneum/product partition coefficient K is defined as $C_{sc(o)}/C_v$, $C_{sc(i)}$ is assumed to be much less than $C_{sc(o)}$, and the permeability coefficient (k_p) is KD/h, equation 4 is equivalent to equation 3. The lag time is normally defined by Fick's law as $h^2/6D$. The importance of equation 4 is well illustrated by the work of Rougier and Lotte (1993) in which it was shown that the *in vivo* percutaneous absorption ($= J_s$) of a series of compounds was directly related to their concentration in stripped stratum corneum, irrespective of their structure, concentration or site of application. In theory, drug transport could go via a polar pathway, with a permeability coefficient $k_{p,polar}$, as well as through the intercellular lipid pathway, with a permeability coefficient $k_{p,lipid}$, although the existence of a polar pathway remains controversial. As indicated previously, for lipophilic drugs, an aqueous boundary layer is likely to be present at the stratum corneum-viable epidermis interface with a $k_{p,aqueous}$. Thus

$$k_p = \left(\frac{1}{k_{p,lipid} + k_{p,polar}} + \frac{1}{k_{p,aqueous}}\right)^{-1} \tag{5}$$

For most drugs, $k_{p,\text{lipid}} \gg k_{p,\text{polar}}$ and $k_{p,\text{lipid}} \ll k_{p,\text{aqueous}}$ so that $k_p \sim k_{p,\text{lipid}}$ and hence drug lipophilicity favours skin permeability. The model proposed by Kasting and his colleagues (Kasting et al. 1992) advocated two main determinants for $k_{p,\text{lipid}}$: lipophilicity, as defined by the logarithm of the octanol-water partition coefficient $\log K_{\text{oct}}$ and molecular size, as defined by molecular weight MW:

$$\log k_{p,\text{lipid}} = \log K_{\text{oct}} - \left(\frac{0.018}{2.303}\right) MW - 2.87 \tag{6}$$

Substitution of equation 6 into equation 5, together with the expressions for $k_{p,\text{polar}}$ and $k_{p,\text{aqueous}}$ as a function of MW, provides a simple model for predictions of k_p in terms of octanol-water partition coefficients and MW. An expression similar to equation 6 was also developed by Potts and Guy (1992):

$$\log k_p = 0.711 \log K_{\text{oct}} - 0.0061 MW - 2.72 \tag{7}$$

Of particular interest in pharmaceutical delivery is the maximum flux J_{max} attainable for a selected drug. Assuming that the maximal concentration of drug possible in the stratum corneum is defined by the solubility of the drug in the stratum corneum lipids S_{sc} and that sink conditions apply, equation 4 can be re-expressed in the form:

$$J_{\text{max}} = \frac{DA}{h} S_{sc} \tag{8}$$

Thus, when the lipid pathway predominates, as defined by equation 6, J_{max} is defined by the maximum solubility of the drug in octanol S_{oct} and the MW. Therefore, applying the Kasting et al. (1992) equation:

$$\log J_{\text{max}} = \log S_{\text{oct}} - \left(\frac{0.018}{2.303}\right) MW - 2.87 \tag{9}$$

or applying the Potts and Guy (1992) equation:

$$\log J_{\text{max}} = 0.71 \log S_{\text{oct}} - 0.0061 MW - 2.72 \tag{10}$$

Interrelating equations 9 and 10 with equation 8 suggests that the highest maximal flux in any series of drugs will correlate with the highest possible S_{sc}, as characterized by S_{oct} and the most rapid D corresponding to the smallest drug (lowest MW). The observation that the maximum flux is related to S_{sc} would suggest that a drug substantially more polar, or substantially more lipophilic, than stratum corneum will have a lower maximal flux than a drug with a polarity in the vicinity of octanol. Since octanol has a $\log K_{\text{oct}}$ of 3.15 (Leo et al. 1971), equations 9 and 10 predict maximum flux for any series of drugs at $\log K_{\text{oct}}$ 3.15 and 2.23, respectively (see Figure 14.2, where the data are consistent with a parabolic dependency on lipophilicity with a peak in the vicinity of K_{oct} 2.23 to 3.15). However, it should be noted that the above analysis is confined to data generated for a limited number of compounds which had similar hydrogen-bonding capacity and molecular size.

Figure 14.2 Skin flux, absorption or pharmacodynamic activity as a function of permeant lipophilicity. A: Phenols (Hinz et al. 1991); B: Salicylates (○) and other NSAIDs (●) (Yano et al. 1986); C: Hydrocortisone-21-esters (Flynn 1996).

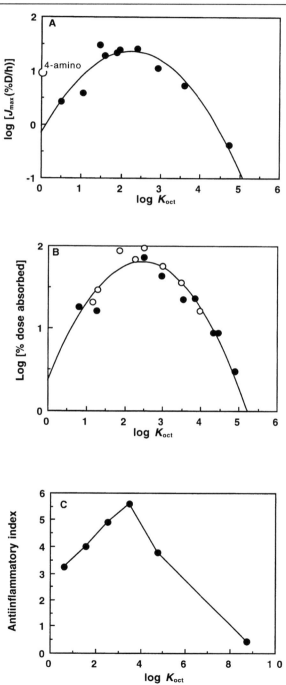

Epidermal Reservoir, Binding and Molecular Size

Equation 4 also suggests that a significant accumulation of drug at the inner surface of the stratum corneum will reduce flux. It is likely that, for most lipophilic drugs, an epidermal reservoir will exist after application for one of two reasons: (1) there is a substantial lag time for the drug to diffuse through the skin (equation 1) and/or (2) the epidermis and dermis do not act as an efficient sink. Historical evidence of reservoir formation is illustrated by the work of Vickers (1963) in which steroid induced vasoconstriction was observed by occluding an area of skin 2 weeks following a single topical application of the drug. Furthermore, the permeability coefficients for a series of phenols, alcohols and steroids was found to be inversely related to the number of hydrogen-bonding groups present (Roberts 1976). It has been shown that, after allowing for molecular size and partitioning into the stratum corneum, the permeability coefficient is related to the number of H-bonding groups in the permeant. Further information on H-binding effects may be found in Pugh et al. (1998).

Another factor potentially limiting diffusion across the stratum corneum is the molecular size of the permeant although, as indicated in equations 6 and 7, molecular size, expressed as MW, appears to have little effect on the diffusion process. It should be noted, however, that these equations were derived from limited data sets (in which MW varied only from 18--~700). It is possible that the diffusion of larger molecules (e.g., polymeric materials) across the stratum corneum will be limited by their molecular size.

The complexity and selectivity of the processes which may be determinants of permeation is well illustrated by the demonstration of differential permeation of isomeric drugs. The mechanisms and significance of this selectivity have been reviewed (Heard and Brain 1995).

Vehicle (Formulation) Thermodynamic Effects

The flux of a drug through the skin is not only dependent on the physicochemical nature of the permeant but also on the nature of the formulation and the vehicle composition. A formulation may alter the properties of the skin and hence enhance or retard the permeation of a drug by increasing or decreasing its diffusivity and/or solubility within the stratum corneum. In the theoretical analysis above, most emphasis was placed on the description of drug absorption from dilute aqueous solution. The historical data, shown in Figure 14.3, illustrate that, whereas the permeability coefficient of alcohols increased with chain length from an aqueous vehicle, the permeability coefficient decreased with chain length when applied in lipophilic vehicles (olive oil and isopropyl palmitate). Similarly, the permeability coefficients for a number of phenolic compounds were reported to increase with lipophilicity for aqueous solutions but decrease with increasing lipophilicity for ethanol and arachis (peanut) oil formulations (Roberts 1991).

Maximal flux has been traditionally defined to be from saturated solutions. However, it is now known that an even higher flux can be achieved using a supersaturated solution (Davis and Hadgraft 1993). Equation 1 is a simplification of the exact physicochemical parameters which control flux. More precisely, the driving force for diffusion is not the concentration but the chemical potential gradient. Higuchi was the first to apply this more rigorous solution (equation 11) to the process of percutaneous penetration (Higuchi 1960).

$$J = \frac{Da}{h(\gamma_{sc})} \tag{11}$$

Figure 14.3 Effect of application vehicle on alcohol (expressed in terms of number of carbons present) permeability coefficients through human skin. The vehicles used were saline (○), isopropyl palmitate (●) and olive oil (▲) (adapted from Blank 1964).

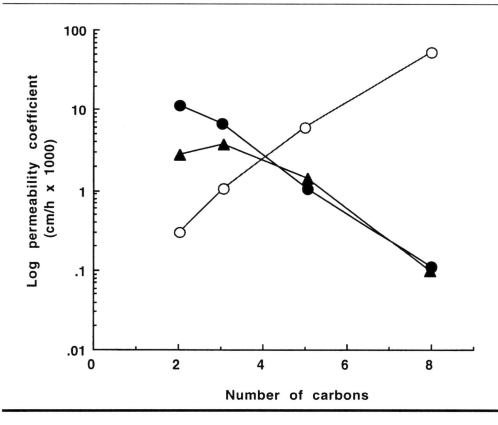

where a is the thermodynamic activity of the permeant in the vehicle (and, assuming equilibrium, also in the outer layer of the stratum corneum) and γ_{sc} is the permeant activity coefficient in the stratum corneum (a/γ_{sc} is equivalent to $C_{sc(o)}$). From this, Higuchi predicted that supersaturation of a drug in a vehicle would increase its percutaneous absorption. The effect may be described as an increase in "push" of the permeant into the stratum corneum. Supersaturation causes an increase in permeant solubility in the stratum corneum beyond and independent of saturated solubility. From this, vehicle systems affecting $C_{sc(o)}$ and/or D and supersaturated vehicle systems, affecting $C_{sc(o)}$, should work independently (and possibly in synergy) and may be capable of multiplicative increases in penetration.

Megrab et al. (1995) measured the uptake of estradiol into stratum corneum from saturated and supersaturated solutions in various propylene glycol-water vehicles. As propylene glycol content in saturated solutions increased, so did uptake of estradiol. As degree of supersaturation increased, so also did the uptake ratio. In addition, the flux of estradiol across the epidermal membranes was linearly proportional to the degree of supersaturation for up to approximately 12-fold saturation systems. Pellett et al. (1997) demonstrated that application of supersaturated solutions of piroxicam to human skin gave rise to proportionally higher drug levels in tape-stripped stratum corneum and viable epidermal/dermal compartments.

Removal from the Epidermis

The clearance of a drug from the epidermis is an important determinant of dermal absorption and can influence therapeutic activity in both dermatological and transdermal therapy. The steady-state ratio of the concentrations of drug in the epidermis ($C_{epidermis}$) and in the applied vehicle ($C_{vehicle}$) may be related (Roberts 1991) as:

$$\frac{C_{epidermis}}{C_{vehicle}} = \frac{k_p}{k_p + CL^*_{dermis}} \tag{12}$$

where k_p is the permeability coefficient of the drug and CL^*_{dermis} is the clearance into the dermis per unit area of application. Equation 12 shows that the epidermal concentration $C_{epidermis}$ depends upon the relative magnitude of dermal clearance, which is determined mainly by blood flow, and the permeability coefficient k_p. Situations which enable k_p to be of a similar order of magnitude to clearance, such as disruption of the barrier or vasoconstriction, will enable blood flow to play a greater role in determining topical absorption. When blood flow is much higher than k_p, epidermal clearance will be the determinant of epidermal concentration. In this situation, equation 12 reduces to:

$$\frac{C_{epidermis}}{C_{vehicle}} = \frac{k_p}{CL^*_{dermis}} \tag{13}$$

There is evidence of altered topical absorption due to changing blood flow as a consequence of elevated temperature or exercise or co-administration of vasoactive drugs (Rogers and Riviere 1994; Singh and Roberts 1994).

Prediction of Skin Permeation

In an ideal world, a large body of historical absorption data would allow a reasonably accurate prediction of the behaviour of a new drug based on previous experimental observations. However, after several decades of research and data accumulation, it is still only possible to make a rather limited approximation of the magnitude of the percutaneous absorption of a new drug from the permeability coefficient predicted using physicochemical properties (as described above). From this approximation, it is further necessary to approximate the potential total absorption for a given application regimen.

Many of the models are based on experiments in which permeants were applied in aqueous solution and, therefore, their value in prediction of permeation from actual formulations applied under in-use conditions is compromised. For example, whilst the predicted K_p for nitrosodiethanolamine is 1.5×10^{-4} cm/h, the experimentally determined value from isopropyl myristate (IPM) was 3.5×10^{-3} cm/h (Franz et al. 1993). The predicted value for octyl salicylate is 1.35×10^{-7} cm/h, whilst the experimental values from a hydroalcoholic lotion were 4.7×10^{-6} cm/h (infinite dose) and 6.6×10^{-7} cm/h (finite dose) and from an oil-in-water emulsion 1.7×10^{-5} cm/h (infinite dose) and 6.6×10^{-7} cm/h (finite dose) (Walters et al. 1997a). The discrepancy between predicted and experimental skin permeation values for methyldodecyl nitrosamine was highly relevant to toxicological considerations of inadvertent exposure, as the predicted value of 12.6×10^{-2} cm/h is four orders of magnitude greater than experimentally determined values 9.0×10^{-6} cm/h (IPM solution) and 4.2×10^{-6} cm/h (oil-in-water emulsion vehicle) (Walters et al. 1997b).

Despite all their limitations, such predictions of skin permeability may be valuable and have several important potential uses. Ranking of drugs in order of potential dermal penetration is probably the most valuable use in the pharmaceutical field. For example, in situations where it is necessary to predict the dermal penetration potential for a series of homologous or closely related drugs, it is possible to rank the compounds using theoretical calculations. However, in order to validate the calculated values, it is essential to experimentally determine the skin permeation properties of several representative compounds of the group in a relevant vehicle.

It is important to appreciate that predictive estimates are of limited value even when the estimates and assumptions within the model are rigorous. Many variables associated with actual product use will significantly alter the extent of skin penetration. For example, reapplication of a formulation, drug release from a formulation and the presence of "inactive" excipients may all affect skin permeability. If these complicating parameters could be factored into the overall calculations, then the predictive values could perhaps provide a closer approximation to the actual skin permeability under "in-use" conditions.

Biological Factors Affecting Percutaneous Absorption

Anatomical Site Variations

Feldman and Maibach (1967) found that the permeation of hydrocortisone decreased in the following order: scrotum > jaw > forehead > scalp > back > forearm > palm (Figure 14.4), and Roberts et al. (1982) found the abdomen was more permeable to methyl salicylate than the arms or feet. Perhaps the clearest data available on variation in skin permeability deal with anatomical site-to-site variation. Site-to-site variation of skin permeability was examined using the tape stripping method (Rougier 1987b) and correlated with corneocyte diameter (Rougier 1991) and hence diffusional path length. Although skin permeation of compounds may follow a different pattern in different skin regions, it is generally agreed that some body sites (the head and genital region) are uniformly more permeable than others (extremities).

Intrasubject and Intersubject Variability

The degree and nature of the distribution patterns of skin permeabilities was addressed to some extent by Southwell et al. (1984) who investigated both *in vitro* and *in vivo* variation in the permeability of human skin between different individuals (interspecimen) and the same individuals (intraspecimen). Based on permeation characteristics for a series of compounds, they concluded that *in vitro* interspecimen variation was 66 ± 25 percent and intraspecimen variation 43 ± 25 percent. The pattern *in vivo* was similar, although the overall level of variation was somewhat smaller. This analysis has been extended by assessing the statistical distribution of human skin permeabilities. Williams et al. (1992) examined the permeation of 5-fluorouracil and estradiol through human abdominal skin. Here, where the possibility of

Figure 14.4 Regional variation in the absorption of hydrocortisone through human skin *in vivo*. Absorption was normalized to that through ventral forearm. Hydrocortisone was applied in acetone to a marked site (redrawn from Feldman and Maibach 1967).

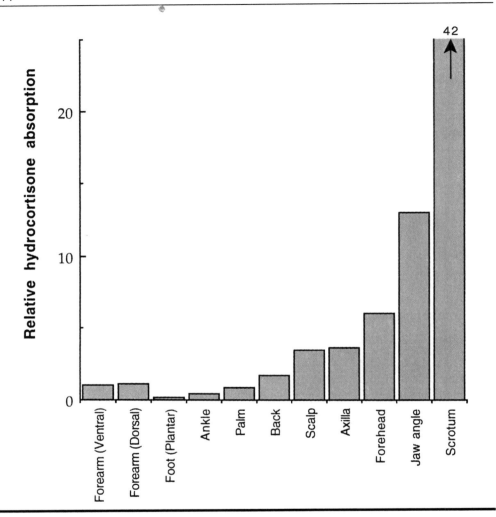

site variability was excluded, the data were log-normally distributed. A log-normal distribution implies that the use of normal Gaussian statistics is inappropriate, and that use of geometric (rather than arithmetic) means should be considered.

Sex and Age Variability

The questions of how age and sex affect the permeability of human skin have been rather poorly addressed to date. Some studies have concluded that, *in vitro* in man, there was no discernible dependence of skin permeability on age, sex or storage conditions (Harrison et al.

1984; Marzulli and Maibach 1984; Bronaugh et al. 1986). The literature on the effect of age and sex on percutaneous absorption in other species, where more data are available, is confused. For example, it was reported (Banks et al. 1990) that the dermal absorption of certain marker compounds was lower in older rats but that, for different compounds, the reverse was the case (Hall et al. 1992) or indeed that age did not influence dermal absorption in rats (Dick and Scott 1992). Skin permeation in the hairless mouse generally increases with age, corresponding to the single hair cycle, but decreases with a return to the hairless state (Behl et al. 1984a,b).

The effect of age on percutaneous absorption has been examined *in vivo* in man with variable results. It was postulated (Roskos et al. 1989) that reduced hydration levels and lipid content of older skin may be responsible for a demonstrated reduction in skin permeability where the permeants were hydrophilic in nature (no reduction was seen for model hydrophobic compounds) (Table 14.2). The reduced absorption of benzoic acid demonstrated in the elderly (Rougier 1991) was in line with this suggestion, but not the reduction in absorption of testosterone (lipophilic) (Roskos et al. 1986), or lack of change in the absorption of methyl nicotinate (more hydrophilic) with age (Guy et al. 1983). There are a number of potential physiological changes which may be responsible for age-related alterations, including an increase in the size of individual stratum corneum corneocytes, increased dehydration of the outer layers of the stratum corneum with age, decreased epidermal turnover and decreased microvascular clearance (reviewed in Roskos and Maibach 1992). The issue of age-related variability, however, is far from resolved.

Racial Differences

Caucasian skin has been reported to be slightly more permeable than black skin (Corcuff et al. 1991; Kompaore and Tsuruta 1993; Leopold and Maibach 1996) which correlates with observations that black skin has both more cell layers within the stratum corneum (Weigand et al. 1974) and a higher lipid content (Rienertson and Wheatley 1959). More recently, Lotte et

Table 14.2
Age-related differences in percutaneous absorption.

Permeant	log K^{*a}	% Applied Dose Permeated over 7 Days[b]	
		22–40 years	>65 years
Testosterone	3.32	19.0 ± 4.4	16.6 ± 2.5
Estradiol	2.49	7.1 ± 1.1	5.4 ± 0.4
Hydrocortisone	1.61	1.5 ± 0.6	0.54 ± 0.15
Benzoic acid	1.83	36.2 ± 4.6	19.5 ± 1.6
Acetylsalicylic acid	1.26	31.2 ± 7.3	13.6 ± 1.9
Caffeine	0.01	48.2 ± 4.1	25.2 ± 4.8

[a]Octanol/water partition coefficient.
[b]Compounds (4 μg/cm^2) were applied in 20 μL acetone to ventral forearm ($n = 3$–8).
Source: Roskos et al. (1989).

al. (1993) determined the penetration and permeation of benzoic acid, caffeine or acetylsalicylic acid into and through Asian, Black and Caucasian skin and found no statistical differences between the races (Table 14.3). The equivocal findings in this area highlight the necessity for further systematic research.

Skin Metabolism

It is widely established that there is potential for biotransformation of molecules within the skin (Bronaugh et al. 1989; Noonan and Wester 1989; Sharma 1996; Merk et al. 1996; Hotchkiss 1998), but the nature of skin enzymes differs quantitatively and qualitatively from those in the liver. In general, the activities of many metabolic processes are much lower in skin than in liver, although certain enzymes, such as N-acetyltransferases and those involved in reductive processes, have demonstrated fairly high activity (Table 14.4).

The majority of metabolic work on skin has employed epidermal homogenates or cell cultures, which are useful for the study of enzyme activity per se, but have little predictive value for the *in vivo* situation where drugs may not contact cellular systems during permeation. A more useful *in vitro* model uses metabolically active fresh skin mounted in a diffusion cell under conditions which maintain viability. For example this technique has been used to investigate *in vitro* permeation and metabolism of several compounds such as estradiol and testosterone (Collier et al. 1989).

Enhancement and Retardation of Skin Absorption

Because of the very extensive barrier properties of the stratum corneum, it is often necessary to increase the intrinsic rate of dermal or transdermal drug delivery to achieve the required therapeutic drug levels. In these instances, skin penetration and permeation enhancement

Table 14.3
Race-related differences in percutaneous absorption.

| Permeant | Race | Amount of Permeant Recovered (nmol/cm^2) | |
		Urine at 24 h	Stratum Corneum at 30 min[a]
Benzoic acid	Caucasian	9.0 ± 1.5	6.8 ± 1.0
	Black	6.4 ± 0.9	6.1 ± 1.0
	Asian	9.7 ± 1.2	8.1 ± 1.5
Caffeine	Caucasian	5.9 ± 0.6	5.5 ± 0.6
	Black	4.5 ± 1.0	5.8 ± 1.0
	Asian	5.2 ± 0.8	6.1 ± 0.9
Acetylsalicylic acid	Caucasian	6.2 ± 1.9	11.9 ± 1.9
	Black	4.7 ± 0.9	9.0 ± 1.7
	Asian	5.4 ± 1.7	10.1 ± 1.7

[a]Amount in stratum corneum determined by tape-stripping ($n = 6$–9).
Source: Lotte et al. (1993).

Table 14.4
Comparison between specific activities of cutaneous enzymes
compared with hepatic enzymes.

Enzyme System	Substrate	Cutaneous Specific Activity (% hepatic)
Cytochrome P450s	Aldrin	0.4–2.0
	Aminopyrine	1.0
	Diphenyloxazole	2.0–3.0
	Ethylmorphine	0.5
	7-Pentoxyresorufin	20–27
Epoxide hydrolases	*cis*-Stilbene oxide	9–11
	trans-Stilbene oxide	24–25
	Styrene oxide	6.0
Glutathione transferases	*cis*-Stilbene oxide	49
	Styrene oxide	14
Glucuronosyl transferases	Bilirubin	3.0
	1-Naphthol	2–50
Sulfotransferases	1-Naphthol	10
Acetyltransferases	*p*-Aminobenzoic acid	18
	2-Aminofluorene	15

Source: Hotchkiss (1998).

strategies must be evaluated. The therapeutic target may be the skin, the local subcutaneous tissues or the microvasculature, depending on the requirement for local, regional or systemic therapy. In some cases, for example, the use of sunscreen agents, insect repellents and drugs whose therapeutic target is the epidermis, skin permeation retardation would be an attractive option from a toxicological standpoint. Both enhancement and retardation of skin permeation can be achieved using either particular formulation strategies or the co-application of specific chemicals designed to modify stratum corneum barrier function. Other chemical and physical mechanisms for enhancement, including prodrugs with more suitable physicochemical properties, liposomes, iontophoresis, electroporation and ultrasound, have been fully reviewed elsewhere (Walters and Hadgraft 1993; Smith and Maibach 1995; Korting 1996; Prausnitz 1996) and will not be discussed here.

Formulation Strategies

As discussed earlier, it is well established that a principle driving force for diffusion across the skin is the thermodynamic activity of the permeant in the donor vehicle. This activity is reflected by the concentration of the permeant in the donor vehicle as a function of its saturation solubility within that medium. The closer to saturation concentration, the higher is the thermodynamic activity and the greater is the escaping tendency of the permeant from the vehicle. This principle has been extensively and successfully utilized in pharmaceutical formulations in attempts to enhance percutaneous absorption of drugs (Davis and Hadgraft 1993; Pellett et al. 1997). Supersaturated systems can be created using a binary mixture in which one component is a good solvent for the solute and the other component is a non-solvent. Slow addition of the non-solvent to the solvent (both presaturated with solute) creates a supersaturated solution. Because of the high potential for crystal growth in these systems, it is necessary to add an appropriate antinucleant polymer such as hydroxypropylmethyl cellulose.

Supersaturated transdermal delivery devices have also been described, although, in these cases, stability considerations limit the degree to which the systems can be supersaturated. Supersaturated systems containing nitroglycerine or isosorbide dinitrate have been formed in polymer films. Jenkins (1992) described the development of saturated and supersaturated transdermal drug-in-adhesive systems and demonstrated their use with norethisterone and estradiol. In the preparation of these systems, the active agent was dissolved in a mixture of solvents, at least one of which had a boiling point above that of the solvent used as a vehicle for the adhesive. The degree of saturation or supersaturation was dictated by the selected solvent mix and, because there are a large number of suitable solvents, the system is suitable for a wide range of drugs. Also embodied in the patent application is the suggestion that at least one of the remaining solvents may act as a skin permeation enhancer, and in this respect propylene glycol-diethyltoluamide and *n*-methyl-pyrrolidone-diethyltoluamide are included in the preferred solvent systems. It would be interesting to evaluate the potential for development of systems in which both the drug and the permeation enhancer were in the supersaturated state.

Penetration Enhancers

Chemical penetration and permeation enhancers comprise a diverse group of compounds including water, organic solvents, phospholipids, simple alkyl esters, long-chain alkyl esters, fatty acids, urea and its derivatives and pyrrolidones (for reviews, see Walters and Hadgraft 1993; Smith and Maibach 1995). In some cases molecules with specific potential as skin penetration enhancers have been designed and synthesised. Of the latter, 2-*n*-nonyl-1,3-dioxolane (SEPA®, Gyurik et al. 1996; Gauthier et al. 1998), 1-dodecylazacycloheptan-2-one (Azone®, Hadgraft et al. 1993), 1-[2-(decylthio)ethyl]azacyclopentan-2-one (HPE-101, Yano et al. 1992), 4-decyloxazolidin-2-one (Dermac™ SR-38, Rajadhyaksha 1990) and dodecyl-N,N-dimethylamino isopropionate (NexACT 88, Büyüktimkin et al. 1993) have all been shown to possess enhancing properties on the skin penetration and permeation of a variety of permeants. Hoogstraate et al. (1991) demonstrated that several linear alkyl chain analogues of Azone were less effective in enhancing the human skin penetration rate of desglycinamide arginine vasopressin than the parent molecule (Figure 14.5). Many derivatives of Azone have been synthesised and evaluated for skin penetration enhancement activity (Phillips and Michniak 1996).

Although Azone has been shown to be a useful skin penetration enhancer for many compounds, it does not appear to be appropriate in all cases. For example, Baker and Hadgraft (1995) evaluated the effectiveness of Azone in vehicles containing the antiviral agent Arildone and found that penetration through human skin was not increased above levels found with a propylene glycol vehicle. Azone enhancement activity is believed to occur in the stratum corneum intercellular lipid lamellae. Since a similar mechanism of action is proposed for a number of related compounds, it follows that the skin permeation of highly lipophilic compounds would also not be expected to be enhanced using these compounds alone.

Figure 14.5 Influence of Azone and analogues on the permeation rate (expressed as the permeability coefficient) of 9-desglycin-amide-8-arginine vasopressin through human stratum corneum *in vitro* (data from Hoogstraate et al. 1991).

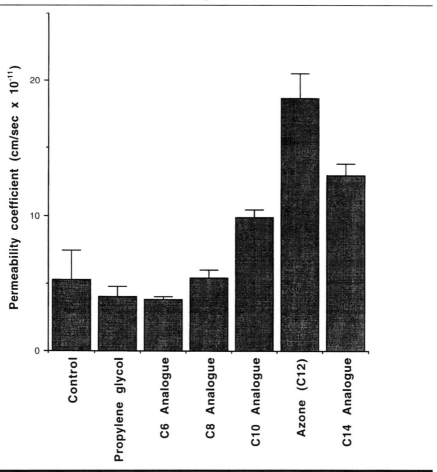

On the other hand, SEPA (2-*n*-nonyl-1,3-dioxolane) has been shown to be a more versatile penetration enhancer in terms of its ease of formulation, chemical stability and its ability to enhance the skin penetration of a wide variety of compounds of varying physicochemical characteristics. Permeants that have been evaluated include indomethacin, ibuprofen, minoxidil, acyclovir, caffeine, econazole, papaverine, progesterone and estradiol. The degree of skin penetration enhancement using SEPA is dependent on the physicochemical characteristics of the permeant. For example, following application of indomethacin in a simple ethanol-propylene glycol vehicle to human skin *in vitro*, cumulative absorption over 24 h amounted to 0.7 percent of the applied dose. The addition of 2 percent SEPA to the vehicle increased the 24 h absorption value to 23 percent of the applied dose (Marty et al. 1989). Furthermore, in comparative studies between SEPA and Azone, SEPA was shown to be a more effective human skin permeation enhancer for indomethacin (Figure 14.6, Marty et al. 1989).

Figure 14.6 Influence of the penetration enhancers SEPA and Azone on the permeation of indomethacin through human skin *in vitro*. The permeant and enhancers were applied in a hydroalcoholic solution (data courtesy of Dr C. M. Samour).

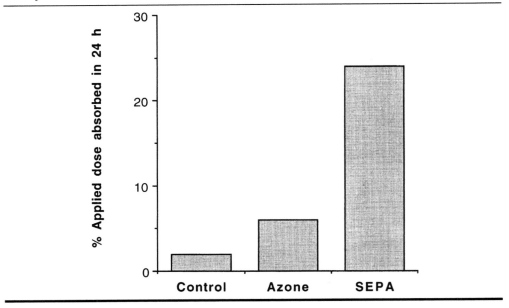

SEPA has been shown to enhance the penetration of econazole into human skin *in vitro* (Gyurik et al. 1995). Levels of econazole, in both the epidermis (stratum corneum and viable epidermis) and dermis, were significantly increased when SEPA was incorporated into gel vehicles at 5 percent and 10 percent. Following application of econazole in a 5 percent SEPA gel, approximately 12 percent of the applied dose was recovered from the epidermis following 24 h exposure. Interestingly, the 5 percent SEPA gel was more effective than the 10 percent SEPA gel, suggesting a concentration dependency in SEPA activity (Figure 14.7). The concentration dependency may be the result of a saturable phenomenon within the skin or a decrease in the thermodynamic activity of econazole in the SEPA gels as a consequence of increased solubility of the permeant in the vehicle.

DRUG CANDIDATE SELECTION AND PREFORMULATION

Drug Candidate Selection

While it may appear to be a simple task, based on therapeutic rationale and compound safety/efficacy, to select lead compounds for pharmaceutical product development, the practicality of this procedure is somewhat more complex. For the most part, therapeutic efficacy is dependent on the ability of the compound to cross biological barriers to reach the target site. However, as pointed out and excellently reviewed by Flynn (1996), in topical therapy it is more appropriate, in many instances, to select compounds based on their inability to cross relevant

Figure 14.7 Influence of SEPA on the *in vitro* human skin uptake of econazole. The permeant and enhancer were applied in a hydroalcoholic gel and the skin content assessed following 24 h exposure (data from Gyurik et al. 1996).

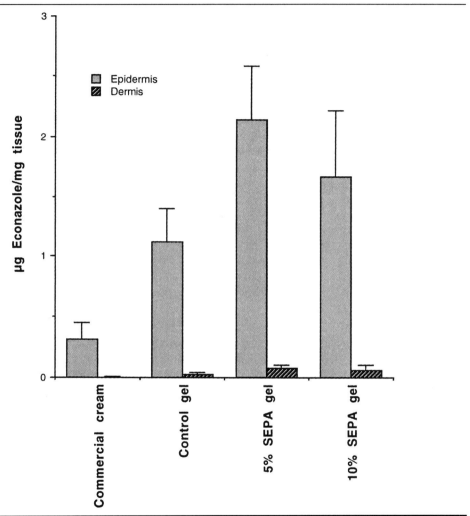

biological barriers. Since the site of action may be the skin surface, the stratum corneum, the viable epidermis, the appendages, the dermis or, the local subcutaneous tissues that may require systemic distribution, the rules of candidate selection will vary. For the purposes of this discussion, it will be assumed that the therapeutic rationale for dermal or transdermal drug delivery has been established, and that a series of compounds with appropriate pharmacological activity has been identified. It will also be assumed that each compound within the series possesses equivalent chemical and physical stability. In other words, drug candidate selection need only be made on the basis of the ability to deliver the compound to its site of action.

In the section "Skin Permeability," the physicochemical determinants of the ability of a compound to permeate the skin were addressed. It was shown that the primary requirement for a compound to penetrate into the skin was the ability to leave the delivery vehicle and diffuse into the stratum corneum. This characteristic has been shown to be dependent on the compound's stratum corneum-vehicle partition coefficient, for which the octanol-water partition coefficient is often used as a surrogate. What is immediately apparent is that a high value for this parameter will favour delivery of the drug into the stratum corneum, but it will not favour diffusion to the more hydrophilic regions of the viable epidermis. Furthermore, the rate of diffusion though the stratum corneum and lower layers of the skin is linked to the molecular volume of the permeant. From this, it is evident that a compound with a high octanol-water partition coefficient and a relatively high molecular volume will possess a high affinity for the stratum corneum (i.e., be substantive to the stratum corneum). This principle is used extensively in the design of sunscreen agents, where it is not uncommon to add a medium length or branched alkyl chain to the ultraviolet (UV) reflective molecule to increase residence time in the skin.

At the other end of the spectrum, however, in transdermal systemic delivery, the molecular attributes required are rather different. In this case, compounds are required to partition into the relatively lipophilic stratum corneum, diffuse rapidly across the stratum corneum and partition easily into the more hydrophilic viable epidermis and dermis prior to vascular removal. The intrinsic requirements of compounds for transdermal delivery are, therefore, a medium polarity (a log octanol-water partition coefficient of 1–3), a low molecular volume and a lack of potential to bind to skin components (e.g., via hydrogen bonding).

Preformulation

Preformulation encompasses those studies that should be carried out before the commencement of formulation development. The major goal of the preformulation process is to permit the rational development of stable, safe and efficacious dosage forms and it is mainly concerned with the characterization of the physicochemical properties of the drug substance. At the preformulation stage, the final route of drug administration is usually undecided and, as such, any protocols must be able to cover all required aspects. As with any development programme, progression can be limited by several factors, including

- project objectives,

- priority rating,

- compound availability and

- availability of analytical procedures.

For the purposes of this discussion, we will assume that the project objectives are known, that priority has been established, that there are sufficient amounts of raw materials to carry out the investigations and that initial analytical procedures have been developed. A fundamental point that must be kept in mind throughout the early stages is that for New Chemical Entities (NCEs) the toxicological profile will not normally have been established at the preformulation stage. It is of paramount importance, therefore, to take all due precautions throughout the study. The preformulation study has several distinct phases (in approximate chronological order):

- General description of the compound

- Calorimetry

- Polymorphism

- Hygroscopicity

- Analytical development

- Intrinsic stability

- Solubility and partitioning characteristics

- Drug delivery characteristics

A detailed description of most of the studies that form part of the preformulation stage are given elsewhere in this volume and will not be considered here. In addition, the importance of preformulation studies in the overall development of transdermal drug delivery systems has recently been excellently reviewed and discussed by Roy (1997). The only aspect of preformulation which is specific to and important for dermatological and transdermal formulations that will be discussed in depth in this chapter concerns drug delivery characteristics.

Measurement of Skin Penetration, Distribution and Permeation in Vitro

In dermatological and transdermal drug delivery, there is a need to optimize the delivery of the drug into and through various skin strata to provide maximum therapeutic effect. The requirement for such data, produced under reproducible and reliable conditions, using relevant membranes, has led to an increase in the development and the standardisation of *in vitro* and *in vivo* test procedures. There have been numerous recommendations on *in vitro* and *in vivo* methodologies, and many of these have been collated as guidelines. Perhaps the most widely known of these guidelines was produced following an FDA/AAPS workshop on the performance of *in vitro* skin penetration studies (Skelly et al. 1987). However, more recent publications also contain useful information; for example, see the European Centre for the Validation of Alternative Methods (ECVAM) workshop report on "Methods for Assessing Percutaneous Absorption" (Howes et al. 1996), the documents from the European Centre for Ecotoxicology and Toxicology of Chemicals (ECETOC 1993) and the European Cosmetic Toiletry and Perfumery Association (Diembeck et al. 1999).

In many respects, *in vitro* techniques have advantages over *in vivo* testing. For example, permeation through the skin is measured directly *in vitro* where sampling is carried out immediately below the skin surface. This contrasts with most *in vivo* methods which rely on the measurement of systemic (or at least non-local) levels of permeant. Some form of *in vitro* diffusion cell experiment is, therefore, the most appropriate method for assessment of skin penetration, distribution and permeation in a transdermal or topical drug developmental programme.

The major advantage of *in vitro* investigation is that the experimental conditions can be controlled more precisely, such that the only major variables are the skin and the test material. Although a potential disadvantage is that little information on the metabolism, distribution and effects of blood flow on permeation may be obtained, it has been reported that such procedures were more effective than several other methods for the assessment of differential delivery of hydrocortisone from commercial formulations (Lehman et al. 1996). *In vitro* systems range in complexity from a simple two-compartment "static" diffusion cell (Franz 1975) to multi-jacketed "flow-through" cells (Bronaugh and Stewart 1985a) (Figure 14.8). Construction materials must be inert; glass is most common, although other materials (Walters et al. 1981) are also used. In all cases, excised skin, preferably human, is mounted as a barrier between a donor chamber and a receptor chamber, and the amount of compound permeating from the donor to the receptor side is determined as a function of time. Efficient mixing of the receptor phase (and sometimes the donor phase) is essential, and sample removal should be simple. Neither of these processes should interfere with diffusion of the permeant

Static diffusion cells are usually of the upright ("Franz") or side-by-side type. The main difference in the application of these two static cell types is that side-by-side cells can be used for the measurement of permeation from one stirred solution, through a membrane and into another stirred solution. Upright cells are particularly useful for studying absorption from semi-solid formulations spread on the membrane surface and are optimal for simulating *in vivo* performance. The donor compartments can be capped, to provide occlusive conditions, or left open, according to the objectives of the particular study. Flow-through cells can be useful when the permeant has a very low solubility in the receptor medium, and designs are continuously improving (Tanojo et al. 1997). Sink conditions are maximized as the fluid is continually replaced (Bronaugh 1996). However, the dilution produced by the continuous flow can raise problems with analytical sensitivity, particularly if the permeation is low. Flow-through and static systems have been shown to produce equivalent results (Hughes et al. 1993; Clowes et al. 1994).

To summarise, a well-designed skin diffusion cell should

- be inert,

- be robust and easy to handle,

- allow the use of membranes of different thicknesses,

- provide thorough mixing of the receptor chamber contents,

- ensure intimate contact between membrane and receptor phase,

- be maintainable at constant temperature,

- have precisely calibrated volumes and diffusional areas,

- maintain membrane integrity,

- provide easy sampling and replenishment of receptor phase and

- be available at reasonable cost.

The receptor phase of any diffusion cell should provide an accurate simulation of the *in vivo* permeation conditions. The permeant concentration in the receptor fluid should not exceed ~10 percent of saturation solubility (Skelly et al. 1987), as excessive receptor phase concentration can lead to a decrease in absorption rate and result in an underestimate of bioavailability. The most common receptor fluid is pH 7.4 phosphate-buffered saline (PBS), although if a compound has a water solubility below ~10 μg/mL, then a wholly aqueous receptor phase is unsuitable, and addition of solubilizers becomes necessary (Bronaugh 1985).

Receptor fluids described in the literature range from water alone to isotonic phosphate buffers containing albumin, which increases solubility (Dick et al. 1996). Microbial growth can produce problems due to partitioning of the permeant into, or metabolism of the

Figure 14.8 Basic diffusion cell designs. Static horizontal cells may be jacketed (as in the Franz-type) or unjacketed (and temperature controlled using water bath or heating block). Flow-through cells usually have a small receptor chamber to maximize mixing. Side-by-side cells are used mainly for solution vehicles.

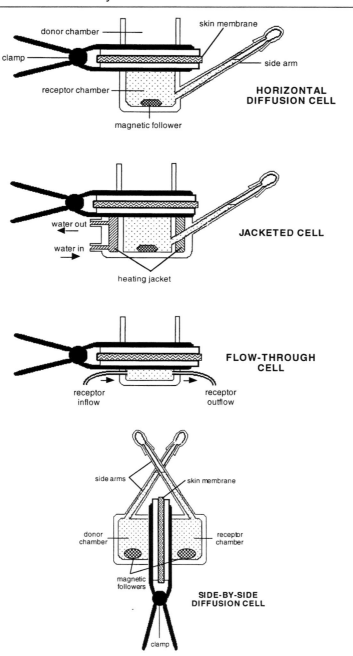

permeant by, the microbes, and preservatives may be required. One particularly useful fluid is 25 percent (v/v) aqueous ethanol, which provides a reasonable "sink" for many permeants, whilst removing the need for other antimicrobial constituents. Other receptor phase modifiers include Volpo N20, rabbit serum, bovine serum albumin, methanol, Triton-X100 and Poloxamer 188 (Bronaugh 1996). Formal protocols for determination of suitability of receptor phases have been proposed (Sclafani et al. 1995). It is important to appreciate that the pH of an aqueous receptor solution may affect the apparent "flux" of a weakly ionizable compound. The pH of the hydrophilic viable epidermal layers may be "altered", and this can result in modulation of the partitioning tendencies of ionizable species (Kou et al. 1993).

It is also important to select an appropriate membrane for use during *in vitro* skin permeation studies. Attempts have been made to model human skin permeation characteristics using artificial membranes and laboratory animal skin. These investigations have been fully discussed elsewhere (Brain et al. 1998). The consensus of opinion is that, whereas animal models may be useful alternatives in the early stages of development, there is no substitute for human skin when definitive values are required. Although the most appropriate scenario would involve experimentation directly on freshly excised surgical skin samples, this is not always practically feasible. In reality, most *in vitro* human skin permeation investigations are carried out on cadaver or surgical specimens which have been frozen prior to experimental use. It is not clear whether the proposed log-normal distribution observed *in vitro* (described in section "Intrasubject and Intersubject Variability") is an experimental artefact due to freezing. Although some authors have concluded that freezing had no measurable effect on permeability (Harrison et al. 1984; Kasting and Bowman 1990), Wester et al. (1998) have cautioned against the use of frozen stored human skin for studies in which cutaneous metabolism may be a contributing factor. It is important to appreciate that the state of hydration of the tissue prior to freezing may influence subsequent permeation characteristics (Fares and Zatz 1997). As a general rule, tissues should not be deliberately hydrated prior to frozen storage.

Several different methods can be used to prepare human skin. The most commonly used membranes are as follows:

-   Full-thickness skin, incorporating the stratum corneum, viable epidermis and dermis

-   Dermatomed skin, in which the lower dermis has been removed to a definite depth

-   Epidermal membranes, comprising the viable epidermis and the stratum corneum (prepared by heat separation)

-   Stratum corneum alone (prepared from epidermal membranes by enzyme treatment)

The most suitable type of membrane is dependent on the nature of the permeant. For example, the relatively aqueous environment of the dermis will inhibit the penetration of lipophilic compounds *in vitro*, whereas *in vivo* this barrier is largely circumvented by the capillary bed. Thus the use of dermatomed, epidermal or stratum corneum membranes is most appropriate for particularly lipophilic permeants. Other considerations may justify the use of epidermal membranes even where the dermis does not present an artificial barrier to a permeant. For example, if a study involves an assessment of the skin content of permeant, it is much easier to extract or solubilize epidermal membranes than full-thickness skin. The disadvantages inherent to the use of epidermal membranes are that preparation is time consuming and that the necessary processing increases the possibility of damage to skin integrity.

For human skin, the separation of the dermis from the epidermis (stratum corneum and viable epidermis) is a relatively simple technique (Scheuplein 1965; Bronaugh et al. 1986). Following removal of the subcutaneous fat, the skin is totally immersed in water at 60°C for ~45 sec. The tissue is then removed from the water, pinned (dermal side down) to a dissecting board and the epidermis gently peeled back using forceps. The epidermal membrane is floated onto warm water, taken onto a support membrane (paper filter or aluminium foil) and air dried before storage in a freezer. To mount previously frozen skin membranes in a diffusion cell, they are thawed and then floated from the support membrane. Isolation of the stratum corneum from the epidermal membrane is achieved by placing the latter into trypsin solution (0.0001 percent), incubating at 37°C for 12 h, rubbing (with a cotton bud) to remove the digested "viable" epidermal cells, rinsing in distilled water and air drying on a surface from which the residual stratum corneum can be easily removed (Boddé et al. 1993).

There are two basic approaches to applying substances to the skin: infinite dose (which involves application of sufficient permeant to make any changes in donor concentration during the experiment negligible) and finite dose (which involves application of a dose that may show marked depletion during an experiment). The infinite dose technique may be useful if the experimental objectives include calculation of diffusional parameters, such as permeability coefficients, or investigation of mechanisms of penetration enhancement. The finite dose technique is normally used for the evaluation of materials in prototype formulations and should be used with a regime that mimics as closely as possible the proposed "in-use" situation (see, e.g., Walters et al. 1997). With finite dosing, the permeation profile usually exhibits a characteristic plateauing effect that is the result of donor depletion (Figure 14.9). There are several published recommendations regarding the amount of formulation which should be applied to correspond with an "in-use" dose level. For example, the FDA/AAPS guidelines (Skelly et al. 1987) suggested a universal application weight of approximately 5 mg/cm^2 of formulation. COLIPA (1993) proposed 5 μL/cm^2 for liquid formulations and 2 mg/cm^2 for semi-solid formulations (or 5 mg/cm^2 if these are being compared to a liquid). Given the high intrasubject and intersubject variability in human skin permeability, a large number of replicates for each dosage regimen is recommended. The most widely quoted recommendation for numbers of replicates in *in vitro* studies on human skin is 12 (Skelly et al. 1987) and donor samples should be distributed throughout the test groups so that comparisons are matched. Skin lipids undergo major phase transitions between 40 and 70°C (Bouwstra et al. 1992), and there is a considerable temperature-dependent modulation of permeation rates, which is probably a manifestation of heat-induced alterations of lipid fluidity. *In vitro* finite dose skin permeation experiments are usually conducted with a constant skin temperature of 32°C. Prior to carrying out *in vitro* experiments, the integrity of each skin sample should be evaluated. This may be a qualitative determination, e.g., by simple visual examination of specimens or, more quantitatively, by measurement of transepidermal water loss or the flux of marker compounds such as tritiated water or sucrose (Hood et al. 1996; Benech-Kieffer et al. 1998; Pendlington et al. 1998). The generally accepted normal permeability coefficient for water diffusion through human skin is $\leq 1.5 \times 10^{-3}$ cm/h, although an upper limit of 2.5×10^{-3} cm/h has also been used (Bronaugh et al. 1986). Samples showing particularly high permeability are often rejected as outliers with questionable integrity, but may actually represent the real population spread if their distribution is indeed log-normal (see earlier discussion).

The ideal sampling and analytical procedures provide accurate assessment of both the quantity and nature of the material present at a given time point, and the sensitivity of the method must be capable of producing data of practical significance. Preliminary prediction from existing data or physicochemical modelling can give "ballpark" estimates of the likely

Figure 14.9 Sample cumulative skin permeation patterns following finite and infinite dosing regimes. With infinite dose, permeation normally reaches a steady-state flux region, from which it is possible to calculate permeability coefficients and diffusional lag times. In finite dosing the permeation profile normally exhibits a plateauing effect as a result of donor depletion.

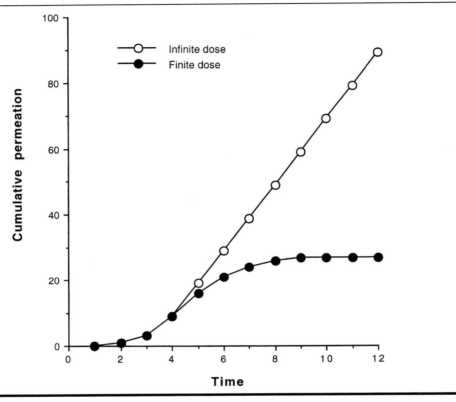

amount of permeant. As replication and multiple time point sampling are common, analysis should not be unnecessarily complex. High performance liquid chromatography (HPLC) is particularly useful, as relatively large (~200 µL) aqueous samples can often be handled without preliminary processing or concentration. Determination of permeants in tissue samples necessitates some form of extraction or solubilization process. When radiolabelled permeants are used, tissue samples are routinely taken up in commercially available solubilisers. Such aggressive products are often not applicable in other cases where more traditional extraction methods are required. Recovery of permeant from stratum corneum tape strips is less demanding and can often be accomplished by vortexing and sonicating with relatively small volumes of appropriate solvent.

A typical *in vitro* permeation experiment will involve analysis of receptor samples at intervals up to 24–72 h. At the termination of the exposure period, the remaining formulation on the skin surface is often removed using a suitable rinsing procedure (which will depend on the nature of the applied formulation). This removed material is analysed to determine the amount of permeant remaining on the skin. The epidermal membranes or skin samples are removed from the diffusion cells, and the stratum corneum may be tape-stripped 15–20 times and the tape strips extracted and analysed for permeant content. Tape-stripping of the stratum corneum is a comparatively new technique which is under evaluation by the U.S. Food and Drug Administration (FDA) as a potential method for determining relative bioavailability of dermatological products. Following the tape-stripping, the remaining epidermal membranes or skin samples may be homogenised, extracted and analysed for permeant content. The results of these studies demonstrate how the developed prototype formulations compare in terms of *in vitro* skin penetration, distribution and permeation. The criteria for determining the preferred formulation using an *in vitro* skin model will depend on the particular circumstances. For example, preferred formulations for dermatological activity may demonstrate rapid uptake of drug into the epidermal layers together with limited transfer of the drug through the skin. On the other hand, preferred vehicles for transdermal systemic delivery will be those demonstrating both rapid penetration into and rapid permeation across the skin.

FORMULATION

In the previous sections, the theoretical aspects of dermatological and transdermal drug delivery, together with some aspects of product preformulation, have been discussed. This section concentrates on the formulation development of dermatological and transdermal products and will take into account several important factors in the development process. In many companies, the first stage of product development is the formation of a Project Team. At the inaugural meeting of this team, it is essential that all members be aware of what is required from both a medical and a marketing point of view. Realistic time schedules should be drawn up with well-defined decision points, and due allowance should be made for the inevitable slippage time.

In the early stages of product development, there is usually a bottleneck in the analytical department. Most companies work on the basis of allowing two analysts per formulator, but this ratio is often inadequate. It is of paramount importance that the analytical department be involved in the early stages of the formulation process. These are the people who will have to analyse the prototype formulations and look for evidence of stability problems as soon as possible. They are, of course, capable and equipped to do this, but time will be saved if they know precisely what materials the formulator is putting into the prototypes. There is no substitute for a fully validated stability indicating assay, but initial "rough" analytical methods can be extremely useful for determining what excipients to avoid and what conditions, such as pH, are critical to the formulation.

Although the medical and marketing departments will have defined targets in terms of disease to be treated, and territories in which the product is to be launched, it is up to the formulator to specify and identify the optimum formulation. Often, however, the formulator is hindered by the fact that, for an NCE, the dose level is unknown and will remain so until a dose ranging study has been carried out. This leads to the unsatisfactory, but unavoidable, situation of the formulator trying to obtain a formulation containing a "hypothetical" maximum dose.

Throughout the development process, it is important to maintain a high level of quality. The application of systematic quality assurance (QA) in the research and development (R&D) portion of topical product development is necessary to facilitate registration and also acts as a safeguard should any problems arise during scale-up and manufacture. The QA/quality control (QC) systems for topical product development are exactly the same as for any new drug development and can be achieved only by the systematic applications of Good Laboratory Practice (GLP), Good Clinical Practice (GCP) and Good Manufacturing Practice (GMP).

Formulation Type

The selection of formulation type for systemic transdermal products, which are designed for application to intact non-diseased skin, is guided by the requirement of the system, be it a semi-solid or patch preparation, to deliver therapeutic amounts of drug into the systemic circulation. On the other hand, the selection of formulation type for dermatological products is influenced more by the nature of the skin lesion. As pointed out by Kitson and Maddin (1998): "It is idle to pretend that the therapy for skin diseases, as currently practiced, has its origins in science". To this day a practicing dermatologist would prefer to apply a "wet" formulation (ranging from simple tap water to complex emulsion formulations—with or without drug) to a wet lesion and a "dry" formulation (e.g., petrolatum) to a dry lesion. For these reasons, the dermatological and transdermal formulator must be skilled in the art and knowledgeable in the science of a variety of formulation types.

In general, the preparation of such formulations as poultices and pastes is extemporaneous, and it is unlikely that the industrial pharmaceutical formulator will be required to develop stable, safe and efficacious products of this type. Solutions and powders lack staying power (retention time) on the skin and can only afford transient relief. In modern-day pharmaceutical practice, semi-solid formulations are preferred vehicles for dermatological therapy because they remain *in situ* and deliver their drug payload over extended periods. In the majority of cases, therefore, the developed formulation will be an ointment, emulsion or a gel. Typical constituents for these types of formulations are shown in Table 14.5.

Ointments

In its strictest definitive form, an ointment is classified as any semi-solid containing fatty material and intended for external application (U.S. Pharmocopeia, USP). In this discussion, ointments will be defined as semisolid anhydrous external preparations. In the nineteenth century, ointments were based on lard, a compounding material, the usefulness of which was severely limited by its tendency to turn rancid. Early in the twentieth century, lard was replaced by petrolatum (white or yellow soft paraffin or petroleum jelly). In present practice, nonmedicated ointments (ointment bases) are used alone, for emollient or lubricating purposes, or in combination with a drug for therapeutic purposes.

There are four types of ointment base (classified in the USP as hydrocarbon bases, absorption bases, water-removable bases, and water-soluble bases), but only the hydrocarbon bases are completely anhydrous. The anhydrous hydrocarbon bases contain straight or branched hydrocarbon chain lengths ranging from C_{16} to C_{30} and may also contain cyclic alkanes. They are used principally in nonmedicated form as described above. A typical formulation contains fluid hydrocarbons (mineral oils, liquid paraffins) mixed with longer alkyl chain, higher melting point hydrocarbons (white and yellow soft paraffin, petroleum jelly). The difference between white and yellow soft paraffin is simply that the white version has been bleached. Hard paraffin and microcrystalline waxes are similar to the soft paraffins except that they contain no liquid components. These anhydrous mixtures tend to produce formulations which are greasy and unpleasant to use. The addition of solid components, such as microcrystalline cellulose, can reduce the greasiness. Improved skin feel can also be attained by the

**Table 14.5
Constituents of semi-solid formulations.**

Function	Sample Ingredients		
Polymeric thickeners	**Gums** Acacia Alginates Carageenan Chitosan Collagen Tragacanth Xantham **Celluloses** Sodium carboxymethyl Hydroxyethyl Hydroxypropyl Hydroxypropylmethyl		**Acrylic acids** Carbomers Polycarbophil **Colloidal solids** Silica Clays Microcrystalline cellulose **Hydrogels** Polyvinyl alcohol Polyvinylpyrrolidone **Thermoreversible polymers** Poloxamers
Oil phase	Mineral oil Isopropyl myristate Beeswax Cottonseed oil Cetostearyl alcohol Lanolin (and derivatives)	White soft paraffin Yellow soft paraffin Canola oil Cetyl alcohol Arachis (peanut) oil Oleic acid	Isopropyl palmitate Castor oil Stearyl alcohol Jojoba oil Stearic acid Silicone oils
Surfactants	**Nonionic** Sorbitan esters Polysorbates Polyoxyethylene alkyl ethers Polyoxyethylene alkyl esters Polyoxyethylene aryl ethers Glycerol esters Cholesterol		**Anionic** Sodium dodecyl sulphate **Cationic** Cetrimide Benzalkonium chloride
Solvents	**Polar** Water Propylene glycol Glycerol Sorbitol Ethanol Industrial methylated spirit Polyethylene glycols Propylene carbonate Triacetin		**Nonpolar** Isopropyl alcohol Medium chain triglycerides
Preservatives	**Antimicrobial** Benzalkonium chloride Benzyl alcohol Chlorhexidine Imidazolidinyl urea Phenol Potassium sorbate	Benzoic acid Bronopol Chlorocresol Paraben esters Phenoxyethanol Sorbic acid	**Antioxidants** α-Tocopherol Ascorbic acid Ascorbyl palmitate Butylated hydroxyanisole Butylated hydroxytoluene Sodium ascorbate Sodium metabisulphite **Chelating agents** Citric acid Edetic acid
pH adjusters	Diethanolamine Lactic acid Monoethanolamine Triethanolamine	Sodium hydroxide Sodium phosphate	

incorporation of silicone materials, such as polydimethylsiloxane oil or dimethicones. Silicones are often used in barrier formulations which are designed to protect the skin against water-soluble irritants.

Although the non-medicated anhydrous ointments are extremely useful for emolliency, their value as topical drug delivery platforms is limited by the relative insolubility of many drugs in hydrocarbons and silicone oils. However, it is possible to increase drug solubility within the formulation by incorporating hydrocarbon-miscible solvents, such as isopropyl-myristate or propylene glycol, into the ointment. Although increasing the solubility of a drug within a formulation may often decrease the release rate, it does not necessarily decrease the therapeutic effect. It is well accepted that simple determination of release rates from formulations may not be predictive of drug bioavailability. For example, when formulated in a simple white petrolatum/mineral oil ointment, the release rate of betamethasone dipropionate was shown to be considerably higher than when the drug was formulated at the same concentration (0.05 percent) in an augmented, and more clinically effective, ointment containing propylene glycol (Figure 14.10) (Zatz et al. 1996). It is also important to appreciate that various grades of petrolatum are commercially available and that the physical properties of these materials will vary depending on the source and refining process. Slight variations in physical properties of the constituents of an ointment may have significant effects on drug release behaviour (see, for example, Kneczke et al. 1986).

The preparation of ointment formulations may, at first sight, appear a simple matter of heating all of the constituents to a temperature higher than the melting point of all of the excipients and cooling with constant mixing. The reality, however, is that the process is somewhat more complex and requires careful control over various parameters, especially the cooling rate. Rapid cooling, for example, creates stiffer formulations in which there are numerous small crystallites. On the other hand, a slow cooling rate results in the formation of fewer, but larger, crystallites and a more fluid product. Further information regarding temperature effects and ointment phase behaviour can be found in Osborne (1992, 1993) and Pena et al. (1994).

Gels

The common characteristic of all gels is that they contain continuous structures which provide solid-like properties (Barry 1983). Depending on their constituents, gels may be clear or opaque, and be polar, hydroalcoholic or non-polar. The simplest gels contain water thickened with either natural gums (e.g., tragacanth, guar, xanthan), semi-synthetic materials [e.g., methylcellulose (MC), carboxymethylcellulose (CMC), hydroxyethylcellulose (HEC)], synthetic materials (e.g., carbomer-carboxyvinyl polymer) or clays (e.g., silicates, hectorite). Gel viscosity is generally a function of the amount and molecular weight of the added thickener.

There are a variety of semisynthetic celluloses in use as thickeners in gel formulations. These include MC, CMC, HEC, hydroxypropyl cellulose (HPC) and hydroxypropyl methylcellulose (HPMC). These celluloses are obtainable in diverse molecular weight grades, and the higher molecular weight moieties are used at 1–5 percent (w/w) for gellation. In the preparation of aqueous gels, the cellulose is dissolved in a preheated portion of the required water. Upon dispersion of the cellulose in the hot water, the remainder of the water is added, cold, and stirred to form the gel. When polar organic solvents (e.g., ethanol, propylene glycol) form part of the formulation, the cellulose should be dispersed or dissolved in the organic phase and the aqueous phase subsequently added. It is useful, when developing prototype gel formulations, to evaluate a variety of different types of cellulose. If a major requirement is for clarity of the gel, for example, HPMC is preferable to MC. It is also important to appreciate

Figure 14.10 Release rates of betamethasone dipropionate from ointments into various receptor fluids. (1), 5% hexane in acetonitrile; (2), octanol; (3), acetonitrile; (4), 60% acetonitrile in water; (5), 95% ethanol (data from Zatz et al. 1996).

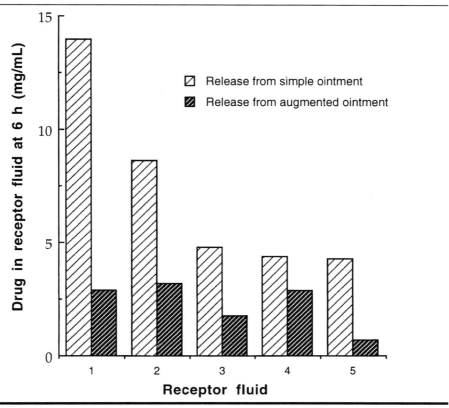

that some celluloses may exhibit specific incompatibilities with other potential formulation ingredients. For example, HEC is incompatible with several salts, and MC and HPC are incompatible with parabens. This latter incompatibility will limit the choice of preservative for gel formulations based on MC and HPC. Finally, the presence of oxidative materials (e.g., peroxides or other ingredients containing peroxide residues) in formulations gelled with celluloses should be avoided because oxidative degradation of the polymer chains may cause a rapid decrease in formulation viscosity (Dahl et al. 1998).

Because they are of naturally occurring plant origin, the branched chain polysaccharide gums, such as tragacanth, pectin, carrageenan and guar, will have widely varying physical properties depending on their source. They are incorporated into formulations at concentrations of between 0.5 and 10 percent contingent upon the required viscosity. Viscosity may be enhanced synergistically by the addition of inorganic suspending agents such as magnesium aluminium silicate. Tragacanth, a mixture of water-insoluble and water-soluble polysaccharides, is negatively charged in aqueous solution and therefore incompatible with many preservatives when formulated at a pH of 7 and above. Similarly, xanthan gum, which is produced by bacterial fermentation, is incompatible with some preservatives. Alginic acid is a hydrophilic colloidal carbohydrate obtained from seaweed. The sodium salt, sodium alginate, is used at 5–10 percent as a gelling agent, and firm gels may be obtained by incorporating small amounts of soluble calcium salts (e.g., tartrate, citrate). Many gums are ineffective in hydroalcoholic gels containing greater than 5 percent alcohol. Nonetheless, ethanol or glycerin are often used as wetting agents to ease aqueous dispersion of the gums.

The natural clay thickeners (e.g., bentonite and magnesium aluminium silicate) are useful for thickening aqueous gels containing co-solvents, such as ethanol, isopropanol, glycerin and propylene glycol. These materials possess a lamellar structure that can be extensively hydrated. The flat surfaces of bentonite are negatively charged, whereas the edges are positively charged. The clays swell in the presence of water because of hydration of the cations and electrostatic repulsion between the negatively charged faces. Thixotropic gels form at high concentrations because the clay particles combine in a flocculated structure in which the edge of one particle is attracted to the face of another. The rheological properties of these clay dispersions are, therefore, particularly sensitive to the presence of salts. Bentonite, a native colloidal hydrated aluminium silicate (mainly montmorillonite), can precipitate under acidic conditions, and formulations must be at pH 6 or above. A synthetic clay (colloidal silicon dioxide) is also useful for thickening both aqueous and non-polar gels. The usual concentrations of clay required to thicken formulations is from 2 to 10 percent.

By far the most extensively employed gelling agent in the pharmaceutical and cosmetic industries are the carboxyvinyl polymers known as carbomers. These are synthetic high molecular weight polymers of acrylic acid cross-linked with either allylsucrose or allyl ethers of pentaerythritol. Pharmaceutical grades of carbomers are available (e.g., Carbopol 981NF, BFGoodrich Performance Materials). In the dry state, a carbomer molecule is tightly coiled. When dispersed in water, the molecule begins to hydrate and partially uncoil. This uncoiling exposes free acidic moieties. In order to attain maximum thickening, the carbomer molecule must be fully uncoiled, and this can be achieved by one of two mechanisms (Figure 14.11). The most common way is to convert the acidic molecule to a salt by the addition of an appropriate neutralizing agent. For aqueous or polar solvent containing formulations, carbomer gellation can be induced by the addition of simple inorganic bases, such as sodium or potassium hydroxide. Less polar or non-polar solvent systems may be neutralized with amines, such as triethanolamine or diethanolamine. A number of alternative amine bases (e.g., diisopropanolamine, aminomethyl propanol, tetrahydroxypropyl ethylenediamine and tromethamine) may be employed. For example, clear and stable hydroalcoholic gels containing 40 percent ethanol can be thickened with triethanolamine or tromethamine. Neutralization ionizes the carbomer molecule, generating negative charges along the polymer backbone, and the resultant electrostatic repulsion creates an extended three-dimensional structure. Care must be taken not to under- or overneutralize the formulation as this will result in viscosity or thixotropy changes (Planas et al. 1992). Overneutralization will reduce viscosity because the excess base cations screen the carboxy groups and reduce electrostatic repulsion. Hydrated molecules of carbomer may also be uncoiled in aqueous systems by the addition of 10–20 percent of a hydroxyl donor, such as a non-ionic surfactant or a polyol (Figure 14.12), which is able to hydrogen bond with the polymer. Using this mechanism, maximum thickening will not be instantaneous, as it is with base neutralization, and may take several hours. Heating will accelerate the process, but the system should not be heated above 70°C.

A typical carbomer gel can be prepared as follows. The carbomer resin (0.5–1.0 percent) is dispersed in water to form a lump-free mixture which is allowed to stand to free entrapped air. A small proportion (~2 percent) of 10 percent aqueous NaOH is added using moderate

Figure 14.11 A tightly coiled carbomer molecule will hydrate and swell when dispersed in water (a). The molecule will completely uncoil to achieve maximum thickening when it is converted from the acid form to the salt form upon neutralization (b).

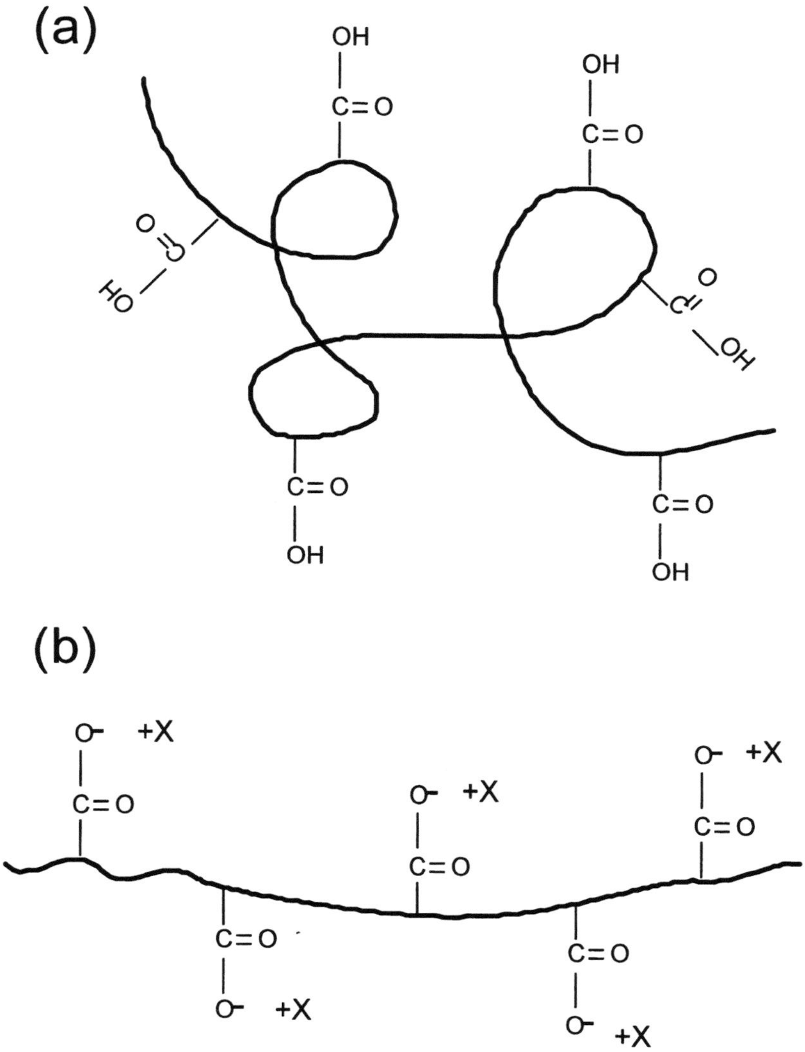

agitation to form the gel. The dispersion process may take some time, and many formulators prepare a concentrated stock dispersion of carbomer for dilution. The exact quantity of neutralizing agent to be added depends upon the type and equivalent weight (carbomer resins have an approximate equivalent weight of 76). Because they are synthetic, carbomer bases vary little from lot to lot. However, differences in batch to batch mean molecular weight may result in variations in the rheological characteristics of aqueous dispersions (Pérez-Marcos et al. 1993).

Figure 14.12 Hydrated carbomer molecules may be uncoiled in water by adding hydroxyl donors such as propylene or polyethylene glycols (PEG).

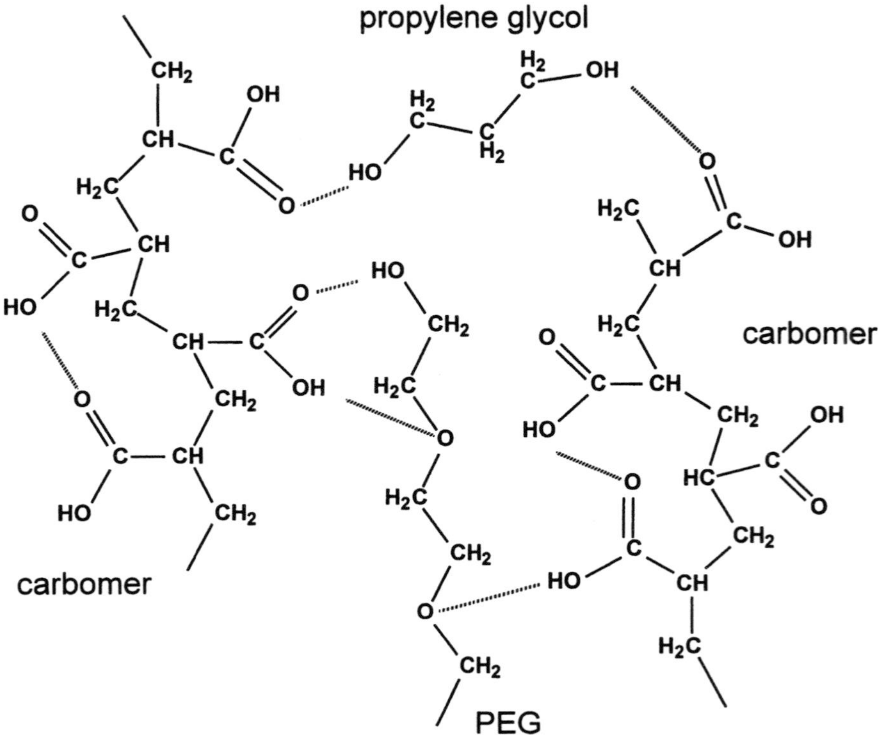

The carbomers have an excellent safety profile, are generally regarded as essentially non-toxic and non-irritant materials and have been extensively used by the pharmaceutical and cosmetic industries. In addition, there is no evidence of hypersensitivity or allergic reactions in humans as a result of topical application.

Emulsions

The most common emulsions used in dermatological therapy are creams. These are two-phase preparations in which one phase (the dispersed or internal phase) is finely dispersed in the other (the continuous or external phase). The dispersed phase can be either hydrophobic based (oil-in-water creams, O/W) or aqueous based (water-in-oil creams, W/O). Whether a cream is O/W or W/O is dependent on the properties of the system used to stabilize the interface between the phases. Given the fact that there are two incompatible phases in close conjunction, the physical stability of creams is always tenuous, but may be maximised by the judicious selection of an appropriate emulsion stabilizing system. In most pharmaceutical emulsions, stabilizing systems are comprised of either surfactants (ionic and/or non-ionic), polymers (non-ionic polymers, polyelectrolytes or biopolymers) or mixtures of these. The most commonly used surfactant systems are sodium alkyl sulphates (anionic), alkylammonium halides (cationic) and polyoxyethylene alkyl ethers or polysorbates (non-ionic). These are often used alone or in conjunction with non-ionic polymerics, such as polyvinyl alcohol or poloxamer block copolymers, or polyelectrolytes, such as polyacrylic/polymethacrylic acids.

The physicochemical principles underlying emulsion formulation and stabilization are extremely complex and will not be covered in depth here. The interested reader is referred to the volume edited by Sjöblom (1996). Briefly, an emulsion is formed when two immiscible liquids (in most cases oil and water) are mechanically agitated. When this occurs in the absence of any form of interfacial stabilization during agitation, both liquids will form droplets which rapidly flocculate and coalesce into two phases on standing. Flocculation is the term used to describe the close accumulation of two or more droplets of dispersed phase without loss of the interfacial film and is largely the result of Van der Waals forces. The flocculated droplets may then coalesce into one large droplet with the loss of the interfacial film. In reality, there is a brief period where one of the phases becomes the continuous phase because the droplets of this liquid coalesce more rapidly than the droplets of the other. Physical stability of an emulsion is determined by the ability of an additive to counteract the Van der Waals attractions, thereby reducing flocculation and coalescence of the dispersed phase. This may be achieved in two ways: an increase in the viscosity of the continuous phase, which will reduce the rate of droplet movement, and/or the establishment of an energy barrier between the droplets. While it is true that increasing the viscosity of the continuous phase will reduce the rate at which droplets flocculate, in pharmaceutical shelf-life terms, a stable system will be generated in this way only when the continuous phase is gelled and the droplet diameter is <0.1 μm.

In pharmaceutical emulsions, it is more common to develop stability using the energy barrier technique and to complement this stabilization, if necessary, by increasing the viscosity of the continuous phase. The basis of the energy barrier is that droplets experience repulsion when they approach each other. Repulsion can be generated either electrostatically, by the establishment of an electric double layer on the droplet surface, or sterically, by adsorbed non-ionic surfactant or polymeric material. Electrostatic repulsion is provided by ionic surfactants which, when adsorbed at the oil-water interface, will orient such that the polar ionic group faces the water. Some of the surfactant counterion (e.g., the sodium ion of sodium dodecyl sulphate) will separate from the surface and form a diffuse cloud surrounding the droplet. This diffuse cloud, together with the surface charge from the surfactant, forms the electric double layer. Electrostatic repulsion will occur when two similarly charged droplets approach each other. For obvious reasons, this method of emulsion stabilization is only appropriate for O/W formulations. In addition, it is important to appreciate that emulsions stabilized by electrostatic repulsion are extremely sensitive to additional electrolytes which will disrupt the electrical double layer.

Steric repulsion may be produced using non-ionic surfactants or polymers, such as polyvinyl alcohol or poloxamers. The specific distribution of the polyethoxylated non-ionic surfactants and block copolymers (Figure 14.13a, b) results in the formation of a thick hydrophilic shell of polyoxyethylene chains around the droplet. Repulsion is then afforded by both mixing interaction (osmotic repulsion) and entropic interaction (volume restriction), the latter as a result of a loss of configurational entropy of the polyoxyethylene chains when there is a significant overlap. For polymeric materials without definitive hydrophobic and hydrophilic regions, the adsorption energy is critical to generation of steric repulsion. The adsorption energy should not be so low as to result in no polymer adsorption, nor so high as to result in complete polymer adsorption to the droplet. In either case, there will be none of the loops or tails (Figure 14.13c) which are essential to steric repulsion. For this reason, polymeric steric repulsion is usually achieved using block copolymers such as poloxamers, which consist of linked polyoxyethylene and polyoxypropylene chains. More recently, polyacrylic acid

Figure 14.13 Oil-in-water emulsions may be stabilized by (A) non-ionic surfactants, (B) poloxamer block copolymers or (C) polymeric materials. The hydrophilic chains produce repulsion by mixing interaction (osmotic) or volume restriction (entropic).

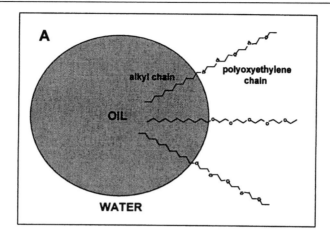

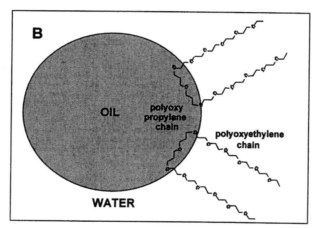

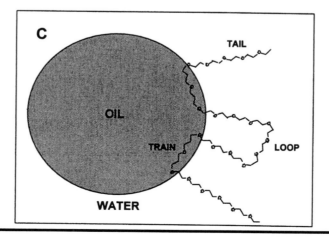

polymers linked to hydrophobic chains (Pemulen™, BFGoodrich) have been used as primary emulsification systems in O/W formulations and are listed in the USP as carbomer 1342. These materials form very stable emulsions because the polyacrylic acid chain, anchored to the oil droplet by the alkyl methacrylate moieties, considerably increases the surface charge on the oil droplet, forming a strong electrical barrier at the interface. Furthermore, emulsion stability is enhanced by an increase in the viscosity of the continuous phase.

In most cases for O/W emulsions, and all cases for W/O emulsions, it is necessary to select an emulsification system based on surfactants. Whilst we have already seen that ionic surfactants can only be used for O/W emulsions, non-ionic surfactants may be used for both O/W and W/O formulations. Although, at first glance, the choice of surfactant system appears limitless (there are hundreds to choose from), there are some basic guidelines to aid the formulator. In the first instance, use of pharmaceutically approved surfactants (or those having a Drug Master File in place with the Regulatory Authority) will save a considerable amount of regulatory justification time. Very often, guidelines are provided by the raw material supplier, although these will obviously be biased toward the use of their products. Nonetheless, it should be appreciated that the suppliers have considerable experience in the applications and uses of their products, and they provide a very useful resource. In addition, a rough and ready guide is provided by the hydrophilic-lipophilic balance (HLB) system which generates an arbitrary number (usually between 0 and 20) which is assigned to a particular surfactant. The HLB value of a polyoxyethylene based non-ionic surfactant may be derived from

$$\text{HLB} = \frac{\text{mol\% hydrophobic group}}{5} \tag{14}$$

and the HLB of a polyhydric alcohol fatty acid ester (e.g., glyceryl monostearate) may be derived from

$$\text{HLB} = 20\left(1 - \frac{S}{A}\right) \tag{15}$$

where S is the saponification number of the ester and A the acid number of the fatty acid. When it is not possible to obtain a saponification number (e.g, lanolin derivatives), the HLB can be calculated from:

$$\text{HLB} = \frac{E + P}{5} \tag{16}$$

where E is the weight percentage of the polyoxyethylene chain and P the weight percentage of the polyhydric alcohol group in the molecule.

It is immediately obvious from the above equations that hydrophilic surfactants will have high HLB values and lipohilic surfactants low values. It is generally recognised that surfactants with HLB values between 4 and 6 are W/O emulsifiers, and those with HLB values between 8 and 18 are O/W emulsifiers. It is also generally recognised, though poorly understood, that mixtures of surfactants create more stable emulsions than the individual surfactants. The overall HLB of a surfactant mixture (HLB_M) can be calculated from

$$\text{HLB}_M = f\text{HLB}_A + (1 - f)\text{HLB}_B \tag{17}$$

where f is the weight fraction of surfactant A. The required emulsifier HLB values for several oils and waxes are given in Table 14.6. It is important to appreciate, however, that the HLB system can only be used as an approximation in emulsion design, and that stability of an emulsion cannot be guaranteed by the use of an emulsifier mix with the appropriate HLB value. As an example, creaming of an emulsion, a typical physical stability problem, is much more dependent on the viscosity of the continuous phase than the characteristics of the interfacial film.

As mentioned above, it is recognised that mixtures of surfactants create more stable emulsions that the individual surfactants. A reasonable and coherent explanation for this is given by the gel network theory (Eccleston 1990, 1997). Briefly, the theory relates the consistencies and stabilities of O/W creams to the presence or absence of viscoelastic gel networks in the continuous phase. These networks form when there is an amount of mixed emulsifier, in excess of that required to stabilize the interfacial film, that can interact with the aqueous continuous phase. In its simplest form, a cream consists of oil, water and mixed emulsifier. Official emulsifying waxes may be cationic (Cationic Emulsifying Wax BPC; a mixture of cetostearyl alcohol and cetyltrimethylammonium bromide, 9:1), anionic (Emulsifying Wax BP; a mixture of cetostearyl alcohol and sodium dodecyl sulphate, 9:1) or non-ionic (Non-ionic Emulsifying Wax BPC; a mixture of cetostearyl alcohol and cetomacrogol, 4:1). The theory dictates that when the cream is formulated, it is composed of at least four phases (Figure 14.14):

1. bulk water

2. a dispersed oil phase

3. a crystalline hydrate

4. a crystalline gel phase composed of bilayers of surfactant and fatty alcohol separated by layers of interlamellar fixed water.

Examination of ternary systems (containing the emusifying wax and water but no oil phase) by X-ray diffraction indicates that, for all emulsifying systems, addition of water causes swelling of the interlamellar spaces. Ionic emulsifying systems possess a greater capacity to swell than non-ionic systems. Swelling in ionic systems is an electrostatic phenomenon, whereas that

---

Table 14.6
Hydrophilic–lipophilic balance (HLB) values for several oils and waxes.

Constituent	Emulsion Type	
	O/W	W/O
Liquid paraffin	12	4
Hard paraffin	10	4
Stearic acid	16	–
Beeswax	12	5
Castor oil	14	–
Cottonseed oil	9	–

in non-ionic systems is due to hydration of the polyoxyethylene chains and is limited by the length of this chain. The gel network theory also offers an explanation for the observation that non-ionic O/W creams thicken on storage. This change is related to the formation of additional gelation in the continuous phase as a result of slow hydration of the polyoxyethylene chains of the surfactant. This process reduces the amount of free water in the formulation.

A relatively stable emulsion formulation may be prepared from a simple four component mixture: oil, water, surfactant and fatty amphiphile. In practice, however, things are never this straightforward. In addition to the four principle components, a pharmaceutical emulsion

Figure 14.14 The gel network theory suggests that when a cream is formulated, it is composed of four phases: bulk water, a dispersed oil phase, a crystalline hydrate and a crystalline gel composed of bilayers of surfactant and fatty alcohol separated by layers of interlamellar fixed water (courtesy of Dr. G. M. Eccleston).

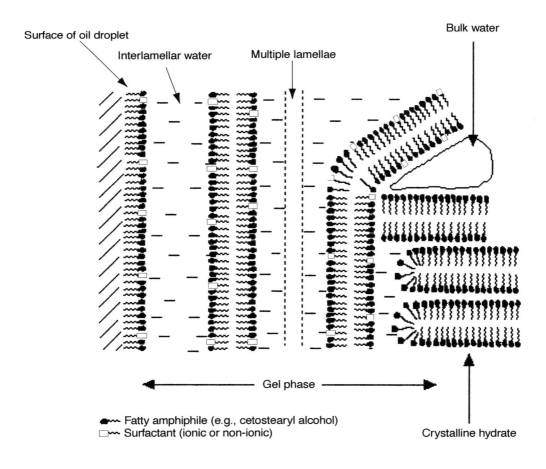

formulation will also contain the drug, and is likely to contain a co-solvent for the drug, a viscosity enhancer, a microbiological preservative system, a pH adjusting/stabilizing buffer and an antioxidant system. All of the additional components are related to the requirement that the formulation must be capable of delivering the correct amount of drug to the therapeutic application site in a formulation that is free from microbial contamination and is essentially physically unchanged from the day of manufacture.

Other Semi-solid Formulations

In addition to the traditional dermal delivery formulations discussed above, several other pharmaceutical semi-solid and liquid formulation types have been the subject of a considerable amount of R&D. These include sprays, foams, multiple emulsions, microemulsions, liposomal formulations, niosomes, cyclodextrins, glycospheres, dermal membrane structures and microsponges. Although some of these formulations form part of the pharmaceutical armamentorium, they are yet to achieve widespread application and are not within the scope of this chapter. The interested reader is referred to the excellent coverage by Osborne and Amann (1990), Kreuter (1994) and Liu and Wisniewski (1997).

Drug Release from Semi-Solid Formulations and SUPAC-SS

Determination of the ability of a semi-solid formulation to release a drug, the pattern of release and the rate at which this release occurs are important aspects of formulation development and optimization. However, it is also important to appreciate that the data obtained should not be overinterpreted. Release studies normally involve the measurement of drug diffusion out of a mass of formulation into a receiving medium which is separated from the formulation by a synthetic membrane (Shah et al. 1991; Chattaraj and Kanfer 1995). Detailed study of the data obtained using this type of system will generate invaluable data concerning the physical state of the drug in the formulation. For example, an examination of the early models, and their refined updates, derived to describe drug release from semi-solids reveals that release patterns are different depending on whether the drug is present as a solution or suspension within the formulation (Higuchi 1960; 1961; Bunge 1998). These subtle differences, together with differences in the rate of release, may be used to determine such parameters as drug diffusivity within the matrix of a formulation, the particle size of suspended drug and the absolute solubility of a drug within a complex formulation (Flynn et al. [in press]). It is generally agreed that drug release rate data cannot be used to predict skin permeation or bioavailability. When a formulation is applied to the skin, the situation is ephemeral. The formulation will undergo considerable shearing forces, and solvents will evaporate. There may be excipients in the formulation that will interact with the skin and potentially modulate bioavailability. Nonetheless, release rate determinations are important for purposes other than formulation development and characterization.

The FDA has issued a guidance document (FDA 1997) which recommends the use of *in vitro* drug release testing in the scale-up and post-approval changes for semi-solids (SUPAC-SS). The FDA intends to promote the use of this test as a QA tool to monitor minor differences in formulation composition or changes in manufacturing sites, but not at present as a routine batch-to-batch QC test. Thus, the FDA is suggesting *in vitro* release rate data for Level 2 and Level 3 changes in formulation components and composition, but such data are not required for a Level 1 change. In the former, the *in vitro* release rate of the new or modified formulation should be compared to a recent batch of the original formulation and the

90 percent confidence limit should fall within the limits of 75 to 133 percent. Similarly, *in vitro* release testing is suggested for Level 2 changes in manufacturing equipment, processes and scale-up, and Level 3 changes in manufacturing site. Recently the use of *in vitro* testing as a QA tool has been questioned, especially in the case of a hydrophilic formulation containing the highly water-soluble drug, ammonium lactate (Kril et al. 1999). The method was found not to be specific enough to differentiate between small differences in drug loading or minor compositional and processing changes.

Bioequivalence of Dermatological Formulations

Bioequivalence of dermatological dosage forms presents particular difficulties, mainly because it is difficult to determine the very low blood levels of a specific drug following dermal application. The FDA has, therefore, suggested the use of alternative methods such as determining dermatopharmacokinetics by the tape-stripping method. The use of *in vivo* skin stripping in dermatopharmacokinetic evaluation was discussed at an AAPS/FDA workshop on bioequivalence of topical dermatological dosage forms (Bethesda, Md., USA, September 1996). Although opinion was divided, it was concluded that stratum corneum skin stripping "may provide meaningful information for comparative evaluation of topical dosage forms" (Shah et al. 1998). Furthermore, it was established that a combination of dermatopharmacokinetic and pharmacodynamic data may provide sufficient proof of bioequivalence "in lieu of clinical trials". However, much remains to be validated in skin-stripping protocols. The *in vivo* tape-stripping technique is based on the dermal reservoir principle (Dupius et al. 1984; Rougier 1987b; Tojo and Lee 1989). It is hypothesised that if a compound is applied to the skin for a limited time (for example 0.5 h) and then removed, the amount of drug in the upper layers of the stratum corneum will be predictive of the overall bioavailability of the compound. It follows that determination of the stratum corneum content of a permeating material following a short-term application will predict *in vivo* bioavailability from a corresponding administration protocol. Data obtained in studies of this type have shown reasonable predictability for several compounds.

An outline protocol for skin-stripping bioequivalence studies has been suggested (Shah et al. 1998). The basic protocol has two phases: uptake and elimination.

1. Uptake:

   a. Test and reference drug products are applied concurrently at multiple sites.

   b. After exposure for a suitable time (determined by a pilot study), excess drug is removed by wiping three times with tissue or cotton swab.

   c. The adhesive tape is applied with uniform pressure. The first strip is discarded (skin surface material). Repeat if necessary to remove excess surface material.

   d. Collect nine successive tape strips from the same site. If necessary collect more than nine strips.

   e. Repeat the procedure for each site at designated time intervals.

   f. Extract the drug from the combined tape strips for each time point and site and determine the content of drug using an appropriate validated analytical method.

   g. Express the data as amount of drug per cm^2 of tape.

2. Elimination:

    a. As for a, b and c above.

    b. After a predetermined time interval (e.g., 1, 3, 5 and 21 h post-drug removal), perform steps d) through g) as above.

The results are then expressed as the amount of drug recovered from the tape strips against time. Uptake and elimination phases are observed and "bioavailability" may be predicted from the area under the curve (AUC). There are several sources of variability in such studies, all of which must be considered in standard operating procedures. The major causes of concern are variability in

- drug application procedure,
- type of tape,
- size of tape,
- pressure applied by investigator,
- duration of application of pressure,
- drug removal procedure,
- drug extraction procedure,
- analytical methodology,
- temperature,
- relative humidity,
- skin type and
- skin surface uniformity.

Nonetheless, following further validation, the technique will have several advantages. For example, basic pharmacokinetic parameters such as AUC, C_{max}, T_{max} and half-life may be approximated from the data obtained. In addition, the approach could be applicable to all types of topical preparation.

Pershing and colleagues (Pershing et al. 1992) validated an *in vivo* skin-stripping protocol by correlating the stratum corneum strip data obtained for betamethasone dipropionate with a skin bioassay blanching experiment. Skin blanching was assessed at 1, 24 and 48 h following removal of formulations applied under occlusion for 24 h. The correlation between the amount of betamethasone dipropionate in skin and skin blanching score was good ($r = 0.994$), although the skin blanching scores were not entirely objective because they were assessed visually rather than using a chromameter. Nonetheless, differences in responses between formulations (cream and ointment) and manufacturers could be discerned with both the pharmacokinetic and the pharmacodynamic techniques. Further details of the dermatological drug product bioequivalence, including the proposed protocol, may be obtained from the FDA draft guidance document (FDA 1998).

Preservation of Semi-Solid Formulations

All pharmaceutical semi-solid formulations which are not sterilized unit dose products can support the growth of micro-organisms. Preservatives are ingredients which prevent or retard microbial growth and thus protect formulations from spoilage. The use of preservatives is required to prevent product damage caused by micro-organisms during manufacture, storage and inadvertent contamination by the patient during use. Similarly, preservatives serve to protect consumers from possible infection from contaminated products. The characteristics of an ideal preservative system are shown in Table 14.7. Unfortunately, no single preservative meets all of these characteristics for all formulations (Orth 1993), and it is often necessary to use a preservative system containing a combination of individual preservatives. It is also important to appreciate that preservatives are intrinsically toxic materials, and a balance must be found between antimicrobial efficacy and dermal toxicity.

The most commonly used preservatives in pharmaceutical products are the parabens (alkyl esters of *p*-hydroxybenzoic acid, such as methyl- and propylparaben). These compounds are highly effective against both gram-positive bacteria and fungi at low concentrations (e.g., at concentrations of 0.1–0.3 percent, paraben combinations provide effective preservation of most emulsions). Because of their widespread use, the toxicological profile of the parabens has been extensively researched, and the safety in use of the lower esters (methyl, ethyl, propyl and butyl) has been established (Cosmetic Ingredient Review 1984). Other preservatives that have been used widely in topical pharmaceutical formulations include benzoic acid, sorbic acid, benzyl alcohol, phenoxyethanol, chlorocresol, benzalkonium chloride and cetrimide. All have particular advantages and disadvantages, which makes combination preservatives particularly effective. For example, although methylparaben is highly active against Gram-positive bacteria and moderately active against yeasts and moulds, it is only weakly active against Gram-negative bacteria. A combination of methylparaben with phenoxyethanol generates a preservative system that is also highly active against Gram-negative species. The acid preservatives, benzoic and sorbic, are only active as free acids, and it is therefore necessary to ensure that formulations containing these preservatives are buffered to acid pH values (pH < 5). A list of pharmaceutical preservatives useful in topical formulations is given in Table 14.8, together with their microbiological and physicochemical properties. More

Table 14.7
Characteristics for an ideal preservative.

1	Effective at low concentrations against a wide spectrum of microbes
2	Soluble in the formulation at the required concentration
3	Non-toxic and non-sensitizing to the consumer at in-use concentrations
4	Compatible with other formulation components
5	No physical effect on formulation characteristics
6	Stable over a wide range of pH and temperature
7	Inexpensive

Adapted from Takruri and Anger (1989).

information on preservatives and preservative systems may be found in the British Pharmaceutical Codex (The Pharmaceutical Press) and in the excellent text by Orth (1993).

It is interesting to note that, despite their widespread use and excellent safety profile, there is an increasing interest in the potential systemic exposure to preservatives following application in pharmaceutical and cosmetic products. In many cases, however, skin penetration data for preservatives are not available in the literature. In addition, much of the data that are publicly available have been obtained under conditions inappropriate to risk assessment. By far the most available data concerns the parabens.

Although most studies on the skin permeation of parabens have evaluated one or two of the homologous series, Dal Pozzo and Pastori (1996) reported their results on the *in vitro* human skin permeation of six parabens (methyl, ethyl, propyl, butyl hexyl and octyl esters). The permeants were applied to abdominal epidermal membranes, mounted in diffusion chambers, either as solid compounds (deposited in acetone) or as saturated solutions in various vehicles, including three typical emulsion formulations (two O/W and one W/O emulsion). Following application of the unformulated pure substance, maximum flux decreased with increasing lipophilicity, from 65.0 μg/cm^2/h for methyl paraben to 13.7 μg/cm^2/h for hexyl paraben. Similarly, when applied as saturated aqueous solutions, the maximum flux decreased with increasing lipophilicity. In the latter case, however, when flux was normalised to the vehicle concentration of the permeant, the permeability coefficient increased with increasing lipophilicity. Addition of 50 percent propylene glycol or 20 percent polyethylene glycol 400 to the aqueous solutions did not alter the profile of permeation, although the permeability coefficients were somewhat reduced. On the other hand, when the parabens were dissolved in liquid paraffin, the relationship between the permeability coefficient and lipophilicity appeared parabolic, and the maximum flux occurred for the butyl ester, and the highest permeability coefficient occurred for the propyl ester. The results described above are

Table 14.8
Microbiological and physicochemical properties of selected preservatives.

Preservative	Gram +	Antimicrobial Activity[a] Gram −	Moulds	Yeasts	In-Use Conc. (%)	pH Range[b]	O/W[c]
Benzoic acid	1	2	3	3	0.1	2–5	3–6
Sorbic acid	2	2	2	1	0.2	<6.5	3.5
Phenoxyethanol	2	1	3	3	1.0	Wide	–
Methylparaben	1	3	2	2	0.4–0.8	3.0–9.5	7.5
Propylparaben	1	3	2	2	0.4–0.8	3.0–9.5	80
Butylparaben	1	3	2	2	0.4–0.8	3.0–9.5	280
Chlorocresol	1	2	3	3	0.1	<8.5	117–190
Benzalkonium Cl	1	2	3	2	0.01–0.25	4–10	<1
Cetrimide	1	2	3	2	0.01–0.1	4–10	<1

[a]1, highly active; 2, moderately active; 3, weakly active.
[b]Optimal pH range for activity.
[c]Oil-water partition coefficient.

consistent with theory and demonstrate that the vehicle of application can significantly affect the skin permeability characteristics of compounds.

In emulsion systems, the existence of two distinct phases (oil and water) results in a distribution of the parabens according to their physicochemical characteristics. This distribution can be influenced by the presence of other ingredients, such as co-solvents and surfactants. Furthermore, these excipients may also affect skin barrier properties. Thus, Dal Pozzo and Pastori (1996) found that permeation of the parabens from two O/W emulsions was higher than expected, based on their data using simple vehicles (described above), and that permeation from the O/W emusions was higher than that from the W/O emulsion. These results were rationalised on the basis of permeant release from the formulation, and it was assumed that the external lipid phase of the W/O emulsion retained the parabens.

It is difficult, however, to relate this data to conditions of actual consumer exposure because, in the DalPozzo and Pastori study, the formulations were applied at infinite dose (which effectively generated occlusive conditions) and at an artificially high permeant concentration (0.7 percent w/w). When applied to the skin surface at low finite doses, the vehicle is continually changing. Whether the vehicle is O/W or W/O, the water content will be released by the shear forces generated by application to the skin, and most of the water will evaporate. On the basis of the argument above, this should tend to reduce the skin penetration of these preservatives.

It is theoretically possible to reduce the skin absorption of the parabens by formulation manipulation. This manipulation may be achieved by altering the distribution pattern of the preservative within the formulation or by complexation. Care must be taken, however, to ensure that any formulation modification does not interfere with the antimicrobial activity of the preservative system (Evans 1964; Kurup et al. 1995). One such modification involved the complexation of methylparaben with 2-hydroxypropyl-β-cyclodextrin (Tanaka et al. 1995). Although the aqueous solubility of methyparaben was increased considerably in the presence of the cyclodextrin, the percutaneous penetration of the preservative through hairless mouse skin *in vivo* over 24 h was reduced by 66 percent. While clearly this system had benefit in terms of potential reduction in systemic absorption of the preservative, there was no indication of any possible alteration of preservative efficacy. Incorporation of butylparaben into liposomes prepared from phosphatidylcholine-cholesterol-diacetyl-phosphate was shown to have no effect on preservative efficacy, although the antimicrobial effect was shown to be proportional to the free, and not the total, concentration of the preservative (Komatsu et al. 1986a). However, further study by the same authors demonstrated that incorporation of butylparaben in some liposomal systems had little effect on the permeation of the preservative across guinea pig skin either *in vivo* or *in vitro* (Komatsu et al. 1986a,b), although incorporation of increasing amounts of lipid into the liposome did tend to decrease the overall percutaneous absorption of this preservative.

In summary, although there is considerable evidence that parabens can penetrate into the skin, permeation and systemic availability of intact compounds are likely to be considerably reduced by transcutaneous and systemic metabolism. Furthermore, since these preservatives are present at concentrations of 0.1–0.2 percent w/w in topical pharmaceutical formulations, in-use dermal exposure to these compounds will be relatively low. In the cosmetic industry, there is a trend toward preservative-free and self-preserving formulations (Kabara and Orth 1997). However, before starting down this road, the pharmaceutical formulator must consider the potential implications on the efficacy and safety of the product.

Transdermal Drug Delivery Systems

The skin was not commercially or scientifically exploited as a route of delivery into the systemic circulation until the 1950s. Development of therapeutically effective ointments containing agents such as nitroglycerin and salicylates dispelled the notion that the skin was largely impermeable. It was shown that angina, for example, could be controlled for several hours by applying an ointment containing 2 percent nitroglycerin (Reichek et al. 1974). Similarly, topical salicylates could be absorbed through the skin into arthritic joints and more recently non-steroidal anti-inflammatory agents, such as ibuprofen and ketoprofen, estradiol and testosterone, have been developed and marketed in semi-solid preparations. A major problem with semi-solid preparations, however, is that of control of drug delivery. Drug concentrations in plasma and duration of action are not reliably predictable for several reasons, many of which are patient dependent. Quantity and area of application and dosage frequency obviously affect therapeutic efficacy, but the most significant factors are inter- and intraindividual variations in skin permeability. The seminal work of Scheuplein and Blank (1971) opened a floodgate of research into skin permeation, which has ultimately resulted in the development of modern controlled transdermal drug delivery.

The particular advantages of transdermal therapy have been fully discussed elsewhere (Cleary 1993a). Briefly, transdermal devices are easy to apply, can remain in place for up to 7 days (depending on the system) and are easily removed following or during therapy. Reduced dosing frequency and production of controllable and sustained plasma levels tend to minimize risks of undesirable side-effects which may be observed after oral dosage. Although viable epidermis contains enzyme systems which may be capable of catabolizing drugs (Hotchkiss 1998), the avoidance of hepatic first-pass metabolism is an obvious advantage. The intrinsic barrier property of the skin is the major limitation to transdermal drug delivery, a problem which is discussed later. Marketed patch type transdermal delivery systems are currently available for only a few drugs (chiefly scopolamine, nitroglycerin, clonidine, estradiol, fentanyl, testosterone and nicotine), although several other candidates are at various stages of development. Many drugs under investigation do not intrinsically possess a great ability to cross the skin and ways must be found, therefore, to enhance their transdermal delivery. For example, prodrugs can be designed with properties which result in more rapid absorption than the parent compound but are subsequently metabolized to the active species before reaching the receptor site (Anderson 1993; Ahmed et al. 1995). Permeation enhancement strategies should increase the number of successful candidate drugs for transdermal delivery in the near future. Another important factor that must be taken into account during transdermal product development is the potential for allergic or irritant responses to the drug and/or other formulation constituents (Schmidt 1989; Sutinen et al. 1993).

Current patch type transdermal delivery systems utilise one of three basic design principles: drug in adhesive, drug in matrix (usually polymeric) or drug in reservoir (Figure 14.15). In the latter case, the reservoir is separated from the skin by a rate-controlling membrane. Several features are common to all systems, including the release liner, pressure-sensitive adhesive and backing layer, all of which must be compatible (Baker and Heller 1989; Cleary 1993b; Sugibayashi and Morimoto 1994). In a system where the drug is intimately mixed with adhesive, or diffuses from a reservoir through adhesive, the potential for interaction between drug and adhesive, which can lead to either reduction of adhesive effectiveness or formation of a new chemical species, must be fully assessed. Similarly, residual monomers, catalysts, plasticizers and resins may react to give new chemical species, and it is possible that excipients (including enhancers) and/or their reaction products may interfere with adhesive systems.

Figure 14.15 Typical transdermal drug delivery system designs.

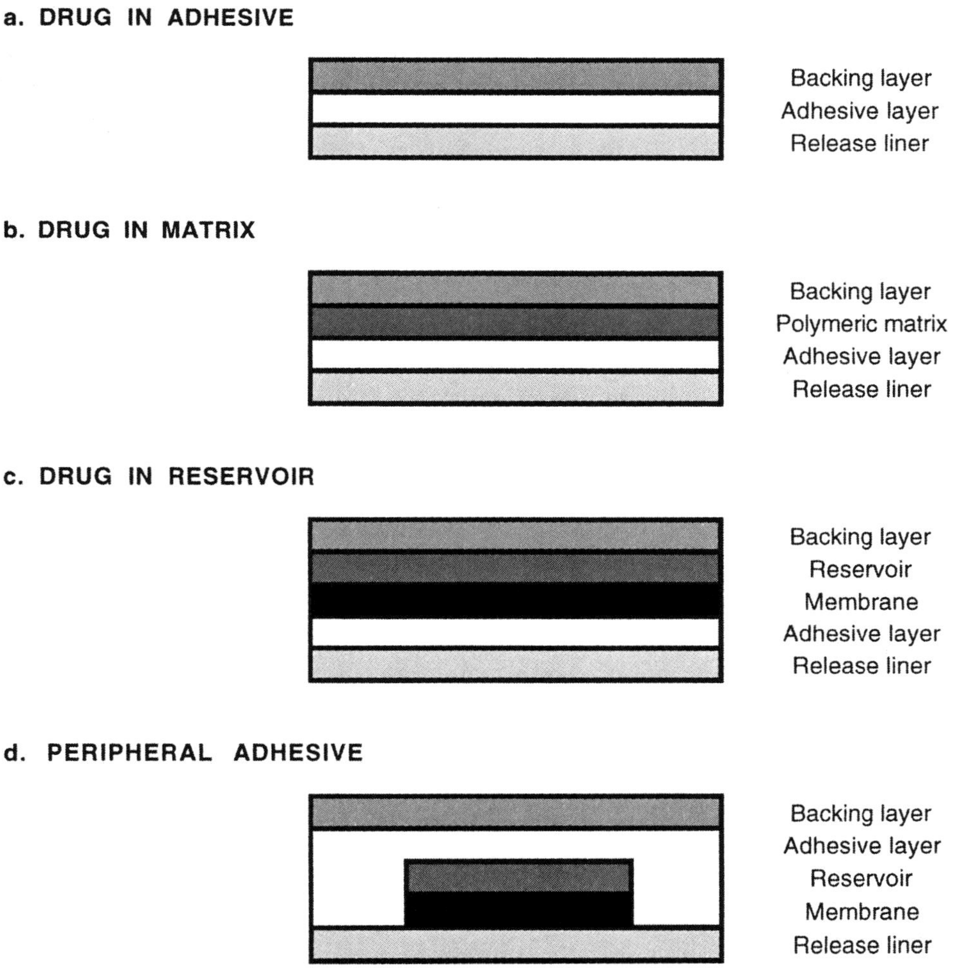

a. DRUG IN ADHESIVE

Backing layer
Adhesive layer
Release liner

b. DRUG IN MATRIX

Backing layer
Polymeric matrix
Adhesive layer
Release liner

c. DRUG IN RESERVOIR

Backing layer
Reservoir
Membrane
Adhesive layer
Release liner

d. PERIPHERAL ADHESIVE

Backing layer
Adhesive layer
Reservoir
Membrane
Release liner

Incompatibilities between the adhesive system and other formulation excipients may be circumvented by designs in which the adhesive is remote from the drug delivery area of the system (Figure 14.15d). Three critical considerations in system selection are: adhesion to skin, compatibility with skin and physical/chemical stability of the total formulation and components.

Devices are secured to the skin by use of a skin-compatible pressure-sensitive adhesive, usually based on silicones, acrylates or polyisobutylenes. These adhesives are evaluated by shear-testing and assessment of rheological parameters (Musolf 1987). Standard rheological tests include creep compliance (measurement of the ability of the adhesive to flow into surface irregularities), elastic index (the extent of stretch or deformation as a function of load and time) and recovery following deformation. Skin-adhesion performance is described by properties such as initial and long-term adhesion, lift and residue. The adhesive must be soft enough to ensure initial adhesion, yet have sufficient cohesive strength to remove cleanly, leaving no residue. Premature lift will interfere with drug delivery, and therefore, the cohesive and adhesive properties must be carefully balanced and maintained over the intended period of application. This must be evaluated by wear-testing using placebo patches applied to the skin.

Adhesion to the skin is affected by shape, conformability and occlusivity. Round patches tend to be more secure than those of more sharply angled geometry. A patch which is able to conform to the contours of the skin will resist buckling and lifting during movement. Water may affect adhesive properties, and therefore, the occlusivity of the system must be taken into consideration. Occlusion for prolonged periods can lead to excessive hydration and microbial growth, which may increase the possibilities of irritation or sensitization.

The backing material and release liner can be fabricated from a variety of materials including polyvinylchloride, polyethylene, polypropylene, ethylene-vinyl acetate and aluminium foil. The most important property of these materials is that they are impervious to both drug and formulation excipients. The most useful backing materials conform with the skin and provide a balanced resistance to transepidermal water loss, which will allow some hydration of the stratum corneum, yet maintain a healthy subpatch environment. The release liners are usually films or coated papers and must separate easily from the adhesive layer without lifting off any of the pressure-sensitive adhesive. Silicone release coatings are used with acrylate and rubber-based adhesive systems, and fluorocarbon coatings with silicone adhesives.

The three principal methods of incorporation of active species into a transdermal system have led to the loose classification of patches as membrane, matrix or drug-in-adhesive types. Combinations of the main types of patch can also be fabricated, for example, by placing a membrane over a matrix or using a drug-in-adhesive with a membrane/matrix device in order to deliver an initial bolus dose. Membrane patches contain delivery rate-controlling membranes between the drug reservoir and the skin (Komerska 1987; Friend et al. 1988; Yuk et al. 1991a). These may be microporous membranes, which control drug flux due to the size and tortuosity of pores in the membrane, or dense polymeric membranes, through which the drug permeates by dissolution and diffusion. Examples of rate-controlling membranes are ethylene-vinyl acetate copolymers, silicones, high-density polyethylene, polyester elastomers and polyacrylonitrile. Ideally, the membrane should be permeable only to the drug and enhancer (if present) and retain other formulation excipients. Membranes have been designed which allow differential permeation of enhancer and drug (Yuk et al. 1991b; Okabi et al. 1994), and this type (sometimes designated as a one-way membrane) is useful when the drug is located in the adhesive, whilst the enhancer is formulated into a reservoir.

A variety of materials are used in the drug reservoir, ranging from mineral oil to complex formulations, such as aqueous/alcoholic gels. A reservoir system should provide zero-order release of the drug over the entire delivery period which requires that the reservoir material remains saturated with the drug over the period of product application, which can usually be achieved by formulating the drug as a suspension.

The second type is the matrix transdermal system where the drug is uniformly dispersed in a polymeric matrix through which it diffuses to the skin surface (Leuenberger et al. 1995). The polymeric matrix (which may be composed of silicone elastomers, polyurethanes, polyvinyl alcohol, polyvinylpyrrolidones, etc.) may be considered as the drug reservoir. A series of steps are involved in the drug delivery process: dissociation of drug molecules from the crystal lattice, solubilization of the drug in the polymer matrix and diffusion of drug molecules through the matrix to the skin surface. Many factors can affect dissolution and diffusion rates, making it particularly difficult to predict release rates from experimental or prototype formulations. It is fundamental, however, that for a drug to be released from the matrix under zero-order kinetics it must ideally be maintained at saturation in the fluid phase of the matrix, and the diffusion rate of the drug within the matrix must be much greater than the diffusion rate of the drug in the skin.

The release rate of a drug or an enhancer from a polymeric matrix can be modified in several ways (Pfister et al. 1987; Ulman et al. 1989a,b,; Ulman and Lee 1989; Gelotte and Lostrito 1990), some of which are illustrated by a study of release of several drugs from silicone matrices (Pfister et al. 1987). Silicone medical-grade elastomers (polydimethylsiloxanes) are flexible, lipophilic polymers with excellent compatibility with biological tissues. They can be co-formulated with hydrophilic excipients, such as glycerol, and inert fillers, such as titanium dioxide, in order to alter release kinetics. Increasing the level of glycerol in the matrix increases the release rates of indomethacin, propranolol, testosterone and progesterone, whilst the presence of the inert fillers, titanium dioxide or barium sulphate, tends to reduce release rates. Release rates for hydrophilic drug from polydimethylsiloxane matrices can be increased by up to three orders of magnitude using polydimethyl siloxane/polyethylene oxide graft copolymers (Ulman et al. 1989b). These examples demonstrate the relative ease with which release rates of drugs can be tailored to produce a desired profile.

The microsealed delivery device is a variation of the matrix-type transdermal system in which the drug is dispersed in a reservoir phase which is then immobilized as discrete droplets in a cross-linked polymeric matrix. Release can be further controlled by inclusion of a polymeric microporous membrane. This system therefore combines the principles of both the liquid reservoir and matrix-type devices. Rate of release of a drug from a microsealed delivery system is dependent on the partition coefficient between the reservoir droplets and the polymeric matrix; the diffusivity of the drug in the reservoir, the matrix and the controlling membrane; and on the solubility of the drug in the various phases. There are, obviously, many ways to achieve the desired zero-order release rate, but only nitroglycerin has been commercially formulated into this type of delivery device (Karim 1983).

The simplest form of transdermal drug delivery device, most commonly employed at present, is the drug-in-adhesive system where the drug (and enhancer if present) is formulated in an adhesive mixture which is coated onto a backing membrane to produce an adhesive tape. The apparent simplicity is, however, deceptive, and a number of factors which arise from potential interactions between drug or enhancer and adhesive must be considered (Viegas et al. 1988; Toddywala et al. 1991; Kokubo et al. 1991, 1994; Morimoto et al. 1992; Hille 1993). Chemical interactions may interfere with adhesive performance, cause breakdown of the active species, or formation of new chemical entities. The variability in physicochemical characteristics of drugs and adhesive systems will result in different release rates for hydrophilic and hydrophobic drugs: for example, silicone adhesives are typically lipophilic, which markedly limits the solubility of hydrophilic drugs within the adhesive matrix.

Incorporation of additional excipients, such as skin permeation enhancers, into a drug-in-adhesive system may alter drug release rates and adhesive properties. For example, addition of 1 percent urea to a polyacrylate type pressure-sensitive adhesive resulted in a loss of adhesion so that skin contact could not be maintained over the required period (Hille 1993). Reduction of the influence of both drug and enhancer on adhesive properties has been achieved by design of transdermal systems where there is no contact between these constituents and the adhesive (for example, where the adhesive is present in a boundary laminate surrounding a drug/enhancer releasing layer). A disadvantage of this type of system is that the drug/enhancer releasing layer may not remain in intimate contact with the skin. Where high levels of liquid skin-penetration enhancers are incorporated into drug-in-adhesive transdermal patches, there is often a loss in cohesiveness which results in patch slipping and skin residues following patch removal. Cohesive strength can be increased by high levels of cross-linking in acrylate adhesives, but this may alter both long-term bonding and drug release rates. These problems have been overcome by the development of grafted copolymer adhesives such as ARcare® ETA Adhesive Systems where reinforcement is mainly achieved through phase separation of the side chain within the continuous polymer network. A variety of side chains are available, and up to 30 percent of enhancers have been incorporated without seriously affecting the adhesive properties. This work involved fatty acid ester type enhancers, and utility with other enhancer types remains to be established. Adhesive properties may also be maintained in the presence of skin-penetration enhancers by using blends of acrylic copolymers with different molecular weights (Ko et al. 1995). It is important to appreciate that it is a fundamental requirement that the enhancer, as well as the drug, be released by the adhesive. It is also probable that an enhancer will increase skin permeation of other formulation excipients, which may have an impact on local toxicity.

Manufacturing processes for reservoir, matrix and drug-in-adhesive transdermal systems are largely similar and involve the following stages:

- Preparing drug;

- Mixing drug (and any other excipients) with reservoir, matrix or adhesive;

- Casting into films and drying (or moulding and curing);

- Laminating with other structural components (e.g., backing layer, rate-controlling membrane and release liner);

- Die-cutting

- Final packaging.

The most critical steps in the manufacturing process are casting and lamination, and tensions and pressures must be carefully controlled to produce a wrinkle-free laminate with uniform drug content and reproducible adhesive-coating thickness (Jenkins 1995).

In common with other controlled-release delivery systems, final product checks include content uniformity, release-rate determination and physical testing. Content-uniformity evaluation involves taking a random sample of patches from a batch and assaying for drug content. Several methods are available for determining drug release rates from controlled-release formulations, but the U.S. PMA Committee (PMA Committee Report 1986) has recommended three: the "Paddle over Disk" (identical to the USP paddle dissolution apparatus, except that the transdermal system is attached to a disk or cell resting at the bottom of the vessel that contains medium at 32°C), the "Cylinder-Modified USP Basket" (similar to the USP basket method, except that the system is attached to the surface of a hollow cylinder immersed in medium at 32°C) and the "Reciprocating Disk" (where patches attached to holders are oscillated in small volumes of medium, allowing the apparatus to be useful for systems delivering low concentrations of drug). In a comparative study using a scopolamine patch, a diffusion cell method was evaluated against the "Paddle over Disk" and "Reciprocating Disk" methods (Mazzo et al. 1986). Although the latter two methods gave equivalent results, these were ~25 percent greater than the steady-state flux determined using the diffusion cell. The "Paddle over Disk" method was preferred on the basis of ease of use and ready availability of equipment. The FDA have developed a modified paddle procedure (essentially the "Paddle over Disk" method) for determining drug release from transdermal systems (Shah et al. 1986). One problem with the original method was the mode of keeping the patch in position in the dissolution beaker, and a device to improve and maintain placement of the patch has been subsequently suggested (Man et al. 1993).

CONCLUDING REMARKS

In this chapter, we have described some of the considerations that we believe to be important in the design and development of pharmaceutical products intended for application to the skin. Space limitations dictated that we could not provide an exhaustive review of all the factors that are essential in pharmaceutical product development. The reader who has read this far will appreciate that preformulation, formulation recipes, scale-up, safety and clinical are not covered. These aspects are fully covered either elsewhere in this volume or in some of the excellent and fully recommended texts listed in the bibliography. What we have attempted to achieve herein is to share our knowledge of the structure of skin and the biological and physicochemical determinants of skin penetration and permeation. We have then descibed the methodologies employed and the usefulness of skin permeation measurement in the development of formulations. Finally, we have described some of the formulation types that are applied to the skin together with their properties. We hope that our comments will provide the novice formulator with some insights borne of experience and the experienced formulator with some novel insights in the field of dermatological and transdermal product development.

BIBLIOGRAPHY

Skin and Skin Permeability

Brain, K. R., V. J. James, and K. A. Walters, eds. 1993. *Prediction of percutaneous penetration*, vol. 3b. Cardiff, UK. STS Publishing.

Brain, K. R., V. J. James, and K. A. Walters. eds. 1996. *Prediction of percutaneous penetration*. vol. 4b. Cardiff, UK. STS Publishing.

Brain, K. R., V. J. James, and K. A. Walters. eds. 1998. *Perspectives in percutaneous penetration*, vol. 5b. Cardiff, UK. STS Publishing.

Bronaugh, R. L., and H. I. Maibach, eds. 1999. *Percutaneous absorption*, 3rd ed. New York: Marcel Dekker.

Marzulli, F. N., and H. I. Maibach, eds. 1996. *Dermatotoxicology*, 5th ed. Washington, D.C.: Taylor & Francis.

Roberts M. S., and K. A. Walters, eds. 1998. *Dermal absorption and toxicity assessment*. New York: Marcel Dekker.

Schaefer, H., and T. E. Redelmeier. 1996. *Skin barrier—Principles of percutaneous absorption*. Basel: Karger.

Scott, R. C., R. H. Guy, and J. Hadgraft, eds. 1990. *Prediction of percutaneous penetration*, vol. 1. London: IBC Technical Services.

Scott, R. C., R. H. Guy, J., Hadgraft, and H. E. Boddé, eds. 1991. *Prediction of percutaneous penetration*, vol. 2. London: IBC Technical Services.

Shah, V. P., and H. I. Maibach, eds. 1993. *Topical drug bioavailability, bioequivalence, and penetration*. New York: Plenum Press.

Shroot, B., and H. Schaefer, eds. 1987. *Skin pharmacokinetics*, Basle: Karger.

Zatz, J. L., ed. 1993. *Skin permeation, fundamentals and application*. Wheaton, Ill., USA: Allured Publishing.

Methods

Bronaugh, R. L., and H. I. Maibach, eds. 1991. *In vitro percutaneous absorption: Principles, fundamentals, and applications*. Boca Raton, Fla., USA: CRC Press.

Kemppainen, B. W., and W. G. Reifenrath, eds. 1990. *Methods for skin absorption*. Boca Raton, Fla., USA: CRC Press.

Skin Penetration Enhancement

de Boer, A. G., ed. 1994. *Drug absorption enhancement*. Chur, Switzerland: Harwood Academic Publishers.

Hsieh, D. S., ed. 1994. *Drug permeation enhancement, theory and applications*. New York: Marcel Dekker.

Smith, E. W., and H. I. Maibach, eds. 1995. *Percutaneous penetration enhancers*. Boca Raton, Fla., USA: CRC Press.

Walters, K. A., and J. Hadgraft, eds. 1993. *Pharmaceutical skin penetration enhancement*. New York: Marcel Dekker.

Dermatological Formulations

Barry, B. W. 1983. *Dermatological formulations: Percutaneous absorption*. New York: Marcel Dekker.

Ghosh, T. K., W. R. Pfister, and S. I. Yum, eds. 1997. *Transdermal and topical drug delivery systems*. Buffalo Grove, Ill., USA: Interpharm Press, Inc.

Lieberman, H. A., M. M. Rieger, and G. S. Banker, eds. 1998. *Pharmaceutical dosage forms: Disperse systems*, 2nd ed., vols. 1–3. New York: Marcel Dekker.

Osborne, D. W., and A. H. Amann, eds. 1990. *Topical drug delivery formulations*. New York: Marcel Dekker.

Sjöblom, J., ed. 1996. *Emulsions and emulsion stability*. New York: Marcel Dekker.

Transdermal Drug Delivery

Chien, Y. W. ed. 1987. *Transdermal controlled systemic medications*. New York: Marcel Dekker.

Hadgraft, J., and R. H. Guy, eds. 1989. *Transdermal drug delivery, developmental issues and research initiatives*. New York: Marcel Dekker.

Potts, R. O., and R. H. Guy, eds. 1997. *Mechanisms of transdermal drug delivery*. New York: Marcel Dekker.

Tyle, P., ed. 1988. *Drug delivery devices—Fundamentals and applications*. New York: Marcel Dekker.

REFERENCES

Ahmed, S., T. Imai, and M. Otagiri. 1995. Stereoselective hydrolysis and penetration of propranolol pro-drugs: In vitro evaluation using hairless mouse skin. *J. Pharm. Sci.* 84:877–883.

Anderson, B. D. 1993. Prodrugs and their topical use. In *Topical drug bioavailability, bioequivalence, and penetration*, edited by V. P. Shah, and H. I. Maibach. New York: Plenum Press, pp. 69–89.

Aszterbaum, M., G. K. Menon, K. R. Feingold, and M. L. Williams. 1992. Ontogeny of the epidermal bar-rier to water loss in the rat: Correlation of function with stratum corneum structure and lipid con-tent. *Pediatr. Res.* 31:308–317.

Baden, H. P. 1979. Keratinization in the epidermis. *Pharm. Ther.* 7:393–411.

Baker, E. J., and J. Hadgraft. 1995. In vitro percutaneous absorption of arildone, a highly lipophilic drug, and the apparent no-effect of the penetration enhancer Azone in excised human skin. *Pharm. Res.* 12:993–997.

Baker, R. W., and J. Heller. 1989. Materials selection for transdermal delivery systems. In *Transdermal drug delivery*, edited by J. Hadgraft, and R. H. Guy. New York: Marcel Dekker, pp. 293–311.

Banks, Y. B., D. W. Brewster, and L. S. Birnbaum. 1990. Age-related changes in dermal absorption of 2,3,7,8-tetrachlorodibenzo-p-dioxin and 2,3,4,7,8-pentachlorodibenzofuran. *Fundam. Appl. Toxi-col.* 15:163–173.

Barry, B. W. 1983. *Dermatological formulations, percutaneous absorption.* New York: Marcel Dekker.

Behl, C. R., G. L. Flynn, M., Barrett, K. A., Walters, E. E., Linn, Z., Mohamed, T., Kurihara, N. F. H., Ho, W. I., Higuchi, and C. L. Pierson. 1981. Permeability of thermally damaged skin II: Immediate influences of branding at 60°C on hairless mouse skin permeability. *Burns* 7:389–399.

Behl, C. R., G. L. Flynn, T., Kurihara, W. M., Smith, N. H., Bellantone, O. Gatmaitan, W. I., Higuchi, N. F. H. Ho, and C. L. Pierson, 1984a. Age and anatomical site influences on alkanol permeation of skin of the male hairless mouse. *J. Soc. Cosmet. Chem.* 35:237–252.

Behl, C. R., G. L. Flynn, E. E., Linn, and W. W. Smith. 1984b. Percutaneous absorption of corticosteroids: Age, site, and skin-sectioning influences on rates of permeation of hairless mouse skin by hydro-cortisone. *J. Pharm. Sci.* 73:1287–1290.

Benech-Kieffer, F., Wegrich, P., and H. Schaefer. 1998. Transepidermal water loss as an integrity test for skin barrier function in vitro: Assay standardization. In *Perspectives in percutaneous penetration*, vol. 5b. Edited by K. R. Brain, V. J. James, and K. A. Walters. Cardiff, UK: STS Publishing, pp. 125–128.

Blank, I. H. 1964. Penetration of low-molecular weight alcohols into the skin. I. The effect of concentra-tion of alcohol and type of vehicle. *J. Invest. Dermatol.* 43:415–420.

Boddé, H. E., M. Ponec, A. P. IJzerman, A. J. Hoogstraate, M. A. I. Salomons, and J. A. Bouwstra. 1993. *In vitro* analysis of QSAR in wanted and unwanted effects of azacycloheptanones as transdermal pen-etration enhancers. In *Pharmaceutical skin penetration enhancement*, edited by K. A. Walters, and J. Hadgraft. New York: Marcel Dekker, pp. 199–214.

Bond, J. R., and B. W. Barry. 1988. Damaging effect of acetone on the permeability barrier of hairless mouse skin compared with that of human skin. *Int. J. Pharmaceut.* 41:91–93.

Bouwstra, J. A., G. S. Gooris, M. A. Salomons-de Vries, J. A. van der Spek, and W. Bras. 1992. Structure of human SC as a function of temperature and hydration: A wide-angle X-ray diffraction study. *Int. J. Pharmaceut.* 84:205–216.

Brain, K. R., K. A. Walters, and A. C. Watkinson. 1998. Investigation of skin permeation in vitro. In *Dermal absorption and toxicity assessment*, edited by M. S. Roberts and K. A. Walters. New York: Marcel Dekker. pp. 161–187.

Bronaugh, R. L. 1985. *In vitro* methods for the percutaneous absorption of pesticides. In *Dermal exposure to pesticide use*, edited by R. Honeycutt, G. Zweig, and N. N. Ragsdale. Washington, D.C.: American Chemical Society, pp. 33–41.

Bronaugh, R. L. 1996. Methods for *in vitro* percutaneous absorption. In *Dermatotoxicology*, 5th ed. Edited by F. N. Marzulli, and H. I. Maibach. Washington, D.C.: Taylor and Francis, pp. 317–324.

Bronaugh, R. L., and R. F. Stewart. 1985a. Methods for *in vitro* percutaneous absorption studies. IV: The flow through diffusion cell. *J. Pharm. Sci.* 74:64–67.

Bronaugh, R. L., and R. F. Stewart. 1985b. Methods for *in vitro* percutaneous absorption studies. V: Permeation through damaged skin. *J. Pharm. Sci.* 74:1062–1066.

Bronaugh, R. L., R. F. Stewart, and M. Simon. 1986. Methods for *in vitro* percutaneous absorption studies. VII: Use of excised human skin. *J. Pharm. Sci.* 75:1094–1097.

Bronaugh, R. L., R. F. Stewart, and J. E. Storm. 1989. Extent of cutaneous metabolism during percutaneous absorption of xenobiotics. *Toxicol. Appl. Pharmacol.* 99:534–543.

Bunge, A. L. 1998. Release rates from topical formulations containing drugs in suspension. *J. Contr. Rel.* 52:141–148.

Büyüktimkin, S., N. Büyüktimkin, and J. H. Rytting. 1993. Synthesis and enhancing effect of dodecyl 2-(N,N-dimethylamino)-propionate (DDAIP) on the transepidermal delivery of indomethacin, clonidine, and hydrocortisone. *Pharm. Res.* 10:1632–1637.

Chattaraj, S. C., and I. Kanfer. 1995. Release of acyclovir from semi-solid dosage forms: A semi-automated procedure using a simple plexiglass flow-through cell. *Int. J. Pharmacal.* 125:215–222.

Cleary, G. W. 1993a. Transdermal delivery systems: A medical rationale. In *Topical drug bioavailability, bioequivalence, and penetration*, edited by V. P. Shah, and H. I. Maibach. New York: Plenum Press, pp. 17–68.

Cleary, G. W., 1993b. Transdermal drug delivery. In *Skin permeation, fundamentals and application*, edited by J. L. Zatz. Wheaton, Ill., USA: Allured Publishing, pp. 207–237.

Clowes, H. M., R. C. Scott, and J. R. Heylings. 1994. Skin absorption: Flow-through or static diffusion cells. *Toxicol. In Vitro* 8:827–830.

COLIPA. 1993. *Cosmetic ingredients: Guidelines for percutaneous absorption/penetration.* The European Cosmetic, Toiletry and Perfumery Association.

Collier, S. W., N. M. Sheikh, A. Sakr, J. L. Lichtin, R. F. Stewart, and R. L. Bronaugh. 1989. Maintenence of skin viability during in vitro percutaneous absorption/metabolism studies. *Toxicol. Appl. Pharmacol.* 99:522–533.

Corcuff, P., C. Lotte, A. Rougier, and H. I. Maibach. 1991. Racial differences in corneocytes. A comparison between black, white and oriental skin. *Acta Derm. Venereol.* 71:146–148.

Cosmetic Ingredient Review. 1984. Final report on the safety assessment of methylparaben, ethylparaben, propylparaben, and butylparaben. *J. Amer. Col. Toxicol.* 3:147–209.

Dahl, T., He, G-X., and G. Samuels. 1998. Effect of hydrogen peroxide on the viscosity of a hydroxyethylcellulose-based gel. *Pharm. Res.* 15:1137–1140.

Dal Pozzo, A., and N. Pastori. 1996. Percutaneous absorption of parabens from cosmetic formulations. *Int. J. Cosmet. Sci.* 18:57–66.

Davis, A. F., and J. Hadgraft. 1993. Supersaturated solutions as topical drug delivery sytems. In *Pharmaceutical skin penetration enhancement*, edited by K. A. Walters and J. Hadgraft. New York: Marcel Dekker, pp. 243–268.

Dick, I. P., and R. C. Scott. 1992. The influence of different strains and age on in vitro rat skin permeability to water and mannitol. *Pharm. Res.* 9:884–887.

Dick, I. P., P. G. Blain, and F. M. Williams. 1996. Improved in vitro skin absorption for lipophilic compounds following the addition of albumin to the receptor fluid in flow-through cells. In *Prediction of percutaneous penetration*, vol. 4b. edited by K. R. Brain, V. J. James, and K. A. Walters. Cardiff, UK: STS Publishing, pp. 267–270.

Diembeck, W., H. Beck, F. Benech-Kieffer, P. Courtellemont, J. Dupuis, W. Lovell, M. Paye, J. Spengler, and W. Steiling. 1999. Test guidelines for in vitro assessment of dermal absorption and percutaneous penetration of cosmetic ingredients. *Food Chem. Toxicol.* 37:191–205.

Dupuis, D., A. Rougier, R. Roguet, C. Lotte, and G. Kalopissis. 1984. *In vivo* relationship between horny layer reservoir effect and percutaneous absorption in human and rat. *J. Invest. Dermatol.* 82:353–358.

Durrheim, H. H., G. L. Flynn, W. I. Higuchi, and C. R. Behl. 1980. Permeation of hairless mouse skin. I. Experimental methods and comparison with human epidermal permeation by alkanols. *J. Pharm. Sci.* 69:781–786.

Eccleston, G. M. 1990. Multiple phase oil-in-water emulsions. *J. Soc. Cosmet. Chem.* 41:1–22.

Eccleston, G. M. 1997. Functions of mixed emulsifiers and emulsifying waxes in dermatological lotions and creams. *Colloids Surfaces* 123:169–182.

ECETOC 1993. *Percutaneous absorption*, Monograph No. 20. Brussels: European Centre for Ecotoxicology and Toxicology of Chemicals.

Elias, P. M. 1981. Lipids and the epidermal permeability barrier. *Arch. Dermatol. Res.* 270:95–117.

Elias, P. M., and K. R. Feingold. 1992. Lipids and the epidermal water barrier: Metabolism, regulation, and pathophysiology. *Sem. Dermatol.* 11:176–182.

Evans, W. P. 1964. The solubilization and inactivation of preservatives by nonionic detergents. *J. Pharm. Pharmacol.* 16:323–331.

Fares, H. M., and J. L. Zatz. 1997. Dual-probe method for assessing skin barrier integrity: Effect of storage conditions on permeability of micro-Yucatan pig skin. *J. Soc. Cosmet. Chem.* 48:175–186.

Fartasch, M., and T. L. Diepgen. 1992. The barrier function in atopic dry skin. *Acta Derm. Venereol.* 176 (Suppl.):26–31.

FDA. 1997. *SUPAC-SS—Nonsterile semisolid dosage forms*. Rockville, Md., USA: Food and Drug Adiminstration, U.S. Department of Health and Human Services.

FDA. 1998. *Topical dermatological drug product NDAs and ANDAs—In vivo bioavailability, bioequivalerce, in vivo release, and associated studies*. Rockville, Md., USA: Food and Drug Adminstration, U.S. Department of Health and Human Services.

Feldman, R. J., and H. I. Maibach. 1967. Regional variation in the percutaneous penetration of ^{14}C cortisol in man. *J. Invest. Dermatol.* 48:181–183.

Flynn, G. L. 1996. Cutaneous and transdermal delivery: Processes and systems of delivery. In *Modern pharmaceutics*, 3rd ed., edited by G. S. Banker and C. T. Rhodes. New York: Marcel Dekker, pp. 239–298.

Flynn, G. L., C. R. Behl, K. A. Walters, O. G. Gatmaitan, A. Wittkowsky, T. Kurihara, N. F. H. Ho, W. I. Higuchi, and C. L. Pierson. 1982. Permeability of thermally damaged skin. III: Influence of scalding temperature on mass transfer of water and n-alkanols across hairless mouse skin. *Burns* 8:47–58.

Flynn, G. L., P. A. Caetano, R. S. Pillai, L. M. Abriola, and G. E. Amidon. (in press) Recent perspectives in percutaneous penetration: In vitro drug release and its relationship to drug delivery. In *Perspectives in percutaneous penetration*, vol. 6b, Edited by K. R. Brain, and K. A. Walters. Cardiff, UK: STS Publishing.

Flynn, G. L., and S. H. Yalkowski. 1972. Correlation and prediction of mass transport across membranes. I: Influence of alkyl chain length on flux-determining properties of barrier and diffusant. *J. Pharm. Sci.* 61:838–852.

Franz, T. J. 1975. On the relevance of *in vitro* data. *J. Invest. Dermatol.* 64:190–195.

Franz, T. J., P. A. Lehman, S. F. Franz, H. North-Root, J. L. Demetrulias, C. K. Kelling, S. J. Moloney, and S. D. Gettings. 1993. Percutaneous penetration of N-nitroso-diethanolamine through human skin (in vitro): Comparison of finite and infinite dose application from cosmetic vehicles. *Fundam. Appl. Toxicol.* 21:213–221.

Frazier, C. N., and I. H. Blank. 1954. *A formulary for external therapy of the skin. Springfield, Ill., USA: Charles C. Thomas.*

Friend, D. R., J. Heller, and M. Okagaki. 1988. Evaluation of membranes for transdermal delivery of levonorgestrel. *Proc. Int. Symp. Contr. Rel. Bioact. Mat.* 15:428–429.

Gauthier, E. R., R. J. Gyurik, S. F., Krauser, E. P. Pittz, C. M. Samour, and K. A. Walters. 1998. SEPA® absorption enhancement of polar and non-polar drugs. In *Perspectives in percutaneous penetration*, Vol. 5b, edited by K. R. Brain, V. J. James, and K. A. Walters. Cardiff, UK: STS Publishing, pp. 270–272.

Gelotte, K. M., and R. T. Lostritto. 1990. Solvent interaction with poly-dimethylsiloxane membranes and its effects on benzocaine solubility and diffusion. *Pharm. Res.* 7:523–529.

Guy, R. H., E. Tur, S. Bjerke, and H. I. Maibach. 1983. Are there age and racial differences to methyl nicotinate-induced vasodilation in human skin? *J. Amer. Acad. Dermatol.* 12:1001–1006.

Gyurik, R. J., S. F. Krauser, E. R. Gauthier, C. R. Reppucci, and C. M. Samour. 1996. SEPA® penetration enhancement of econazole in human skin. In *Prediction of percutaneous penetration*, vol. 4b. Edited by K. R. Brain, V. J. James, and K. A. Walters. Cardiff, UK: STS Publishing, pp 124–126.

Hadgraft J., D. G. Williams, and G. Allan. 1993. Azone, mechanism, of action and clinical effect. In *Pharmaceutical skin penetration enhancement*, edited by K. A. Walters and J. Hadgraft. New York: Marcel Dekker, pp. 175–197.

Hall, L. L., H. L. Fisher, M. R., Sumler, M. F. Hughes, and P. V. Shah. 1992. Age-related percutaneous penetration of 2-sec-butyl-4,6-dinitrophenol (dinoseb) in rats. *Fundam. Appl. Toxicol.* 19:258–267.

Harrison, S. M., B. W. Barry, and P. H. Dugard. 1984. Effects of freezing on human skin permeability. *J. Pharm. Pharmacol.* 36:261–262.

Heard, C. M., and K. R. Brain. 1995. Does solute stereochemistry influence percutaneous penetration? *Chirality* 7:305–309.

Higuchi, T. 1960. Physical chemical analysis of percutaneous absorption process from creams and ointments. *J. Soc. Cosmet. Chem.* 11:85–97.

Higuchi, T. 1961. Rate of release of medicaments from ointment bases containing drugs in suspension. *J. Pharm. Sci.* 50:874–875.

Hille, T. 1993. Technological aspects of penetration enhancers in transdermal systems. In *Pharmaceutical skin penetration enhancement*, edited by K. A. Walters, and J. Hadgraft. New York: Marcel Dekker. pp. 335–343.

Hinz, R. S., C. R. Lorence, C. D. Hodson, C. Hansch, L. L. Hall, and R. H. Guy. 1991. Percutaneous penetration of para-substituted phenols in vitro. *Fundam. Appl. Toxicol.* 47:869–892.

Hood, H. L., R. R. Wickett, and R. L. Bronaugh. 1996. *In vitro* percutaneous absorption of the fragrance ingredient musk xylol. *Food Chem. Toxicol.* 34:483–488.

Hoogstraate, A. J., J. Verhoef, J. Brussee, A. P. IJzerman, F. Spies and H. Boddé. 1991. Kinetics, ultrastructural aspects and molecular modelling of transdermal peptide flux enhancement by N-alkylazacyclo-heptanones. *Int. J. Pharmaceut.* 76:37–47.

Hotchkiss, S. A. M. 1998. Dermal metabolism. In *Dermal absorption and toxicity assessment*, edited by M. S. Roberts, and K. A. Walters. New York: Marcel Dekker, pp. 43–101.

Howes, D., R. Guy, J. Hadgraft, J. Heylings, F. Hoeck, H. Maibach, J-P. Marty, H. Merk, J. Parra, D. Rekkas, I. Rondelli, H. Schaefer, U. Täuber, and N. Verbiese. 1996. Methods for assessing percutaneous absorption. *ECVAM Workshop Report 13, ALTA* 24:81–106.

Hughes, M. F., S. P. Shrivasta, H. L. Fisher, and L. L. Hall. 1993. Comparative in vitro percutaneous absorption of p-substituted phenols through rat skin using static and flow-through diffusion systems. *Toxicol. In Vitro* 7:221–227.

Idson, B. 1975. Percutaneous absorption. *J. Pharm. Sci.* 64:901–924.

Jenkins, A. W. 1992. Transdermal device. UK Patent GB 2,249,956A.

Jenkins, A. W. 1995. Developing the Fematrix transdermal patch. *Pharm. J.* 255:179–181.

Kabara, J. J., and D. S. Orth, eds. 1997. *Preservative-free and self-preserving cosmetics and drugs—Principles and practice*. New York: Marcel Dekker.

Karim, A. 1983. Transdermal absorption of nitroglycerin from microseal drug delivery (MDD) system. *Angiology* 34:11–22.

Kasting, G. B., R. L. Smith, and B. D. Anderson. 1992. Prodrugs for dermal delivery: Solubility, molecular size, and functional group effects. In *Prodrugs*, edited by K. B. Sloan. New York: Marcel Dekker, pp. 117–161.

Kasting, G. B., and L. A. Bowman. 1990. Electrical analysis of fresh excised human skin: A comparison with frozen skin. *Pharm. Res.* 7:1141–1146.

Kitson, N., and S. Maddin. 1998. Drugs used for skin diseases. In *Dermal absorption and toxicity assessment*, edited by M. S. Roberts, and K. A. Walters. New York: Marcel Dekker, pp. 313–326.

Kneczke, M., L. Landersjö, P. Lundgren, and C. Führer. 1986. In vitro release of salicylic acid from two different qualities of white petrolatum. *Acta Pharm. Suec.* 23:193–204.

Ko, C. U., S. L. Wilking, and J. Birdsall. 1995. Pressure sensitive adhesive property optimizations for the transdermal drug delivery systems. *Pharm. Res.* 12:S-143.

Kokubo, T., K. Sugibayashi, and Y. Morimoto. 1991. Diffusion of drug in acrylic-type pressure-sensitive adhesive matrices. I. Influence of physical property of the matrices on the drug diffusion. *J. Contr. Rel.* 17:69–78.

Kokubo, T., K. Sugibayashi, and Y. Morimoto. 1994. Interaction between drugs and pressure-sensitive adhesives in transdermal therapeutic systems. *Pharm. Res.* 11:104–107.

Komatsu, H., K. Higaki, H. Okamoto, K. Miyagawa, M. Hashida, and H. Sezaki. 1986a. Preservative activity and *in vivo* percutaneous penetration of butyl paraben entrapped in liposomes. *Chem. Pharm. Bull.* 34:3415–3422.

Komatsu, H., H. Okamoto, K. Miyagawa, M. Hashida, and H. Sezaki. 1986b. Percutaneous absorption of butyl paraben from liposomes *in vitro*. *Chem. Pharm. Bull.* 34:3423–3430.

Komerska, J. F. 1987. Urethane films—Transdermal opportunities. *J. Plastic Film Sheet* 3:58–64.

Kompaore, F., and H. Tsuruta. 1993. *In vivo* differences between Asian, Black and White in the stratum corneum barrier function. *Int. Arch. Occup. Environ. Health* 65:S223-S225.

Korting, H. C. ed., 1996. The skin as a site for drug delivery: The liposome approach and its alternatives. *Adv. Drug Del. Rev.* 18 (3):271–425.

Kou, J. H., S. D. Roy, J. Du, and J. Fujiki. 1993. Effect of receiver fluid pH on *in vitro* skin flux of weakly ionizable drugs. *Pharm. Res.* 10:986–990.

Kreuter, J., ed. 1994. *Colloidal drug delivery systems*. New York: Marcel Dekker.

Kril, M. B., P. V. Parab, S. E. Genier, J. E. DiNunzio, and D. Alessi. 1999. Potential problems encountered with SUPAC-SS and the in vitro release testing of ammonium lactate cream. *Pharm. Tech.* (March):164–174.

Kurup, T. R. R., L. S. C. Wan, and L. W. Chan. 1995. Interaction of preservatives with macromolecules. Part II. Cellulose derivatives. *Pharm. Acta. Helv.* 70:187–193.

Lazo, N. D., J. G. Maine, and D. T. Downing. 1995. Lipids are covalently attached to rigid corneocyte protein envelopes existing predominantly as β-sheets: A solid-state nuclear magnetic resonance study. *J. Invest. Dermatol.* 105:296–300.

Lehman, P. A., I. N. Agrawa, T. J. Franz, K. J. Miller, and S. Franz. 1996. Comparison of topical hydrocortisone products: Percutaneous absorption vs. tape stripping vs. vasoconstriction vs. membrane rate of release. *Pharm. Res.* 13:S310.

Leo, A., C. Hansch, and D. Elkins. 1971. Partition coefficients and their uses. *Chem. Rev.* 71:525–616.

Leopold, C. S., and H. I. Maibach. 1996. Effect of lipophilic vehicles on in vivo skin penetration of methyl nicotinate in different races. *Int. J. Pharmaceut.* 139:161–167.

Leuenberger, H., J. D. Bonny, and M. Kolb. 1995. Percolation effects in matrix-type controlled drug release systems. *Int. J. Pharmaceut.* 115:217–224.

Liu, J-C. and S. J. Wisniewski. 1997. Recent advances in topical drug delivery systems. In *Transdermal and topical drug delvery systems*, edited by T. K. Ghosh, W. R. Pfister, and S. I. Yum. Buffalo Grove, Ill., USA: Interpharm Press, pp. 593–612.

Lotte, C., R. C. Wester, A. Rougier, and H. I. Maibach. 1993. Racial differences in the *in vivo* percutaneous absorption of some organic compounds: A comparison between black, Caucasian and Asian subjects. *Arch. Dermatol. Res.* 284:456–459.

Man, M., C. Chang, P. H. Lee, C. T. Broman, and G. W. Cleary. 1993. New improved paddle method for determining the in vitro drug release profiles of transdermal delivery systems. *J. Contr. Rel.* 27:59–68.

Marty, J-P., A. M. Dervault, J. F. Chanez, O. Doucet, and C. M. Samour. 1989. Effect of dioxolanes on indomethacin in vitro percutanteous absorption enhancement. *Proc. Int. Symp. Contr. Rel. Bioact. Mater.* 16:179–180.

Marzulli, F. N., and H. I. Maibach. 1984. Permeability and reactivity of skin as related to age. *J. Soc. Cosmet. Chem.* 35: 95–102.

Mazzo, D. J., E. K. F. Fong, and S. E. Biffar. 1986. A comparison of test methods for determining in vitro drug release from transdermal delivery dosage forms. *J. Pharmaceut. Biomed. Anal.* 4:601–607.

Megrab, N. A., A. C. Williams, and B. W. Barry. 1995. Oestradiol permeation through human skin and silastic membrane: Effects of propylene glycol and supersaturation. *J. Contr. Rel.* 36: 277–294.

Merk, H. F., F. K. Jugert, and S. Frankenburg. 1996. Biotransformations in the skin. In *Dermatotoxicology*, 5th ed. Edited by F. N. Marzulli, and H. I. Maibach. Washington, DC: Taylor and Francis, pp. 61–73.

Morimoto, Y., T. Kokubo, and K. Sugibayashi. 1992. Diffusion of drug in acrylic-type pressure-sensitive adhesive matrices. I. Influence of interaction. *J. Contr. Rel.* 18:113–122.

Musolf, M. C. 1987. Pressure-sensitive adhesives: science and engineering. In *Transdermal controlled systemic medications*, edited by Y. C. Chien. New York: Marcel Dekker, pp. 93–112.

Noonan, P. K., and R. C. Wester. 1989. Cutaneous metabolism of xenobiotics. In *Percutaneous absorption: Mechanisms, methodology, drug delivery*, 2nd ed. Edited by R. L. Bronaugh, and H. I. Maibach. New York: Marcel Dekker, pp. 53–75.

Okabe, H., E. Suzuki, T. Saitoh, K. Takayama, and T. Nagai. 1994. Development of novel transdermal system containing d-limonene and ethanol as absorption enhancers. *J. Contr. Rel.* 32:243–247.

Orth, D. S. 1993. *Handbook of cosmetic microbiology*. New York: Marcel Dekker.

Osborne, D. W. 1992. Phase behavior characterization of propylene glycol, white petrolatum, surfactant ointments. *Drug Dev. Ind. Pharm.* 18:1883–1894.

Osborne, D. W. 1993. Phase behavior characterization of ointments containing lanolin or a lanolin substitute. *Drug Dev. Ind. Pharm.* 19:1283–1302.

Osborne, D. W. and A. H. Amann, eds. 1990. *Topical drug delivery formulations*. New York: Marcel Dekker.

Pellett, M. A., M. S. Roberts, and J. Hadgraft. 1997. Supersaturated solutions evaluated with an in vitro stratum corneum tape stripping technique. *Int. J. Pharm.* 151:91–98.

Pena, L. E., B. L. Lee, and J. F. Stearns. 1994. Structural rheology of a model ointment. *Pharm. Res.* 11:875–881.

Pendlington, R. U., D. J. Sanders, K. J. Cooper, D. Howes, and W. W. Lovell. 1998. The use of sucrose as a standard penetrant in in vitro percutaneous penetration experiments. In *Perspectives in percutaneous penetration*, vol. 5b. Edited by K. R. Brain, V. J. James, and K. A. Walters. Cardiff, UK: STS Publishing, pp. 123–124.

Pérez-Marcos, B., R. Martínez-Pacheco, Gómez-Amoza, C. Souto, A. Concheiro, and R. C. Rowe. 1993. Interlot variability of carbomer 934. *Int. J. Pharm.* 100:207–212.

Pershing, L. K., B. S. Silver, G. G. Krueger, V. P. Shah, and J. P. Skelly. 1992. Feasibility of measuring the bioavailability of topical betamethasone dipropionate in commercial formulations using drug content in skin and a skin blanching bioassay. *Pharm. Res.* 9:45–51.

Pfister, W. R., M. A. Sheeran, D. E. Watters, R. P., Sweet, and P. Walters. 1987. Methods for altering release of progesterone, testosterone, propranolol, and indomethacin from silicone matrices: Effects of co-solvents and inert fillers. *Proc. Int. Symp. Contr. Rel. Bioact. Mat.* 14:223–224.

Phillips, C. A., and B. Michniak. 1996. Transdemal delivery of drugs with differing lipophilicities using Azone analogs as dermal penetration enhances. *J. Pharm. Sci.* 84:1427–1433.

Planas, M. D., F. G. Rodriguez, and M. H. Dominguez. 1992. The influence of neutralizer concentration on the rheological behaviour of a 0.1% Carbopol® hydrogel. *Pharmazie* 47:351–355.

PMA Committee Report. 1986. Transdermal drug delivery systems. *Pharmacop. Forum* 12:1798–1807.

Potts, R. O., and R. H. Guy. 1992. Predicting skin permeability. *Pharm. Res.* 9:663–669.

Prausnitz, M. R. 1996. The effects of electric current applied to skin: A review for transdermal drug delivery. *Adv. Drug Del. Rev.* 18:395–425.

Pugh, W. J., J. Hadgraft, and M. S. Roberts. 1998. Physicochemical determinants of stratum corneum permeation. In *Dermal absorption and toxicity assessment*, edited by M. S. Roberts, and K. A. Walters. New York: Marcel Dekker, pp. 245–268.

Rajadhyaksha, V. J. 1990. Oxalodinone penetration enhancing compounds, U.S. Patent 4,960,771.

Raykar, P. V., M. C. Fung, and B. D. Anderson. 1988. The role of protein and lipid domains in the uptake of solutes by human stratum corneum. *Pharm. Res.* 5:140–150.

Reichek, N., R. E. Goldstein, and D. R. Redwood. 1974. Sustained effects of nitroglycerin ointment in patients with angina pectoris. *Circulation* 50:348–352.

Rienertson, R. P., and V. R. Wheatley. 1959. Studies on the chemical composition of human epidermal lipids. *J. Invest. Dermatol.* 32:49–59.

Roberts, M. S. 1976. Percutaneous absorption of phenolic compounds. PhD thesis, University of Sydney.

Roberts, M. S. 1991. Structure-permeability considerations in percutaneous absorption. In *Prediction of Percutaneous Penetration*, vol. 2. Edited by R. C. Scott, R. H. Guy, J. Hadgraft, and H. E. Boddé. London: IBC Technical Services, pp. 210–228.

Roberts, M. S., R. A. Anderson, and J. Swarbrick. 1977. Permeability of human epidermis to phenolic compounds. *J. Pharm. Pharmacal.* 29:677–683.

Roberts, M. S., W. A. Favretto, A. Meyer, M. Reckmann, and T. Wongseelashote. 1982. Topical bioavailability of methyl salicylate. *Aust. NZ J. Med.* 12:303–305.

Roberts, M. S., and K. A. Walters., eds. 1998. *Dermal absorption and toxicity assessment.* New York: Marcel Dekker.

Rogers, R. A., and J. E. Riviere. 1994. Pharmacological modulation of the cutaneous vasculature in the isolated perfused porcine skin flap. *J. Pharm. Sci.* 83:1682–1689.

Roskos, K. V., R. H. Guy, and H. I. Maibach. 1986. Percutaneous absorption in the aged. *Dermatol. Clin.* 4:455–465.

Roskos, K. V., and H. I. Maibach. 1992. Percutaneous absorption and age: Implications for therapy. *Drugs and Aging* 2: 432–449.

Roskos, K. V., H. I. Maibach, and R. H. Guy. 1989. The effect of aging on percutaneous absorption in man. *J. Pharm. Biopharm.* 17:617–630.

Rougier, A. 1987a. An original predictive method for *in vivo* percutaneous absorption studies. *J. Soc. Cosmet. Chem.* 38:397–417.

Rougier, A. 1987b. In vivo percutaneous penetration of some organic compounds related to anatomic site in humans: Stripping method. *J. Pharm. Sci.* 76:451–454.

Rougier, A. 1991. Percutaneous absorption-transepidermal water loss relationship in man in vivo. In *Prediction of percutaneous penetration*, vol. 2. Edited by R. C. Scott, R. H. Guy, J. Hadgraft, and H. E. Boddé. London: IBC Technical Services, pp. 60–72.

Rougier, A., and C. Lotte. 1993. Predictive approaches. I. The stripping technique. In *Topical drug bioavailability, bioequivalence and penetration*, edited by V. P. Shah, and H. I. Maibach. New York: Plenum Press, pp. 163–182.

Roy, S. D. 1997. Preformulation aspects of transdermal drug delivery systems, In *Transdermal and topical drug delivery systems*, edited by T. K. Ghosh, W. R. Pfister, and S. I. Sum. Buffalo Grove, Ill., USA: Interpharm Press, pp. 139–166.

Schaefer, H., and T. E. Redelmeir. 1996. *Skin barrier, principles of percutaneous* absorption. Basel: Karger.

Scheuplein, R. J. 1965. Mechanism of percutaneous absorption. I. Routes of penetration and the influence of solubility. *J. Invest. Dermatol.* 45:334–346.

Scheuplein, R. J., and I. H. Blank. 1971. Permeability of the skin. *Physiol. Rev.* 51:702–747.

Scheuplein, R. J., and I. H. Blank. 1973. Mechanism of percutaneous absorption. IV. Penetration of nonelectrolytes (alcohols) from aqueous solutions and from pure liquids. *J. Invest. Dermatol.* 60:286–296.

Schmidt, R. J. 1989. Cutaneous side effects in transdermal drug delivery: Avoidance strategies. In *Transdermal drug delivery*, edited by J. Hadgraft and R. H. Guy. New York: Marcel Dekker, pp. 83–97.

Sclafani, J., P. Liu, E. Hansen, M. G. Cettina, and J. Nightingale. 1995. A protocol for the assessment of receiver solution additive-induced skin permeability changes. An example with gamma-cyclodextrin. *Int. J. Pharmaceut.* 124:213–217.

Scott, R. C., P. H. Dugard, and A. W. Doss. 1986. Permeability of abnormal rat skin. *J. Invest. Dermatol.* 86:201–207.

Scott, R. C. 1991. In vitro absorption through damaged skin. In *In vitro percutaneous absorption, principles, fundamentals and applications*, edited by R. L. Bronaugh and H. I. Maibach. Boca Raton, Fla., USA: CRC Press, pp. 129–135.

Shah, V. P., J. Elkins, J. Hanus, C. Noorizadeh, and J. P. Skelly. 1991. In vitro release of hydrocortisone from topical preparations and automated procedure. *Pharm. Res.* 8:55–59.

Shah, V. P., G. L. Flynn, A. Yacobi, H. I. Maibach, C. Bon, N. M. Fleischer, T. J. Franz, S. A. Kaplan, J. Kawamoto, L. J. Lesko, J-P., Marty, L. K. Pershing, H. Schaefer, J. A. Sequeira, S. P. Shrivastava, J. Wilkin, and R. L. Williams. 1998. AAPS/FDA workshop report: Bioequivalence of topical dermatological dosage forms—methods of evaluation of bioequivalence. *Pharm. Res.* 15:167–171.

Shah, V. P. and H. I. Maibach, eds. 1993. *Topical drug bioavailability, bioequivalence, and penetration*. New York: Plenum Press.

Shah, V. P., N. W. Tymes, L. A. Yamamoto, and J. P. Skelly. 1986. In vitro dissolution profile of transdermal nitroglycerin patches using paddle method. *Int. J. Pharmaceut.* 32:243–250.

Sharma, R. 1996. Xenobiotic metabolizing enzymes in skin. In *Prediction of percutaneous penetration*, vol. 4b. Edited by K. R. Brain, V. J. James, and K. A. Walters. Cardiff, UK: STS Publishing, pp. 14–18.

Singh, P., and M. S. Roberts. 1994. Effects of vasoconstriction on dermal pharmacokinetics and local tissue distribution of compounds. *J. Pharm. Sci.* 83:783–791.

Sjöblom, J., ed. 1996. *Emulsions and emulsion stability*. New York: Marcel Dekker.

Skelly, J. P., V. P. Shah, H. I. Maibach, R. H. Guy, R. C. Wester, G. L. Flynn, and A. Yacobi. 1987. FDA and AAPS report of the workshop on principles and practices of *in vitro* percutaneous penetration studies: Relevance to bioavailability and bioequivalence. *Pharm. Res.* 4:265–267.

Smith, E. W., and H. I. Maibach, eds. 1995. *Percutaneous penetration enhancers*, Boca Raton, Fla., USA: CRC Press.

Southwell, J. D., B. W. Barry, and R. Woodford. 1984. Variations in permeability of human skin within and between specimens. *Int. J. Pharmaceut.* 18:299–309.

Sugibayashi, K., and Y. Morimoto. 1994. Polymers for transdermal drug delivery systems. *J. Contr. Rel.* 29:177–185.

Surber, C., K-P. Wilhelm, and H. I. Maibach. 1993. In vitro and in vivo percutaneous absorption of structurally related phenol and steroid analogs. *Eur. J. Pharm. Biopharm.* 39:244–248.

Sutinen, R., A. Urtti, V. Saano, and P. Paronen. 1993. Water-activated and pH-controlled transdermal patch: Drug absorption and skin irritation. In *Prediction of percutaneous penetration*, vol. 3b. Edited by K. R. Brain V. J. James, and K. A. Walters. Cardiff, UK: STS Publishing, pp. 554–557.

Takruri, H., and C. B. Anger. 1989. Preservation of dispersed systems. In *Pharmaceutical dosage forms: Disperse systems*, vol. 2. Edited by H. A. Lieberman, M. M. Rieger, and G. S. Banker. New York: Marcel Dekker, pp. 73–114.

Tanaka, M., Y. Iwata, Y. Kouzuki, K. Taniguchi, H. Matsuda, H. Arima, and S. Tsuchiya. 1995. Effect of 2-hydroxypropyl-β-cyclodextrin on percutaneous absorption of methyl paraben. *J. Pharm. Pharmacol.* 47:897–900.

Tanojo, H., P. E. H. Roemelé, G. H. van Veen, H. Stieltjes, H. E. Junginger, and H. E. Boddé. 1997. New design of a flow-through permeation cell for studying *in vitro* permeation studies across biological membranes. *J. Contr. Rel.* 45: 41–47.

Toddywala, R. D., K. Ulman, P. Walters, and Y. W. Chien. 1991. Effect of physicochemical properties of adhesive on the release, skin permeation and adhesiveness of adhesive-type transdermal drug delivery systems containing silicone-based pressure-sensitive adhesives. *Int. J. Pharmaceut.* 76:77–89.

Tojo, K., and A. C. Lee. 1989. A method for predicting steady-state rate of skin penetration *in vivo*. *J. Invest. Dermatol.* 92:105–110.

Turpeinen, M. 1991. Absorption of hydrocortisone from the skin reservoir in atopic dermatitis. *Br. J. Dermatol.* 124:358–360.

Turpeinen, M., O. P. Salo, and S. Leisti. 1986. Effect of percutaneous absorption of hydrocortisone on adrenocortical responsiveness in infants with severe skin disease. *Br. J. Dermatol.* 115:475–484.

Ulman, K. L., G. A. Gornowicz, K. R. Larson, and C-L. Lee. 1989a. Drug permeability of modified silicone polymers. I. Silicone-organic block copolymers. *J. Contr. Rel.* 10:251–260.

Ulman, K. L., K. R. Larson, C-L. Lee, and K. Tojo. 1989b. Drug permeability of modified silicone polymers. II. Silicone-organic graft copolymers. *J. Contr. Rel.* 10:261–272.

Ulman, K. L., and C-L. Lee. 1989c. Drug permeability of modified silicone polymers. III. Hydrophilic pressure-sensitive adhesives for transdermal controlled drug release applications. *J. Contr. Rel.* 10:273–281.

van der Valk, P. G. M., J. P. Nater, and E. Bleumink. 1985. Vulnerability of the skin to surfactants in different groups of eczema patients and controls as measured by water vapour loss. *Clin. Exp. Dermatol.* 10:98–103.

Vickers, C. F. H. 1963. Existence of reservoir in stratum corneum. Experimental proof. *Arch. Dermatol.* 88:21–23.

Viegas, T. X., A. H. Hikal, and G. W. Cleary. 1988. Formulation of penetration enhancers in polymers. *Drug Dev. Ind. Pharm.* 14:855–866.

Walters, K. A., and J. Hadgraft, eds. 1993. *Pharmaceutical skin penetration enhancement.* New York: Marcel Dekker.

Walters, K. A., K. R. Brain, D. Howes, V. J. James, A. L. Kraus, N. M. Teetsel, M. Toulon, A. C. Watkinson, and S. D. Gettings. 1997a. Percutaneous penetration of octyl salicylate from representative sunscreen formulations through human skin in vitro. *Food Chem. Toxicol.* 35:1219–1225.

Walters, K. A., K. R. Brain, W. E. Dressler, D. M. Green, D. Howes, V. J. James, C. K. Kelling, A. C. Watkinson, and S. D. Gettings. 1997b. Percutaneous penetration of N-nitroso-N-methyldodecylamine through human skin in vitro: Application from cosmetic vehicles. *Food Chem. Toxicol.* 35:705–712.

Walters, K. A., G. L. Flynn, and J. R. Marvel. 1981. Physicochemical characterization of the human nail. I. Pressure sealed apparatus for measuring nail plate permeabilities. *J. Invest. Dermatol.* 76:76–79.

Watkinson, A. C., K. R. Brain, K. A. Walters, and J. Hadgraft. 1992. Prediction of the percutaneous penetration of ultra-violet filters used in sunscreen formulations. *Int. J. Cosmet. Sci.* 14:265–275.

Weigand, D. A., C. Haygood, and J. R. Gaylor. 1974. Cell layers and density of Negro and Caucasian SC. *J. Invest. Dermatol.* 62:563–568.

Wertz, P. W., and D. T. Downing. 1982. Glycolipids in mammalian epidermis: Structure and function in the water barrier. *Science* 217:1261–1262.

Wertz, P. W., and D. T. Downing. 1989. Stratum corneum: Biological and biochemical considerations. In *Transdermal drug delivery*, edited by J. Hadgraft, and R. H. Guy. New York: Marcel Dekker, pp. 1–22.

Wester, R. C., J. Christoffel, T. Hartway, N. Poblete, H. I. Maibach, and J. Forsell. 1998. Human cadaver skin viability for *in vitro* percutaneous absorption: Storage and detrimental effects of heat-separation and freezing. *Pharm. Res.* 15:82–84.

Williams, A. C., P. A. Cornwell, and B. W. Barry. 1992. On the non-Gaussian distribution of human skin permeabilities. *Int. J. Pharmaceut.* 86:69–77.

Yano, T., N. Higo, K. Furukawa, M. Tsuji, K. Noda, and M. Otagiri. 1992. Evaluation of a new penetration enhancer 1-[2-(decylthio)-ethyl]aza-cyclopentan-2-one (HPE-101). *J. Pharmacobio-Dyn.* 15:527–533.

Yano, T., A. Nakagawa, T. Masayoshi, and K. Noda. 1986. Skin permeability of non-steroidal antiinflammatory drugs in man. *Life Sci.* 39:1043–1050.

Yuk, S. H., S. J. Lee, T. Okano, B. Berner, and S. W. Kim. 1991a. One-way membrane for transdermal drug delivery systems. I. Membrane preparation and characterization. *Int. J. Pharmaceut.* 77:221–229.

Yuk, S. H., S. J. Lee, T. Okano, B. Berner, and S. W. Kim. 1991b. One-way membrane for transdermal drug delivery systems. II. System optimization. *Int. J. Pharmaceut.* 77:231–237.

Zatz, J. L., J. Varsano, and V. P. Shah. 1996. In vitro release of betamethasone dipropionate from petrolatum-based ointments. *Pharm. Dev. Technol.* 1:293–298.

INDEX

ABPI Compendium of Data Sheets and Summaries of Product Characteristics, 298
absorption (physiological). *See also* percutaneous absorption
 biopharmaceutics classification system (BCS), 29, 105
 diffusion, passive, 120
 dissolution and, 100–102, 104–106
 enhancers, 140–141
 fractional amount, 268–269
 GI luminal interactions, 111–116
 high-throughput screening (HTS) for, 141–143
 in vitro simulation methods, 118–132
 in vivo dissolution/absorption time profiles, 265–268
 in vivo methods, 135–139
 in vivo simulation methods, 131
 IVIVC correlation, 270–276
 log *P* and, 26–27
 model dependent analysis, 264
 moment analysis, 264–265
 nasal, 494, 508–509
 non-biological evaluation, 120–121
 optimal criteria for, 98–99
 process of, 97–98, 117–118
 skin, 518–527
 solvents and vehicles for testing, 139–141
 surfactants, effect on, 140
acacia, 427, 428, 545
accelerated stress stability studies, 39, 314, 479, 480
Accuhaler™, 362
AccuSpray™, 501
ACDpKa software, 25
acetabulol, 134
acetaminophen, 85, 86, 400, 423, 429
acetate buffer, 333–334
acetate salt, 52, 53, 56
acetazolamide, 480
acetic acid, 44, 498
acetohexamide, 73
acetone, 24, 436
acetonitrile, 29, 43, 547
acetylcysteine, 203, 476
acetylsalicylic acid, 529, 530
acetyltransferases, 531

acid-base catalysis. *See* specific acid-base catalysis
acid-base degradation, 35
Acid Brilliant Green BS, 417
Acid Fuschin D, 416
acids, used in salt formation, 53, 53–54
Acid Yellow G, 416
acitazanolast, 461
acrylic acids, 545
active transport, 136–137
actuators, 368, 504, 508
acyclovir, 460, 466, 533
additives. *See* excipients
adequate water, 39
adhesives, 303, 562–564, 565–566
ADL-2-1294, 461
administration of parenteral products, 350
adsorption, 302–303
adsorption-desorption, 186–187
adverse effects, of excipients, 198, 339
Aerosil, 409
Aerosizer, 186
Afrin®, 492
agar gum, 420
age factors, 528–529
agglomerates and agglomeration, 424–427, 429–431
agitation, 247
airflow and aerosolisation, 362
albendazole, 215
albuterol, 217–218. *See also* salbutamol
alcohol group, 224
alcohols, 436, 523–524
aldrin, 531
alginates, 476, 545
alginic acid, 420, 548
aliphatics, 35
alkylammonium halides, 550
allergic conjunctivitis, 462
Allura red, 416
alprostadil, 339
alteplase, 350
aluminum-EDTA chelate, 207
aluminum salt, 52
Amaranth, 416
American Association of Pharmaceutical Scientists (AAPS), 374
amethocaine, 460

amides, 35
4-amidinoindanone guanylhydrazone, 46
amiloride hydrochloride, 44
amine hydrochlorides, 224, 225
3-amino-1-hydroxypropylidine-1,1-diphosphonate, 141
amino acids, 30, 343
p-aminobenzoic acid, 531
2-aminofluorene, 531
amino group, 224
aminopyrine, 531
ammonium buffer, 334
amorphous compounds, 39, 45, 60, 81–82, 212–213
amoxicillin, 58
amphotericin B, 343
ampicillin, 58
ampoules, 204–205, 347
Anderson-Graseby impactor, 358–359
angle of repose, 388, 447
animal membranes, 452
animal models, 132–134, 276–279, 347, 528–529
annular shear testers, 386
antacids, 113, 287
Anthocyanin, 416
antiadherent lubricants, 410–411, 414
antibiotics, 57–58, 82, 460, 461
antiglaucoma agents, 485
anti-inflammatory agents, 460, 461, 462, 522–523
antimicrobial preservatives, 476–477, 559–561
antioxidants, 203–206, 216, 341, 343, 476
antipyrine, 476
antivirals, 460
apparent particle density, 382
aprotic solvents, 29
Aquasol A, 339
arachis (peanut) oil, 524, 545
Aradigm, 371
ARcare® ETA Adhesive Systems, 566
area under the curve, 139. *See also* AUC
arginine, 343
arildone, 532
Arrhenius relationship, 37, 39, 314
artificial tear preparations, 460
ascorbate buffer, 334
ascorbate salt, 53